DEDICATION

To my wife, Helene; my children, Allison (and her husband Ted), Mitchell (and his wife Deborah), Jessica (and her husband Zac), and Gregory; and my beautiful grandchildren, Lindsey and Eli. Without their love and support I could never have accomplished as much as I have as a physician and a teacher.

Richard A. Polin, MD

This book is dedicated to my wife, Elaine; my children, Steve, Jen, Sara, Kevin, and Lauren; and especially to my two premie grandchildren, Jacob and Matthew Spitzer; who never fail to amaze us each and every day. Their survival and their remarkable outcomes are a great testimony to the specialty of neonatal-perinatal medicine.

This book is also dedicated to the two "mothers" that I have had in my life—my true mother, Florence Spitzer, to whom I owe so much, and to my "neonatology mother," Maria Delivoria-Papadopoulos, whose ceaseless quest for knowledge continues to inspire us all.

Alan R. Spitzer, MD

CONTENTS

CONTRIBUTORS

K.J.S. Anand, MBBS, DPhil
Professor of Pediatrics, Anesthesiology, Neurobiology, and Pharmacology, University of Arkansas for Medical Sciences, Little Rock, Arkansas

David A. Bateman, MD
Associate Professor of Pediatrics, Director of Network Nurseries, Columbia University Medical Center; Morgan Stanley Children's Hospital of New York–Presbyterian, New York, New York

Wendy K. Chung, MD, PhD
Department of Pediatrics, Columbia University College of Physicians and Surgeons, New York, New York

Reese H. Clark, MD
Director of Research, Pediatrix Medical Group, Inc., Sunrise, Florida

Elizabeth Alvarez Connelly, MD
Assistant Clinical Professor, Division of Pediatric Dermatology, Department of Dermatology, University of Miami School of Medicine, Miami, Florida

Lawrence F. Eichenfield, MD
Professor of Pediatrics and Medicine; Chief, Pediatric and Adolescent Dermatology, University of California at San Diego School of Medicine; Children's Hospital, San Diego, California

Christiana R. Farkouh, MD, MPH
Assistant Clinical Professor of Pediatrics, Columbia University College of Physicians and Surgeons; Morgan Stanley Children's Hospital of New York–Presbyterian, New York, New York

T. Ernesto Figueroa, MD
Clinical Associate Professor of Urology, Jefferson Medical College of Thomas Jefferson University, Philadelphia, Pennsylvania; Chief, Division of Urology, A.I. duPont Hospital for Children, Wilmington, Delaware

Mary Pat Gallagher, MD
Assistant Professor of Clinical Pediatrics, Division of Pediatric Endocrinology, Columbia University College of Physicians and Surgeons, New York, New York

Thomas J. Garite, MD
Department of Obstetrics and Gynecology, University of California, Irvine, College of Medicine, Orange, California; Director of Research, Obstetrix Medical Group, Sunrise, Florida

Julie S. Glickstein, MD
Associate Professor of Clinical Pediatrics, Columbia University College of Physicians and Surgeons; Morgan Stanley Children's Hospital of New York–Presbyterian, New York, New York

Richard W. Hall, MD
Associate Professor of Pediatrics, University of Arkansas for Medical Sciences, Little Rock, Arkansas

Mary Catherine Harris, MD
Professor, Division of Neonatology, Department of Pediatrics, University of Pennsylvania School of Medicine; Division of Neonatology, Children's Hospital of Philadelphia, Philadelphia, Pennsylvania

Karen D. Hendricks-Muñoz, MD, MPH
Associate Professor, Department of Pediatrics, Division of Neonatology, New York University School of Medicine, New York, New York

Joshua E. Hyman, MD
Assistant Professor, Orthopedic Surgery, Morgan Stanley Children's Hospital of New York–Presbyterian, New York, New York

Kent R. Kelley, MD
Assistant Clinical Professor of Pediatrics and Neurology, Children's Memorial Epilepsy Center, Feinberg School of Medicine of Northwestern University, Chicago, Illinois

M. Richard Koenigsberger, MD
Professor of Clinical of Neurology and Pediatrics, Columbia University College of Physicians and Surgeons; Director of Pediatric Neurology Clinic, Morgan Stanley Children's Hospital of New York–Presbyterian, New York, New York

Jane S. Lee, MD, MPH
Assistant Professor of Pediatrics, Columbia University College of Physicians and Surgeons; Morgan Stanley Children's Hospital of New York–Presbyterian, New York, New York

John M. Lorenz, MD
Professor of Clinical Pediatrics, Columbia University College of Physicians and Surgeons; Morgan Stanley Children's Hospital of New York–Presbyterian, New York, New York

Kimberly D. Morel, MD, FAAD, FAAP
Assistant Professor of Clinical Dermatology and Clinical Pediatrics, Columbia University College of Physicians and Surgeons; Morgan Stanley Children's Hospital of New York–Presbyterian, New York, New York

David A. Munson, MD
Clinician, Division of Neonatology, Department of Pediatrics, University of Pennsylvania School of Medicine; Division of Neonatology, Children's Hospital of Philadelphia, Philadelphia, Pennsylvania

Sharon E. Oberfield, MD
Professor of Pediatrics, Director, Division of Pediatric Endocrinology, Columbia University College of Physicians and Surgeons, New York, New York

Carol Prendergast, EdD
Assistant Professor, Department of Pediatrics, Division of Neonatology, New York University School of Medicine, New York, New York

Roy Proujansky, MD
Chairman, Department of Pediatrics, A.I. duPont Hospital for Children, Wilmington, Delaware

Sujit Sheth, MD
Assistant Professor of Pediatrics, Morgan Stanley Children's Hospital of New York–Presbyterian, New York, New York

Helen M. Towers, LRCP&SI, MB
Assistant Professor of Pediatrics, Columbia University Medical Center; Morgan Stanley Children's Hospital of New York–Presbyterian, New York, New York

Peter C. Wilmot, DO
Department of Pediatrics, Jefferson Medical College of Thomas Jefferson University, Philadelphia, Pennsylvania; GI Fellow, Division of Pediatric Gastroenterology and Nutrition, A.I. duPont Hospital for Children, Wilmington, Delaware

Philip J. Wolfson, MD
Professor of Surgery, Jefferson Medical College of Thomas Jefferson University, Philadelphia, Pennsylvania; Attending Surgeon, A.I. duPont Hospital for Children, Wilmington, Delaware

PREFACE

From the time we become physicians until the time we retire from medicine, we are guided by the phrase widely attributed to Hippocrates: *primum non nocere*, "first do not harm." Although the origins of that exact phrase are unclear, Hippocrates certainly conveyed that meaning in his oath: "I will prescribe regimen for the good of my patients according to my ability and my judgment and never do harm to anyone." Fundamental to the concept of "doing good" is the acquisition of medical knowledge that allows each of us to practice according to the highest possible standards. In the first two years of medical school, knowledge is transferred predominantly by large group lectures and required readings. Once we enter the clinical years, the process of acquiring new information begins to change. We continue to read textbooks, but journal articles become increasingly important sources of the newest information, and much information is transmitted to us through "personal communications" by individuals who are further along in their training. For the medical student, that often means an intern or resident, and for the senior resident, a fellow or an attending. This apprenticeship aspect of medicine has been an intrinsic part of the field since its inception. Even in this era of rapidly intensifying technologic advances, "see one, do one, teach one" remains a cornerstone of bedside medical education.

With this concept in mind, *Fetal and Neonatal Secrets*, is designed to serve as a primer for the bedside teaching that remains such an important part of medical education. While it can be read from cover to cover (e.g., to prepare for a certifying examination), we believe that the information in the book should be shared wherever health care providers congregate to provide care to the fetus and newborn infant (inpatient service, clinics, operating room). Although the word *secrets* connotes a sense of privacy, we hope that this book reveals rather than obscures secrets, and that the cumulative wisdom shared by the many experienced contributors serves to enlighten the reader. Furthermore, we would love to see these secrets used by the youngest members of the health care team to challenge those more experienced, as well as by professors to make their residents and students think. We fear that we may need to tote around a copy of this book on rounds ourselves, as our house staff, fellows, and nurse practitioners may throw down the gauntlet to test us on a daily basis! Although we have tried to make this book as comprehensive and practical as possible, the reader will encounter many facts that might be considered trivial (e.g., what is the ductus of Botallo?), but we hope that the reader is forgiving in this respect. The retention of important information has always seemed to be enhanced by its association with interesting, but less essential information (the Mary Poppins approach—"a spoonful of sugar helps the medicine go down"). Where would medicine be without mnemonics? In any event, we hope you find this book useful in your daily practice, but more importantly, we want you to have some fun along the way.

Richard A. Polin, MD
Alan R. Spitzer, MD

ACKNOWLEDGMENTS

In my development as a physician, I have been exposed to many wonderful teachers, scientists, and physicians. However, because of the enormous influence they have had on my career, I would like to acknowledge five individuals by name: Bill Speck (my lifelong friend—no one has ever cared more about resident and student education), David Cornfield (the consummate general pediatrician who helped shape my career in academic medicine), John Driscoll (the person who first excited me about neonatology and my role model for the warm, caring physician), Bill Fox (my coeditor for *Fetal and Neonatal Physiology*, who shared with me his infectious excitement about research), and Mark Ditmar (my coeditor for *Pediatric Secrets*, whose combination of humor, knowledge, and compassion has allowed me to achieve a balance in medicine and who has shown me how "academic" and wonderful the practice of general pediatrics can be). I am indebted to all of them.

Finally, I would like to thank my publisher, Linda Belfus, for hooking me on the Secrets series and allowing me to put my love of education into print.

Richard A. Polin, MD

In the 5 years since the first edition of this book was published, much has happened in the world and in the specialty of neonatal-perinatal medicine. Although the Cold War is over, the war on terrorism, which emerged in its place, seems uncomfortably ominous and creates an environment in which the future is even less certain than it was during the years of the Cold War. With this background to our lives, we still strive to find better ways to care for the newborn infants who, hopefully, will someday create a world that is more at peace with itself than the world of today.

The births of my grandchildren, Jacob and Matthew, both premature infants, have allowed me to experience neonatology from a very different perspective. After 30 years in newborn medicine, I still continue to learn more each day. While this book professes to offer answers to many questions in this field, I have come to realize that, with my grandchildren as my teachers, my knowledge only begins to scratch the surface of this specialty. Therefore, I feel very privileged to be working in an environment in which my ideas are constantly being tested and expanded by my colleagues in Pediatrix Medical Group. From the leadership of the company, Roger Medel, Joe Calabro, Karl Wagner, and Tom Hawkins, to our more than 800 practicing neonatologists, perinatologists, pediatric cardiologists, pediatric intensivists, and hospitalists, I am surrounded by people who never settle for anything less than the best. Our extraordinary advanced practice nurses also bring a special level of expertise and caring to their patients. I am also particularly indebted to Reese Clark and Tom Garite, the Directors of Research at Pediatrix and Obstetrix and contributors to this book, whose work represents the pinnacle of sound scientific investigation in neonatal and perinatal medicine. All of these individuals are constantly challenging accepted notions and working to improve the health care of women and infants. I am deeply grateful for the opportunity to call them colleagues and friends.

I am also most indebted to the editorial staff at Elsevier, especially Linda Belfus and Trevor MacDougall, whose tireless efforts in seeing this book to publication cannot be overemphasized. My extraordinary executive assistant, Janet Graff, helped keep my daily life well-coordinated so I could finish this book.

Lastly, no effort would be possible without the ongoing support of my wife, Elaine. After 35 years of marriage, she is still my greatest inspiration and my best friend. She is also the finest teacher that I have ever seen. She and my children—my son Stephen and my daughter-in-law Jennifer, my daughter Sara and my new son-in-law Kevin, my daughter Lauren, and my wonderful grandchildren, Jacob and Matthew—make everything in this life worthwhile.

Alan R. Spitzer, MD

TOP 100 SECRETS

These secrets are 100 of the top board alerts. They summarize the concepts, principles, and most salient details of fetal and neonatal medicine.

1. A normal biophysical profile (BPP) is never associated with fetal acidemia.

2. Fetal hydrops is a harbinger of fetal demise.

3. Primary complications of fetal surgery are premature labor and preterm delivery.

4. Liver position and lung-to-head ratio relate to prognosis in congenital diaphragmatic hernia, whereas in congenital cystic adenomatoid malformation, morphology is a better prognostic indicator than histology. Mortality from sacrococcygeal teratoma is inversely related to gestational age at diagnosis.

5. Selective laser photocoagulation is the only potentially curative intervention in twin-twin transfusion syndrome.

6. The fastest way to obtain results of chromosomal analysis for genetic testing of amniotic fluid is through fluorescent in situ hybridization (FISH).

7. Cigarette smoking and cocaine are important causes of placental abruption.

8. A Kleihauer-Betke test remains the best way to determine fetal-maternal bleeding.

9. The absence of fetal fibronectin in cervicovaginal secretions has excellent negative predictive value in ensuring that delivery is not imminent.

10. Multiple courses of antenatal steroids (>3) may be associated with subsequent reduction of brain growth in the fetus and neonate.

11. Progesterone administration appears to be the most effective way to prevent premature delivery at present.

12. The BPP consists of fetal movement, fetal breathing movements, fetal tone, amniotic fluid volume, and fetal heart rate monitoring. A BPP score <6 is worrisome and needs careful attention.

13. Flow reversal through the umbilical artery during diastole is a critical measure of impending fetal demise, especially in a growth-retarded infant.

14. Developmental care such as paying attention to light, sound, handling, and touch in the neonatal intensive care unit (NICU) can improve the medical outcome of critically ill infants.

15. Including parents as part of the care team reduces infant pain and stress and improves the medical outcome. Also pay attention to infant responses or cues. Premature infants who shield their face with their hands are not saying hello; they are letting you know they have had enough stress.

16. The senses continue to develop in the NICU, beginning with touch and ending with vision. Neuronal connections will be affected by negative and positive environmental influences.

17. The brain of the premature infant is primed to respond to pain in the NICU. Shield the infant from light and provide containment with pacifiers before, during, and after procedures. Premature infants have a greater sensitivity to pain than term infants.

18. The recommended light (<60 fc) and sound standards (<50 dB) decrease hearing loss and poor developmental outcome in critically ill infants. Hearing deficit is the most common sensory deficit in newborns.

19. Fetal abnormalities and congenital malformations remain the most common causes of fetal death.

20. The use of waterless, alcohol-based hand gels reduces infection rates and maintains better skin integrity.

21. Retinopathy of prematurity is responsible for more blindness among children in the United States than all other causes combined.

22. Catch-up growth may be associated with an increased risk of childhood obesity.

23. Proper positioning will prevent infants from developing positional deformities of the cranium, torso, and pelvis. These deformities interfere and delay subsequent development. Infants cannot easily move around. Pay attention to their position.

24. The absence of a murmur in the neonatal period does not rule out congenital heart disease. An abnormal electrocardiograph in the newborn period warrants a cardiology evaluation.

25. Maintaining patency of the ductus arteriosus is important in both severe right and left heart obstructive lesions. The physiologic effects and clinical manifestations of certain left-sided obstructive lesions (i.e., coarctation of the aorta) may not be apparent until after the ductus arteriosus closes.

26. The most common cyanotic congenital heart lesion in the newborn period is d-transposition of the great vessels. Tetralogy of Fallot is the most common cyanotic lesion presenting outside the newborn period.

27. The physical examination is still the most important procedure in making a diagnosis of congenital heart disease, although the echocardiogram will confirm the diagnosis. If a diagnosis of congenital heart disease is made, look for other anatomic lesions and consider the possibility of genetic and/or chromosomal abnormalities as well.

28. In neonates with visible midline lumbosacral lesions (e.g., sacral pits, hypertrichosis, lipomas), imaging of the spine should be performed to search for occult spinal dysraphism.

29. Hemangiomas in a "beard distribution" may be associated with internal airway hemangiomas. Certain neonatal malignancies can mimic the appearance of a "congenital hemangioma."

30. Premature infants born before 34 weeks' gestation are at increased risk for transepidermal water loss. They are also at increased risk for toxic side effects of topically applied substances.

31. If you strongly suspect an inborn error of metabolism, you should make the baby NPO (fed nothing by mouth) and give nutritional support with sufficient glucose to keep the baby anabolic.

32. The most common cause of hypercalcemia during the neonatal period is excessive administration of calcium. The most common cause of hypermagnesemia during the newborn period is excessive maternal administration of magnesium.

33. Treatment for congenital hypothyroidism should begin as soon as possible after birth to prevent neurologic impairment. The in utero effects of hypothyroidism are variable and may have severe adverse consequences, even with early treatment. Early neonatal screening is therefore essential for optimal outcome.

34. The most common cause of congenital adrenal hyperplasia and sexual ambiguity at birth is 21-hydroxylase deficiency.

35. Many of the diseases screened for at birth with expanded neonatal screening can be treated with dietary alteration with good outcome. In addition, sudden death can be avoided by knowing the presence of metabolic abnormalities such as medium- or long-chain fatty acid oxidation deficiencies in some infants.

36. Ninety-seven percent of infants will void during the first day of life and 100% by 48 hours of age. Any infant who fails to pass urine by this time should be evaluated.

37. A neonate requires approximately 4–8 mg/kg/min of glucose for maintenance of blood glucose levels. Under certain stress conditions, even higher rates may be necessary.

38. Because urine output is so low and insensible water loss is high, it is exceedingly rare for a neonate to need supplemental sodium on the first day of life; early administration of sodium may actually result in hypernatremia.

39. An infant cannot overcorrect for a metabolic acid-base disorder. In examining a blood gas result, the primary disturbance is always defined by the pH. A pH below 7.35 means that the primary disturbance is an acidosis (metabolic or respiratory), whereas a pH above 7.45 indicates that the primary disorder is an alkalosis. One cannot have, for example, a compensatory respiratory alkalosis that elevates a pH *above* 7.45 in response to metabolic acidosis.

40. At term, about 40% of amniotic fluid comes from the fetal urinary tract. The remainder comes from the placenta and the lung.

41. The serum creatinine level at the time of birth reflects the mother's renal status, not that of the neonate. After 24–48 hours, the creatinine level is a reflection of the neonatal kidney function.

42. Neonatal polyuria always reflects either an abnormality in renal function or excessive administration of free water to the infant.

43. Although neonates tend to run higher serum potassium levels than older children or adults, iatrogenically induced hyperkalemia is one of the most common safety errors in the NICU and is a life-threatening emergency.

44. In a male infant, the presence of hydronephrosis should be considered diagnostic for posterior urethral valves until proven otherwise. Posterior urethral valves are virtually never seen in a female infant.

45. Hypertension in the low-birth-weight patient is most commonly caused by either an umbilical artery catheter or volume changes in the intravascular space associated with chronic disease states such as bronchopulmonary dysplasia.

46. Peripheral eosinophilia is extremely common in the growing premature infant. It should not be considered an indicator of allergic gastrointestinal disease in an infant without other features to suggest such a diagnosis.

47. The ophthalmologic examination is an extremely useful adjunct in the evaluation of the infant with cholestatic jaundice to examine for evidence of congenital infection or genetic etiology.

48. Significant hepatic synthetic dysfunction that is disproportionate to the degree of transaminase elevation should lead to serious consideration of underlying metabolic disease (e.g., galactosemia, neonatal iron storage disease, tyrosinemia).

49. Inadequate caloric intake continues to be the most common cause of failure to thrive for the infant recovering from a complicated neonatal medical course.

50. For an infant needing a very high calorie formula, the use of additional carbohydrate to increase calories can be associated with diarrhea; the use of additional fat calories may be associated with recurrent emesis.

51. Bloody diarrhea is the hallmark of colitis (e.g., allergic colitis, infection, Hirschsprung enterocolitis). Rectal bleeding without diarrhea should lead to the consideration of a focal source of bleeding (e.g., localized ulceration, arteriovenous malformation).

52. Cholestatic jaundice associations include:
    - **Cholestatic jaundice and a murmur:** Think Alagille syndrome.
    - **Cholestatic jaundice and ascites:** Think metabolic etiologies of hepatic failure and spontaneous perforation of the bile duct.
    - **Cholestatic jaundice and sepsis:** Think urinary infection or metabolic disease, especially galactosemia.
    - **Cholestatic jaundice with low gamma-glutamyl transferase:** Think bile salt transport defects.

53. Patchy alternations in skin pigmentation in females suggest the possibility of genetic mosaicism or X-linked disorders that result from differential lyonization.

54. Thumb and radial ray abnormalities with or without café-au-lait spots may be the first indication of Fanconi anemia, a condition that may ultimately require carefully timed bone marrow transplant. The condition is autosomal recessive and more common in Jewish families.

55. Half of all babies diagnosed with nonsyndromic deafness have autosomal mutations in connexin 26 with a 25% risk of recurrence in future siblings.

56. All *genetic* problems in the child are not necessarily *inherited* from the parents. Many genetic problems are *de novo*, or new, to the child and suggest a low risk of recurrence for future pregnancies. However, such genetic problems can be passed on to the children of the child with the *de novo* mutation.

57. Although the risk of Down syndrome is highest in mothers above the age of 35 years, the majority of cases occur in women below age 35, since they have the majority of pregnancies.

58. Most deaths from Potter's syndrome are due to lung hypoplasia, even though the primary disorder evolves from the genitourinary tract. The lung needs adequate amniotic fluid production to develop normally in utero.

59. FISH testing is most helpful for disorders that emerge from the subtelomeric ends of the chromosomes, where there is great genetic density that may not be resolved by standard genetic testing.

60. Minor chromosomal abnormalities are quite common, affecting nearly one in seven infants.

61. The most common cause of anemia in the newborn is excessive blood drawing.

62. Whereas Rh isoimmunization usually occurs in a second pregnancy, neonatal alloimmune thrombocytopenia may occur in the first.

63. Neonates should always be transfused with cytomegalovirus (CMV)-negative, irradiated, leukocyte-depleted blood products.

64. Disseminated intravascular coagulation (DIC) is always pathologic and always secondary to another process. DIC will resolve when that process is treated appropriately. Neonates require higher doses of heparin to achieve therapeutic anticoagulation.

65. The most common tumor presenting as an abdominal mass is a neuroblastoma.

66. Universal screening for group B *Streptococcus* colonization is now recommended for all pregnant women.

67. Neonatal meningitis can occur in the setting of negative blood culture results; therefore, a lumbar puncture should be strongly considered during a sepsis evaluation.

68. Zidovudine treatment of expectant HIV-positive mothers and their infants remains the primary intervention for decreasing the risk of vertical transmission. However, additional antiretroviral agents may be indicated for infants born to mothers without antiretroviral treatment.

69. Fluconazole prophylaxis for infants weighing less than 1000 gm has been demonstrated to decrease the incidence of candidemia in these high-risk patients.

70. The clinician should have a high suspicion for herpes simplex virus as a causative organism in the ill-appearing neonate. A child with fever in the first 24 hours of life should be considered to have herpes infection until proven otherwise.

71. Six weeks of ganciclovir can improve the preservation of hearing in infants with congenital CMV infection and evidence of central nervous system involvement.

72. Eye discharges in the neonate should always be approached with great caution. What initially seems to be a simple infection may be gonococcal in etiology.

73. Neonatal HIV infection may present in myriad ways and should always be part of the differential diagnosis when answers are not immediately forthcoming.

74. Ampicillin and gentamicin appear to be a more effective and safer therapy for neonatal sepsis than ampicillin and cefotaxime.

75. Observation of the newborn infant is the key to the neurologic examination. Look at the baby for at least 2 minutes before touching him or her.

76. The grade IV hemorrhage classification may be misleading, particularly since not all grade IVs are equivalent. Hemorrhage into the substance of the brain can be small, with a relatively better

prognosis, or quite large, with a guarded prognosis in terms of mortality or serious morbidity. When the size and location of the parenchymal bleed(s) are not carefully documented, misleading therapeutic decisions and prognostic statements can ensue.

77. Clonus, one of the most common movements confused with seizures, may be initiated by stimulation or stopped by holding or repositioning an involved extremity.

78. Neonatal seizures are a red flag for neurologic dysfunction and injury and require emergent evaluation and treatment.

79. When evaluating a "floppy infant," the most important single diagnostic step is to interview and carefully examine the mother.

80. The clinician should ask whether the process causing hypotonia is central (brain-related) or peripheral (caused by lower motor unit dysfunction). Rarely, both are involved.

81. The complex factors that result in periventricular leukomalacia (PVL) are usually operative in utero before the neonatologist ever sees the infant. Proinflammatory cytokines appear to be an important part of the pathophysiology of PVL and, ultimately, cerebral palsy.

82. All newborn babies should be examined for evidence of hip dysplasia, spinal dysraphism, and lower and upper extremity deficiencies and/or deformities. The hip examination consists of the Ortolani, Barlow, and Galeazzi tests.

83. The majority of club feet can be treated effectively with manipulation and casting. Treatment should begin as soon as possible after birth. Because club foot may be associated with other congenital conditions, a thorough evaluation of the entire infant is necessary.

84. Newborn children with a bone or joint infection may present with pseudoparalysis of the affected extremity. A fever is not a prerequisite for a bone or joint infection. Treatment of joint infections requires aspiration and antibiotics.

85. Although children may not directly recall painful experiences from their NICU stay, they may demonstrate altered behavioral states from painful experiences that were not well managed. Morphine and fentanyl appear to be equally effective for pain relief in neonates and have similar outcomes in follow-up studies.

86. Methadone and some of the newer narcotic agonists (e.g., buprenorphine), as well as a number of other agents, appear to be optimal treatments for narcotic withdrawal in neonates. Paregoric and phenobarbital are no longer drugs of choice.

87. If a patient is easy to oxygenate but impossible to ventilate, airway disease should be considered as the most likely pulmonary problem. If a patient is easy to ventilate but impossible to oxygenate, cyanotic congenital heart is the most likely cause for the gas exchange problem. If both oxygenation and ventilation are problems, intrinsic lung disease is the most likely problem.

88. Airway, airway, airway—the most important aspect of neonatal resuscitation is managing the airway! Most neonates who require support in the delivery room respond to stimulation, opening the airway, and gentle ventilation with a bag and mask.

89. Most infants with cerebral palsy do not have a history to suggest an intrapartum event as the primary cause. The use of the term *asphyxia* should be avoided. It is much more useful and appropriate to describe the events and symptoms and assign more definitive diagnoses.

90. Prevention is better than rescue treatment in promoting a healthy outcome of a neonate with respiratory distress syndrome. The most studied and effective way to improve outcomes of neonates with respiratory distress syndrome is instilling surfactant into the trachea.

91. Vigorous meconium-stained infants do not need to be intubated and suctioned in the delivery room. Those who have an initial heart rate >100 bpm, good respiratory effort, and reasonable tone will not benefit from intubation and suctioning. In fact, some vigorous infants may be injured in the process of suctioning because they are so difficult to restrain.

92. The most studied and effective therapy for neonates with pulmonary hypertension is inhaled nitric oxide. Ventilator-induced alkalosis, bicarbonate infusions, and prostaglandin products have not been adequately studied and should be avoided. Inhaled nitric oxide does not, however, reduce the need for extracorporeal membrane oxygenation (ECMO) in neonates with congenital diaphragmatic hernia.

93. Both intrinsic defects in the larynx or trachea and extrinsic compression of the trachea can cause airway obstruction syndrome. Lung function is normal in most of these disorders so that airway management, which relieves the obstruction, usually normalizes gas exchange.

94. The most effective ways to avoid lung injury in neonates who require mechanical ventilation are to optimize oxygen delivery and avoid hyperoxia and hypoxia (by carefully adjusting fractional concentration of oxygen in inspired gas [FiO_2] levels), to normalize functional residual capacity to prevent lung collapse (by giving surfactant to patients with respiratory distress syndrome and using end-expiratory pressure to maintain lung volume), and to avoid volutrauma (by limiting the tidal volume used to support ventilation).

95. The type of high-frequency ventilation device may be less important than the ventilatory strategy with which it is used. If the lung is poorly inflated, a strategy of lung recruitment (increased mean airway pressure compared with that of a conventional ventilator) is appropriate. If an air leak is present or if the lung is overinflated, a strategy that minimizes intrathoracic pressure is important, and a lower mean airway pressure may be the most appropriate approach.

96. Survival of critically ill neonates with intractable respiratory failure is better in those offered ECMO than in those receiving conventional care. ECMO is one of the few therapies shown to save the lives of critically ill neonates.

97. The sudden infant death syndrome (SIDS) rate in the United States has dropped precipitously from about 2 deaths per 1000 births in 1992 to the present 0.75 per 1000 births. This rapid decline followed the discovery that the simple act of changing infants' sleeping positions from the stomach to the back dramatically reduced the SIDS rate.

98. Infants born with isolated esophageal atresia (i.e., without a distal tracheoesophageal fistula) characteristically have a very long gap between esophageal segments, such that a primary esophageal anastomosis at the initial surgical procedure is rarely possible.

99. If a baby has an incarcerated hernia, the gonad is at even more risk for sustaining injury than the intestine. In boys, the herniated bowel compresses the delicate spermatic vessels in the inguinal canal and can render the testicle ischemic; in girls, the ovary itself—more often than the intestine—is usually the structure that is actually herniated.

100. Bilious vomiting that develops suddenly in an otherwise healthy infant should always be considered a potential emergency due to the possibility of midgut volvulus, and an upper gastrointestinal tract contrast study must be obtained immediately to rule it out.

CHAPTER 1

FETAL DEVELOPMENT AND GROWTH

Jane S. Lee, MD, MPH, and Christiana R. Farkouh, MD, MPH

1. **What features constitute the biophysical profile score (BPS)?**
   The BPS is a scoring system developed by Frank Manning to assess fetal well-being before birth. Five parameters are assessed:
   - Fetal breathing movements
   - Gross body movements
   - Fetal tone
   - Reactive fetal heart rate
   - Qualitative amniotic fluid volume

   The presence of a normal assessment is scored as 2 points, and the absence of the finding is scored as 0. The maximum score is 10, and the minimum score is 0. If all of the ultrasound measurements are normal (i.e., BPS = 8), fetal heart monitoring may be omitted since it will not improve the test's predictive accuracy. If oligohydramnios is detected, further fetal evaluation is necessary, regardless of the BPS.

2. **Can one really detect breathing movements before birth?**
   A regular pattern of fetal breathing movements is observed by 20–21 weeks' gestation. Fetal breathing movement is controlled by centers on the ventral surface of the fourth ventricle. As a result, the presence of fetal breathing indicates an intact central nervous system. Fetal breathing movements appear to assist the movement of fetal lung fluid into the amniotic cavity and also tone the respiratory muscles for the assumption of breathing at the time of birth.

3. **How does one differentiate pathologic absence of fetal breathing movements from periodic breathing that occurs during fetal sleep?**
   To account for the possibility of fetal sleep during an observation period, the observer must scan the mother for a minimum of 30 minutes. It is exceedingly rare for a fetus to go beyond this time limit without fetal breathing movements.

4. **Why are fetal heart rate reactivity and gross body movements part of the BPS?**
   The acute fetal response to a hypoxemic event is a centrally mediated suppression of a series of biophysical activities such as fetal heart rate and movements. By decreasing these activities, the fetus can significantly reduce oxygen requirements by 19% and raise the fetal venous partial pressure of oxygen as much as 30%.

5. **When should the BPS be used?**
   The BPS is applicable in cases of acute or chronic intrauterine hypoxia. In response to hypoxia, the individual components of the BPS theoretically disappear in the inverse of their appearance. Nonreactive fetal heart rate activity should be the first sign of fetal compromise, followed by fetal breathing movements, gross body movement, and, lastly, tone. Whereas the other BPS parameters reflect more acute changes, amniotic fluid volume assessment is a measure of chronic fetal status. Oligohydramnios may be seen in response to impaired uteroplacental perfusion.

6. **How does the BPS relate to the umbilical venous pH?**
   Figure 1-1 reveals the relationship between the fetal BPS and mean umbilical venous pH.

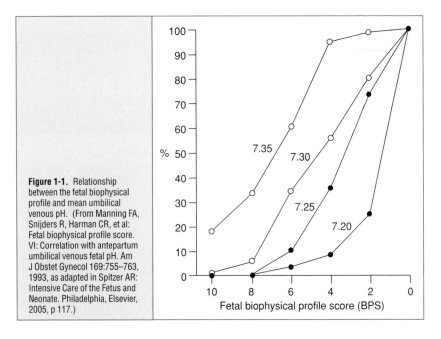

Figure 1-1. Relationship between the fetal biophysical profile and mean umbilical venous pH. (From Manning FA, Snijders R, Harman CR, et al: Fetal biophysical profile score. VI: Correlation with antepartum umbilical venous fetal pH. Am J Obstet Gynecol 169:755–763, 1993, as adapted in Spitzer AR: Intensive Care of the Fetus and Neonate. Philadelphia, Elsevier, 2005, p 117.)

7. **What is the relationship between the fetal BPS and neonatal outcome?**
   Figure 1-2 depicts the relationship between the fetal BPS and risk of any perinatal morbidity, meconium aspiration, and major congenital anomaly. A normal BPS is never associated with fetal acidemia. The perinatal mortality rate is 0.8 per 1000 live births after a normal BPS. However, a BPS of 0 is almost always associated with fetal compromise.

8. **When do the five senses develop in the fetus?**
   - **Touch:** Between 8 and 15 weeks' gestational age (GA), the fetal somatosensory system develops in a cephalocaudal pattern. By 32 weeks' GA, the fetus consistently responds to temperature, pressure, and pain.
   - **Taste:** Taste buds are morphologically mature by 13 weeks' GA. By 24 weeks' GA, gustatory responses may be present.
   - **Hearing:** Auditory function begins at 20 weeks' GA when the cochlea becomes functional. By 25 weeks' GA, response to intense vibroacoustic stimuli can be elicited. Sensitivity and frequency resolution approach adult level by 30 weeks' GA and are indistinguishable from the adult by term.
   - **Sight:** Pupillary response to light appears as early as 29 weeks' GA and is present consistently by 32 weeks' GA.
   - **Smell:** By 28–32 weeks' GA, premature infants appear to respond to concentrated odor.

9. **What is the normal rate of postnatal head growth in the preterm infant?**
   Head growth is categorized in three phases: an initial growth arrest or suboptimal growth, rapid catch-up growth, and stable growth following standard reference curves. During the first 2–4 months of age, the appropriate rate of head growth is 0.5–1.0 cm per week. Head growth >1.0 cm per week during the first 6 weeks of age may indicate possible central nervous system pathology (e.g., hydrocephalus). The ratio of head circumference (HC) to body length may also help distinguish normal from pathologic head growth. HC typically follows the same percentile

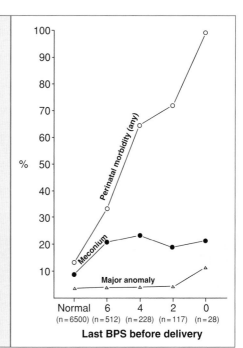

Figure 1-2. Relationship between the fetal biophysical profile score (BPS) and neonatal outcome. (From Manning FA, Harman CR, Morrison I, et al: Fetal assessment based on fetal biophysical profile scoring. VI: An analysis of perinatal morbidity and mortality. Am J Obstet Gynecol 162:703–709, 1990, as adapted in Spitzer AR: Intensive Care of the Fetus and Neonate. Philadelphia, Elsevier, 2005, p 118.)

curve as the length. If the HC differs from the length by more than one quartile, further investigation is warranted.

10. **How does postmaturity differ from dysmaturity?**
    Postmaturity refers to an infant born of a post-term pregnancy (i.e., >42 weeks' GA).
    Dysmaturity describes an infant who exhibits characteristics of placental insufficiency such as loss of subcutaneous fat and muscle mass or meconium staining of the amniotic fluid, skin, and nails. The gestation may be term or preterm.

11. **What screening is available for fetal growth assessment?**
    The best screening tool to assess fetal growth is fundal height, which is measured from the upper edge of the symphysis pubis to the top of the uterine fundus. Between 20 and 34 weeks' GA, fundal height measurements (in cm) approximate GA (in weeks). A discrepancy between measured and expected fundal height measurements of 3 cm or more is suggestive of fetal growth restriction.

12. **Once fetal growth restriction is suspected based on history and clinical assessment of fundal height, what is the next step in determining the degree of impaired fetal growth?**
    Fetal biometry should be performed to evaluate possible inappropriate fetal growth.
    Ultrasonographic measurements of fetal growth are as follows:
    - Biparietal diameter
    - HC
    - Abdominal circumference
    - Femur length

Abdominal circumference is the most sensitive single measurement. These individual growth parameters are commonly input into standard formulas to calculate the estimated fetal weight. When estimated fetal weight is <10th percentile, serial ultrasounds at regular intervals are necessary to monitor growth over time.

13. **Is there a difference between growth retardation and growth restriction? Define fetal growth restriction.**
Because of the pejorative nature of the term *retardation*, the term *restriction* has been substituted. There is no difference between the terms. Intrauterine growth restriction (IUGR) is a deviation in the rate of growth of a fetus that is less than its genetically predetermined growth potential.
- *Symmetric IUGR* is characterized by equal reduction in head, abdominal, and skeletal dimensions. It is indicative of an insult during the period of most active cell division, as seen in chromosomal or congenital abnormalities.
- *Asymmetric IUGR* is distinguished by a reduction in abdominal circumference but sparing of head and skeletal growth. It most likely represents an insult during cell growth from extrinsic factors such as uteroplacental insufficiency or maternal vascular disease.

14. **How do you differentiate a growth-restricted infant from a small-for-gestational-age (SGA) infant and a low-birth-weight (LBW) infant?**
The critical distinction is the fetal growth potential.
- An *IUGR infant* has failed to meet his or her own growth potential. The term *intrauterine growth restriction* is frequently used interchangeably, but incorrectly, with *SGA*.
- *SGA* refers to an infant whose birth weight is below a preset weight cutoff, typically the 10th percentile for GA, when compared with reference population norms.
- The *LBW* classification refers to any infant who weighs less than 2500 gm at birth, independent of GA. This category includes term (≥37 weeks' gestation) SGA infants as well as premature infants who may be SGA or of appropriate size relative to their GA.

KEY POINTS: EXTREMES OF FETAL GROWTH

1. IUGR: failure to meet growth potential
2. SGA: <10th percentile for GA based on population norms
3. LBW: birth weight <2500 gm
4. Prematurity: normal or altered growth at <37 weeks' GA

15. **Name the major risk factors for fetal growth restriction.**
Factors that affect fetal growth are typically categorized as fetal, placental, or maternal in origin and are summarized in Table 1-1. Common examples include the following:
- **Prior maternal history of fetal growth restriction**
- **Maternal history of immunologic or collagen vascular disease**
- **Maternal TORCH infection:** **T**oxoplasmosis, **o**ther (syphilis and other viruses), **r**ubella, **c**ytomegalovirus, and **h**erpes simplex virus
- **Maternal hypertension or preeclampsia**
- **Genetic syndromes in the fetus:** Trisomy 21, 18, or 13, Turner syndrome
- **Teratogens:** Cigarette smoke, retin-A, warfarin, alcohol
- **Advanced maternal diabetes**
- **Placental insufficiency**
- **Placental infarction**
- **Idiopathic factors**

TABLE 1-1. RISK FACTORS FOR INTRAUTERINE GROWTH RESTRICTION

Maternal	Placental	Fetal
Poor or inadequate nutritional intake	**Mosaicism**	**Chromosomal abnormalities**
Medical disease	**Abnormal implantation**	Trisomy 13, 18, and 21
Preeclampsia	Previa	Turner syndrome
Chronic hypertension	Accreta	**Genetic syndromes**
Collagen vascular disease	**Abnormal morphology**	Russell-Silver
Diabetes mellitus with vascular disease	Small size	Cornelia de Lange
Thrombophilia (congenital or acquired)	Bilobed, battledore, or circumvallate	**Congenital malformations**
Asthma	Velamentous cord insertion	Anencephaly
Cyanotic heart disease	**Lesions**	Congenital heart defect
Genetic disorder	Chorioangiomata	Congenital diaphragmatic hernia
Environment	**Abruptio placentae**	Gastroschisis
High altitude	**Infarction**	Omphalocele
Emotional or physical stress	Secondary to maternal chronic disease	Renal abnormalities
Medications and drugs	Chronic abruption	Multiple malformations
Warfarin	**Infection**	**Multiple gestation**
Anticonvulsants	Chorionitis	Twin-twin transfusion syndrome
Retin-A	Chorioamnionitis	**Infection**
Cigarette smoking	Funistis	TORCH infections: Toxoplasmosis, other (syphilis and
Alcohol		other viruses), rubella, cytomegalovirus, and herpes
Cocaine		simplex virus
Heroin		
Prior obstetric complications		
Spontaneous abortion		
Stillbirth		
IUGR, LBW, or premature offspring		

16. **Describe the "brain-sparing effect."**

    The brain-sparing effect observed in asymmetric IUGR refers to the fetal adaptive response to chronic hypoxia, in which the fetus preferentially redistributes its blood flow to the brain, myocardium, and adrenal glands. Although still investigational, low middle cerebral artery pulsatility on Doppler ultrasound may provide direct evidence of brain sparing.

17. **What is the ponderal index (PI)?**

    The PI is a widely used measurement of the infant's relative thinness or fatness independent of race, gender, and GA:

    $$PI = \frac{weight\ (gm) \times 100}{(length\ [cm])^3}$$

    Normal PI values range between 2.32 and 2.85. The PI is normal in symmetric IUGR, low in asymmetric IUGR, and high in the macrosomic fetus.

18. **What is the initial work-up when fetal growth restriction is suspected?**
    - Perform fetal karyotyping.
    - Obtain maternal serology (i.e., TORCH studies) for evidence of recent seroconversion and thrombophilia studies.
    - Evaluate the mother for preeclampsia.
    - Consider amniotic fluid viral DNA testing.

19. **How should one follow up a fetus at risk for growth retardation?**
    - Once IUGR is suspected, fetal well-being should be closely monitored with serial antenatal monitoring tests such as the nonstress test and BPP.
    - Qualitative assessment of the amniotic fluid level gives an estimate of the chronicity of the insult.
    - The timing of delivery is based on fetal maturity, signs of fetal distress, and worsening maternal disease. Evaluation of placental Doppler blood flow may be helpful in this decision.
    - Electronic fetal monitoring during labor is essential in the care of an IUGR fetus. Intrapartum fetal acid-base status is another indicator that can be used to confirm electronic fetal monitoring findings.

20. **What role does Doppler ultrasonography have in the management of a growth-restricted fetus?**

    In pregnancies at risk for IUGR, Doppler analysis is used to evaluate placental disease and fetal compromise and may improve fetal and neonatal outcomes. Normal umbilical arterial Doppler flow is reassuring and rarely associated with significant morbidity. Absence of end-diastolic flow in the umbilical artery is indicative of fetal hypoxia. Reversal of flow is suggestive of worsening fetal status and impending demise. Abnormalities in venous circulation (e.g., ductus venosus pulsatility) represent worsening circulatory compromise and may reflect a greater risk of imminent fetal demise than abnormalities in the arterial circulation.

21. **What are the delivery implications for a growth-restricted fetus?**
    - The timing of delivery is determined by the GA and clinical status of the fetus.
    - For an IUGR fetus at term or near term with documented pulmonary maturity, delivery is indicated if fetal distress is present, minimal fetal growth is observed over serial ultrasounds, or maternal status is worsening (e.g., hypertension).
    - For an IUGR fetus <32 weeks' GA, optimal timing of delivery is still unresolved. If the indication for delivery is uncertain, the fetus should undergo continuous monitoring.
    - The IUGR fetus is at increased risk of metabolic acidosis, hypoxia, and mortality during labor because of a reduced capability to withstand insults.

22. **List the primary short-term and long-term morbidities observed in growth-restricted infants.**
    - An IUGR infant is initially at risk for perinatal asphyxia, intraventricular hemorrhage, meconium aspiration, respiratory distress syndrome, impaired thermoregulation, fasting and alimented hypoglycemia, hyperviscosity-polycythemia syndrome, immunodeficiency, and necrotizing enterocolitis.
    - The potential long-term complications are cerebral palsy, behavioral and learning problems, and altered postnatal growth.

KEY POINTS: SEQUELAE OF IUGR

1. Pulmonary pathology: meconium aspiration, respiratory distress syndrome

2. Metabolic derangement: impaired thermoregulation, hypoglycemia, altered postnatal growth

3. Hematologic abnormalities: hyperviscosity, polycythemia, thrombocytopenia, leukopenia

4. Neurodevelopment outcomes: cerebral palsy, behavioral and learning problems

23. **Describe the "fetal origins hypothesis" of adult disease (Barker hypothesis).**
    David Barker and colleagues postulated that impaired fetal growth may be a key determinant of later development of adult diseases such as obesity, insulin resistance, type 2 diabetes mellitus, and cardiovascular disease. Poor fetal nutrition results in developmental adaptations that permanently alter subsequent postnatal physiology and thereby "program" an infant's future predisposition to disease.

24. **Define twin-twin transfusion syndrome (TTTS).**
    Historically, TTTS was defined as a growth discordance of 20% or greater between twins and a hemoglobin difference of 5 gm/dL or more. TTTS is currently defined as the presence of oligohydramnios in one amniotic sac and polyhydramnios in the other sac ("oligopolyhydramnios sequence") in a monochorionic diamniotic twin gestation. TTTS results from an unbalanced interfetal transfusion from a net unidirectional flow through arteriovenous anastomoses deep within the shared cotyledon of the placenta. The severity of clinical presentation is probably modulated by the degree of bidirectional flow from superficial anastomoses.

25. **What is the Quintero staging system? How does it aid in the management of TTTS?**
    The Quintero staging system grades the severity of TTTS and may aid in determining the prognosis and selection of treatment modalities.
    - **Stage I:** Oligo-polyhydramnios sequence and visible donor twin bladder
    - **Stage II:** "Stuck twin" phenomenon and empty (nonvisible) donor twin bladder
    - **Stage III:** Critically abnormal Doppler flow studies in either twin
    - **Stage IV:** Fetal hydrops in one or both twins
    - **Stage V:** In utero fetal demise of one or both twins

    Early-stage disease may be treated with conservative therapies such as amnioreduction, whereas advanced disease may be more effectively treated with selective laser ablation of critical vessels.

26. **What are the complications of TTTS?**
    - Complications specific to the recipient twin are polycythemia, systemic hypertension, biventricular cardiac hypertrophy, and congestive heart failure.
    - The donor twin is at risk for growth failure, anemia, high-output cardiac failure, and hydrops.
    - Both twins are at increased risk of congenital anomalies, in utero demise, and cerebral palsy.

27. **What are the available treatment modalities for TTTS?**
    - Serial amnioreduction of the recipient twin amniotic sac increases perfusion to the "stuck twin" by decreasing pressure on the donor amniotic sac.
    - Selective laser photocoagulation of connecting arteriovenous anastomoses decreases the intertwin transfusion (Fig. 1-3). This is the only intervention that may be potentially curative.
    - Amniotic intertwin septostomy restores normal amniotic fluid pressure gradient by allowing hydrostatic flow of amniotic fluid from the recipient to the donor.
    - Selective feticide by cord occlusion is reserved for severe or refractory cases and imminent in utero fetal demise of one twin to improve the survival of the co-twin.
    - Immediate delivery should be strongly considered if there is fetal demise of one twin because there is risk of acute transfusion, disseminated intravascular coagulation, or infarction in the surviving twin.

28. **Which twin is the better candidate for feticide in TTTS?**
    The choice of candidate for this procedure is unclear. Current evidence favors the selection of the recipient twin due to the ease of cord visualization and access, decreased risk of intraoperative uterine wall injury, and increased risk of developing cardiac dysfunction and hydrops. The donor

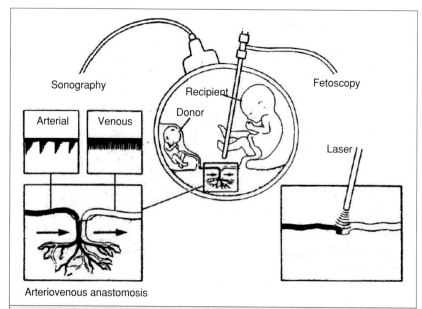

Figure 1-3. Selective laser photocoagulation of connecting arteriovenous anastomoses. (From Cortes RA, Farmer DL: Recent advances in fetal surgery. Semin Perinatol 28:199–211, 2004, with permission.)

twin may be the better candidate for feticide in the presence of a severe cardiac anomaly or brain injury in the donor or increased thickness of the recipient's cord. If the donor is selected, amnioinfusion will most likely need to be performed to enable cord access.

29. **What pathophysiologic factors prompt treatment for fetal arrhythmias? What are the possible fetal interventions?**

The major concern in fetuses with arrhythmia (e.g., supraventricular tachycardia and complete heart block) is compromised cardiac output leading to the development of hydrops. When cardiac output is compromised, maternal antiarrhythmic therapy may be initiated. If fetal arrhythmia remains refractory, direct fetal therapy with antiarrhythmic medications may be considered.

30. **Which disease entities may be treated with fetal surgical intervention? What treatment options are available?**

The major neonatal diseases that may benefit from fetal intervention are listed in Table 1-2. In utero repair has been successfully performed for diseases such as congenital cystic adenomatoid malformation (CCAM), primary fetal pleural effusion, sacrococcygeal teratoma, and lower urinary tract obstruction. Fetal intervention for neural tube defects is currently investigational. To date, interventions for other thoracic anomalies such as congenital diaphragmatic hernia have not proved to be more efficacious than postnatal treatment.

31. **What are the major considerations for fetal intervention in cases of congenital cardiac lesions?**
    - To preserve cardiac structure and function by reversing the pathologic process.
    - To modify or prevent the development of major postnatal disease.

32. **Which congenital cardiac lesions show promise for fetal intervention?**

Left-sided lesions
    - **Severe aortic stenosis:** Fetal aortic valvuloplasty may reverse left ventricular dysfunction, thereby improving flow through the left heart and left ventricular growth, andpossibly preventing the development of hypoplastic left heart syndrome (HLHS).
    - **HLHS and intact/restrictive atrial septum:** In utero balloon septostomy may increase in utero pulmonary blood flow, thereby decreasing or preventing pathologic pulmonary parenchymal remodeling and possibly reducing the degree of subsequent postnatal pulmonary hypertension.

Right-sided lesions
    - **Pulmonary atresia/severe pulmonary valve stenosis with intact ventricular septum:** In utero balloon valvuloplasty may preserve cardiac function by decompressing the right ventricular load and ensuring adequate right heart blood flow and right ventricular growth.

33. **What are the key principles in determining the potential value of a fetal surgical intervention?**
    - The nature and history of the underlying disease should be amenable to fetal surgical intervention.
    - Prenatal repair appears to offer advantages above and beyond postnatal correction.
    - Failure to intervene is likely to result in permanent injury or death to the fetus.
    - Maternal risk is low.

TABLE 1-2. AVAILABLE FETAL INTERVENTIONS

Fetal Diagnosis	Pearls	Fetal Intervention
Myelomeningocele	Incidence: 1:2000 live births Associated with Arnold-Chiari malformation (ACM) type II 70–85% require ventricular shunt ⅔ have normal intelligence; ½ can live independently Overall mortality: 14%; higher if associated with ACM type II	Unclear benefit at this time
Congenital diaphragmatic hernia	Incidence: 1:3000–4000 live births 90% are left sided Associated with chromosomal or congenital abnormalities If isolated, morbidity is related to degree of pulmonary hypoplasia Overall mortality: 26–68%; higher if associated with other defects	No fetal intervention is currently recommended
Congenital cystic adenomatoid malformation (CCAM)	Incidence: 1:25,000–1:35,000 pregnancies Multilobar or bilateral lesions are rare Types: ■ Macrocystic ≥5 mm (single or multiple cysts) ■ Microcystic <5 mm ("solid" appearance) ■ Mixed 10–15% undergo spontaneous reduction or resolution 10–40% progress to hydrops Morbidity is related to size of defect Mortality: ~100% if hydrops develops	Consider in cases of immature fetus with hydrops Options based on fetal maturity and CCAM type Possible options ■ Fetal resection for microcystic lesion ■ Thoracoamniotic shunt for macrocystic lesion

Primary fetal pleural effusion	Incidence: 1:15,000 pregnancies 70% are unilateral, usually on the right Good prognostic indicators: isolated, unilateral, or small volume Poor prognostic indicators: hydrops, chromosomal abnormalities, or multiple congenital malformations Overall mortality: 15–20%	Consider in cases of fetal hydrops Possible options ■ Thoracocentesis (in mature fetus) ● Shunt placement (in immature fetus with unilateral lesion)
Sacrococcygeal teratoma	Incidence: 1:35,000–40,000 live births Types: cystic, solid, or mixed High risk: high output cardiac failure, hydrops, or placentomegaly Malignancy risk increases with delay in excision Morbidity is related to risk of tumor hemorrhage, rupture, or dystocia Overall mortality: 45–100%	Consider in immature high-risk fetus Possible options ■ Amnioreduction for polyhydramnios ■ Cyst aspiration if risk of tumor rupture or mass dystocia ■ Open fetal resection if high output cardiac failure or hydrops
Lower urinary tract obstruction	Incidence: 1% of pregnancies Complications: oligohydramnios, pulmonary hypoplasia, renal dysplasia, and deformational structural anomalies Morbidity is related to timing and duration of obstruction Mortality is correlated with the severity of pulmonary hypoplasia	Consider in fetus who has poor predicted outcome based on ultrasound and urinary fetal electrolyte findings Possible options ■ Vesicoamniotic shunt ■ Open vesicostomy

KEY POINTS: TYPE OF FETAL DEFECT AND TYPE OF INTERVENTION

1. Prevention of the development of defect: correct in utero

2. With progressive worsening: early delivery or in utero correction

3. Presence of dystocia: cesarean section

4. Correctable at term: deliver at term

34. **What major management considerations arise when evaluating a fetus for possible surgical intervention?**
    - Success of surgical options (e.g., survival rate associated with fetal and postnatal repair)
    - Fetal diagnosis capabilities and limitations
    - Degree of antenatal maternal-fetal monitoring
    - Timing of fetal surgery
    - Perioperative maternal risks (e.g., uterine dehiscence, uterine irritability, preterm labor)
    - Obstetric risks in future pregnancies (e.g., uterine rupture and hysterectomy)
    - Timing and mode of delivery
    - Ethical or religious considerations

35. **What is the EXIT procedure?**
    As shown in Fig. 1-4, the ex utero intrapartum treatment (EXIT) is a technique by which a mother undergoes partial cesarean delivery so that placental support to the fetus can be maintained while airway identification, stabilization, and, if necessary, mass resection is performed. The procedure is currently used for the delivery and management of fetal airway compromise from extrinsic mass compression or intrinsic airway defect.

36. **List the congenital malformations that may be indications for the EXIT procedure.**
    - Cervical/oral teratoma compressing the airway
    - Cervical cystic hygroma compressing the larynx/airway
    - Lung mass preventing chest expansion (e.g., CCAM)
    - Less common lesions include fetal goiter, hemangioma, epignathus, neuroblastoma, and congenital high-airway obstruction sequence

KEY POINTS: SURGICAL CONDITIONS THAT MAY WARRANT FETAL INTERVENTION

1. CCAM

2. Primary pleural effusion

3. Sacrococcygeal teratoma

4. Lower urinary tract obstruction

37. **Describe the pathophysiologic effects of large fetal lung masses.**
    - Esophageal compression interferes with fetal swallowing and results in polyhydramnios.
    - Mediastinal shift causes cardiac compression and obstruction of the great vessels and the development of fetal hydrops.

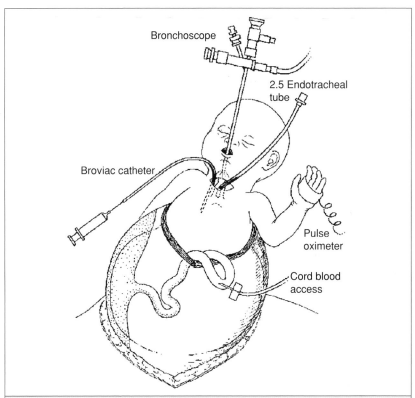

Figure 1-4. The ex utero intrapartum treatment (EXIT). (From Cortes RA, Farmer DL: Recent advances in fetal surgery. Semin Perinatol 28:199–211, 2004, with permission.)

38. **What is the lung-to-head ratio (LHR)?**
    This is an ultrasonographic measurement used in fetuses between 24 and 26 weeks' GA with congenital diaphragmatic hernia.

    $$LHR = \frac{\text{longest right lung length (in mm)} \times \text{perpendicular line to right lung length (in mm)}}{\text{fetal HC (in mm)}}$$

39. **Does the LHR correlate with neonatal outcome?**
    There is a degree of unpredictability in the clinical course despite an accurate LHR measurement.
    - LHR ≥1.4 is considered a good prognostic indicator.
    - LHR <1.0 is associated with poor outcomes.

40. **What is a congenital cystic adenomatoid malformation volume ratio (CVR)?**
    This is an ultrasonographic measurement used as a prognostic tool in the management of CCAM.

    $$CVR = \frac{[\text{mass length (in cm)} \times \text{mass height (in cm)} \times \text{mass width (in cm)}] \times 0.52}{\text{fetal HC (in cm)}}$$

41. **How does the CVR assist the clinician in determining prognosis of infants with CCAM?**
    The CVR identifies fetuses at high risk for developing hydrops. These infants may benefit from closer surveillance and possible fetal intervention.
    - CVR >1.6 is associated with an 80% risk of developing hydrops.
    - Neonatal survival approaches 100% in the absence of hydrops.

42. **What is maternal mirror syndrome?**
    Maternal mirror syndrome is a preeclampsia-like state during pregnancy that "mirrors" the hydropic state of the fetus. When identified, immediate delivery is generally indicated. However, this syndrome may persist after delivery. Although the symptoms are similar to true preeclampsia, mothers with this syndrome typically exhibit anemia from hemodilution and do not commonly develop thrombocytopenia. "Triple edema" (fetus, placenta, and mother) is pathognomonic for maternal mirror syndrome. Other terms that are used interchangeably are *Ballantyne syndrome* and *pseudotoxemia*.

BIBLIOGRAPHY

1. ACOG Practice Bulletin: Antepartum fetal surveillance. Number 9, October 1999 (replaces Technical Bulletin Number 188, January 1994). Clinical management guidelines for obstetrician-gynecologists. Int J Gynaecol Obstet 68:175-185, 2000.

2. Arca MJ, Teich S: Current controversies in perinatal care: Fetal versus neonatal surgery. Clin Perinatol 31:629–648, 2004.

3. Baschat AA: Pathophysiology of fetal growth restriction: Implications for diagnosis and surveillance. Obstet Gynecol Surv 59:617–627, 2004.

4. Bernstein I, Gabbe SG, Reed KL: Intrauterine growth restriction. In Gabbe SG, Niebyl JR, Simpson JL (eds): Obstetrics: Normal and Problem Pregnancies, 4th ed. Philadelphia, Churchill Livingstone, 2002, pp 869–891.

5. Bianchi DW, Cromblehome TM, D'Alton ME: Fetology: Diagnosis and Management of the Fetal Patient. New York, McGraw Hill, 2000.

6. Cortes RA, Farmer DL: Recent advances in fetal surgery. Semin Perinatol 28:199–211, 2004.

7. Cromleholme TM, Coleman B, Hedrick H, et al: Cystic adenomatoid malformation volume ratio predicts outcome in prenatally diagnosed cystic adenomatoid malformation of the lung. J Pediatr Surg 37:331–338, 2002.

8. Degani S: Fetal biometry: Clinical, pathological, and technical considerations. Obstet Gynecol Surv 56:159–167, 2001.

9. Druzin ML, Gabbe SG, Reed KL: Antepartum fetal evaluation. In Gabbe SG, Niebyl JR, Simpson JL (eds): Obstetrics: Normal and Problem Pregnancies, 4th ed. Philadelphia, Churchill Livingstone, 2002, pp 313–349.

10. Harrison MR, Evans MI, Adzick NS, Holzgrieve W: The Unborn Patient: The Art and Science of Fetal Therapy, 3rd ed. Philadelphia, W.B. Saunders, 2001.

11. Harkness UF, Mari G: Diagnosis and management of intrauterine growth restriction. Clin Perinatol 31:743–764, 2004.

12. Jain V, Fisk NM: The twin-twin transfusion syndrome. Clin Obstet Gynecol 47:181–202, 2004.

13. Lasky RE, Williams AL: The development of the auditory system from conception to term. NeoReviews 6:141–152, 2005.

14. Laudy JAM, Van Gucht M, Van Dooren MF, et al: Congenital diaphragmatic hernia: An evaluation of the prognostic value of the lung-to-head ratio and other prenatal parameters. Prenat Diagn 23:634–639, 2003.

15. Lecanuet JP, Schaal B: Fetal sensory competencies. Eur J Obstet Gynecol 68:1–23, 1996.

16. Lin CC, Santolaya-Forgas J: Current concepts of fetal growth restriction. Part I: Causes, classification, and pathophysiology. Obstet Gynecol 92:1045–1055, 1998.

17. Manning FA, Harman CR, Morrison I, et al: Fetal assessment of fetal biophysical profile scoring. IV: An analysis of perinatal morbidity and mortality. Am J Obstet Gynecol 162:703–709, 1990.

18. Manning FA, Snijders R, Harman CR, et al: Fetal biophysical profile score. VI: Correlation with antepartum umbilical venous fetal pH. Am J Obstet Gynecol 169:755–763, 1993.

19. Quintero RA: Twin-twin transfusion syndrome. Clin Perinatol 20:591–600, 2003.
20. Resnick R: Intrauterine growth restriction. Obstet Gynecol 99:490–496, 2002.
21. Rurak DW, Cooper C: The effect of relative hypoxemia on the pattern of breathing movements in fetal lambs. Respir Physiol 55:23–37, 1984.
22. Tworetzky W, Marshall AC: Fetal interventions for cardiac defects. Pediatr Clin North Am 51:1503–1513, 2004.

CHAPTER 2

OBSTETRIC ISSUES, LABOR, AND DELIVERY

Thomas J. Garite, MD

1. **What is amniocentesis?**

   Amniocentesis is a procedure that involves the aspiration of amniotic fluid from the amniotic sac during pregnancy. It is generally carried out with a spinal needle (20–22 gauge) in a transabdominal approach, using a sterile technique under continuous ultrasound guidance.

2. **How is amniocentesis classified?**

   Amniocentesis can be classified by the time in the pregnancy when it is done and by its indication. Early amniocentesis is performed for genetic indications before 15 weeks' gestation, and 1 mL of amniotic fluid per week of gestation is obtained. However, this technique is gradually being abandoned because it is associated with a high rate of subsequent amniotic fluid leakage (premature rupture of membranes). The majority of amniocenteses for prenatal diagnosis are done between 15 and 20 weeks' gestation.

   At viable gestational ages, amniocentesis is most often performed for fetal lung maturity testing. It can also be done for special diagnostic procedures such as polymerase chain reaction for cytomegalovirus in the setting of intrauterine growth restriction (IUGR) or hydrops. Amniocentesis can be helpful in reducing amniotic fluid volume in the setting of polyhydramnios with either premature labor or maternal respiratory difficulty. It is also used for twin-to-twin transfusion associated with polyhydramnios in one fetus. This type of amniocentesis is often called *reduction amniocentesis.*

   In Rh and other blood group isoimmunizations, amniocentesis has traditionally been used for bilirubin assessment using ΔOD 450, but it is being done far less frequently now because middle cerebral artery Doppler has been found to be extremely accurate in predicting the degree of fetal anemia. In this setting, amniocentesis is used to determine whether the fetus is Rh positive or positive for the sensitized antigen so that testing can be avoided if the fetus is not at risk.

3. **What are the complications of amniocentesis?**
   - Miscarriage and fetal loss occurring in 0.5–1.0% of cases above the background rate of spontaneous loss (1.5–3.0%), although more recent studies place the risk substantially lower with continuous ultrasound guidance.
   - Premature rupture of the membranes (about 1%).
   - Infection (rare).
   - Fetal trauma (rare).
   - Failure to achieve diagnosis (i.e., cell culture failure, which occurs in 1% of cases).
   - Increased rhesus isoimmunization, especially if the placenta is transversed. In Rh-negative women, RhoGAM is given to prevent sensitization.

4. **If genetic studies are indicated, how quickly can the results be obtained?**

   Immediate and preliminary (1–3-day) results can be obtained for cytogenetics using fluorescence in situ hybridization. Definitive chromosome studies require cultured amniocytes (cells from amniotic fluid) and, therefore, usually require 10–14 days.

5. **What options, aside from amniocentesis, are available for prenatal diagnosis?**
    - **Chorionic villus sampling:** Done in the first trimester (9–12 weeks). This procedure involves either transvaginal or transabdominal ultrasound-guided needle aspiration of a small amount of placental tissue and can be used for cytogenetic, biochemical, or DNA testing. The procedure-related loss rate is 0.8%.
    - **Preimplantation diagnosis:** When there is a risk of genetic disease because the parents are carriers of an adverse genetic trait, this obviates the need for screening during the pregnancy, since only unaffected embryos are transferred to the uterus. In this technique, one or more cells are removed from the developing embryo 2–4 days after fertilization and then analyzed. The embryo(s) without the defect are then transferred back to the uterus.
    - **Maternal serum screening:** This screening for α-fetoprotein (AFP) is done at 15–20 weeks' gestation. AFP can detect 85% of open neural tube defects. Adding two more analytes (estriol and human chorionic gonadotropin [HCG], called the *triple screen*) detects 60% of fetuses with trisomy 21 syndrome at a false-positive rate of 5%. This test is routinely offered to all pregnant women.
    - **Second-trimester ultrasound:** Many structural fetal defects (e.g., anencephaly, omphalocele) can routinely be seen in patients who undergo ultrasound scanning during the second trimester. Other defects, such as major cardiac defects, can be seen most of the time depending on the sophistication of the center, type of equipment, patient body habitus, and other factors. In addition, many fetuses with chromosome abnormalities including trisomy 13, 18, and 21 syndromes will have defects observed that will lead to subsequent amniocentesis to confirm the diagnosis.
    - **First-trimester screening for trisomy 21 syndrome:** This is about to become routine. This procedure includes either transvaginal ultrasound for nuchal lucency (which has a high rate of detection for trisomy 21 syndrome) or maternal serum screening using HCG and inhibin (or both).

KEY POINTS: AMNIOCENTESIS AND GENETIC DIAGNOSIS

1. Before conception: preimplantation diagnosis (in in vitro fertilization pregnancies)

2. 9–12 weeks: chorionic villus sampling, nuchal translucency, maternal serum HCG, and inhibin

3. <15 weeks: amniocentesis

4. 15–20 weeks: α-fetoprotein screening, ultrasound of the fetus

6. **How is third-trimester hemorrhage defined and classified?**
    Third-trimester hemorrhage refers to any bleeding from the genital tract during the third trimester of pregnancy. In practice, it refers to any bleeding that occurs from the time of viability, (i.e., 23–24 weeks' gestation). The common causes are classified as placenta previa (7%), placental abruption (13%), and other bleeding (80%), including local lesions of the lower genital tract, vasa previa, early labor, trauma, neoplasia, and marginal placental separation. Such bleeding complicates about 6% of pregnancies.

7. **How is placenta previa diagnosed?**
    Ultrasound visualization is the method of choice for this diagnosis. Multiple reports show a transvaginal approach to be safe and superior in its accuracy when compared with transabdominal ultrasound.

8. **Should a vaginal examination be performed if there is vaginal bleeding?**
    Digital vaginal examination should be avoided when bleeding occurs until placenta previa is excluded by performing an ultrasound examination.
    Clinical pearl: If ultrasound is not available in late pregnancy, a useful approach is the double setup examination in which two teams prepared to administer anesthesia are in the operating room. A vaginal examination is performed. If bleeding occurs from a placenta previa, an emergency cesarean section is performed by the second team.

9. **How is placenta previa classified?**
    - **Complete:** The placenta symmetrically covers the entire internal os of the cervix.
    - **Partial:** The placenta lies asymmetrically toward one wall of the uterus and crosses part of the internal os.
    - **Marginal:** The placental edge just reaches the edge of the internal cervical os.
    If the lower margin on ultrasound scan is >2–3 cm from the internal os, it is not a placenta previa but a low-lying placenta.

10. **What is the incidence of placenta previa?**
    Placenta previa occurs in 1 in 200 deliveries at term. Complete placenta previa is detected in 5% of second-trimester gestations, with 90% resolving by term; partial placenta previa is seen in 45% of second-trimester gestations and resolves in more than 95% of cases. This apparent resolution is most likely related to the growth of the lower uterine segment in late pregnancy, so the placenta appears to move away from the os.

11. **What are the risk factors for placenta previa?**
    - Previous placenta previa (8-fold risk)
    - Previous uterine surgery (1.5–15-fold risk)
    - Multiparity (1.7-fold risk)
    - Advanced age, >35 years (4.7-fold risk)
    - Advanced age, >40 years (9-fold risk)
    - Cigarette smoking (1.4–3.0-fold risk)
    - Multiple-birth pregnancy

12. **What are the complications of placenta previa?**
    - **Premature delivery:** 50%—the vast majority of increased perinatal mortality with placenta previa is due to prematurity
    - **Cesarean delivery**
    - **Placenta accreta:** When the placenta infiltrates the uterine wall (1–5%; 25% with one previous uterine surgery; 45% if more than one previous surgery)
    - **Increased risk of postpartum hemorrhage**
    - **Fetal growth restriction:** Studies are inconsistent, and the majority show no increased rates of IUGR with placenta previa
    - **Increased fetal malformations:** Twofold risk

13. **What is placental abruption? How often does it occur?**
    Placental abruption is the separation of the normally implanted placenta before the birth of the fetus. It results from bleeding from a small arterial vessel into the decidua basalis. It is termed a *revealed* abruption when vaginal bleeding is present (90%) and a *concealed* abruption if no bleeding is visible (10%). It is uniquely dangerous to the fetus and the mother because of its serious pathophysiologic sequelae. The incidence varies but averages about 0.83% or 1 in 120 deliveries. Abruption severe enough to cause fetal death is less common (approximately 1 in 420 deliveries).

14. **What are the main risk factors for a placental abruption? Is placental abruption a recurrent disease?**
    - Maternal hypertension and preeclampsia

- Increasing maternal age and parity
- Cigarette smoking
- Cocaine use
- Trauma
- Uterine anomalies/fibroids
- Premature rupture of the membranes
- Spontaneous or artificial rupture of the membranes
  The risk of placental abruption is between 6% and 16%; after two consecutive abruptions, the subsequent risk is 25%. Women who have a placental abruption severe enough to cause fetal death have a 7% risk of a similar outcome in a subsequent pregnancy.

15. **What maternal and fetal complications occur with placental abruption?**
Maternal complications
- **Premature labor and delivery**
- **Hypovolemic shock**
- **Maternal mortality:** <1%
- **Acute renal failure**
- **Disseminated intravascular coagulation**
- **Postpartum hemorrhage**
- **Severe rhesus isoimmunization:** Occurs unless there is adequate treatment with anti-D immunoglobulin

Fetal and neonatal complications
- **IUGR:** Especially in preterm deliveries
- **Increased risk of congenital malformations:** 4.4%
- **Neonatal anemia**
- **Greater incidence of abnormal neurodevelopment at 2 years**
- **Perinatal mortality:** 14.4–67% higher rates occur at earlier gestations; high rate of stillbirth, fetal distress, and asphyxia. Most mortality is due to prematurity
- **Fetal-maternal hemorrhage with resultant fetal anemia:** More common in abruption associated with maternal trauma

16. **What is fetal-maternal hemorrhage? What are the complications?**
Fetal-maternal hemorrhage is caused by a disruption of the normal barrier at the placental-decidual interface. It may occur with abruptio placentae; however, it occurs more commonly with abruptio placentae associated with maternal trauma, with maternal trauma without abruptio placentae, or spontaneously without an apparent precipitating event. Approximately 5% of stillbirths without apparent cause are due to fetal-maternal hemorrhage. The diagnosis is made by performing a Kleihauer-Betke test on maternal blood, which allows quantification of fetal cells in maternal serum. In patients with spontaneous fetal-maternal hemorrhage, the presenting

KEY POINTS: THIRD-TRIMESTER HEMORRHAGE

1. Bleeding at any time during pregnancy is cause for concern and should always be carefully investigated.

2. During the third trimester, however, onset of hemorrhage may be particularly ominous.

3. Some of the diagnoses that should be entertained include placenta previa, placental abruption, marginal placental separation, and lesions of the lower genital tract.

4. About 6% of all pregnancies, however, will have some bleeding.

symptom is decreased fetal movement. If the fetus is still alive and the hemorrhage is severe enough, the diagnosis is often made because of a sinusoidal fetal heart rate (FHR) tracing. Treatment can consist of immediate delivery if the fetus is near term, or intrauterine transfusion if the fetus is premature and no abruption is apparent.

17. **A 32-year-old, G_2P_{1001} woman at term gestation presents in labor. Her membranes are intact, she is afebrile, and the fetal heart tracing is reassuring. Reviewing her prenatal records, you notice that she had a positive Group B Streptococcal culture obtained at 34 weeks' gestation. She is allergic to penicillin and "had difficulty breathing and swelled up" when she received it many years ago. What therapy is appropriate?**
The Centers for Disease Control and Prevention (CDC) protocol, as well as the American Academy of Pediatrics (AAP) and American College of Obstetricians and Gynecologists (ACOG) guidelines, recommend prophylactic treatment with penicillin or ampicillin for women in labor who are positive for Group B Streptococcus (GBS). Erythromycin or clindamycin are appropriate alternatives for penicillin-allergic patients. Recent in vitro data demonstrate an 18% rate of resistance to erythromycin (compared with 1/85 from isolates before the CDC recommendations). Of 100 isolates tested for antibiotic resistance, 5 were resistant to both erythromycin and clindamycin. The clinical implications of this remain unclear. There has been a 50% reduction in the rate of neonatal GBS infection in institutions since the CDC protocols were introduced, which underscores the usefulness of appropriate chemoprophylaxis.

18. **What are the major risk factors for preterm labor?**
     - Low socioeconomic status
     - Smoking
     - Chorioamnionitis
     - Prior preterm birth
     - Preterm premature rupture of membranes
     - Maternal age <18 years
     - Urinary tract infection
     - Diethylstilbestrol (DES) exposure
     - Bacterial vaginosis
     - Uterine anomalies
     - Polyhydramnios
     - Hemorrhage
     - Prior cervical surgery
     - Congenital anomalies
     - Poor nutritional status

KEY POINTS: PRETERM LABOR

1. One of the most difficult problems with preterm labor is simply making the diagnosis.

2. Many women, believing that they are not yet due to deliver, ignore subtle symptoms of preterm labor until it is too late to intervene.

3. In some women, however, cervical dilation may occur in the absence of contractions, eliminating the possible use of tocolytic agents.

4. One of the most important new therapies for preventing preterm labor appears to be the use of progesterone for women who have previously delivered a preterm infant.

- Fetal demise
- Abruptio placentae
- Placenta previa
- Advanced maternal age

19. **What are absolute contraindications to tocolysis?**
    - Severe pregnancy-induced hypertension preeclampsia
    - Acute abruptio placentae
    - Chorioamnionitis
    - Fetal death
    - Nonreassuring fetal status (fetal distress)
    - Fetal anomaly incompatible with life (e.g., anencephaly)

20. **How is the diagnosis of premature labor made?**
    Premature labor is defined as regular painful uterine contractions associated with a change in cervical dilation and effacement. Often, there is concern that by waiting for substantial cervical change before implementing treatment, the delay will result in failed treatment. Furthermore, regular contractions are not uncommon in patients who later go on to deliver at term. Thus, in randomized series, as many of 50% of preterm labor does not progress with placebo treatment, and in practice as many as 80% of patients who are treated are not truly in preterm labor.

21. **What is fetal fibronectin?**
    Fetal fibronectin is an extracellular matrix protein, the presence of which in cervicovaginal secretions is a predictor of preterm labor. This predictor has a high negative predictive accuracy (>99%; the absence of fetal fibronectin indicates delivery is *not* imminent) but only a mediocre positive predictive accuracy.

22. **How is fetal fibronectin used?**
    Most commonly, this test is used in patients with preterm contractions in which the diagnosis of preterm labor is uncertain. A negative test result allows >99% reassurance that the patient will not deliver in the next week and often avoids unnecessary treatment.

23. **What are the common pharmacologic agents used for the inhibition of preterm labor and their mechanisms of action?**
    See Table 2-1.

TABLE 2-1. COMMON PHARMACOLOGIC AGENTS USED FOR THE INHIBITION OF PRETERM LABOR

Pharmacologic Agent	Mechanism of Action
β-adrenergic agonists	Adenyl cyclase inhibitor—sequesters intracellular calcium (e.g., terbutaline, ritodrine)
Magnesium sulfate	Uncertain—magnesium suppresses muscle contraction of myometrial strips in vitro, decreases intracellular calcium, and affects acetylcholine release
Prostaglandin synthase inhibitors (indomethacin)	Inhibition of the cyclooxygenase enzyme responsible for prostaglandins that promote uterine contractions
Calcium antagonists (nifedipine)	Inhibition of influx of calcium through the cell membrane

24. **What are the main adverse effects of tocolytic agents on the fetus and neonate?**
See Table 2-2.

TABLE 2-2. ADVERSE EFFECTS OF TOCOLYTIC AGENTS ON THE FETUS AND NEONATE	
Pharmacologic Agent	**Adverse Effects**
β-adrenergic agonists	Fetal tachycardia, neonatal hypoglycemia, hypocalcemia, and hypotension
Magnesium	Fetal demineralization with prolonged use, neonatal respiratory and motor depression at higher serum levels, ileus
Prostaglandin synthase inhibitors	Constriction of fetal ductus arteriosus leading to pulmonary hypertension, oligohydramnios, decreased fetal urine production, and spontaneous intestinal perforation
Calcium antagonists	No known human effects—decreases fetal arterial PO_2 and pH in animal studies

25. **Is tocolysis effective?**
There is no question that tocolysis is effective over short-term intervals; however, clinical trials have not consistently demonstrated that gestation can be prolonged significantly or that respiratory distress syndrome can be consistently prevented.

26. **What is premature rupture of membranes (PROM)? Why is it important?**
The obstetric definition of PROM is rupture of membranes before the onset of labor. It does not imply at what gestational age this phenomenon occurs. Prolonged rupture of membranes (>24 hours) in the term patient is associated with an increased risk of neonatal infection and mortality; however, the duration of membrane rupture does not alter the rate of infection or mortality in the preterm patient. Complications of PROM include:
- **Premature labor:** PROM accounts for 25–50% of premature deliveries
- **Maternal and neonatal infections**
- **Increased rates of fetal distress and stillbirth**
- **Fetal deformation syndrome:** In the very premature gestation, this includes pulmonary hypoplasia, IUGR, and limb deformities.

KEY POINTS: PREMATURE RUPTURE OF MEMBRANES

1. The factors that lead to premature rupture of membranes may also invoke increased production of cytokines in both the fetus and the mother.

2. Cytokines appear to adversely affect neonatal outcome and to predispose the neonate to both neurologic and pulmonary problems, especially after a preterm birth.

27. **A patient makes inquiries regarding multiple courses of steroids to enhance fetal lung maturity. What should you tell her about this approach?**
Multiple doses of antenatal steroids (more than three) are associated with suppression of the fetal adrenal gland and the response to stress in a critically ill neonate. In addition, animal and

human data suggest less brain growth and developmental delay in childhood after multiple doses of steroids. The benefit of more than one course of antenatal steroids is controversial. As a result, a second National Institutes of Health consensus conference on antenatal steroids recommended that only a single course of steroids be used and that the use of subsequent courses be limited to patients in research studies that address this question.

28. **During a review of the perinatal outcomes for premature infants at your hospital, the nurse manager for the intensive care nursery inquires whether there is an effective method to detect women at risk for premature delivery before they present in active preterm labor. What do current data indicate?**
Many strategies have been used to identify patients who are destined to deliver prematurely. Risk assessment scoring using the modified Creasy score (Table 2-3) or other similar systems work well in some populations but not in others. The Creasy score looks at a series of variables in an attempt to define clinical indicators that are likely to result in preterm labor. Other tools in common use include endovaginal ultrasound to detect cervical shortening and fetal fibronectin testing. Unfortunately, except for progesterone therapy, therapies for prevention of premature delivery have not been consistently effective.

TABLE 2-3.   RISK FACTORS IN THE PREDICTION OF SPONTANEOUS PRETERM LABOR (MODIFIED CREASY SCORE)

Major Risk Factors	Minor Risk Factors
Multiple gestation	Febrile illness
DES exposure	Bleeding after 12 weeks' gestation
Hydramnios	History of pyelonephritis
Uterine anomaly	Cigarette smoking >10 cigarettes/day
Cervix dilated >1 cm at 32 weeks' gestation	Second-trimester abortion × 1
Second-trimester abortion × 2	More than two first-trimester abortions
Previous preterm delivery	
Previous preterm labor, term delivery	
Abdominal surgery during pregnancy	
History of cone biopsy	
Cervical shortening <1 cm at 32 weeks' gestation	
Uterine irritability	
Cocaine abuse	

29. **Are there any promising therapies to prevent premature delivery?**
Two recent large trials of progesterone (one using weekly 17-OH progesterone caproate injections and one using daily vaginal progesterone suppositories) in patients with a history of previous premature deliveries resulted in a marked reduction of premature delivery and complications of prematurity in the treatment groups. The ACOG has endorsed this therapy in such patients, and other trials are ongoing to evaluate its effectiveness in other at-risk groups (e.g., women carrying multiple gestations).

30. **What are some of the increased risks of twin pregnancies?**
   - Premature birth
   - Spontaneous abortion

- Intrauterine growth retardation, including discordant growth (which may occur in up to one third of twin pregnancies)
- Fetal malposition
- Placental abnormalities (abruptio placentae, placenta previa)
- Birth asphyxia
- Increased perinatal mortality, especially for premature, monozygotic, and discordant twins
- Twin-to-twin transfusion syndrome
- Polyhydramnios

31. **Why are monozygotic twins considered to be at higher risk for complications than dizygotic twins?**

Monozygotic twins (identical twins) arise from the division of a single fertilized egg. Depending on the timing of the division of the single ovum into separate embryos, the amnionic and chorionic membranes can be shared (if division occurs >8 days after fertilization), separate (if <72 hours after fertilization), or mixed (separate amnion, shared chorion if 4–8 days after fertilization). Sharing of the chorion and/or amnion is associated with potential problems of vascular anastomoses (and possible twin-twin transfusions), cord entanglements, and congenital anomalies. These problems increase the risk of intrauterine growth retardation and intrauterine death. They also increase the risk of premature delivery. Dizygotic twins, however, result from two separately fertilized ova and, as such, usually have a separate amnion and chorion.

32. **What are the varieties of conjoined twins?**

Conjoined twins are classified according to the degree and nature of their union. These are listed below in order of decreasing frequency:

- **Thoracopagus:** Joined at the thorax
- **Xiphopagus:** Joined at the anterior abdominal wall (from the xiphoid to the umbilicus)
- **Pygopagus:** Joined at the buttocks or rump
- **Ischiopagus:** Joined at the ischium
- **Craniopagus:** Joined at the head

KEY POINTS: TWIN PREGNANCIES AND MULTIPLE BIRTHS

1. Multiple births are associated with an increased risk of problems during pregnancy.

2. The higher the number of fetuses, the greater the risk.

3. Preterm labor, twin-twin transfusion, developmental abnormalities, discordant growth, congenital malformations, fetal crowding syndrome, and several other abnormalities are all more common.

4. Monozygotic twins appear to be at greater risk than fraternal twins.

33. **What is perinatal asphyxia?**

Few terms evoke more trepidation from obstetricians and neonatologists (particularly in a court room, not to mention the delivery room) than perinatal asphyxia. The term *perinatal asphyxia,* however, is so vague and so arbitrarily applied that it is virtually meaningless. In actuality there are two definitions. One is strictly the presence of hypoxia and metabolic acidosis, and the other includes the presence of metabolic acidosis and organ damage. ACOG has suggested that the term not be used, except when all of the following criteria are clearly met:

- Arterial cord pH sample <7.0
- Apgar scores of 4 or less for at least 5 minutes

- Evidence of altered neurologic status (e.g., obtundation, seizures, altered level of consciousness)
- Multisystem organ injury or failure

34. **Why has the term *nonreassuring fetal status* been used to replace the term *fetal distress* in practice?**
In labor, electronic FHR monitoring is the primary modality used to determine fetal oxygenation. Although this method is quite reliable when results are normal, when marked abnormalities occur on the FHR tracing, the infant is more often vigorous and not acidotic at birth. Thus, the term *fetal distress* is more often than not inaccurate. A more accurate expression is that the FHR is no longer reassuring and that either other information must be used to establish fetal well-being or, failing that option, the fetus must be delivered.

35. **What is the purpose of antepartum fetal testing?**
Certain fetuses are at risk for antepartum fetal death and asphyxial injury. The purpose of evaluating fetal well-being before labor is to prevent such adverse outcomes by first identifying hypoxia and impending damage/death and then either reversing the process if possible or, failing that, executing delivery in the hope that the baby will do better in the nursery.

KEY POINTS: PERINATAL ASPHYXIA

1. The term *perinatal asphyxia* applies to relatively few pregnancies, yet it commonly makes its way into medical records with some degree of regularity.

2. Delineation of the physiologic abnormalities seen in the fetus and neonate should be used instead of the term *perinatal asphyxia,* which appears to be an exceedingly uncommon event as defined by the ACOG-AAP criteria.

36. **What methods of fetal evaluation are in common use in *at-risk* patients?**
- Fetal movement counting
- Nonstress testing (NST)
- Contraction stress testing (CST)
- Biophysical profile (BPP) testing
- Modified BPP
- Doppler umbilical artery flow analysis

37. **How is fetal movement counting done?**
Ideally, all patients should be educated to assess fetal movement on a regular basis in the latter half of pregnancy. There is no consensus regarding the best method to count fetal movements. However, when fetal movement reaches an alarmingly low level (e.g., fewer than two in an hour), the mother should come in for an immediate biophysical test to assess the fetus.

38. **What is an NST?**
The FHR accelerates in response to fetal activity. This responsiveness forms the basis of one of the most widely used assessments of fetal well-being, the NST. In the NST, the presence of fetal movement and an intact, responsive central nervous system is evaluated by determining the presence of FHR accelerations that occur in response to fetal movement. The NST is usually performed in an outpatient setting, and the patient is connected to a standard tocodynamometer while the FHR is monitored (by Doppler ultrasound transduction). In general, one looks for at least two accelerations of the FHR of >15 bpm amplitude lasting at least 15 seconds in a

20-minute period of monitoring. If reactivity standards are not met, the tracing is considered nonreactive, although a second period of 20 minutes may be observed to eliminate the possibility of fetal sleep. If the study is deemed nonreactive, it should be followed by a CST or a BPP to further assess fetal well-being.

39. What is a CST?

A CST, or oxytocin challenge test, was one of the earliest techniques to assess fetal well-being. In this test, the mother receives an infusion of oxytocin until adequate uterine contractions have started, while being monitored on a tocodynamometer and a fetal ultrasound transducer. In a negative test result, there are three uterine contractions within 10 minutes with no late decelerations of the FHR. In a positive test result, in which there are late decelerations, the risk of mortality and morbidity for the fetus increases, with some reports of mortality as high as 15%. There are, however, many false-positive instances of CST results. In such situations, the obstetrician often faces a difficult decision of how aggressively to proceed with delivery of the fetus because the cervix may not be in a favorable condition at that time, and a cesarean section may be required. If the test results are equivocal, it may be reasonable to wait for an additional 24 hours to repeat the test.

An alternative to the use of oxytocin is the use of nipple stimulation by the mother. With this approach, the test may be over more rapidly, with no intravenous infusion required. Results are similarly interpreted. At present, the CST is primarily used to back up a nonreactive NST. When the NST is persistently nonreactive, and the CST result is positive, the false-positive rate is virtually nil, and intervention is almost always warranted.

40. What is the BPP?

The BPP is a more extensive biophysical assessment of fetal well-being. It includes five parameters that are scored as 2 points each as normal or present, or 0 as abnormal or absent:

- Fetal movement
- Fetal breathing movements
- Fetal tone
- Amniotic fluid volume
- NST assessed by the usual external FHR method

Scores of 8 or 10 are considered normal and reassure the clinician that the fetus will not die or experience damage due to a chronic process for the next week. A score of 6 is equivocal and requires repeat testing in 1 day. Scores of 0–4 require further evaluation and consideration of delivery.

41. What is the modified BPP?

In large trial it became apparent that the NST alone was associated with a false-negative rate (fetal death within a week of a normal test) that was considerably higher than that of the CST or BPP (1% as opposed to 0.2%). The reason for this is that the loss of fetal movement, and thus reactivity, occurs very late in the process of fetal deterioration and death. Amniotic fluid volume generally declines well before reactivity is lost. Thus, the combination of amniotic fluid volume assessment by ultrasound and the NST done weekly has become the test used by the vast majority of clinicians in testing fetal well-being; the more complete BPP or the CST is used when the modified BPP result is abnormal.

42. What is the value of measuring umbilical arterial flow?

Waveform analysis of umbilical artery flow using ultrasound-guided Doppler warns the clinician of increased resistance to flow within the placenta. This test is expressed as systolic-to-diastolic ratio. When the situation is severe enough, the flow during diastole either becomes absent or goes in the reverse direction, indicating marked resistance to flow. This form of testing is principally of value in the severely growth-restricted fetus and can give a very early warning of impending fetal demise.

43. **What are the indications for obtaining a scalp PH?**
A nonreassuring FHR monitoring optimally requires a backup method, except in extreme circumstances where the pattern is clearly indicative of hypoxia and acidosis. Scalp pH has been the gold standard. For various reasons, however (especially the technical difficulties involved in the procedure), recent surveys have indicated that fewer than 5% of clinicians in practice actually use this procedure and choose to err on the side of operative intervention when the FHR pattern is nonreassuring.

44. **Who should have umbilical cord blood gas testing? Why not all patients?**
Neonatal depression is not always due to hypoxia and acidosis. Furthermore, given the litigious environment surrounding the issue of perinatal brain damage, the issue of documenting the fetal blood gas status at birth is critical to objectively assessing the baby's condition. The following are indications for assessing blood gas status at birth:
- Operative intervention for nonreassuring fetal status
- Low Apgar score
- Thick meconium
- Fetuses that had nonreassuring fetal status but did not have operative intervention
- Premature babies <32 weeks' gestation
- Infants with major congenital anomalies

   Although some clinicians believe that all babies should have cord pH determinations, there is little medical value (babies with normal Apgar scores but low pH cord values have normal nursery and follow-up outcome), and it can be argued that a low pH with a normal Apgar could be more harmful than helpful in a medicolegal setting.

KEY POINTS: FETAL EVALUATION

1. The goal of all pregnancies is the preservation of maternal well-being while delivering a healthy neonate.

2. To this end, assessment of the fetus is one of the most important aspects of care during pregnancy.

3. Although techniques for fetal evaluation have added immensely to improving outcomes, no technique is infallible and each should be considered only as a single additional piece of information.

4. Reliance on any single test can potentially be hazardous to both mother and fetus.

45. **Which drugs that cross the placenta can produce problems in the neonate?**
Virtually all drugs cross the placenta to some degree, but few produce any significant problems for either the fetus or the neonate. Large organic ions such as heparin and insulin do not cross the placenta and are therefore safe. There are some drugs taken by the mother, however, that can be problematic.
- **Anticonvulsants:** Infants of mothers using anticonvulsants have twice the risk of malformations compared with the general population, especially cleft lip and palate and congenital cardiac defects. Valproic acid may cause neural tube defects, and diphenylhydantoin is associated with fetal hydantoin syndrome (i.e., microcephaly, developmental delay, growth failure, mental retardation, dysmorphic facies, and nail hypoplasia). Carbamazepine may also produce dysmorphism.
- **Psychoactive medications:** Lithium has been associated with a slightly increased risk of cardiac defects. In addition, lithium can produce polyhydramnios and fetal diabetes insipidus.

Hypotonia, lethargy, and feeding problems are also seen in some infants. The effects of other psychotropic agents on the fetus appear minimal, but some cases of teratogenesis have been reported, especially with some benzodiazepines. The critical issue that remains unresolved, however, is whether these drugs alter the development of the maturing fetal central nervous system.

- **Anticoagulants:** Warfarin is known to produce teratogenic effects in the fetus. About 5% of pregnancies result in fetal warfarin syndrome (i.e., mental retardation, bone stippling, dysmorphic characteristics, ophthalmologic abnormalities). If necessary, warfarin should be replaced by heparin during pregnancy.
- **Antihypertensive medications:** Angiotensin-converting enzyme inhibitors may cause fetal renal failure in later stages of gestation, leading to oligohydramnios, pulmonary hypoplasia, and fetal deformities.
- **Thyroid drugs:** Propylthiouracil and methimazole (Tapazole) cross the placenta and can cause a fetal goiter and fetal hypothyroidism. Use of thyroid hormone appears, generally, to be safe. Maternal Graves' disease can result in neonatal thyroid storm and hyperthyroidism in rare cases.
- **Acne medications:** Isotretinoin (Accutane) is a significant human teratogen that should be avoided in women planning to become pregnant. It is associated with a high risk of both structural abnormalities and mental retardation in the newborn. The use of topical tretinoin (Retin-A) appears to be safe.
- **Antineoplastic drugs:** The anticancer drugs that appear to have the greatest significance for teratogenesis are methotrexate and cyclophosphamide. Both can cause malformations of the skull and bones, as well as mental retardation.
- **Steroids:** The value of steroids for lung maturation is well established. Chronic exposure to steroids has been reported to inhibit neuronal development. Prednisone and prednisolone cross the placenta to a small degree and, therefore, are the drugs of choice during gestation.
- **Antibiotics:** Tetracycline is the most notorious drug for producing both skeletal and dental abnormalities in pregnant women. Sulfa drugs may accentuate hyperbilirubinemia during the neonatal period by displacing bilirubin from binding sites. Sulfamethoxazole/trimethoprim has been associated with congenital cardiac defects. Kanamycin and streptomycin (rarely used today) have produced congenital deafness. It is unclear whether gentamicin has the same potential. Careful drug monitoring appears to reduce the likelihood of hearing loss. Some cephalosporins (e.g., cefaclor, cephalexin, and cephradine) have been associated with congenital defects, but the association is weak. Most other antibiotics (including acyclovir) appear to be safe for use during pregnancy.
- **Prostaglandin synthase inhibitors:** Aspirin, ibuprofen, and naproxen may cause in utero constriction of the ductus arteriosus in rare cases and probably should be avoided if possible. Indomethacin has been used frequently as a tocolytic agent and is also reported to produce ductal closure, but it appears to be reasonably safe with careful fetal monitoring. These drugs do not appear to be teratogens; however, platelet aggregation is also reduced by many of these agents and may increase the potential for bleeding.
- **Alcohol:** Fetal alcohol syndrome may occur with even minimal ingestion of alcohol. Symptoms include mental retardation, craniofacial abnormalities, and growth failure.
- **Narcotics:** The use of narcotics results in significant problems for the neonate, of which the most classic is neonatal drug withdrawal. Withdrawal typically begins in the immediate newborn period and lasts for days to weeks. With some narcotics, such as methadone, withdrawal may not be seen for several days. Babies of mothers who use narcotics appear to have an increased risk of abortion, prematurity, and growth failure.
- **Cocaine:** Cocaine use appears to result in a higher risk of abortion and stillbirth. Birth weight is generally slightly lower than normal, and there is an increased risk of prematurity. Microcephaly does occur in rare instances with cocaine use during pregnancy. Organ infarction may lead to bowel atresia, porencephaly, and limb maldevelopment.

- **Nicotine:** Exposure to cigarette smoke in utero reduces birth weight by an average of 300 gm if the mother consistently smokes throughout gestation. The risk of apnea and sudden infant death syndrome is increased. The incidence of abruptio placentae also increases.

  Although this list is relatively complete for many of the drugs known to produce significant fetal problems, the practitioner should always review the most recent medical literature for any updates that might reflect changes in awareness of potential risks of drugs during pregnancy. As was demonstrated by the maternal DES story, the full teratogenic potential of some medications may not be known for many years.

KEY POINTS: MATERNAL DRUGS AND MEDICATIONS DURING PREGNANCY

1. Virtually all drugs cross the placenta to some extent.

2. The same is true of breast milk: most medications enter maternal milk to some degree.

3. Few drugs, however, appear in sufficient concentration to have an adverse effect on the fetus or neonate.

BIBLIOGRAPHY

1. Ananth CV, Berkowitz GS, Savitz DA, Lapinski RH: Placental abruption and adverse perinatal outcome. JAMA 17:1646–1651, 1999.

2. Ananth CV, Savitz DA, Luther ER: Maternal cigarette smoking as a risk factor for placental abruption, placental previa and uterine bleeding in a pregnancy. Am J Epidemiol 144:881–887, 1996.

3. Banks BA, Cnaan A, Morgan MA, et al, and North American Thyrotropin-Releasing Hormone Study Group: Multiple courses of antenatal steroids and the outcome of premature neonates. Am J Obstet Gynecol 181:709–717, 1999.

4. Canadian Early and Mid-trimester Amniocentesis Trial (CEMAT) Group: Randomised trial to assess safety and fetal outcome of early and mid-trimester amniocentesis. Lancet 351:242–247, 1998.

5. Clarke SL: Placenta previa and abruptio placenta. In Creasy RK, Resink R (eds): Maternal-Fetal Medicine. Philadelphia, W.B. Saunders, 1999, pp 616–631.

6. Creasy RK, Resnik R, Iams JD: Maternal Fetal Medicine: Principles and Practices, 5th ed. Philadelphia, W.B. Saunders, 2003.

7. El-Sayed YY, Holbrook RH Jr, Gibson R, et al: Diltiazem for maintenance tocolysis of preterm labor: Comparison to nifedipine in a randomized trial. J Maternal Fetal Med 7:217–221, 1998.

8. El-Sayed YY, Riley ET, Holbrook RH Jr, et al: Randomized comparison of nitroglycerin and magnesium sulfate for treatment of preterm labor. Obstet Gynecol 93:79–83, 1999.

9. Farine D, Peisner DB, Timor-Tritch IE: Placenta previa: Is the traditional diagnostic approach satisfactory? J Clin Ultrasound 18:328, 1990.

10. Freeman RK, Garite, TJ, Nageotte MP: Fetal Heart Rate Monitoring, 3rd ed. Philadelphia, Lippincott, Williams & Wilkins, 2003.

11. Ghidini A, Salafia CM, Minior VK: Repeated courses of steroids in preterm membrane rupture do not increase the risk of histologic chorioamnionitis. Am J Perinatol 14:309–313, 1997.

12. Goldenberg RL, Andrews WW, Guerrant RL, et al: The preterm prediction study: Cervical lactoferrin concentration, other markers of lower genital tract infection, and preterm birth. National Institute of Child Health and Human Development Maternal-Fetal Medicine Units Network. Am J Obstet Gynecol 182:631–635, 2000.

13. Goldenberg RL, Andrews WW, Mercer BM, et al: The preterm prediction study: Granulocyte colony-stimulating factor and spontaneous preterm birth. National Institute of Child Health and Human Development Maternal-Fetal Units Network. Am J Obstet Gynecol 182:625–630, 2000.

14. Goldenberg RL, Iams JD, Das A, et al: The preterm prediction study: Sequential cervical length and fetal fibronectin testing for the prediction of spontaneous preterm birth. National Institute of Child Health and Human Development Maternal-Fetal Medicine Units Network. Am J Obstet Gynecol 182:636–643, 2000.

15. Guinn DA, Goepfert AR, Owen J, et al: Terbutaline pump maintenance therapy for prevention of preterm delivery: A double blind trial. Am J Obstet Gynecol 179:874–878, 1998.

16. Hamersley SL, Landy HJ, O'Sullivan MJ: Fetal bradycardia secondary to magnesium sulfate therapy for preterm labor: A case report. J Reprod Med 43:206–210, 1998.

17. Hammerman C, Glaser J, Kaplan M, et al: Indomethacin tocolysis increases postnatal patent ductus arteriosus severity. Pediatrics 102:E56, 1998.

18. Heine RP, McGregor JA, Dullien VK: Accuracy of salivary estriol testing compared to traditional risk factor assessment in predicting preterm birth. Am J Obstet Gynecol 180:5214–5218, 1999.

19. Huang WL, Beazley LD, Quinlivan JA, et al: Effect of corticosteroids on brain growth in fetal sheep. Obstet Gynecol 94:213–218, 1999.

20. Joffe GM, Jacques D, Bernis-Heys R, et al: Impact of the fetal fibronectin assay on admissions for preterm labor. Am J Obstet Gynecol 180:581–586, 1999.

21. Konje JC, Walley RJ: Bleeding in late pregnancy. In James DK, Steer PJ, Weiner CP, Gonik B (eds): High Risk Pregnancy: Management Options. Philadelphia, W.B. Saunders, 1994, pp 119–136.

22. Medical Research Council: An assessment of the hazards of amniocentesis. Br J Obstet Gynaecol 85:1–41, 1978.

23. Morales WJ, Dickey SS, Bornick P, Lim DV: Change in antibiotic resistance of group B streptococcus: Impact on intrapartum management. Am J Obstet Gynecol 181:310–314, 1999.

24. National Institutes of Child Health and Human Development National Registry for Amniocentesis Study Group: Amniocentesis for prenatal diagnosis: Safety and accuracy. JAMA 236:1471–1476, 1976.

25. NIH Consensus Statement: Effect of Corticosteroids for Fetal Maturation on Perinatal Outcomes. NIH Consensus Statement, volume 12. February 28–March 2, 1994.

26. Pearlman MD, Pierson CL, Faix RG: Frequent resistance of clinical group B streptococci isolates to clindamycin and erythromycin. Obstet Gynecol 92:258–261, 1998.

27. Ramsay PA, Fisk NM: Amniocentesis. In James DK, Steer PJ, Weiner CP, Gonik B (eds): High Risk Pregnancy: Management Options. Philadelphia, W.B. Saunders, 1994, pp 19–136.

28. Sameshima H, Ikenoue T, Kamitomo M, Sakamoto H: Effects of 4 hours magnesium sulfate infusion on fetal heart rate variability and reactivity in a goat model. Am J Perinatol 15:535–538, 1998.

29. Sanchez-Ramos L, Kaunitz AM, Gaudier FL, Delke I: Efficacy of maintenance therapy after acute tocolysis: A meta-analysis. Am J Obstet Gynecol 181:484–490, 1999.

30. Schorr SJ, Ascarelli MH, Rust OA, et al: A comparative study of ketorolac (Toradol) and magnesium sulfate for arrest of preterm labor. South Med J 91:1028–1032, 1998.

31. Schuchat A, Whitney C, Zangwill K: Prevention of perinatal group B streptococcal disease: A public health perspective. MMWR 45:1–24, 1996.

32. Scioscia AL: Prenatal genetic diagnosis. In Creasy RK, Resink R (eds): Maternal-Fetal Medicine. Philadelphia, W.B. Saunders, 1999, pp 735–744.

33. Simpson NE, Dallaire L, Miller JR, et al: Prenatal diagnosis of genetic disease in Canada: Report of a collaborative study. Can Med Assoc J 115:739–746, 1976.

34. Sundberg K, Bang J, Smidt-Jensen S, et al: Randomised study of risk of fetal loss related to early amniocentesis versus chorionic villus sampling. Lancet 350:697–703, 1997.

35. Wenstrom KD, Andrews WW, Hauth JC, et al: Elevated second-trimester amniotic fluid interleukin-6 levels predict preterm delivery. Am J Obstet Gynecol 178:546–550, 1998.

36. Wright JW, Ridgway LE, Wright BD, et al: Effect of MgSO4 on heart rate monitoring in the preterm fetus. J Reprod Med 41:605–608, 1996.

FAMILY-CENTERED AND DEVELOPMENTAL CARE IN THE NEONATAL INTENSIVE CARE UNIT

Karen D. Hendricks-Muñoz, MD, MPH, and Carol Prendergast, EdD

CHAPTER 3

1. **What is patient-and family-centered care?**
   Patient- and family-centered care is an approach to planning, delivery, and evaluation of health care that supports partnerships among patients, families, and health care practitioners. It is founded on the principle that the family plays a vital role in ensuring the health and well-being of the infant. Family-centered care provides care to families in a manner that involves respect and empowerment and responds to individual diversity and strengths.

2. **What are the four guiding principles of patient-and family-centered care?**
   According to the American Hospital Association and Institute for Family Centered Care:
   - **Dignity and respect:** Health care practitioners listen to and honor patient and family perspectives and choices. Patient and family knowledge, values, beliefs, and cultural backgrounds are included in the planning and delivery of health care.
   - **Information sharing:** Health care practitioners communicate and share complete and unbiased information with patients and families in ways that are affirming and useful. Patients and families receive timely, complete, and accurate information to effectively participate in care and decision making.
   - **Participation:** Patients and families are encouraged and supported in participating in care and decision making at the level they choose.
   - **Collaboration:** Patients, families, health care practitioners, and hospital leaders collaborate in policy and program development, implementation and evaluation, health care facility design, and professional education.

3. **What are the different approaches to health care delivery?**
   - **System centered:** The needs of the system drive the delivery of care.
   - **Patient centered:** Staff focus on the needs of the infant but do not see him or her within the context of the family.
   - **Family focused:** The family is the focus or unit of care. Interventions are done to and for them instead of with the patient.
   - **Patient and family centered:** The priorities and choices of the patient and family are respected. It is a collaborative approach to decision making.

   Adapted from Hospitals Moving Forward with Patient- and Family-Centered Care. Seminar Institute of Family-Centered Care, Bethesda, MD, Capabilities Statement, 2005, p 50.

4. **Why is it important to form a partnership in care with a family?**
   - To foster the parents' confidence as the role of "expert" in relationship to their infant
   - To support the parent-infant attachment and bonding
   - To help stabilize and strengthen the family unit
   - To equip parents with the necessary skills to be their child's advocate once they leave the neonatal intensive care unit (NICU)

In this way, the best opportunity for developmentally sound outcomes is enhanced, and families become essential partners for staff. This approach takes time and commitment by all health care providers in the NICU environment, yet it yields immeasurable dividends.

5. **Why is patient- and family-centered care a necessary component of care in the NICU?**
Patient- and family-centered care improves and enhances outcomes for infants by providing appropriate support for families as they cope with the challenges of caring for their hospitalized premature and critically ill infants. In addition, it has been observed that:
- Parent-infant attachment is increased.
- Breast-feeding is enhanced.
- Parent-provider communication and parent satisfaction with care are improved.
- Medical professionals' satisfaction with their work is increased.
- Collaboration between families and providers leads to increased parental confidence.
- There are better health outcomes and fewer readmissions.

6. **What should a patient- and family-centered NICU acknowledge?**
- Over time, the family has the greatest influence on an infant's health and well-being.
- All families bring important strengths to their infant's health care experiences.
- It is important to nurture the strong bonds that begin between infants and their families at birth and to support those relationships throughout the intensive care experience.
- Innovative facility design and patient- and family-centered environments should be available.

KEY POINTS: FAMILY-CENTERED CARE IN THE NICU

1. Integrates families in the care process

2. Is respectful of family values

3. Supports families' unique differences and diversity

4. Improves parent-infant attachment

5. Enhances breast-feeding

6. Improves parent satisfaction

7. Improves parent-provider communication

8. Improves parent confidence in the care of their infant

7. **How are NICUs changing their approach to health care delivery?**
In patient- and family-centered approaches in the NICU:
- Parents are viewed as collaborators in care.
- Parents are included in medical rounds.
- Families are no longer seen as visitors, and there is 24-hour participation in care.
- Parents and families participate in hospital/NICU advisory boards and design committees.
- Parents are provided with opportunities to learn and practice caregiving.
- Parent-to-parent mentor networks offer support for families.
- Parent information resource centers have been established in the units.

8. **What are the six key steps used to approach families in the NICU to assess their needs in a family-centered care model?**
   Family assessments in the NICU can be performed in as little as 15 minutes and should be done in a way that supports families and minimizes suffering. The following six key steps can be used as a guideline:
   - Introduce yourself to the family.
   - Ask about people at the bedside to determine their relationship to the infant (identify who can receive information other than the parents).
   - Know the gender of the infant and, especially, learn the infant's name.
   - Stop by frequently to update the parents with information.
   - Telephone parents or stop by, if present, to update them with changes.
   - After any explanation, always ask if there are questions. If you do not know an answer, say so and then find out the answer. Do not attempt to "bluff" when you don't know.

9. **What should be included in a patient-and family-centered neonatal practice?**
   - Privacy is provided for parents at the bedside that is personalized for the infant. Health care providers refer to infants and their family members by their names, not with "mommy," "daddy," or "the baby." Such terms are demeaning and disingenuous.
   - Parents, siblings, and families are not visitors and should be encouraged to be with their infants. There is 24-hour access to the NICU.
   - Cultural diversity is respected, and family preferences are honored.
   - Parents are active participants in medical/nursing rounds by asking questions of and responding to medical providers and are partners in decision making about their infant's care.
   - Primary nursing is available. Consistent caregiving is provided.
   - Early holding and "kangaroo care" is encouraged, and breast-feeding is promoted.
   - Parents participate in pain care by providing comfort before, during, and after painful procedures.

INFANT DEVELOPMENTAL CARE IN THE NICU

10. **What is developmental care?**
    Developmental care is a method of care that acknowledges that the developing fetus and infant can react favorably or unfavorably to environmental influences. Developmental care is a process that assesses each infant's individual developmental needs and responds to those needs to optimize neurodevelopmental outcome.

11. **A premature infant is really a fetus. Is a premature infant capable of reacting or responding to the environment?**
    Absolutely. A premature infant's neurosensory and musculoskeletal development is primed to react to all exposed environments. In the womb, unlike the NICU, a fetus is sheltered from light, sound, and noxious touch.

12. **What is the critical biologic aim of developmental care?**
    The aim is to reduce stress and improve or preserve neurodevelopmental outcome. Understanding infant vulnerabilities and responses to stress can lead to a systematic method to support the infant's strengths to alleviate the stress response. Calm infants require less oxygen (and fewer changes in mechanical ventilation), expend less energy, have improved feeding tolerance, and have a shortened duration of hospitalization.

13. **What are the key components of infant developmental care?**
    Infant developmental care is care responsive to an individual infant's developmental needs. The key components are as follows:

- **Management of the environment:** Decreasing noise and visual stimulation, providing appropriate bedding
- **Collaboration with parents and promotion of infant-parent bonding**
- **Activities that promote self-regulation and state regulation:** Nonnutritive sucking, kangaroo care, cobedding of multiples
- **Fixed midline positioning and containment**
- **Clustering of care:** To promote rest

KEY POINTS: GOALS OF DEVELOPMENTAL CARE IN THE NICU

1. To improve respiratory function

2. To enhance feeding and promote weight gain

3. To support brain and psychological development

4. To prevent muscular skeletal deformities

5. To shorten length of hospitalization

14. **How is developmental care different from the care that is currently provided in the NICU?**
In current care practices, the caregiver has a set treatment plan that is performed regardless of the responses of the infant. In the practice of developmental care, the caregiver responds to infant behavior to alter or manage the infant's environment before, during, and after the treatment. The caregiver individualizes the treatment process based on infant behavioral observations.

15. **How long have we known that the NICU environment can affect infant outcome?**
The theory of impact of the environment on infant outcome is not new. As early as 1973, during the "infancy" of neonatal intensive care, environmental effects such as sound, light, and positioning were noted to have a negative impact on infant medical outcomes.

KEY POINTS: COMMON CHARACTERISTICS OF DEVELOPMENTAL CARE

1. An environment supportive of the needs of the child

2. Caregiving staff and families who identify and respond to the needs of the infant

3. Caregiving staff and families who collaborate in care

4. Specific supportive techniques, such as kangaroo care, swaddling, and pacifier use to support development

16. **How is the Newborn Individualized Developmental Care and Assessment Program (NIDCAP) different from other methods of providing developmental care training?**
NIDCAP is a model of care that emphasizes the behavioral individuality of each infant. Caregivers receive intensive specialized training in neurobehavioral and environmental infant observations that result in a behavioral profile that can be used in the plan of care. This method seeks to diminish the infant's stress experience and to enhance the infant's strengths. Wee Care, another developmental care program, incorporates developmental care training of the entire NICU care team to increase awareness of the importance of the environment and developmental care responses needed to address the needs of high-risk infants.

17. **Does developmental care for critically ill infants improve outcomes?**
Yes. Developmental care has been shown to accomplish the following:
- Facilitate the transition to independent feeding
- Promote weight gain
- Shorten hospitalization
- Reduce hospital charges
- Improve neurobehavioral outcomes
- Reduce parental stress and improve parent perception of the infant
    In addition, developmental care methods such as containment, facilitated tuck, and kangaroo care have been shown to reduce infant stress and pain.

18. **What neuronal changes occur in the brain of the premature infant in the NICU environment?**
Neuronal changes occurring during 23–40 weeks' gestation include the following:
- Cell migration
- Cell differentiation
- Myelination
- Reorientation of cells
- Axonal growth
- Apoptosis
- Cell proliferation
- Formation of dendrites
- Formation of synapses

KEY POINTS: ONGOING NEURONAL CHANGES IN THE NICU

1. Cell migration and proliferation

2. Reorientation and differentiation of cells

3. Axonal growth and formation of dendrites

4. Myelination, apoptosis, and formation of synapses

19. **How critical is the environment for brain development?**
During this critical period of brain development, sensory and environmental influences can regulate wiring of neuronal networks, which can be permanently altered by early abnormal sensory input. In rats, pain experienced during the neonatal period is associated with persistent accentuated stress responses, learning deficits, and behavioral changes. In addition, chronic interference with rapid-eye-movement (REM) sleep has been associated with decreased size of the cerebral cortex.

20. **What is the order of development of the fetal senses?**
The senses develop in the following order: touch > balance > taste > smell > hearing > sight.

21. **What happens when sensory exposure occurs out of sequence?**
Animal studies have identified abnormal physiologic and brain development when the senses are stimulated out of order. Quail hatchlings cannot discriminate their mothers' cry if exposed to light before hatching. Premature human infants may be at risk of "executive dysfunction" and hearing loss when sensory systems have been stimulated out of order.

22. **When does tactile or touch sensation develop in an infant?**
Tactile sensory development occurs by 12–14 weeks' gestation. It is the first sensory system to develop and plays an important role in overall development. By 14 weeks, all sensory connections are present in the fetus.

23. **What are the most sensitive areas of the body in a fetus and premature infant?**
The areas that are the most sensitive for the fetus and premature infant are the mouth and extremities, especially the hands and feet.

24. **What are the physiologic responses to noxious stimuli in premature infants?**
Premature infants are very sensitive to what they perceive as noxious touch. When they experience these events they respond with tachycardia, agitation, hypertension, apnea, a decrease in oxygen saturation, disorganization, and sleep deprivation.

25. **What is the normal position of an infant in the womb?**
In the buoyant conditions of the womb, the infant remains in a flexed, contained, and midline position at all times. The head, back, and feet are contained by the uterine boundaries. This position allows for soothing and self-regulation by touching of the face and sucking on fingers.

26. **How does the loss of the uterine environment affect muscular development in an infant?**
Muscular development in the womb is critically dependent on the buoyancy and contained uterine space. The constant give and take of the uterine push against the fetal body is imperative for proper development of flexion and extension muscular tone in the infant.

27. **In the NICU, why is it important to provide boundaries for muscular development in a premature infant?**
Synaptic connections are stimulated with repeated use, and they weaken with disuse. Once outside the womb, the loss of uterine containment cannot support muscular development. A weak, premature infant is unable to counteract the effects of gravity and assumes a flattened posture with extremity extension, abduction, and external rotation on the bed surface. Over time, this position will lead to abnormal developmental tone and positional deformities.

28. **Why is it important to turn a premature infant every few hours?**
Premature infants in the womb are buoyant and turn easily, equalizing pressure stimuli. In the NICU, the impact of gravity inhibits any movement by the infant, who must rely on caregivers for proper positioning. Infants who are not turned are fixed in one position for prolonged periods and are at risk for development of muscular skeletal deformities that negatively affect the infant's future motor development and ability to explore, play, and develop social and other skills.

29. **Premature infants often have misshapen heads. Why does this happen?**
A progressive lateral flattening of the skull, called *scaphocephaly* or *dolichocephaly,* results in a narrow and elongated infant head. This occurs because the skull of the premature infant is thinner, softer, and at greater risk for postural deformities. Although this deformity appears to have

KEY POINTS: WHAT PROPER INFANT POSITIONING CAN PREVENT

1. Cranial flattening (scaphocephaly)

2. Torso deformities

3. Scapular deformities

4. Frog leg pelvic deformities

5. Facial deformities from endotracheal tubes

no effect on brain development, lateral flattening has implications for infant attractiveness and may affect parental social attachment. With good care, this appearance can be significantly minimized.

30. **When is the vestibular system developed in a premature infant?**
By 14–16 weeks' gestation the vestibular system, situated in the nonauditory labyrinth of the inner ear, is in place, allowing the fetus and infant to maintain balance in the womb. The vestibular system is important for movement, gravity, and directional balance.

31. **How should an infant be turned to support the vestibular system?**
The infant should be turned slowly and gradually, maintaining a midline flexed position.

32. **When is taste developed in an infant?**
The chemoreceptors for taste are developed in a fetus by 16–18 weeks' gestation. Taste buds appear early, at 8–9 weeks' gestation, with receptors fully present by 16 weeks.

33. **What kinds of tastes do infants prefer?**
Infant tongue taste buds prefer sweet tastes and withdraw from bitter tastes.

34. **When is smell developed in infants?**
The olfactory system develops early and is thought to be functioning in a fetus at 16–18 weeks' gestation.

35. **What is the rationale for non-nutritive sucking (e.g., pacifier)?**
Non-nutritive sucking facilitates the development of sucking behavior and improves digestion of enteral feeds. Controlled studies have demonstrated that non-nutritive sucking resulted in improved gavage tube-to-bottle transition, improved behavior (including improvement in sleep states), decreased stress behavior, and decreased length of hospital stay.

36. **When is an infant capable of responding to sound?**
A fetus is capable of responding to sound by 25 weeks' gestation. All major auditory structures are in place at this time. Both cortical and brain stem auditory-evoked responses can be elicited at 24–28 weeks' gestation, although the morphology and latency is different than in the term infant.

37. **Is noise associated with permanent long-term sequelae for a premature infant?**
Yes. Preterm infants are at risk for sensorineural hearing loss, which occurs at a rate of 10% compared with 0.5% for term infants. Noise may interfere with the development of auditory pathways necessary for communication and language skills. Premature infants are at risk for

KEY POINTS: PREDETERMINED ORDER FOR DEVELOPMENT ✔ OF SENSES

1. Tactile/touch
2. Vestibular/balance
3. Gustatory/ taste
4. Olfactory/smell
5. Auditory/hearing
6. Vision/sight

auditory processing deficits such as speech sound discrimination and other disorders of syntax, semantics, and auditory memory.

38. When is vision fully functioning in a fetus?
Vision is the last sensory system to develop in a fetus. All major structures and visual pathways for vision are complete by 24 weeks' gestation. Visual evoked responses (VERs) have been elicited (but with prolonged latency) as early as 24 weeks' gestation. By 36 weeks' gestation, the VER is similar to that of an infant carried to term.

39. Are closed eyelids enough to shield infants from light exposure in the NICU?
No. A premature infant is unable to guard against light exposure and requires shielding from the common sources of light in the NICU. At least 38% of white light can penetrate the eyelids and disturb an infant. There is also concern that excess light exposure at 32–40 weeks' gestational age may lead to sensory interference. Sensory interference may occur when immature sensory systems are stimulated out of order or are bombarded with inappropriate stimuli.

PAIN AND STRESS

40. How are infant stress and provision of developmental care linked?
Provision of developmental care is a method of care that provides a soothing, supportive, and responsive environment. This type of care decreases infant stress because caregivers and families, instructed in developmental care practices, can identify and provide therapy to relieve stress in infants.

41. Why is stress management so important in the NICU?
Research suggests that stress from the environment can prolong hospitalization and worsen medical conditions such as chronic lung disease. Stress may have long-term consequences on brain development and organization. Use of developmental care is a proactive approach to identify and reduce stress for infants in the NICU.

42. How is environmental stress and pain identified in a fetus or premature infant?
Pain and stress in a fetus are identified by physiologic (e.g., vital sign changes) and behavioral responses (e.g., tremors, crying). Understanding infant states of behavioral organization can assist in identifying pain and stress in infants. The states of organization are as follows:

- **State 1:** Deep sleep
- **State 2:** Light sleep
- **State 3:** Dozing
- **State 4:** Quiet awake
- **State 5:** Active awake
- **State 6:** Crying

43. **What are common daily stressful factors that an infant in the NICU encounters?**
    In addition to light and sound, NICU medical and nursing procedures necessary to ensure the infant's survival are by nature stressful. Suctioning, chest physical therapy, gavage tube insertion and feeding, intravenous line placements, chest radiographs, ultrasound studies, ophthalmologic examinations, daily physical examinations, frequent assessments of vital signs, bathing, and weighing have all been shown to cause significant stress in preterm or critically ill infants.

44. **Are apnea and decreased oxygen saturation common infant stress responses?**
    Yes. In one study, three of four hypoxic or oxygen-desaturation episodes in preterm infants were associated with caregiving procedures. Similarly, increased concentrations of stress hormones have been observed in association with routine nursing procedures.

45. **What are the pain-reducing interventions recommended by the international evidence-based group for neonatal pain?**
    Nonpharmacologic treatments to reduce pain and stress in infants include behavioral and environmental strategies such as non-nutritive sucking, administration of sucrose, swaddling and containment, attention to sound and light, limiting environmental stressors such as clustering of care, and allowing for rest periods.

46. **How is a premature infant different than a term infant in expression of pain and stress?**
    A premature infant is unable to sustain physiologic and behavioral responses to pain for prolonged periods. Infant pain scales may not be as clinically useful because the responses may be dampened or may not be identified by caregivers.

47. **Give examples of stress cues that infants use to communicate with caregivers or parents.**
    Autonomic stress cues can be divided into three categories:
    - **Color change:** Cyanosis, pallor, mottling, flushing
    - **Cardiorespiratory signs:** Irregular respirations, apnea, retractions, nasal flaring, tachycardia, oxygen desaturation, bradycardia
    - **Gastrointestinal signs:** Hiccups, emesis, feeding intolerance

THE NICU ENVIRONMENT

48. **What are the common components of the NICU environment that can be altered by implementation of developmental care?**
    The NICU environment includes sound, light, touch, handling, caregivers, facilities, bedding, positioning, and parents.

49. **What are the sound levels in the NICU?**
    Sound levels in the NICU are often greater than 90 dB. Common sounds in the NICU include intravenous pump alarms (61–78 dB), writing on tops of incubators (59–64 dB), vacuum

sounds (70 dB), bottles being placed on top of incubators (96 dB), metal door cabinet of incuba-tor opening and closing (96 dB), and telephones ringing (80dB).

50. **How is sound measured?**
Sound is a function of frequency and intensity. Intensity of sound is measured in decibels. The decibel (dB) is a unit that logarithmically expresses the pressure of the power of sound. Frequency is measured in hertz (Hz). The adult hearing frequency range is 30–20,000 Hz. Preterm infants generally have a restricted frequency range of 500–1000 Hz compared with term infants, who have a frequency range that is similar to the speech range of 500–4000 Hz.

51. **What level of sound is a fetus exposed to in the womb?**
In the womb, the intensity of sound recorded in the amniotic fluid has been of low frequency, <1000 Hz, and 70–85 dB. There are no peaks in intensity or frequency in the womb. In the NICU, the intensity increases to >90 dB and the frequency ranges from 500–10,000 Hz.

52. **How does the sound stimulus create stress in an infant?**
Sound exposure can increase infant agitation, increase intracranial pressure, decrease oxygen saturations, and affect sensorineural development.

53. **What levels of sound wake infants?**
Sound levels >70 dB are incompatible with sleep in term infants, whereas sound levels of >55 dB arouse an infant from light sleep.

54. **What are the American Academy of Pediatrics' (AAP) recommendations for sound in the NICU?**
Current recommendations from the AAP call for a sound level of <45 dB and a minimization of sound levels of >80 dB to less than 10-minute durations.

55. **What is the easiest and most cost-effective way to decrease sound in the NICU?**
The purchase of a sound meter and measurement of sound levels in the NICU can decrease infant sound exposure by alerting staff to high sound intensity. Incubator covers decrease noise levels inside the incubator. Soft ear plugs/covers have been found to increase oxygen saturation, decrease behavioral state changes, and increase quiet sleep time.

56. **What are other interventions that can be used to decrease sound in the NICU?**
Other interventions include "rounding" away from the bedside, limiting and altering conversation at the bedside, setting beepers to vibration mode, placing signs to remind staff/families to be quiet, and using incubators early in the infant's postnatal course. Removing radios from the NICU treatment areas and padding garbage cans are also helpful in decreasing sound.

57. **Is it true that children can have hearing loss if their mothers have been exposed to high levels of sound?**
Yes. Increased hearing loss has been reported in school-aged children whose mothers were exposed to noise levels of 65–85 dB during working environments 8 h/day during pregnancy.

58. **How can light cause stress and pain in the NICU?**
Bright lights are stressful for neonates and have been shown to increase infant agitation, interfere with weight gain, and cause lower oxygen desaturation. The intrauterine environment is dim with minimal light. The NICU environment has been designed to require light to perform procedures. The NICU overhead light (80–90 fc) is much brighter than the intrauterine environment or light at home, which approaches 50–60 fc.

59. **Should light in the NICU be cycled?**
    Yes. Cycled light (versus near darkness) has a positive effect on the infant. Constant high-intensity light that is usually found in the NICU can interfere with the natural circadian rhythms. Cycling low (1 fc) and normal light levels (60 fc) in the NICU is one way to support the development of normal day and night rhythms and is associated with lower heart and respiratory rates, increased behavioral organization, faster weight gain, and decreased length of hospitalization and ventilator days in infants.

60. **How is light intensity measured?**
    Light intensity is measured in footcandles (fc) or lux. A *footcandle* is a unit of illumination that is produced by a standard candle at the distance of 1 foot. One footcandle is approximately equal to 10 lux. The *lux* is the international unit of illumination. A lux is the illumination on the surface at a distance of 1 meter from a light source.

61. **What are the current AAP hospital recommendations for light intensity in the NICU?**
    The current recommendations are to maintain light levels at 1–60 fc by day and 0.5 fc at night.

62. **What is the easiest and most cost-effective way to decrease light in the NICU?**
    Purchase a light meter and develop guidelines for NICU light-intensity standards. In addition, educate staff regarding the impact of light on infant outcome. Interventions that can be used to decrease light intensity include covering the infant's eyes with protective covers during examination and repositioning incubators or covering incubators to avoid direct natural/sunlight that may come from windows. Windows and overhead light are the two most common sources of increased light intensity. Overhead light intensity can be minimized and individualized for each child. Individual light source controls and dimmers are effective in minimizing overhead light.

KEY POINTS: RECOMMENDED STANDARDS OF NICU DESIGN

1. Adjustable ambient lighting levels through a range of 10–600 lux (1–60 fc)

2. Separate procedural lighting available at each infant's care area

3. At least one source of daylight (60 fc) with shading devices

4. A combination of continuous background sound and transient sound not exceeding an hourly mean of 50 dB, with maximum transient sound not exceeding 70 dB.

63. **How often are infants touched during a routine day in the NICU?**
    It has been estimated that a critically ill infant is handled or manipulated for monitoring or other therapeutic procedures more than 150 times per day with <10 minutes of uninterrupted rest.

64. **What does *containment* mean, and why is it useful?**
    Containment and facilitated tuck are methods to decrease the stress response in infants undergoing a procedure. During containment, the infant is gathered and flexed midline to decrease stress.

65. **What is *clustering of care*, and is it important?**
    Clustering of care is a method used to provide a group of caregiving activities during one time period. It is important in allowing for infant rest between procedures.

66. **What is kangaroo care?**
    Kangaroo care, defined as skin-to-skin contact, originally consisted of placing a diapered infant in an upright position on the mother's bare chest. In Bogota, Columbia, where kangaroo care was initiated, the practice decreased infant mortality. Fathers should also be encouraged to participate in kangaroo care.

67. **What are the benefits of kangaroo care for the infant?**
    Infants who receive kangaroo care exhibit improved growth, had better breast-feeding rates, and had reduced nosocomial infections.

68. **How should kangaroo care be implemented in the NICU?**
    Kangaroo care should be implemented with written guidelines that are agreed on by all caregivers. Guidelines generally include the following:
    - **Eligibility of the infant for kangaroo care:** Multidisciplinary agreement
    - **Preparation of the parents:** Education related to the procedure, expectations
    - **Monitors needed:** Temperature, cardiorespiratory, and saturation monitors
    - **Methods to maintain temperature:** Infant cap and blanket over parent and infant
    - **Recording of the infant's activity during the procedure**

69. **Is kangaroo care widely practiced in NICUs in the United States?**
    Yes. A survey in 2002 found that 82% of NICUs were practicing kangaroo care. Some barriers to its use still exist for infants with certain illnesses.

BIBLIOGRAPHY

FAMILY–CENTERED CARE IN THE NICU

1. Ahmann E, Abraham MR, Johnson BH: Changing the concept of families as visitors: Supporting family presence and participation. Advances: Institute for Family-Centered Care 8:2–15, 2002.

2. Altimier L, Lutes L: Changing units for changing times: The evolution of a NICU. Neonatal Intens Care 13:23–27, 2000.

3. American Hospital Association, Institute for Family Centered Care: Strategies for Leadership: Patient- and Family-Centered Care: A Resource Guide for Hospital Senior Leaders, Medical Staff and Governing Boards. Bethesda, MD, 2004, p 2. Available at http://www.aha.org/aha/key_issues/patient_safety/resources/patientcenteredcare.html

4. Cisneros KA, Coher K, Dubuisson AB, et al: Implementing potentially better practices for improving family-centered care in neonatal intensive care units: Success and challenges. Pediatrics 111:450–460, 2003.

5. Conner JM, Nelson EC: Neonatal intensive care: Satisfaction measured from parent's perspective. Pediatrics 103(Suppl):336–349, 1999.

6. Hospitals Moving Forward with Patient- and Family-Centered Care Seminar Institute of Family-Centered Care, Bethesda, MD, 2004, p 50.

7. Johnson BH, Hanson JL, Jeppson ES: Family-Centered Care: Changing Practice, Changing Attitudes. Newborn Intensive Care: Resources for Family-Centered Practice. Institute for Family-Centered Care, Bethesda, MD, 1997, p 117.

8. Lawon G: Facilitation of parenting the premature infant within the newborn intensive care unit. J Perinatal Neonatal Nurs 16:71–82, 2002.

9. Leahey M, Wright L: Maximizing time, minimizing suffering: The 15-minute (or less) family interview. J Fam Nurs 5:259–274, 1999.

10. Peterson MF, Cohen J, Parsons V: Family-centered care: Do we practice what we preach? J Obstet Gynecol Neonatal Nurs 33:421–427, 2004.

11. Roman LA, Lindsay JK, Boger RP, et al: Parent-to-parent support initiated in the neonatal intensive care unit. Res Nurs Health 18:385–394, 1995.

12. Saunders RP, Abraham MR, Crosby MJ, et al: Evaluation and development of potentially better practices for improving family-centered care in neonatal intensive care units. Pediatrics 111:e437–e449, 2003.

13. Sudia-Robinson TM, Freeman SB: Communication patterns and decision-making among parents and health care providers in the neonatal intensive care unit: A case study. Heart Lung 29:143–148, 2000.

14. Van Ripper M: Family provider relationships and well-being in families with preterm infants in the NICU. Heart Lung 30:74–84, 2001.

15. Weiss SJ, Wilson P, Morrison D: Maternal tactile stimulation and the neurodevelopment of low birth weight infants. Infancy 5:85–107, 2004.

16. White RD: Mother's arms—the past and future locus of neonatal care? Clin Perinatol Jun 31:83–387, 2004.

17. White R, Martin GI, Graven SN: Newborn intensive care unit design: Scientific and practical considerations. In Avery GB, Fletcher MF, MacDonald MG (eds): Neonatology: Pathophysiology and Management of the Newborn. Philadelphia, Lippincott Williams, & Wilkins, 1999, pp 49–59.

INFANT DEVELOPMENTAL CARE IN THE NICU

18. Als H: Reading the premature infant. In Goldson E (ed): Developmental Interventions in the Neonatal Intensive Care Nursery. New York, Oxford University Press, 1999, pp 18–85.

19. Als H, Gibes R: Newborn Individualized Developmental Care and Assessment Program (NIDCAP). Training Guide. Boston, Children's Hospital, 1990.

20. Als H, Gilkerson L, Duffy F, et al: A three-center, randomized, controlled trial of individualized developmental care for very low birth weight preterm infants: Medical, neurodevelopmental, parenting, and caregiving effects. J Dev Behav Pediatr 24:399–408, 2003.

21. Als H, Lawhon G, Brown E, et al: Individualized behavioral and environmental care for the very low birth weight preterm infant at high risk for bronchopulmonary dysplasia: Neonatal intensive care unit and developmental outcome. Pediatrics 78:1123–1132, 1986.

22. Anand KJ, Coskun V, Thrivikraman KV, et al: Long-term behavioral effects of repetitive pain in neonatal rat pups. Physiol Behav 66:627–637, 1999.

23. Anand KJS, Scalzo FM: Can adverse neonatal experiences alter brain development and subsequent behavior? Biol Neonate 77:69–82, 2000.

24. Birnholz JC, Benacerraf BR: The development of human fetal hearing. Science 222:516–518, 1983.

25. Bourgeois JP: Synaptogenesis in the neocortex of the newborn: The ultimate frontier for individuation? In Lagercrantz H, Hanson M, Evrard P, et al (eds): The Newborn Brain. Cambridge, Cambridge University Press, 2002, pp 91–113.

26. Cartilidge PHT, Rutter N: Reduction of head flattening in preterm infants. Archives Dis Child 63:755–757, 1988.

27. Downs JA, Edwards AD, McCormick DC, et al: Effect of intervention on the development of hip posture in very preterm babies. Archives Dis Child 66:197–201, 1991.

28. Evans JC: Incidence of hypoxemia associated with caregiving in premature infants. Neonat Netw 10:17–24, 1991.

29. Gerhardt KJ, Abrams RM: Fetal exposures to sound and vibroacoustic stimulation. J Perinatol 20:S21–S30, 2000.

30. Grenier IR, Bigsby R, Vergara ER, Lester BM: Comparison of motor self-regulatory and stress behaviors of preterm infants across body positions. Am J Occupation Therapy 57:289–297, 2003.

31. Gressens P, Rogido M, Paindaveine B, et al: The impact of neonatal intensive care practices on the developing brain. Pediatrics 140:646–653, 2002.

32. Hendricks-Muñoz KD, Prendergast C, Caprio MC, et al: Developmental care: The impact of Wee Care developmental care training on short-term infant outcome and hospital costs. Newborn Infant Nurs Rev 2:39–45, 2002.

33. Lagercrantz H, Ringstedt T: Organization of the neuronal circuits in the central nervous system during development. Acta Paediatr 90:707–715, 2001.

34. Lai CH, Chan YS: Development of the vestibular system. Neuroembryology 1:61–71, 2002.

35. Lary S, Briassoulis G, de Vries L, et al: Hearing threshold in preterm and term infants by auditory brainstem response. J Pediatr 107:593–599, 1985.

36. Liu D, Caldji C, Sharma S, et al: Influence of neonatal rearing conditions on stress-induced adrenocorticotropin responses and norepinephrine release in the hypothalamic paraventricular nucleus. J Neuroendocrinol 12:5–12, 2000.

37. Long JG, Philip AGS, Lucey JF: Excessive handling as a cause of hypoxemia. Pediatrics 65:203–208, 1980.

38. Lotas M J, Walden M: Individualized developmental care for very low birth-weight infants: A critical review. J Obstet Gynecol Neonat Nurs 25:681–687, 1996.

39. Mennella JA, Beauchamp GK: Early flavor experiences: research update. Nutr Rev 56:205–211, 1998.

40. Mirmiran M, Kok JH: Circadian rhythms in early human development. Early Hum Dev 26:121–124, 1991.

41. Mouradian LE, Als H: The influence of neonatal intensive care unit caregiving practices on motor functioning of preterm infants. Am J Occup Ther 48:527–533, 1994.

42. National Association of Neonatal Nurses Infant and Family-centered Developmental Care: Guideline for Practice. Des Plaines, IL, Byers, 2000.

43. Penn AA, Shatz CJ: Principles of endogenous and sensory activity-dependent brain development: The visual system. In Lagercrantz H, Hanson M, Evrard P, et al (eds): The Newborn Brain. Cambridge, Cambridge University Press, 2002, pp 204–225.

44. Pinelli J, Symington A: Non-nutritive sucking for the promotion of physiologic stability and nutrition in preterm infant. Cochrane Database Syst Rev 3:CD001071, 2001.

45. Rabinowicz T, de Courten-Myers GM, Petetot JM, et al: Human cortex development: Estimates of neuronal numbers indicate major loss late during gestation. J Neuropathol Exp Neurol 55:320–328, 1996.

46. Ruda MA, Ling QD, Hohmann AG, et al: Altered nociceptive neuronal circuits after neonatal peripheral inflammation. Science 289:628–631, 2000.

47. Schaal B, Orgeur P, Rognon C: Odor sensing in the human fetus: Anatomical, functional, and chemeo-ecological bases. In Lecanuet J-P, Fifer WP, Krasnegor NA, Smotherman WP (eds): Fetal Development: A Psychobiological Perspective. Hillsdale, NJ, Lawrence Erlbaum Associates, 1995, pp 205–237.

48. Sweeney JK, Gutierrez P: Musculoskeletal implications of preterm infant positioning in the NICU. J Perinat Neonat Nurs 16:58–70, 2002.

49. Symington A, Pinelli J: Developmental care for promoting development and preventing morbidity in preterm infants. Cochrane Database Syst Rev 4:CD001814, 2003.

50. Tatzer E, Schubert MT, Timischl W, Simbrunger G: Discrimination of taste and preference for sweet in premature babies. Early Hum Dev 12:23–30, 1985.

51. Turkewitz G, Kenny PA: The role of developmental limitations of sensory input on sensory/perceptual organization. J Devel Behav Pediatr 6:302–308, 1985.

52. Vanden Berg KA: Basic principles of developmental caregiving. Neonat Netw 6:69–71, 1997.

PAIN AND STRESS

53. Anand KJS and the International Evidence-Based Group for Neonatal Pain: Consensus statement for the prevention and management of pain in the newborn. Arch Pediatr Adolesc Med 155:173–180, 2001.

54. Blickman JG, Brown ER, Als H, et al: Imaging procedures and developmental outcomes in the neonatal intensive care unit. J Perinatol 10:304–306, 1990.

55. Evans J: Incidence of hypoxia associated with care giving in premature infants. Neonatal Netw 10:17–24, 1991.

56. Field T: Alleviating stress in newborn infants in the intensive care unit. Clin Perinatol 17:1–9, 1990.

57. Field T, Ignatoff, M., Stringer S, et al: Nonnutritive sucking during tube feeding: Effects on preterm neonates in an intensive care unit. Pediatrics 70:381–384, 1982.

58. Franck LS, Lawhon G: Environmental and behavioral strategies to prevent and manage neonatal pain. In Anand KJS, Stevens BJ, McGrath PJ (eds): Pain Research and Clinical Management. Amsterdam, Elsevier Science, 2000, pp 203–216.

59. Gorski PA, Davison ME, Brazelton TB: Stages of behavioral organization in the high risk neonate: theoretical and clinical considerations. Semin Perinatol 3:61–73, 1979.

60. Johnston CC, Steven BJ, Yang F, Herton H: Differential response to pain by very premature neonates. Pain 61:471–479, 1995.

61. Murdock D: Handling during neonatal intensive care. Arch Dis Child 59:957–961, 1984.

62. Peters KL: Does routine nursing care complicate the physiologic status of the premature neonate with respiratory distress syndrome? J Perinat Neonat Nurs 6:67–84, 1992.

63. Peters KL: Neonatal stress reactivity and cortisol. J Perinat Neonat Nurs 11:45–49, 1998.

64. Pickler RH, Frankel HB, Walsh KM, Thompson NM: Effects of nonnutritive sucking on behavioral organization and feeding performance in preterm infants. Nurs Res 45:132–135, 1995.

65. Pinelli J: Nonnutritive sucking in high-risk infants: benign intervention or legitimate therapy? J Obstet Gynecol Neonatal Nurs 31:582–591, 2002.

66. Pinelli J, Symington A: How rewarding can a pacifier be? A systematic review of nonnutritive sucking in preterm infants. Neonatal Netw 19:41–48, 2000.

THE NICU ENVIRONMENT

67. American Academy of Pediatrics, Committee on Environmental Health: Noise: A hazard for the fetus and newborn. Pediatrics 100:724–727, 1997.

68. Appleton SM: "Handle with Care": An investigation of the handling received by preterm infants in intensive care. J Neo Nurs 3:23–27, 1997.

69. Brandon DH, Holditch-Davis D, Belyea M: Preterm infants born at less than 31 weeks' gestation have improved growth in cycled light compared with continuous near darkness. J Pediatrics 140:192–199, 2002.

70. Bremmer T: Noise and the premature infant: Physiological effects and practice implications. J Obstet Gynecol Neonatal Nurs 32:447–454, 2003.

71. Chang YJ, Lin CH, Lin LH: Noise and related events in a neonatal intensive care unit. Acta Paediatr Taiwan 42:212S–217S, 2001.

72. Charpak N, Ruiz-Pelaez JG, Figueroa de CZ, et al: A randomized, controlled trial of kangaroo mother care: Results of follow-up at 1 year of corrected age. Pediatrics 108:1072, 2001.

73. Chow M., Anderson, GC, Good M, et al: A randomized controlled trial of early kangaroo care for preterm infants: Effects on temperature, weight, behavior, and acuity. J Nur Res 10:129–142, 2002.

74. Engler, AJ, Ludington-Hoe SM, Cusson RM, et al: Kangaroo care: National survey of practice, knowledge, barriers and perceptions. Am J Matern Child Nur 27:146–153, 2002.

75. Gayle G, Franck L, Lund C: Skin to skin (kangaroo) holding of the intubated premature infant. Neonat Netw 12:49–57, 1993.

76. Gayle G, VandenBerg KA: Kangaroo care. Neonat Netw 17:69–71, 1998.

77. Graven SN: Sound and the developing infant in the NICU: Conclusions and recommendation for Care. J Perinatol 20:S88–S93, 2000.

78. Graven SN, Bowen FW, Brooten, et al: The high-risk infant environment, Part 1: The role of the neonatal intensive care unit in the outcome of high-risk infants. J Perinatol 12:164–172, 1992.

79. Harrison LL, Williams AK, Berbaum ML, et al: Physiologic and behavioral effects of gentle human touch on preterm infants. Res Nurs Health 23:435–446, 2000.

80. Holditch-Davis D, Torres C, O'Hale A, Tucker B: Standardized rest periods affect the incidence of apnea and rate of weight gain in convalescent preterm infants. Neonatal Netw 15:87, 1996.

81. Korones SB: Disturbances and infant rest. In Moore TD (ed): Iatrogenic Problems in Neonatal Intensive Care. Report of the 69th Ross Conference on Pediatric Research. Columbus, OH, Ross Laboratories, 1976.

82. Lalande NM, Hetu R, Lambert J: Is occupational noise exposure during pregnancy a risk factor of damage to the auditory system of the fetus? Am J Intern Med 10:427–435, 1986.

83. Latas M: Effects of light and sound in the neonatal intensive care unit environment on the low-birth-weight infant. NAACOG Clin Iss 3:3444, 1992.

84. Long JG, Lucey JF, Philip AGS: Noise and hypoxemia in the intensive care nursery. Pediatrics 65:143–145, 1980.

85. Luke B, Mamelle N, Keith L: The association between occupational factors and preterm birth: A United States nurses' study. Am J Obstet Gynecol 173:849–862, 1995.

86. Mirmiran M, Ariagno R: Influence of light in the NICU on the development of circadian rhythms in preterm infants. Sem Perinat 24:247–257, 2000.

87. Neu M: Parents perception of skin-to-skin care with their preterm infants requiring assisted ventilation. J Obstet Gynecol Neonat Nurs 28:157–164, 1999.

88. Porter FL, Wolf CM, Milller JP: The effect of handling and immobilization on the response to acute pain in newborn infants. Pediatrics 102:1383–1389, 1998.

89. Scafidi F, Field T: Massage therapy improves behavior in neonates born to HIV positive mothers. J Pediatr Psychol 21:889–897, 1996.

90. Zahr LK, Balia S: Responses of premature infants to routine nursing interventions and noise in the NICU. Nurs Res 44:179–185, 1995.

91. Zahr LK, de Traversay J: Premature infant responses to noise reduction by earmuffs: Effects on behavioral and physiologic measures. J Perinatol 15:448–455, 1995.

CHAPTER 4

GENERAL NEONATOLOGY

Helen M. Towers, LRCP&SI, MB, and David A. Bateman, MD

NICU ENVIRONMENT: HANDWASHING, HANDWASHING, HANDWASHING

1. **The following quiz is designed to test your knowledge of handwashing. Please wash your hands before taking the quiz and then again before you move on to the next section.**
    A. True or false: Total bacterial counts on the hands are higher when rings are worn.
    B. True or false: Long fingernails are associated with higher gram-negative colony counts on the hands than short fingernails.
    C. True or false: Artificial fingernails are associated with higher colony counts of gram-negative bacteria on the hands compared with natural nails.
    D. What is the recommended duration for hand washing? 30 seconds, 20 seconds, or 10 seconds?
    E. True or false: In a recently published survey, an incorrect answer for each of the above questions was given by about two thirds of neonatal intensive care unit (NICU) personnel who participated.
    F. True or false: Gowning is a useful infection control practice.
    G. True or false: Most neonatologists wash/degerm their hands before handling an infant.
    Answers: A. True; B. True; C. True; D. 20 seconds; E. True; F. False; G. False

    If you missed any of these questions, you must absolutely wash your hands before touching your next patient or anything in your patient's environment, including the Isolette and blankets. You must also wear gloves as directed by the policy of your unit. However, if you answered all the questions correctly, you need merely to wash your hands before touching your next patient or anything in the patient's environment including the Isolette and blankets. You, too, must wear gloves as directed by the policy of your unit.

    Cohen B, Saiman L, Cimiotti J, Larson E: Factors associated with hand hygiene practices in two neonatal intensive care units. Pediatr Infect Dis J 22:494–498, 2003.

    Kennedy AM, Elward Am, Fraser VJ: Survey of knowledge, beliefs, and practices of neonatal intensive care unit healthcare workers regarding nosocomial infections, central venous catheter care, and hand hygiene. Infect Control Hosp Epidemiol 25:747–752, 2004.

NICU ENVIRONMENT: PARENTAL RESPONSES TO THE NICU

2. **What are some of the stresses experienced by parents whose infant is being cared for in a NICU?**
    Parental reactions to a severe, life-altering event run the entire gamut of emotional response. These include shock, denial, grief, fear, sadness, anger, and guilt. Typical parental concerns include:
    - Infant appearance, health, course of hospitalization
    - Separation from infant/not feeling like a parent
    - Disruption of family life: concerns/communication with spouse; concerns for siblings; disruption of family routines, time, household tasks
    - Own health and well-being
    - Difficulty breast-feeding/pumping
    - Communications with or actions of medical staff

- Postdischarge expectations
- NICU environment

It is important to remember that mothers and fathers may prioritize these concerns differently, and that alone may be a source of severe family distress. As one family member put it, "There is no such thing as a good NICU experience." The physician and nurse, however, can have a positive impact on a family's NICU experience simply by acknowledging these stresses.

3. **What are some of the stresses experienced by the family of a preterm infant after hospital discharge?**
The stresses are more dramatic for families of infants with ongoing medical issues and home care needs than for families of healthy preterm infants. The following are some common stresses:
- Insecurity with parenting abilities
- Marital stress and possible discord
- Bonding and attachment issues due to prolonged hospitalization
- Financial stress, especially when there is a loss of income because one parent needs to remain home with the infant
- Inadequate or lack of insurance coverage for home care needs (e.g., nursing, equipment, special formulas and therapies)
- Isolation, reduced contact with family and friends due to concerns about exposure to infection (especially during winter months)
- Resentment felt by siblings because of parent's attention and time spent with new infant

   Hughes MA, McCollum J, Sheftel D, Sanchez G: How parents cope with the experience of neonatal intensive care. Children's Health Care 23:1–14, 1994.

NICU ENVIRONMENT: CONDITIONS

4. **What is the optimal intensity and pattern of ambient light exposure for a preterm infant?**
Although the answer is not really known, current data suggest that relatively dim ambient light (180–200 lux or typical indoor lighting), to be cycled dimmer at night, may be preferable to lighting of unvaried intensity or chaotically varied lighting. The evidence for this is as follows:
- Cycled dim light entrains circadian rhythm in newborn primates.
- Day/night differences in activity are observed during the first 10 days after discharge in preterm infants exposed to diurnal cycled dim ambient light (i.e., the babies are more likely to sleep at night and be awake during the day). These characteristics develop later in infants exposed to continuous dim lighting.
- Day/night light cycling in the NICU may improve postdischarge weight gain compared with chaotic light cycling.
- There is little evidence that newborns born before 35 weeks' gestation establish circadian variations in behavior, temperature, and activity in response to day/night light variation. However, such effects are well documented at term and thereafter.

   Rivkees SA: Emergence and influences of circadian rhythmicity in infants. Clin Perinatol 31:217–228, 2004.

5. **What are the effects of excessive noise on the fetus and newborn?**
Fetal exposure to excessive noise may cause:
- High-frequency hearing loss
- Preterm birth and intrauterine growth retardation

Excessive noise in the NICU may cause:
- Cochlear damage
- Disruption of normal growth and development

6. **How loud is the noise inside an infant's Isolette? Should you ever knock on the Isolette to rouse a child during an apnea spell?**
   Noise usually ranges from about 50 to 90 db. With the slamming of an Isolette door, the level can approach 100 db. By comparison, room conversation is 60–70 db, and louder rock music is 100–120 db. The American Academy of Pediatrics (AAP) recommends newborn exposure to noise be less than 70 db because:
   - Noise >70 db disrupts or awakens sleeping infants.
   - Noise >70 db is associated with cardiovascular changes (e.g., increased heart rate).
   - Ototoxicity resulting from the use of aminoglycoside antibiotics may be potentiated by constant loud noise.
     Hence, those who pound on the Isolette deserve a bit of a pounding themselves!

   American Academy of Pediatrics, Committee on Environmental Health: Noise: A hazard for the fetus and newborn. Pediatrics 100:724–727, 1997.

7. **What are the major etiologies of deafness in the newborn?**
   Hearing screening is now mandatory in many states in the United States. Early intervention can be critical and assists in the development of speech and improved learning. Infants in the following groups are at risk for hearing deficits:
   - Low birth weight
   - Congenital infections (e.g., rubella, toxoplasmosis, cytomegalovirus, syphilis, herpes)
   - Toxins (including ototoxic antibiotics)
   - Hyperbilirubinemia
   - Hypoxic-ischemic encephalopathy
   - Craniofacial anomalies
   - Family history of deafness
   - Term infants ventilated at high pressures for prolonged periods

   Graziani LJ, Desai S, Baumgart S, et al: Clinical antecedents of neurologic and audiologic abnormalities in survivors of neonatal ECMO—a group comparison study. J Child Neurol 12:415–422, 1997.

8. **What is the estimate of visual acuity of a term infant? When does color vision develop?**
   At birth, the newborn has at least 20/150 vision, and color vision develops at 2 months of age.

NICU ENVIRONMENT: THE UMBILICAL CORD

9. **How much fetal blood is in the placenta and umbilical cord?**
   Approximately one third of the total volume of fetal blood (about 120 mL/kg) resides in the placenta and umbilical cord. About two thirds resides in the fetus.

10. **How does the handling of the umbilical cord at birth influence neonatal hemoglobin concentrations?**
    The proportion of fetal-to-placental blood may be altered by:
    - **Perinatal asphyxia:** Increases blood flow away from the fetus to the placenta.
    - **A tight nuchal cord:** Pressure on the umbilical cord may preferentially compress the umbilical vein and inhibit venous return, trapping blood in the placenta at the expense of fetal blood volume. With early cord clamping, blood trapped in the placenta stays there for good.
    - **Infant positioning after birth:** Drainage from the placenta to the infant via the umbilical vein depends on gravity.
    - **Timing of cord clamping:** In general, the longer the cord takes to be clamped, the larger the neonatal blood volume. Larger blood volume may lead to polycythemia as re-equilibration of intravascular fluid volume with the extracellular compartment occurs.
    - **"Stripping the cord":** This may result in plethora and the possible need for partial exchange transfusion.

11. **Describe the best method of umbilical cord care in the immediate neonatal period.**
    - No single method of cord care has been determined to be superior in preventing colonization and infections.
    - Antimicrobial agents such as bacitracin or triple dye have been used but have unproven efficacy.
    - Lately, "dry cord" care has been advocated, consisting of simply keeping the cord clean and dry until it falls off.
    - Alcohol accelerates drying of the cord, but it has not been shown to reduce the rates of colonization or omphalitis.

12. **What is triple dye?**
    Triple dye consists of an aqueous solution of brilliant green proflavine hemisulphate and crystal violet that is bactericidal against *Staphylococcus aureus.* Possible adverse effects include:
    - Toxicity or carcinogenicity
    - Promotion of gram-negative cord colonization
    - Poor parental acceptance
    Triple dye care has also been advocated in underdeveloped areas of the world where sanitation is poor and rates of omphalitis and sepsis are much higher.

13. **Which way does the umbilical cord twist?**
    - The cord twists counterclockwise in approximately 95% of newborns.
    - Spiraling may result from the mobility of the fetus.
    - Noncoiled cords may be associated with an increased likelihood of anomalies.

14. **When should a parent begin to worry if an umbilical cord has not fallen off?**
    The umbilical cord generally dries up and sloughs by 2 weeks of life. Delayed separation can be normal up to 45 days. However, persistence of the cord beyond 30 days should prompt consideration of the following:
    - An underlying functional abnormality of neutrophils (leukocyte adhesion deficiency) or neutropenia, since these cells are involved in cord autolysis.
    - Factor XIII deficiency (see Chapter 11, Hematology).

Janssen PA, Selwood BL, Dobson SR, et al: To dye or not to dye: A randomized, clinical trial of a triple dye/alcohol regime versus dry cord care. Pediatrics 111:15–20, 2003.

Kemp AS, Lubitz L: Delayed cord separation in alloimmune neutropenia. Arch Dis Child 68:52–53, 1993.

Strong TH, et al: Antepartum diagnosis of noncoiled umbilical cords. Am J Obstet Gynecol 170:1729–1733, 1994.

Zupan J, Garner P: Topical umbilical cord care at birth. Update in Cochrane Database Syst Rev 3:CD001057, 2004.

KEY POINTS: NICU ENVIRONMENT

1. The NICU environment is a stressful place for infants, parents, families, and staff.

2. The physical environment of an infant affects biologic function.

3. Hearing deficit is the most common sensory deficit in newborns.

4. Cutting the cord between 30 and 120 seconds after birth allows adequate passage of blood, leading to fewer transfusions.

5. The use of waterless, alcohol-based hand gels reduces infection rates and maintains better skin integrity.

PROCEDURES

15. **What are some good sites for venous access in the neonate?**
Oh, that veins were so visible in babies as they are in Figure 4-1!

16. **What are some common complications of peripheral intravenous (IV) access?**
Common complications of peripheral venous cannulation include:
- **Infiltrates, burns, and sloughs:** Nearly every IV "comes out" because of an infiltrate; the point is not to let a small one progress to a major burn or slough. The most common sites of serious infiltrates are on the dorsum of hands and feet. Hypertonic solutions, especially those containing bicarbonate or calcium, appear to cause the worst IV burns.
- **Inadvertent arterial cannulation:** This may cause severe downstream necrosis when medications or hypertonic fluids are infused. Arteries may sometimes be mistaken for veins in the groin, antecubital fossa, ventral wrist, and scalp.
- **Infection:** Infection control procedures must be strictly followed when cannulating a peripheral vein (especially when inserting a percutaneous central venous line). The ideal of sterile insertion seems to wane as the IV line gets more difficult to insert, and the goal may disappear altogether with multiple attempts. The rate of nosocomial sepsis approaches 40% among very-low-birth-weight infants in some nurseries.

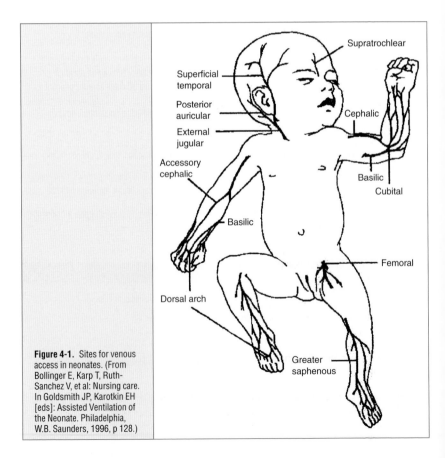

Figure 4-1. Sites for venous access in neonates. (From Bollinger E, Karp T, Ruth-Sanchez V, et al: Nursing care. In Goldsmith JP, Karotkin EH [eds]: Assisted Ventilation of the Neonate. Philadelphia, W.B. Saunders, 1996, p 128.)

17. **How do you estimate the insertion distance necessary for umbilical catheters?**
Measuring the distance from the umbilicus to the shoulder (lateral end of clavicle) allows an estimation of the desired length (Table 4-1).

TABLE 4-1.	INSERTION DISTANCE FOR UMBILICAL CATHETERS		
Shoulder to Umbilicus (cm)	Aortic Catheter to Diaphragm (cm)	Aortic Catheter to Aortic Bifurcation (cm)	Venous Catheter to Right Atrium (cm)
9	11	5	6
10	12	5	6–7
11	13	6	7
12	14	7	8
13	15	8	8–9
14	16	9	9
15	17	10	10
16	18	10–11	11
17	20	11–12	11–12

Adapted from Dunn PM: Localization of umbilical catheters by post mortem measurement. Arch Dis Child 41:69, 1966.

18. **What are the risks of umbilical catheters?**
Short-term risks
- Perforation and development of retroperitoneal hemorrhage (umbilical artery [UA] catheter)
- Decreased femoral pulses and blanching of limbs and/or buttocks (UA catheter)
- Accidental hemorrhage (both UA and umbilical vein [UV] catheters)
- Infection (both UA and UV catheters)
- Cardiac rhythm disturbances (usually UV catheters, if catheter enters the right atrium)
- Hemopericardium (extremely rare, usually right atrial perforation from UV catheter)
- Air embolus (both UA and UV catheters). In a spontaneously breathing baby, do not open a UV catheter to the air if the tip is above the diaphragm!

Long-term risks
- Embolization and infarcts (both UA and UV catheters)
- Thrombosis of hepatic vein (UV catheter)
- Liver necrosis (UV catheter)
- Aortic thrombi and hypertension (UA catheter)
- Renal artery thrombosis (UA catheter)
- Mesenteric thrombosis and necrotizing enterocolitis (UA catheter)
- Infection (both UA and UV catheters)

19. **How do you determine the appropriate length for nasotracheal tube insertion?**
See Table 4-2.

20. **How far should you insert an oral endotracheal tube in an emergency?**
Measuring from the lip to the tip of the endotracheal tube, the baby's weight in kilograms plus 6 is a useful memory tool. Of course, you will need to check tube position by auscultation and x-ray.

TABLE 4-2. DETERMINATION OF APPROPRIATE LENGTH FOR NASOTRACHEAL TUBE INSERTION

Crown Heel Length (cm)	Nasotracheal Length (cm)
30	6.50
32	7.00
34	7.50
36	8.00
38	8.25
40	8.75
42	9.25
44	9.50
46	10.00
48	10.25
50	10.50
52	11.00
54	11.50
56	12.00
58	12.50

Adapted from Coldiron JS: Estimation of nasotracheal tube length in neonates. Pediatrics 41:823–828, 1968.

UNCONJUGATED HYPERBILIRUBINEMIA

21. **Who was Sister Ward?**
    Sister Ward, the nurse in charge of the unit for premature infants at Rochford General Hospital in Essex, England, was responsible for the observation that led to the development of phototherapy. On warm summer days, she would take her charges to the courtyard to give them a little fresh air and sunshine. The account of her discovery, as recorded by R. H. Dobbs, follows:

    One particularly fine summer's day in 1956, during a ward routine, Sister Ward diffidently showed us a premature baby, carefully undressed and with fully exposed abdomen. The infant was pale yellow except for a strongly demarcated triangle of skin very much yellower than the rest of the body. I asked her, "Sister, what did you paint it with—iodine or flavine—and why?" But she replied that she thought it must have been the sun. "What do you mean Sister? Suntan takes days to develop after the erythema has faded." Sister Ward looked increasingly uncomfortable and explained that she thought it was a jaundiced baby, much darker where a corner of the sheet had covered the area. "It's the rest of the body that seems to have faded." We left it at that, and as the infant did well and went home, fresh air treatment of prematurity continued.

22. **How common is hyperbilirubinemia? How do we define its severity?**
    For infants in the first week of life:
    - 90% of healthy term newborns have total serum bilirubin (TSB) levels above 2.0 mg/dL
    - 50% have levels greater than 6.0 mg/dL
    - 5% have levels above 13 mg/dL

    Bhutani et al. constructed a percentile nomogram of TSB values plotted against age in hours, based on serial predischarge and postdischarge blood samples collected from 2840 normal newborns ≥36 weeks' gestation in the first week of life (Fig. 4-2). By the fourth day of life, approximately 95% of TSB values were ≤17 mg/dL, a value they considered indicative of *severe neonatal hyperbilirubinemia.*

23. **What are the primary causes of neonatal hyperbilirubinemia?**
    - Increased bilirubin production from enhanced red cell turnover
    - Decreased bilirubin clearance, due to decreased hepatic clearance or increased enterohepatic circulation

24. **What are the usual causes of increased bilirubin production?**
    Bilirubin is the end product of heme catabolism. In newborns, bilirubin production is distributed as follows:
    - 75% from normal destruction of senescent red blood cells (RBCs)
    - 25% from the breakdown products of ineffective erythropoiesis and from nonhemoglobin sources such as cytochromes and catalyses
    Factors associated with increased bilirubin production include:
    - Normally elevated hemoglobin levels (15–20 gm/dL)
    - Prematurity
    - Blood group incompatibility
    - Breakdown of extravascular blood
    - Maternal diabetes
    - Ethnicity, especially East Asian
    - RBC enzyme defects, such as glucose-6-phosphate dehydrogenase (G6PD) deficiency
    - RBC membrane defects (e.g., hereditary spherocytosis)
    - Hemoglobinopathies
    - Other hemolytic processes, such as sepsis

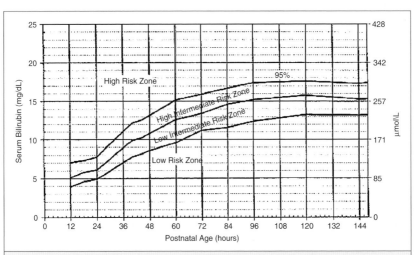

Figure 4-2. Percentile nomogram of TSB values plotted against age in hours. (From Bhutani VK, Johnson L, Sivieri EM: Predictive ability of a predischarge hour-specific serum bilirubin for subsequent significant hyperbilirubinemia in healthy term and near-term newborns. Pediatrics 103:6–14, 1999, with permission.)

25. **What are the common causes of delayed clearance of bilirubin?**
Bilirubin clearance from the body requires hepatic processing (conjugation), biliary excretion, and fecal or urinary elimination of intestinally metabolized bilirubin products. Conditions that may interfere with or delay this process include:
   - **Diminished uptake of bilirubin by the hepatocyte**
   - **Decreased glucuronyl transferase enzyme conjugating activity**
   - **Familial disorders of bilirubin excretion**
   - **Sluggish or obstructed biliary excretion:** This causes an increase in serum direct bilirubin.
   - **Active enterohepatic circulation:** (e.g., with antibiotic treatment, prolonged gut transit time, delayed passage of meconium, and inadequate enteral intake). This increases the level of unconjugated bilirubin.
   - **Prematurity:** All of the systems noted are even less mature.

26. **What are the hematologic manifestations of neonatal hemolysis?**
   - Decrease in hemoglobin concentration
   - Reticulocytosis: >8% at birth, >5% in first 2–3 days, and >2% after first week
   - Changes in the peripheral smear: microspherocytosis, anisocytosis, target cells
   - Elevated carboxyhemoglobin levels

27. **How does carbon monoxide (CO) relate to bilirubin production?**
   - The degradation of heme to biliverdin by heme oxygenase releases equimolar amounts of CO and ferrous iron.
   - Eighty to ninety percent of endogenous CO results from heme degradation.
   - Although CO binds tightly to hemoglobin, producing carboxyhemoglobin, it is liberated by the mass action effect of oxygen and expelled in expired breath. Thus, end-tidal CO can be used as a measure of bilirubin production.

   Stevenson DK, Vreman HJ: Carbon monoxide and bilirubin production in neonates. Pediatrics 100:252–254, 1997.

28. **Do transcutaneous bilirubin (TCB) measurements correlate with TSB measurements regardless of variations in skin pigmentation in newborns?**
Yes. At TSB levels below 15 mg/dL, the correlation coefficient between TcB and TSB is 0.90 or greater, regardless of gestational age and racial-ethnic group, provided that:
   - The device uses multiwavelength spectral reflectance.
   - Measurements are not useful after phototherapy, which bleaches the skin.

   Bhutani V, Gourley GR, Adler S, et al: Noninvasive measurement of total serum bilirubin in a multiracial predischarge newborn population to assess the risk of severe hyperbilirubinemia. Pediatrics 106:E17, 2000.

29. **What are the potential mechanisms of bilirubin neurotoxicity?**
The exact mechanism of bilirubin neurotoxicity remains unknown. Hypotheses include:
   - Bilirubin disruption of cellular enzyme and regulatory function by inhibition of protein/peptide phosphorylation
   - Interference with the phosphorylation of synapsin I, inhibiting neurotransmitter release
   - Interference with protein and DNA synthesis
   - Direct inhibition of exocytic release and synaptic storage of brain catecholamines
   Bilirubin transmission across the blood-brain barrier is probably a dynamic, potentially reversible process rather than an all-or-none phenomenon leading inevitably to toxic cellular disruption. For example, hypercapnia, by increasing cerebral blood flow and altering pH, increases both the influx and efflux of bilirubin across the blood-brain barrier, resulting in high-level, short-term exposure. In hyperosmolality, on the other hand, the cell entry of bilirubin is slower, but efflux is compromised and the level of exposure is lower

but of longer duration. It is not clear which of these processes is more likely to result in lasting neurotoxicity.

Hansen TWR: Bilirubin brain toxicity. J Perinatol 21:S48–S51, 2001.

30. **Which areas of the brain are stained by bilirubin during acute bilirubin encephalopathy?**
The most commonly affected areas are:
- **Basal ganglia:** Particularly, globus pallidus and subthalamic nuclei
- **Hippocampus:** Specifically, sectors H2–3
- **Substantia nigra**
- **Cranial nerve nuclei:** Oculomotor, vestibular, cochlear, and facial
- **Reticular formation of the pons**
- **Inferior olivary nuclei**
- **Cerebellar nuclei:** Especially the dentate
- **Anterior horn cells of the spinal cord**

   The yellow staining may last 7–10 days. The distribution of bilirubin staining often corresponds to the distribution of neuronal injury. However, damage to the basal ganglia and brain stem nuclei (oculomotor and cochlear) are most evident clinically. Involvement of cerebral cortical nuclei is not a prominent feature of kernicterus.

31. **Why do certain parts of the brain have a predilection for bilirubin-related neuronal injury?**
- Neurons are more easily injured than glial cells.
- Neurons have selective regional susceptibility to bilirubin injury.
- The neuronal surface has abundant gangliosides that readily bind to bilirubin.
- Glial cells may be preferentially protected by increased activity of a mitochondrial bilirubin oxidase.

32. **What are the clinical manifestations of acute bilirubin encephalopathy?**
Clinical manifestations of acute bilirubin encephalopathy can be insidious and progress rapidly to severe and life-threatening illness. The signs of bilirubin-induced neurologic dysfunction (BIND) can be grouped as in Table 4-3.

33. **What is the tetrad of clinical signs of *kernicterus*?**
The term *kernicterus* should be reserved for the chronic sequelae of acute bilirubin encephalopathy. Clinical signs include:
- **Motor:** Choreoathetoid cerebral palsy, motor delay
- **Cochlear:** Sensorineural deafness (auditory aphasia)
- **Oculomotor:** Gaze abnormalities, upward gaze paresis
- **Dental enamel dysplasia**

   In kernicterus, intellectual impairment and cognitive dysfunction are variable. Note that preterm infants may not always manifest these classic signs even when the neuropathologic findings are consistent with kernicterus.

34. **Are elevated bilirubin levels potentially beneficial?**
Yes. Unconjugated bilirubin has potent antioxidant and free-radical scavenger properties that may protect cells during the sudden exposure to high ambient oxygen levels at birth. Small intracellular concentrations of bilirubin, continually recycled from oxidized biliverdin, form a highly efficient mechanism to protect cell membranes from lipid peroxidation.

Sedlak TW, Snyder SH: Bilirubin benefits: Cellular protection by a biliverdin reductase antioxidant cycle. Pediatrics 113:1776–1782, 2004.

TABLE 4-3. CLINICAL FEATURES OF BILIRUBIN-INDUCED NEUROLOGIC DYSFUNCTION (BIND)

Signs	Mild	Moderate	Severe
Behavior	Too sleepy Decreased feeding Decreased vigor	Lethargic and/or irritable (state-dependent); very poor feeding	Semi-coma Apnea Seizures Fever
Muscle tone	Slight but persistent decrease in tone	Mild to moderate hypertonicity Mild nuchal/truncal arching	Severe hypotonia or hypertonia Atonia Opisthotonus, posturing, bicycling
Cry pattern	High-pitched	Shrill and piercing (especially when stimulated)	Inconsolable, very weak; cries only with stimulation

35. **Is the incidence of kernicterus increasing?**
    The incidence of kernicterus is unknown. However, case reports of kernicterus have increased in the past decade, as documented in the Kernicterus Registry. The AAP Subcommittee on Hyperbilirubinemia identified the following potentially correctable causes for a "resurgence" of kernicterus:
    1. Early discharge (<48 hours) with no early follow-up (within 48 hours of discharge); this problem is particularly important in near-term infants (35–37 weeks' gestation)
    2. Failure to check the bilirubin level in an infant noted to be jaundiced in the first 24 hours
    3. Failure to recognize the presence of risk factors for hyperbilirubinemia
    4. Underestimating the severity of jaundice by clinical (i.e., visual) assessment
    5. Lack of concern regarding the presence of jaundice
    6. Delay in measuring serum bilirubin level despite marked jaundice or in initiating phototherapy in the presence of elevated bilirubin levels
    7. Failure to respond to parental concern regarding jaundice, poor feeding, or lethargy
    American Academy of Pediatrics, Subcommittee on Hyperbilirubinemia: Neonatal jaundice and kernicterus. Pediatrics 108:763–765, 2001.

36. **What factors potentiate bilirubin deposition in the brain?**
    - Increased free bilirubin due to (1) elevated bilirubin–albumin ratio or hypoalbuminemia, (2) competitive displacement of unconjugated bilirubin bound to albumin by small molecules such as sulfa drugs or benzoate (a preservative in several drugs), or (3) impaired bilirubin–albumin binding
    - Increased proportion of bilirubin as bilirubin acid (in acidosis)
    - Increased transport of bilirubin across the blood-brain barrier (in hypercarbia)
    - Injury to the blood-brain barrier with asphyxia/hypoxia, hyperosmolarity (with use of hypertonic solutions), seizures, meningitis, sepsis with shock, and hypercapnia
    - Loss of cerebral blood flow autoregulation
    - Increased neuronal susceptibility (in hypoxemia-ischemia)

- Increased susceptibility to excitotoxic amino acids and reperfusion injury
- Illness (in respiratory distress syndrome, infection, shock)

37. **At what serum albumin value should there be a concern of bilirubin neurotoxicity?**
The bilirubin-to-albumin (B:A) ratio has been shown by Japanese investigators to predict bilirubin-related abnormalities in auditory brain stem–evoked responses. In an ideal situation, one molecule of albumin is capable of tightly bonding with one molecule of bilirubin, giving a potential equimolar B:A ratio. However, because some of the binding sites on albumin may be unavailable for bilirubin, free bilirubin is anticipated when the molar B:A ratio exceeds 0.80. This translates to 7.0 mg of bilirubin for each 1.0 gm of albumin. A molar ratio of <0.65 (5.5 mg of bilirubin per gram of albumin) could be considered safe in term and near-term babies. Thus, for a baby with a serum albumin level of 3.0 gm/dL, a TSB value >21 mg/dL is likely to exceed the albumin-binding sites available for bilirubin. In preterm and sick babies, the B:A ratio may underestimate the risk of irreversible injury because the binding affinity of albumin for bilirubin is compromised.

38. **What are the common drugs that displace bilirubin from the albumin-binding sites?**
Common drugs that displace bilirubin from the binding sites on albumin, in descending order of effect, include:
- Ceftriaxone
- Sulfisoxazole
- Cefmetazole
- Sulfamethoxazole
- Cefonicid
- Cefotetan
- Moxalactam
- Salicylates
- Carbenicillin
- Ethacrynic acid
- Aminophylline
- Ibuprofen
   Ampicillin, cefotaxime, and vancomycin can be safely given to an infant with jaundice.

39. **At what level of bilirubin should a premature baby receive phototherapy?**
The empiric approach has been to apply phototherapy early at relatively low TSB values. Aggressive use of phototherapy in preterm babies (especially those with a birth weight of <1000 gm) has been associated with near elimination of low-bilirubin kernicterus. Two approaches include:
- In an at-risk or bruised very-low-birth-weight baby, initiate phototherapy by 24 hours of age.
- Initiate phototherapy at 0.5% of body weight. For example, in a baby with a birth weight of 800 gm, phototherapy might be started when the TSB is ≥4 mg/dL.

40. **At what level is bilirubin neurotoxic in the term newborn?**
There are no precise data to correlate a specific bilirubin value with neurotoxicity. The decision to treat hyperbilirubinemia is based on the infant's history, course, physical findings (especially neurologic signs), and increasing levels of bilirubin, as well as a risk-benefit analysis of the disease process and the intervention. The AAP proposes the algorithm in Table 4-4 for healthy term newborns who do *not* have hemolytic jaundice. An alternative paradigm for applying phototherapy in term or near-term newborns (35–37 ⁶/₇ weeks' gestation) is shown in Fig. 4-3.

   American Academy of Pediatrics, Provisional Committee for Quality Improvement and Subcommittee on Hyperbilirubinemia: Practice parameter: Management of hyperbilirubinemia in the healthy term newborn. Pediatrics 94:558–562, 1994.
   American Academy of Pediatrics, Subcommittee on Hyperbilirubinemia: Management of hyperbilirubinemia in the newborn infant 35 or more week's gestation. Pediatrics 114:297–316, 2004.

TABLE 4-4. MANAGEMENT OF HYPERBILIRUBINEMIA IN THE HEALTHY TERM NEWBORN TSB LEVEL (mg/dL [μmol/L])

Age (h)	Consider Phototherapy*	Phototherapy	Exchange Transfusion if Intensive Phototherapy Fails†	Exchange Transfusion and Extensive Phototherapy
≤24‡ (see below)				
25–48	≥12 (200)	≥15 (260)	≥20 (340)	≥25 (430)
49–72	≥15 (260)	≥18 (310)	≥25 (430)	≥30 (510)
>72	≥17 (290)	≥20 (340)	≥25 (430)	≥30 (510)

*Phototherapy at these TSB levels is a clinical option, meaning that the intervention is available and may be used on the basis of individual clinical judgment.
†Intensive phototherapy should produce a decrease of TSB of 1–2 mg/dL within 4–6 hours, and the TSB level should continue to fall and remain below the threshold level for exchange transfusion. If this does not occur, it is considered a failure of phototherapy.
‡Term infants who are clinically jaundiced at ≤24 hours old are not considered healthy and require further evaluation.

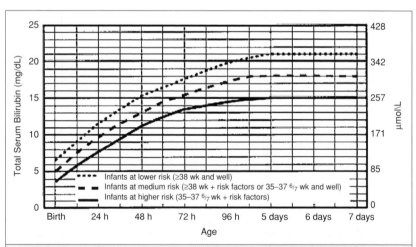

Figure 4-3. Alternative paradigm for applying phototherapy in term or near-term newborns. Use total bilirubin. Do not subtract direct reading or conjugated bilirubin. Risk factors: isoimmune hemolytic disease, G6PD deficiency, asphyxia, significant lethargy, temperature instability, sepsis, acidosis, or albumin level <3.0 gm/dL (if measured). For infants 35–37 % weeks, you can adjust TSB levels for intervention around the median risk line. It is an option to intervene at lower TSB levels closer to 35 weeks and at higher TSB levels for infants closer to 37 % weeks. It is an option to provide conventional phototherapy in hospital or at home at TSB levels 2–3 mg/dL (30–50 mmol/L) below those shown, but home phototherapy should not be used in any infant with risk factors.

41. **What are the major risk factors for severe hyperbilirubinemia in term newborns?**
    - Jaundice within first 24 hours after birth
    - A sibling who had jaundice as a neonate
    - Unrecognized hemolysis such as ABO blood type incompatibility or Rh incompatibility
    - Nonoptimal sucking/nursing
    - Deficiency in G6PD
    - Infection
    - Cephalohematomas/bruising
    - East Asian or Mediterranean descent
    - Maternal diabetes

    Centers for Disease Control and Prevention: Kernicterus in full-term infants—United States, 1994–1998. MMWR 50:491–494, 2001.

42. **Which newborns require a systematic assessment for the risk of severe hyperbilirubinemia prior to hospital discharge?**
    All newborns should have this assessment. Alternative assessment strategies include:
    - Universal predischarge TSB or transcutaneous assessment.
    - TSB assessment based on a combination of risk factor assessment and visual assessment. Note that visual assessment alone is inadequate.

43. **Why is a near-term newborn more likely to have excessive hyperbilirubinemia than the term newborn?**
    Near-term infants weighing more than 2000 gm are generally cared for in "well-baby" nurseries. However, because of their biologic immaturity, they are likely to:
    - Accept feedings more slowly
    - Exhibit slower maturation of hepatic glucuronyl transferase enzyme activity
    - Have delayed passage of meconium
    - Have prolonged enterohepatic circulation

    Near-term babies are often discharged by 48 hours of age (like term babies) and are more likely to be readmitted with dehydration, excessive hyperbilirubinemia, and even kernicterus. In some instances, near-term neonates may be at even greater risk than more premature infants who do enter the NICU, not only for bilirubin problems, but for infection and pulmonary disease as well. *Near-term infants are not term infants!* Predischarge evaluation, risk assessment, nutritional support, diligent plans for follow-up, and mandatory revisits are crucial to ensure the babies' well-being.

44. **How does phototherapy work?**
    The mechanism of phototherapy involves the following steps:
    1. Light absorption by bilirubin molecule
       - In vitro, the unconjugated bilirubin molecule absorbs light maximally in the blue portion of the visible spectrum, at a wavelength of 450 nm.
       - In vivo, because of bilirubin binding to albumin and tissue proteins as well as improved skin penetration at longer wavelengths, incident light in the blue-green spectrum may be more effective.
    2. Photoconversion of bilirubin to water-soluble isomers
       - Absorption of photon energy produces an excited state of bilirubin, leading to photoiso-merization and photo-oxidation.
       - Photoisomerization is the main pathway of bilirubin elimination. Two pathways are (1) configurational isomerization (formation of the 4Z,15E isomer and other photoisomers) and (2) structural isomerization (formation of lumirubin).
       - Photoisomerization disrupts the internal hydrogen bonds of native bilirubin (the 4Z,15Z isomer), making it more polar and increasing its water solubility.
       - Lumirubin, but not the 4Z,15E isomer, is rapidly excreted from the body and accounts for the effectiveness of phototherapy.

3. Excretion of bilirubin
   - The photoisomers are principally excreted in the bile. When cholestasis is present, the photoisomers can be excreted in the urine.
   - Excessive serum concentrations of the photoisomers (lumirubin) may manifest as bronze baby syndrome.

45. **What variables control the effectiveness of phototherapy?**
    - Spectrum of incident light
    - Irradiance of the phototherapy unit
    - Exposed surface area in the infant
    - Distance of the infant from light source

46. **What is the irradiance of phototherapy?**
    Irradiance is the dosage of light (μwatts/cm^2/nm) at the skin surface. The rate of bilirubin decline is proportional to the dose of phototherapy. Devices that measure irradiance accurately are easy to operate. The maximal achievable irradiance is generally between 30 and 40 μwatts/cm^2/nm. The minimally effective irradiance is approximately 5 μwatts/cm^2/nm.

47. **What is "intensive" phototherapy?**
    Maximization of irradiance in the blue-green spectrum by use of:
    - Spectrum-specific bulbs
    - "Double" or "triple" light sources
    - Foil reflectance around the bassinet
    - Close light-infant distances

    If not given with care, intensive phototherapy may generate large amounts of heat, increase insensible water loss, overheat the baby, or burn the baby's skin. Heat generating phototherapy lamps should not be placed closer to the infant than is recommended by the manufacturer.

    Maisels MJ: Phototherapy—Traditional and nontraditional. J Perinatol 21:S93–S97, 2001.

48. **By how much should phototherapy reduce bilirubin levels in the first 24 hours of treatment?**
    - **Intensive phototherapy:** Up to 30–50% decline from initial TSB in term infants with nonhemolytic jaundice
    - **Standard phototherapy:** Approximately 6–20% decline

49. **What are the side effects of phototherapy?**
    These are generally mild and manageable and include:
    - Increased insensible water loss, especially in preterm neonates and those cared for under radiant warmers. Different light sources have variable effects on insensible water loss.
    - Reduced gut transit time, probably related to increased bilirubin and photoproducts in the gut.
    - Decreased platelet counts to <150,000/mm^3 (controversial).
    - Transient riboflavin deficiency that usually resolves within 24 hours of the discontinuation of phototherapy.

50. **Do events during labor and delivery influence the severity of hyperbilirubinemia?**
    No! The following events have *not* been shown to affect the severity or incidence of hyperbilirubinemia:
    - **Pitocin induction**
    - **Epidural anesthesia and maternal anesthetic agents**
    - **Maternal vitamin K levels**

- **Tocolytic agents**
- **Mode of delivery:** No known effect unless associated with bruising or cephalohematoma

51. **Can elevated bilirubin levels be diluted by administering IV fluids or oral glucose water?**
No. However, a severely jaundiced infant with dehydration/oliguria may benefit from receiving IV fluid because poor hydration status and poor feeding compromise the baby's ability to eliminate bilirubin through the urine and stool. It is preferable to continue milk feeding because this interrupts the enterohepatic circulation by colonizing the gut with bacteria and stimulating meconium passage.

52. **Should phototherapy be discontinued in babies with both unconjugated and conjugated hyperbilirubinemia?**
No. Babies with a combined indirect and direct hyperbilirubinemia are prone to acquire long-term "bronzing" of the skin as a result of exposure to phototherapy and accumulation of lumirubin. However, although these infants look unwell, bronzing is not a reason to discontinue phototherapy. Direct bilirubin may compete with indirect bilirubin for albumin-binding sites and increase the risk of kernicterus, although it is not by itself neurotoxic. Furthermore, the concentration of direct-reacting bilirubin *should not* be subtracted from the TSB value to ascertain the potential neurotoxicity of indirect bilirubin. The validity of that practice has never been substantiated.

53. **When should phototherapy be stopped in term and near-term babies?**
When phototherapy is discontinued in a term or near-term baby with nonhemolytic disease, the "rebound hyperbilirubinemia" is generally modest. Some arbitrary recommendations for discontinuing phototherapy include the following:
- Stop phototherapy at bilirubin values <12–15 mg/dL.
- Alternatively, continue phototherapy until bilirubin values have reached to <40th percentile track for the hour-specific bilirubin level.
- Similar recommendations for hemolytic and nonhemolytic jaundice apply.
- Rebound levels in hemolytic jaundice may be higher; recheck bilirubin at 6–12 hours after phototherapy.
- With intensive phototherapy, consider step-wise weaning to avoid a significant rebound effect.

54. **When should phototherapy be stopped in preterm infants?**
There is no consensus or adequate clinical data to address this issue. Phototherapy may be discontinued at the level at which it was considered appropriate to initiate the intervention, generally ≤5 mg/dL for infants weighing <1 kg.

55. **Should exposing the term newborn with hyperbilirubinemia to sunlight (i.e., heliotherapy) be encouraged as the natural source of phototherapy?**
The potential complications of heliotherapy in newborns include:
- Overheating
- Excessive insensible water loss and dehydration
- Unnecessary exposure to ultraviolet light (prevented by window glass)
- Unpredictable dose; seasonal dependence

56. **When should term and near-term infants receive an exchange transfusion for hyperbilirubinemia?**
See Fig. 4-4.

57. **Should intravenous immunoglobulin (IVIG) administration be considered in babies with severe Rh hemolytic disease?**
Yes. Maternal administration of IVIG lessens the severity of fetal hemolysis. Administration of IVIG to neonates with severe Rh hemolytic disease accomplishes the following:

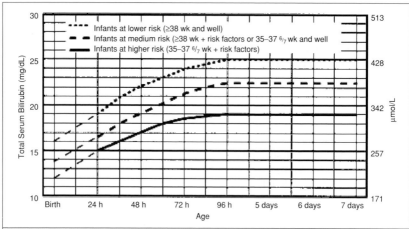

Figure 4-4. Exchange transfusion for hyperbilirubinemia. The dashed lines for the first 24 hours indicate uncertainty due to a wide range of clinical circumstances and a range of responses to phototherapy. Immediate exchange transfusion is recommended if the infant shows signs of acute bilirubin encephalopathy (e.g., hypertonia, arching, retrocollis, opisthotonos, fever, high-pitched cry) or if the TSB level is ≥5 mg/dL (85 μmol/L) above these lines. Risk factors include isoimmune hemolytic disease, G6PD deficiency, asphyxia, significant lethargy, temperature instability, sepsis, and acidosis. Measure serum albumin and calculate B:A ratio. Use total bilirubin. Do not subtract direct reading or conjugated bilirubin. If the infant is well and at 35–37 ⁵/₇ weeks (median risk), you can individualize TSB levels for exchange based on actual gestational age. (From American Academy of Pediatrics Subcommittee on Hyperbilirubinemia: Management of hyperbilirubinemia in the newborn infant 35 or more weeks of gestation. Pediatrics 114:297–316, 2004; and Johnson LH, Bhutani VK, Brown AK: System-based approach to management of neonatal jaundice and prevention of kernicterus. J Pediatr 140:396–403, 2002.)

- Reduces hemolysis (as measured by carboxyhemoglobin levels)
- Lowers bilirubin levels
- Reduces need for exchange transfusion
- Shortens hospital stays

58. **Why has double-volume exchange transfusion been recommended instead of a single-volume or triple-volume exchange transfusion?**
An effective double-volume exchange transfusion (160 mL/kg) reduces the serum bilirubin levels by two time constants (84.5% reduction). With a one-volume exchange transfusion (80 mL/kg), bilirubin is reduced one time constant (63%), and with a three-volume exchange it is reduced by 95%. The three-volume exchange transfusion is not used because it prolongs the procedure and increases the risk of a complication.

59. **What rates of mortality and morbidity are associated with exchange transfusions?**
- **Mortality:** Approximately 3/1000
- **Morbidity:** Approximately 5%; complications include apnea, bradycardia, cyanosis, vasospasm, thrombosis, necrotizing enterocolitis
These rates are probably much lower in term/near-term infants and higher in small preterm infants.

60. **What are some potential causes of death during an exchange transfusion?**
Cardiac/vascular
- Arrhythmia
- Vascular perforation by catheter
- Acute hemorrhage

- Thrombus
- Acute volume overload
- Massive air embolism (Note: Do not open the umbilical venous catheter to the air if the tip is above the diaphragm!)

Metabolic (especially in preterm infants)

- Severe acidosis
- Hyperkalemia
- Hypocalcemia

61. **What are the indications for readmission of an infant with hyperbilirubinemia?**
    - Rate of rise in TSB level >6 mg/24 h
    - Level of bilirubin >95th percentile track (persistent)
    - Level of bilirubin that has jumped tracks from ≤75th percentile track to >95th percentile track
    - Clinical signs of neurotoxicity (see BIND evaluation)
    - B:A ratio (mg/gm) >6.0
      A baby must be hospitalized to receive intensive phototherapy. The bilirubin levels in such infants should be persistently >95th percentile track. In babies with B:A ratio (mg/gm) of <5.5, the decision to administer intensive phototherapy can be delayed as long as the baby is closely watched for clinical signs of BIND (*see* Table 4-3) and is feeding, urinating, and stooling normally. On the other hand, in an infant with a low serum albumin level (concentration <3.4 gm/dL), one needs to be more aggressive in implementing intensive phototherapy.

62. **Is there any reason to discontinue breast-feeding in an excessively jaundiced baby?**
    No. At times, however, it may be helpful to interrupt breast-feeding for approximately 24 hours to diagnose breast milk jaundice. In such cases, the bilirubin levels usually drop precipitously but may rebound when breast-feeding resumes.

63. **What advice should be given to a mother who is breast-feeding her jaundiced baby?**
    - Continue breast-feeding. Evaluate for adequate latching and audible swallowing of milk by the baby and assess the infant's consolability after a feed.
    - Use an electric breast pump to facilitate "let down of milk" and to collect expressed breast milk for extra supplementation.
    - Avoid maternal use of opioid analgesics (e.g., Percocet, Tylenol III, and other codeine preparations) that could have an impact on the newborn's feeding and stooling.
    - Identify ways to reduce maternal stress and anxiety to promote lactation.

    Johnson LH, Bhutani VK, Brown AK: System-based approach to management of neonatal jaundice and prevention of kernicterus. J Pediatr 140:396–403, 2002.

KEY POINTS: KERNICTERUS

1. Kernicterus is associated with early discharge home from the hospital.

2. To avoid kernicterus, all newborns should have early systematic clinical assessment for jaundice by visual inspection and transcutaneous or serum bilirubin level determination.

3. Supplementation with water or glucose will not prevent hyperbilirubinemia or decrease TSB levels in the newborn period. If supplementation is needed, breast milk or formula should be offered.

4. All bilirubin levels should be interpreted according to the infant's age in hours.

5. Planned follow-up after discharge is critical in many infants for appropriate jaundice management.

CIRCUMCISION

64. **What are the indications for routine male circumcision?**
There are no medical indications for routine circumcision of a male infant. Cultural and ethnic traditions have led to the useful mnemonic of 5 Ms:
- **M**oses
- **M**ohammad
- **M**other
- **M**oney
- **M**edicine

Adherents of both the Jewish and Muslim religions routinely circumcise males. The rate of circumcision has been directly linked to the maternal socioeconomic group. Many parents choose to have their son circumcised if the father is circumcised. Medical bills are generated by circumcision. Rarely, medical indications such as recurrent balanitis or secondary phimosis may be indication for circumcision.

65. **What are the complications of neonatal circumcision?**
In 0.2–0.6% of cases there are complications, including the following:
- Bleeding is the most frequent complication, seen in 0.1% of circumcisions.
- Infection, recurrent phimosis, urinary retention, meatitis, meatal stenosis, chordee, wound separation, inclusion cysts, and unsatisfactory cosmesis have been reported.
- Rare complications include scalded skin syndrome, necrotizing fasciitis, sepsis and meningitis, urethral fistula, partial amputation of the glans penis, and penile necrosis.

66. **What analgesia should be used for circumcision?**
Analgesia is essential for the relief of pain associated with circumcision.
- Dorsal penile nerve block is effective in reducing the behavioral and physiologic indicators of pain. A 27-guage needle is used to inject 0.4 mL of 1% lidocaine (without epinephrine) at both the 10- and 12-o'clock positions at the base of the penis. Peak concentrations are achieved at 60 minutes. Bruising at the site is the most frequent complication.
- A subcutaneous ring block of 0.8 mL of 1% lidocaine without epinephrine administered at the midshaft of the penis has also been effective in reducing a pain response.
- The administration of sucrose on a pacifier or acetaminophen is insufficient for the operative pain.

PREMATURITY

67. **What are the differences among gestational age, chronologic age, and calculated (i.e., adjusted) age?**
- **Gestational age:** An obstetric assessment based on the date of the last menstrual period, measured in completed weeks. A term pregnancy usually lasts 40 weeks.
- **Chronologic age:** Based on birth date.
- **Adjusted age:** Chronologic age—number of weeks born prematurely.

For example, a preterm infant of 32 weeks' gestational age at 6 months chronologic age has an adjusted age of 4 months. Adjusted age is used for plotting growth parameters and for developmental assessment until 2–3 years of age.

68. **What is the difference between developmental delay and mental retardation?**
- *Developmental delay* is a term used to describe preschoolers who exhibit some degree of delay in meeting expected milestones of development. It does not indicate that the delay will be permanent.
- *Mental retardation* is defined by a demonstrated delay on standardized assessments of intelligence and adaptive skills. The term is generally not used until the child is approaching school age and it is apparent the delays are not transient.

69. **Can one predict survival in extremely-low-birth-weight (ELBW) infants?**
    Prediction of survival in ELBW infants is difficult, but recent evidence suggests:
    - One half of observed mortality in infants weighing <700 gm occurs by 2 days of life.
    - Half of the observed mortality in infants weighing 901–1000 gm occurs by 12 days of life.
      Survival predictability in the smallest infants improves dramatically during the first few days of life, but there is significant risk for late death in the smallest infants.

    Cooper TR, Berseth CL, Adams JM, Weisman LE: Actuarial survival in the premature infants less than 30 weeks gestation. Pediatrics 101:975–978, 1998.

70. **How do infants born before 25 weeks' gestation fare developmentally?**
    The incidence of early childhood neurodevelopmental handicaps among infants of <25 weeks' gestation is significant, despite advances in perinatal and neonatal treatment. The incidence of major disability (e.g., cerebral palsy, mental retardation, profound hearing loss, blindness) is at least 30%. Multihandicap is common in this population. Infants of 23 and 24 weeks' gestation experienced rates of impairment or disability of 64% and 43%, respectively, at a corrected age of 18 to 24 months.

    Hintz SR, Kendrick DE, Vohr BR, et al: for the National Institute of Child Health and Human Development National Research Network. Changes in neurodevelopmental outcomes at 18 to 22 months' corrected age among infants of less than 25 weeks' gestational age born in 1993–1999. Pediatrics 11:1645–1651, 2005.
    Jacobs SE, O'Brien K, Inwood S, et al: Outcome of infants 23–26 weeks' gestation pre and post surfactant. Acta Paediatr 89:959–965, 2000.

71. **How does one counsel a family about the probable outcome for a preterm infant weighing less than 1500 gm in terms of major disabilities or school-related problems?**
    - The healthy 1500-gm infant is likely to be free of major disabilities.
    - The lower the birth weight of the child, the higher the risk for significant delay.
    - Learning disabilities, attention deficit disorder, and academic delays have been reported in low-birth-weight infants.

72. **What is *catch-up growth*? Is it good for low-birth-weight infants?**
    Catch-up growth refers to a rapid weight gain of preterm infants, allowing comparisons with reference infants by approximately 2 years of age. Recent evidence suggests that it occurs at the expense of fat deposition and may not always be good for a prematurely born infant.

    Ehrenkrantz RA: Growth outcomes of very low birth weight infants in the newborn intensive care unit. Clin Perinatol 27:325–345, 2000.

73. **Should a breast-feeding mother supplement her preterm infant after discharge from the hospital?**
    - Preterm human milk provides insufficient quantities of protein, sodium, calcium, and phosphorus to meet the estimated growth needs of these infants.
    - Large fluid volumes may be required to provide sufficient calories to maintain adequate growth.
    - Although the use of fortification is common practice, the limited data available on outcome do not permit practice recommendations.
    - Preterm infants require long-term monitoring of adequate growth and bone mineralization.

74. **What should be considered in the differential diagnosis of a preterm infant who presents to the office with ongoing problems and inadequate oral intake?**
    - Oral motor dysfunction
    - Central nervous system dysfunction (e.g., secondary to hypoxia)
    - Gastroesophageal reflux
    - Abnormal behavioral response
    - Upper airway compromise

- Chronic microaspiration
- Chronic lung disease (CLD)
- Mechanical problems with either nipple flow or sucking ability
- Caregiver limiting volume of feedings

75. **What are the guidelines for scheduling routine immunizations of preterm infants?**
    - Infants should be immunized according to chronologic age.
    - Infants should be immunized according to the guidelines developed by the AAP Advisory Committee on Immunization Practices.

76. **Which additional immunizations beyond those given routinely should be considered for the preterm infant with CLD?**
    - **Influenza vaccine:** Should be given each fall for infants >6 months chronologic age; also caretakers and other family members.
    - **Palivizumab (Synagis):** This monoclonal antibody against respiratory syncytial virus (RSV) should be given intramuscularly monthly throughout the RSV season to the following categories of infants: (1) those with CLD who are younger than 2 years of chronologic age and who required medical therapy for CLD within 6 months before the onset of RSV season and (2) preterm infants without CLD as summarized in Table 4-5.

TABLE 4-5. PALIVIZUMAB VACCINATION IN PRETERM INFANTS WITHOUT CLD	
Gestational Age (GA)	**Chronologic Age at Start of RSV Season**
<28 weeks	Until 12 months
29–32 weeks	Until 6 months
32–35 weeks	Until 6 months*

*Only if additional risk factors exist (e.g., exposure to smoke, attendance at day care, one of multiple birth, or other siblings at home).

77. **What visual abnormalities are common sequelae of mild-to-moderate stages of retinopathy of prematurity?**
    - Refractive errors
    - Strabismus
    - Amblyopia

KEY POINTS: CEREBRAL PALSY, RETINOPATHY OF PREMATURITY, AND IMMUNIZATIONS

1. The diagnosis of cerebral palsy should generally be delayed until after 12–18 months' corrected age.

2. Immunizations are given according to chronologic age.

3. Retinopathy of prematurity is responsible for more blindness among children in this country than all other causes combined.

4. Palivizumab, the monoclonal antibody against RSV infection, has been shown to be effective in reducing hospital admission in high-risk infants.

DUCTUS ARTERIOSUS

78. Who discovered the ductus arteriosus?

Although widely attributed to Botallo, it was Galen who first described the ductus arteriosus in the second century A.D. Galen's description was as follows: "Nature is neither lazy nor devoid of foresight. Having given the matter thought, she knows in advance that the lung of the fetus does not require the same arrangements of a perfected lung endowed with motion. She has therefore anastomosed the pulmonary artery with the aorta." Botallo (an Italian surgeon) is credited with discovering the foramen ovale.

79. When was postnatal constriction of the ductus arteriosus first recognized?

William Harvey (1578–1657) described constriction of the ductus arteriosus in his famous publication, "Exercitato anatomica de mortu cordis et sanguinis in aminalibus." These are his words: "From the pulmonary artery, a kind of arterial canal is carried obliquely to terminate in the great artery or aorta. The canal shrinks after birth and after time becomes withered."

80. When was the first ductal ligation performed?

In 1938, Robert Gross ligated the patent ductus arteriosus (PDA) in Loraine Sweeney.

> Gross R: Surgical ligation of a patent ductus arteriosus: Report of a first successful case. JAMA 112:729–731, 1939.

81. What is the purpose of the ductus arteriosus in the fetus?

In the fetus, the ductus arteriosus diverts right ventricular blood away from the fluid-filled lungs toward the descending aorta and placenta.

- Ninety percent of fetal right ventricular output shunts via the ductus arteriosus.
- Ten percent flows through the pulmonary vascular bed.

82. When does the ductus arteriosus normally close after birth?

The vast majority of term infants have functional ductal closure by 12–15 hours of life. In preterm infants, functional ductal closure occurs in 90% of infants between 30 and 37 weeks' gestation and in <50% of infants of <30 weeks' gestation. Anatomic obliteration of the ductus arteriosus usually is not complete for several months. A ductus that is functionally open beyond 72 hours postnatally can be considered a persistent PDA.

83. Name the major risk factors for the development of a symptomatic PDA.

- Prematurity
- Respiratory distress syndrome
- Excessive fluid administration in the first few days after birth
- Surfactant therapy (controversial)
- Perinatal asphyxia

84. What is the effect of antenatal steroids on ductal patency?

In experiments involving animals, in utero administration of a wide variety of steroids has caused ductal constriction. Data from human newborn infants exposed to antenatal steroids are controversial but suggest there may be a decreased need for ductal ligation.

> Eronen M, Kari A, Personen E, Hallman M: The hemodynamic effects of antenatal dexamethasone administration on the fetal and neonatal ductus arteriosus. A randomized double-blinded study. Am J Dis Child 147:187–192, 1993.

85. When indomethacin is administered to a mother antenatally, why is ductal constriction less likely to occur in immature fetuses?

When indomethacin is administered antenatally as a tocolytic agent, ductal constriction results in part from decreased blood flow in the vaso vasorum supplying the media. The vaso vasorum does not develop until 28 weeks' gestation. Before that time, luminal blood flow is sufficient to nourish the wall of the ductus arteriosus.

86. **Does antenatal indomethacin increase the probability of ductal patency after birth?**
Once again, the data are controversial; however, recent studies suggest a greater need for postnatal indomethacin or surgical ligation.

> Hammerman C, Glaser J, Kaplan M, et al: Indomethacin tocolysis increases postnatal patent ductus arteriosus severity. Pediatrics 102:E56, 1998.

> Suarez, Thompson LL, Jain V, et al: The effect of *in utero* exposure to indomethacin on the need for surgical closure of a patent ductus arteriosus in the neonate. Am J Obstet Gynecol 187:886–888, 2002.

87. **Does surfactant administration increase the likelihood of a PDA?**
The meta-analysis of prophylactic synthetic surfactant trials suggests a slightly increased risk of a PDA (relative risk [RR], 1.11; confidence interval [CI], 1.0–1.22). A similar analysis of prophylactic synthetic surfactants does not support that association. Despite the lack of convincing data, it must be remembered that surfactant use is associated with a slightly increased incidence of pulmonary hemorrhage.

88. **Does the presence of a PDA in a preterm infant increase morbidity and mortality, or is it merely associated with increased morbidity?**
Once again, this is a controversial topic. A meta-analysis by Clyman in 1996 indicated that prophylactic ligation of a PDA was associated with a decreased incidence of intraventricular hemorrage (IVH). "Early treatment" of a PDA compared with "late treatment" (when signs of congestive heart failure are present) was associated with a significant reduction in the incidence of bronchopulmonary dysplasia (BPD) and necrotizing enterocolitis (NEC). Recent meta-analyses from the Cochrane Collaborative indicate that prophylactic indomethacin does decrease the incidence of grade III/IV IVH without improving long-term neurodevelopmental outcome. The use of prophylactic indomethacin or treatment of an asymptomatic PDA does not decrease the incidences of BPD or NEC. It is uncertain that treatment of a "symptomatic PDA" before signs of congestive heart failure develop reduces pulmonary morbidity.

> Clyman RI: Recommendations for the postnatal use of indomethacin: An analysis of four separate treatment strategies. J Pediatr 128:601–607, 1996.

89. **What are the potential deleterious effects of a symptomatic PDA in the premature infant?**
Pulmonary overperfusion results in an increased risk of:
- Pulmonary hemorrhage
- Bronchopulmonary dysplasia

Cerebral, mesenteric, and renal underperfusion result in an increased incidence of:
- Metabolic acidosis
- Intracranial hemorrhage
- Periventricular leukomalacia
- Necrotizing enterocolitis
- Renal insufficiency and oliguria

90. **What are the clinical manifestations of a PDA?**
- **Cardiac murmur:** Usually systolic, pansystolic murmurs are rare in neonates
- **Apnea**
- **Increased pulse volume and widened pulse pressure:** Bounding pulses, palmar pulses
- **Worsening pulmonary status:** Tachypnea, need for increased respiratory support, failure to wean from respiratory support
- **Congestive heart failure**

- **Radiographic changes:** Including (1) diffuse increase in homogeneous lung density ("wet lungs"), (2) increased prominence of the pulmonary vasculature, perihilar congestion, (3) increase in heart size, and (4) pleural effusions (rare).

91. What murmurs are associated with a PDA?

The classic PDA murmur (a continuous systolic and diastolic "machinery" murmur) is heard infrequently in the neonatal period. Instead, there is usually a systolic murmur, best heard in the pulmonic area, or no murmur. (In 50% of ventilated preterm infants, no ductal murmur is heard and there may be few other obvious signs.)

92. When should an echocardiogram be performed in evaluating for a PDA?

Two-dimensional cardiac echocardiography with pulsed, continuous-wave or color Doppler ultrasound are both sensitive and specific in identifying ductal patency. An echocardiogram should be performed:

- Within the first 3–4 days after birth in all mechanically ventilated infants of <1000 gm birth weight
- When symptoms compatible with PDA develop in preterm infants
- Before giving indomethacin, to confirm the presence of PDA and exclude other cardiac pathology
- Twenty-four to forty-eight hours after indomethacin therapy to document treatment failure and allow for prompt alternative interventions

93. Is ibuprofen safer than indomethacin?

In studies involving human preterm infants, ibuprofen has not been shown to decrease renal, cerebral, or mesenteric blood flow. However, experimental animal data indicate that ibuprofen does have renal effects. The Cochrane Collaborative concluded that ibuprofen caused less of an increase in serum creatinine levels, and the incidence of decreased urine output (<1 mg/kg/h) was less than that seen with indomethacin.

94. Are there any advantages to a prolonged (5–7 day) course of indomethacin versus a short course?

The Cochrane meta-analysis concluded that a prolonged course was associated with a decreased incidence of severe IVH (RR, 0.49; CI, 0.2–0.98) and renal function impairment (evidenced by creatinine; RR, 0.52; CI, 0.34–0.81).

Herrera C, Holberton J, Davis P: Prolonged versus short course of indomethacin for treatment of patent ductus arteriosus in preterm infants. The Cochrane Library, Issue 1, 2006.

95. Do all premature infants with PDA require treatment?

In a premature infant who does not require mechanical ventilation, ductal closure is less urgent:

- The ductus often closes spontaneously over the first few weeks after birth.
- Treatment should be given if signs of significant left-to-right ductal shunting develop.

96. Describe the side effects of indomethacin treatment for PDA in preterm infants.

Side effects of indomethacin treatment for PDA in preterm infants include:

- Compromised platelet function (clinically apparent adverse effects are not well documented)
- Spontaneous gastrointestinal perforation (may be associated with decreased mesenteric perfusion)
- Decreased renal perfusion, resulting in decreased glomerular filtration rates, oliguria, increased serum creatine levels, fluid retention, and hyponatremia
- Decreased cerebral blood flow with decreased reactive postasphyxial hyperemia and accelerated maturation of the germinal matrix microvasculature

- Although indomethacin treatment has been shown to reduce the incidence of IVH/periventricular leukomalacia, long-term beneficial neurodevelopmental effect of treatment has yet to be demonstrated

97. **Does judicious fluid restriction reduce the incidence of PDA in premature newborns?**

Yes! Preterm infants who received restricted fluid intake, compared with liberal fluid intake, are at significantly lower risks for:

- PDA
- NEC
- Death

They are at significantly higher risk for postnatal weight loss and show nonsignificant tendencies toward an increased risk for dehydration and decreased risk for bronchopulmonary dysplasia.

Bell EF, Acarregui MJ: Restricted versus liberal water intake for preventing morbidity and mortality in preterm infants. Art. No. CD000503. DOI:10.1002/14651858.CD000503. Cochrane Database of Systematic Reviews, Issue 3, 2001.

98. **How should preterm infants be evaluated for PDA? What is an appropriate management strategy?**

Figures 4-5 and 4-6 summarize a suggested strategy based on the author's clinical experience. It has not been evaluated in a prospective trial. Needless to say, there is considerable controversy in this area. A symptomatic PDA is defined by the following:

- Signs of congestive heart failure (or reduced cardiac output)
- Increasing oxygen requirements on continuous positive airway pressure or mechanical ventilation
- Failure to wean ventilator settings
- Increased need for ventilator support with no other apparent cause
- Rising serum creatinine

KEY POINTS: INDOMETHACIN USAGE

1. Prophylactic indomethacin usage does not provide long-term neurodevelopmental protection.

2. Indomethacin failure rates may be higher in small-for-gestational age infants.

3. Attention to fluid management in a preterm infant may prevent morbidity and enhance nutritional intake.

4. Remember to exclude ductal-dependent cardiac lesions by echocardiogram before giving indomethacin.

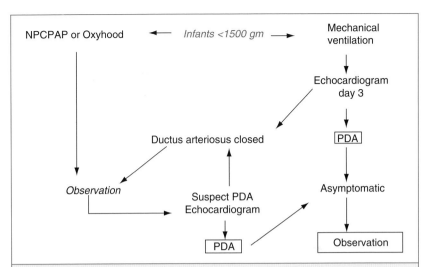

Figure 4-5. Management of patent ductus arteriosus in an infant treated with nasopharyngeal continuous positive airway pressure (NPCPAP).

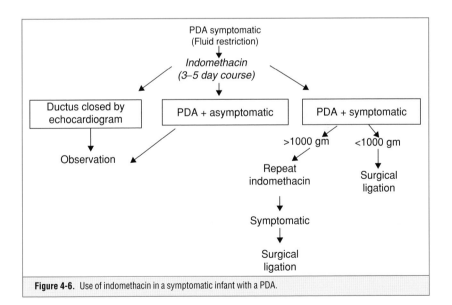

Figure 4-6. Use of indomethacin in a symptomatic infant with a PDA.

CHAPTER 5

CARDIOLOGY

Julie S. Glickstein, MD

1. **When was the first report of a successful ligation of a patent ductus arteriosus (PDA)?**
   The first successful ligation of a PDA was performed by Gross and Hubbard in 1938.

2. **Who was responsible for the first successful treatment of cyanotic congenital heart disease?**
   Alfred Blalock (Professor of Surgery at Johns Hopkins), Helen Taussig (Director of the Pediatric Cardiology Clinic at Johns Hopkins), and Vivien Thomas (Research Assistant for Dr. Blalock at Johns Hopkins). Their tireless work contributed to the successful research and techniques behind the Blalock-Taussig shunt. The first successful operation was in November 1944.

   Neill CA, Clark EB: The Developing Heart: A History of Pediatric Cardiology. London, Kluwer Academic Associates, 1995.

FETAL ECHOCARDIOGRAPHY AND PRENATAL CONDITIONS THAT CAN CONTRIBUTE TO NEONATAL HEART DISEASE

3. **What are the indications for a fetal echocardiogram?**
   Maternal indications
   - Family history of congenital heart disease
   - Metabolic disorders (e.g., diabetes, phenylketonuria)
   - Exposure to teratogens
   - Exposure to prostaglandin synthetase inhibitors (e.g., ibuprofen, salicylic acid)
   - Rubella infection
   - Autoimmune disease (e.g., systemic lupus erythematosus, Sjögren's syndrome)
   - Familial inherited disorders (e.g., Marfan and Noonan syndromes)
   - In vitro fertilization

   Fetal indications
   - Abnormal results of an obstetric ultrasound screening
   - Extracardiac abnormality
   - Chromosomal abnormality
   - Arrhythmia
   - Hydrops fetalis
   - Increased first-trimester nuchal translucency
   - Multiple gestation and suspicion of twin-twin transfusion
   - Genetic syndromes

   Rychik J, Ayres N, Cuneo B, et al: American Society of Echocardiography Guidelines and Standards for Performance of the Fetal Echocardiogram. J Am Soc Echocardiog 17:803–810, 2004.

4. **What is the incidence of congenital heart disease? What is the recurrence risk if a previous child has congenital heart disease?**
The incidence of congenital heart disease is 0.8%. The recurrence risk with a prior sibling who has a cardiovascular anomaly is between 1% and 4%.

Nora JJ: Etiologic aspects of heart disease. In Moss AJ, Adams FH, Emmanouilides GC V (eds): Heart Disease in Infants, Children and Adolescents. Baltimore, Williams & Wilkins, 1995.

5. **What are the common genetic and/or chromosomal syndromes associated with congenital heart disease?**
See Table 5-1.

TABLE 5-1. COMMON GENETIC OR CHROMOSOMAL SYNDROMES ASSOCIATED WITH CONGENITAL HEART DISEASE

Genetic or Chromosomal Syndrome	Common Cardiac Anatomic Lesion
Apert syndrome	Ventricular septal defect, coarctation of the aorta, tetralogy of Fallot
Beckwith-Wiedemann syndrome	Atrial septal defect, ventricular septal defect, cardiomegaly
CHARGE syndrome	Endocardial cushion defect, coarctation of the aorta, ventricular septal defect, tricuspid atresia, double outlet right ventricle, tetralogy of Fallot
DiGeorge syndrome	Ventricular septal defect, coarctation of the aorta, tricuspid atresia, d-transposition of the great vessels, tetralogy of Fallot, interrupted aortic arch, double-outlet right ventricle
Ellis-van Creveld syndrome	Atrial septal defect, single/common atrium
Holt-Oram syndrome	Atrial septal defect, ventricular septal defect
Marfan syndrome	Dilated aortic root, mitral valve prolapse, tricuspid valve prolapse
Neurofibromatosis	Atrial septal defect, coarctation of the aorta, interrupted aortic arch, pulmonic stenosis, ventricular septal defect, complete heart block, hypertrophic cardiomyopathy
Noonan syndrome	Pulmonic stenosis, ventricular septal defect, atrial septal defect, interrupted aortic arch, hypertrophic cardiomyopathy, aortic stenosis, tetralogy of Fallot
Pentalogy of Cantrell	Atrial septal defect, ventricular septal defect, total anomalous pulmonary venous drainage, tetralogy of Fallot, ectopia cordis
Pierre Robin syndrome	Atrial septal defect
Thrombocytopenia-absent radius syndrome	Atrial septal defect, tetralogy of Fallot, dextrocardia
Treacher Collins syndrome	Ventricular septal defect, atrial septal defect

TABLE 5-1. COMMON GENETIC OR CHROMOSOMAL SYNDROMES ASSOCIATED WITH CONGENITAL HEART DISEASE—CONT'D

Genetic or Chromosomal Syndrome	Common Cardiac Anatomic Lesion
Tuberous sclerosis	Rhabdomyoma, angioma, coarctation of the aorta, interrupted aortic arch
VACTERL	Hypoplastic left heart syndrome, ventricular septal defect
Trisomy 13 syndrome	Ventricular septal defect, atrial septal defect, hypoplastic left heart syndrome, endocardial cushion defect, tetralogy of Fallot, coarctation of the aorta, interrupted aortic arch
Trisomy 18 syndrome	Bicuspid aortic valve, pulmonic stenosis, ventricular septal defect, atrial septal defect, endocardial cushion defect, double-outlet right ventricle, coarctation of the aorta, interrupted aortic arch
Trisomy 21 syndrome	Endocardial cushion defect, ventricular septal defect, atrial septal defect, tetralogy of Fallot, coarctation
Turner syndrome	Coarctation of the aorta, bicuspid aortic valve, aortic stenosis, ventricular septal defect, atrial septal defect, endocardial cushion defect, pulmonic stenosis, interrupted aortic arch, total anomalous pulmonary venous drainage

Adapted from Drose J: Fetal Echocardiography. Philadelphia, W.B. Saunders, 1988.

6. **What teratogens are known to cause congenital heart disease?**
   See Table 5–2.

PHYSIOLOGIC VARIABLES IN FETAL AND PERINATAL LIFE

7. **What four shunts are present in the fetal circulation?**
   - **Ductus venosus:** Allows placental blood flow to bypass liver
   - **Fossa ovalis:** Allows venous return to bypass the heart
   - **PDA:** Allows right ventricular blood to bypass the pulmonary circulation
   - **Placenta:** Receives the largest amount of combined ventricular output and has the lowest vascular resistance in the fetus
   The fetal circulation is illustrated in Fig. 5-1.

TABLE 5-2. TERATOGENS THAT CAUSE CONGENITAL HEART DISEASE

Teratogen	Common Cardiac Anatomic Lesion
Fetal alcohol syndrome	Ventricular septal defect, atrial septal defect, tetralogy of Fallot, coarctation of the aorta
Fetal hydantoin (Dilantin) syndrome	Ventricular septal defect, tetralogy of Fallot, pulmonic stenosis, patent ductus arteriosus, atrial septal defect, coarctation of the aorta
Fetal trimethadione syndrome	Ventricular septal defect, d-transposition of the great vessels, tetralogy of Fallot, hypoplastic left heart syndrome, double-outlet right ventricle, pulmonary atresia, atrial septal defect, aortic stenosis, pulmonic stenosis
Fetal carbamazepine syndrome	Ventricular septal defect, tetralogy of Fallot
Valproic acid	Ventricular septal defect, coarctation of the aorta, interrupted aortic arch, tetralogy of Fallot, hypoplastic left heart syndrome, aortic stenosis, atrial septal defect, pulmonary atresia
Retinoic acid embryopathy	Conotruncal malformations
Thalidomide embryopathy	Conotruncal malformations
Maternal phenylketonuria (fetal effects)	Tetralogy of Fallot, ventricular septal defect, coarctation of the aorta
Maternal systemic lupus erythematosus/Sjögren's syndrome (fetal effects)	Complete congenital heart block, dilated cardiomyopathy
Fetal rubella syndrome	Patent ductus arteriosus, peripheral pulmonary artery stenosis, ventricular septal defect, atrial septal defect
Lithium	Ebstein's anomaly of the tricuspid valve, tricuspid atresia
Maternal diabetes	Hypertrophic cardiomyopathy, conotruncal abnormalities

Adapted from Drose J: Fetal Echocardiography. Philadelphia, W.B. Saunders, 1988.

8. **Why does the fossa ovalis close shortly after birth?**
The fossa ovalis is composed of the septum primum overlying the septum secundum in the left atrium. In fetal life, the right atrial pressure is greater than the left atrial pressure, causing the fossa ovalis to remain patent. After birth, with the increase in pulmonary blood flow and pulmonary venous return to the left atrium, the left atrial pressure increases and causes the septum primum to close against the septum secundum, thereby closing the fossa ovalis.

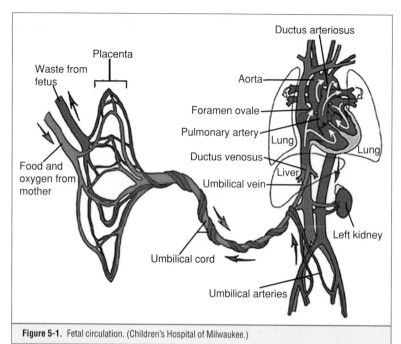

Figure 5-1. Fetal circulation. (Children's Hospital of Milwaukee.)

9. **What are the determinants of pulmonary vascular resistance (PVR)?**

Pulmonary vascular resistance = pulmonary artery pressure/pulmonary blood flow

---

KEY POINTS: PULMONARY VASCULAR RESISTANCE

1. The pulmonary vascular resistance begins to fall after birth and reaches a nadir by 6–8 weeks of age.

2. Oxygen is a potent vasodilator and contributes to the fall in the pulmonary vascular resistance after birth.

---

10. **How does pulmonary vascular resistance change after birth?**
    In fetal life, the pulmonary vascular resistance is high. As the newborn infant expands the lungs at birth and inspires oxygen (a potent vasodilator), the pulmonary vascular resistance falls. The nonmuscular pulmonary arteries dilate, and small muscular arteries are recruited into the circulation. The pulmonary vascular resistance continues to fall as the arterial wall thins and remodels, leading to a normal pulmonary vascular resistance by 6–8 weeks of age. The systemic vascular resistance increases because of the removal of the low-resistance placenta from the circulation.

    Park M: Pediatric Cardiology for the Practitioner, 3rd ed. St. Louis, Mosby, 1996.

ECHOCARDIOGRAPHIC ASSESSMENT OF VENTRICULAR FUNCTION
AND PULMONARY HYPERTENSION

11. **Why is echocardiography particularly useful in the assessment of ventricular function and pulmonary hypertension?**
It can be used for noninvasive assessment of right ventricular/pulmonary artery pressure.

12. **Name three scenarios in which a right-to-left shunt is seen in an infant with a PDA.**
   - A right-to-left shunt in the ductus arteriosus is seen in a healthy newborn during the first 24 hours of life. Usually, this right-to-left shunt occurs in early systole and is brief in duration.
   - Infants with left-sided obstructive lesions (e.g., coarctation of the aorta, severe aortic stenosis, interrupted aortic arch, or hypoplastic left heart syndrome) typically have a right-to-left ductal shunt in systole and a left-to-right shunt beginning in late systole and in diastole. This right-to-left shunt helps bypass the region of obstruction to blood flow, thus contributing to systemic circulation.
   - Infants with a high pulmonary vascular resistance (i.e., persistent pulmonary hypertension of the newborn or congenital heart disease complicated by marked elevation of pulmonary vascular resistance) tend to have continuous right-to-left flow in the ductus arteriosus.

13. **What is the modified Bernoulli equation?**
The modified Bernoulli equation enables one to calculate the relationship between velocity and pressure across either an area of stenosis or two different chambers of the heart:

$$\text{pressure 1} - \text{pressure 2} = 4\,(V2 - V1^2)$$

The pressure gradient is measured in millimeters of mercury (mmHg), and the velocity is measured in meters per second. Because V1 is assumed to be of low velocity (<1 m/sec) it can be ignored, and the formula can be approximated as:

$$\text{pressure 1} - \text{pressure 2} = 4\,(Vmax^2)$$

14. **How can the modified bernoulli equation be useful in interpreting pulmonary artery pressures in a neonate?**
By using this formula, the pulmonary artery pressure can be estimated. Two examples are as follows:
   1. If the velocity across a tricuspid regurgitant jet is 4 m/sec, the calculated right ventricular pressure will be 64 mmHg ($P = 4 \times [V\,max^2]$ which is ($4 \times [4^2] = 64$ mmHg). By adding an estimation of right atrial pressure (usually use 5 mmHg), the estimated right ventricular pressure (as well as a pulmonary artery pressure) would be 69 mmHg. Therefore, this patient has pulmonary hypertension.
   2. If the jet velocity across a ventricular septal defect (VSD) is 4 m/sec, the calculated pressure difference between the right and left ventricles would be 64 mmHg ($P = 4 \times [4^2] = 64$ mmHg). In a patient with a systolic blood pressure of 80 mmHg, the right ventricular pressure can be estimated by subtracting the calculated pressure difference between the ventricles from the systolic blood pressure (systolic arm blood pressure 80 mmHg – 64 mmHg = 16 mmHg (right ventricular pressure). In this patient, the right ventricular pressure and the pulmonary artery pressure would be normal.

15. **What does the echocardiographic term *shortening fraction* mean?**
Shortening fraction (SF) is a measure of the percentage of change in diameter of the left ventricle that occurs during the cardiac cycle. Preload, contractility, and afterload all influence shortening fraction.

16. **How is shortening fraction measured?**
Shortening fraction (SF) is measured using the following formula:

$$\% \text{ SF} = (\text{left ventricular [LV] diastolic diameter} - \text{LV systolic diameter/LV diastolic diameter}) \times 100$$

The normal range is 28–44%.

17. **How does ejection fraction differ from shortening fraction?**
The ejection fraction (EF) measures a change in volume as opposed to a change in diameter of the left ventricle during the cardiac cycle. The ejection fraction is obtained by measuring ventricular volumes on two orthogonal views. The formula is as follows:

$$\% \text{ EF} = (\text{LV diastolic volume} - \text{LV systolic volume/LV diastolic volume}) \times 100$$

The normal range is 64–83%.

18. **Assuming normal circulatory transition occurs, what changes can be expected with respect to the pulmonary artery pressure at 6 weeks of age?**
The principal circulatory change during the transitional circulation is an exponential decrement in pulmonary vascular resistance over the first 6–8 weeks of life.

19. **During postnatal life, as pulmonary vascular resistance falls, what changes can be expected in the magnitude of a left-to-right shunt?**
If there is a large VSD, the right ventricular and pulmonary artery pressures remain high; with a nonrestrictive VSD, right and left ventricular pressures are equal. The volume of the left-to-right shunt increases because there is an inverse relationship between the pulmonary blood flow (PBF) and the pulmonary vascular resistance.

PBF = Δ pressure across the pulmonary vascular bed/pulmonary vascular resistance

As pulmonary vascular resistance declines in the early postnatal period, left-to-right shunt increases.

Snider AR, Serwer GA, Ritter SB: Echocardiography in Pediatric Heart Disease, 2nd ed. St. Louis, Mosby, 1997.

INNOCENT MURMURS

20. **What are electrocardiography (ECG) and chest x-ray findings of all innocent murmurs?**
All innocent murmurs should have normal ECG results and normal cardiac silhouettes on chest x-ray.

21. **What are the common innocent murmurs heard in the newborn period?**
   - **Peripheral pulmonary artery stenosis:** This is a soft, grade 1–2/6 systolic ejection murmur, heard best at the left upper sternal border, with radiation to both axilla and the back.
   - **Transient systolic murmur of a closing PDA:** This is a 1–2/6 systolic ejection murmur, best heard at the left upper sternal border and also in the left infraclavicular area. This murmur usually disappears by day 2 of life in term infants.
   - **Transient systolic murmur of tricuspid regurgitation:** This clinical finding is heard as a 2/6 systolic murmur, which can mimic a VSD murmur and can be seen in neonates with fetal distress or neonatal asphyxia.

22. **What causes the murmur in an infant with peripheral pulmonary artery stenosis?**

Peripheral pulmonary artery stenosis is caused by flow acceleration at the acute angle of the bifurcation of the pulmonary artery into right and left branches. The angle becomes less acute with growth, and the murmur usually disappears by 2–4 months of age.

PHYSIOLOGY OF THE CYANOTIC NEONATE

23. **What is central cyanosis? What are some of the causes in the newborn?**

Central cyanosis occurs when deoxygenated blood (reduced hemoglobin) enters the systemic circulation. Inadequate alveolar ventilation (central nervous system depression, obstruction of the airway, ventilation/perfusion [V/Q] mismatch), intracardiac right-to-left shunt/cyanotic congenital heart disease, and pulmonary arteriovenous (AV) fistula are some causes of central cyanosis.

KEY POINTS: THE CYANOTIC NEONATE

1. The hyperoxia test does not rule out some common mixing congenital heart lesions.

2. Reversed differential cyanosis is seen when the postductal saturations are higher than the preductal saturations.

3. Reversed differential cyanosis can be seen in d-transposition of the great arteries with a coarctation of the aorta, d-transposition of the great arteries with interrupted aortic arch, and d-transposition of the great arteries with pulmonary hypertension.

24. **At what level of desaturation is cyanosis detectable at physical examination in most neonates?**

The perception of cyanosis occurs when there is 5 gm of reduced hemoglobin in the capillaries. In an infant with a normal hemoglobin level, perception of cyanosis typically occurs at an oxygen saturation of 70%. An experienced observer can sometimes detect cyanosis when the saturation falls to 80–85%.

25. **What is peripheral cyanosis?**

Peripheral cyanosis can occur in states of low cardiac output, even when the arterial saturation is normal. When the cardiac output is low, the arteriovenous difference widens, leading to an increased amount of reduced hemoglobin in the capillaries. Low-output cyanosis is commonly referred to as *acrocyanosis*. Polycythemia can also cause cyanosis because of the increased levels of reduced hemoglobin in the circulation.

26. **What is differential cyanosis (i.e., pink upper body and blue lower body), and what are the implications?**

Measuring oxygen saturation at both preductal and postductal sites is part of the initial evaluation in a patient with suspected heart disease. If the preductal oxygen saturation is higher than the postductal oxygen saturation, there is differential cyanosis. This sign occurs when the great arteries are normally related and deoxygenated blood from the pulmonary circulation enters the descending aorta through a PDA (right-to-left shunting). This pattern of cyanosis is seen with persistent pulmonary hypertension of the newborn and with left ventricular outflow obstruction (e.g., aortic arch hypoplasia, interrupted aortic arch, critical coarctation, and critical aortic stenosis).

27. **What is reversed differential cyanosis (i.e., blue upper body and pink lower body)?**
    Reversed differential cyanosis occurs when the postductal saturation is higher than the pre-
    ductal saturation. This occurs in children with transposition of the great arteries, when oxy-
    genated blood from the pulmonary circulation enters the descending aorta through a PDA.
    Reversed differential cyanosis can occur in the following conditions: d-transposition of the
    great arteries with coarctation of the aorta or interrupted aortic arch and d-transposition of
    the great arteries with pulmonary hypertension. In these situations, the descending aorta is
    filled with oxygenated blood from the pulmonary system because of right-to-left shunting
    through the ductus arteriosus.

28. **What are oxygen capacity and oxygen saturation?**
    Oxygen is transported in the blood primarily on hemoglobin. Oxygen capacity is the maxi-
    mum quantity of oxygen that can be bound to each gram of hemoglobin (Hgb) (i.e., 1.39 mL
    × Hgb level; each gram of Hgb combines maximally with 1.39 mL of oxygen). The number
    derived from this equation is the total oxygen-carrying capacity of hemoglobin in a particular
    patient. Oxygen saturation is the amount of oxygen bound to hemoglobin compared with the
    oxygen capacity. It is expressed as a percentage. Oxygen saturation tells how much oxygen
    is carried only if the amount of hemoglobin is known.

29. **What is the oxygen dissociation curve? What influences it?**
    The oxygen dissociation curve (Fig. 5-2) compares the relationship of oxygen saturation (%) to
    the partial pressure of oxygen, PO_2 (mmHg). Blood pH, temperature, PCO_2, 2, 3-diphosphoglyc-
    erate, and the type of hemoglobin influence the relationship between the oxygen saturation and
    the partial pressure of oxygen. Of note, fetal hemoglobin holds more oxygen for a given PO_2
    than adult hemoglobin.

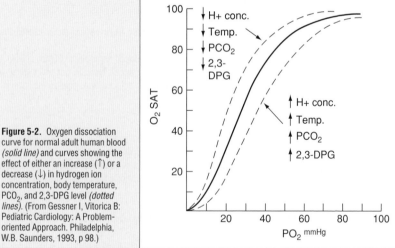

Figure 5-2. Oxygen dissociation curve for normal adult human blood *(solid line)* and curves showing the effect of either an increase (↑) or a decrease (↓) in hydrogen ion concentration, body temperature, PCO_2, and 2,3-DPG level *(dotted lines)*. (From Gessner I, Vitorica B: Pediatric Cardiology: A Problem-oriented Approach. Philadelphia, W.B. Saunders, 1993, p 98.)

30. **What is a hyperoxia test? How is it used in differentiating pulmonary and cardiac causes of cyanosis?**
    A hyperoxia test attempts to differentiate between pulmonary disease with V/Q
    mismatch and cyanotic congenital heart disease. Initially, one measures the oxygen

saturation on room air. If the oxygen saturation is low, the patient should be administered 100% FiO_2. A patient with pulmonary disease will show an increase in PO_2 (to a variable degree). In a patient with a fixed intracardiac mixing lesion, the PO_2 does not change significantly. A preductal and postductal arterial blood gas measurement should be obtained. A preductal arterial blood gas can be obtained from the right radial artery. A postductal arterial blood gas can be obtained either from an umbilical artery or from a lower extremity artery. In pulmonary disease, the preductal arterial PO_2 level in 100% FiO_2 usually exceeds 150 mmHg. If the ductus arteriosus is patent and a right-to-left ductal shunt occurs because of high pulmonary vascular resistance, the postductal PO_2 level will be lower than the preductal PO_2. In addition, the arterial PCO_2 will be elevated relative to the patient's respiratory effort.

In cyanotic congenital heart disease (CHD), the PO_2 in room air is <70 mmHg (usually <50 mmHg) and does not change significantly in 100% oxygen. Typically, the arterial PCO_2 level is normal or low. This is related to the hyperventilation that occurs as a response to the hypoxia. Acidosis is typically of a metabolic nature because of abnormal systemic perfusion, tissue hypoxia, or both.

In some cases, the hyperoxia test must be done with the administration of positive-pressure ventilation to expand atelectatic lung adequately to exchange gas.

31. **Which critical cyanotic lesions may not be excluded if the hyperoxia test yields a PO_2 of >150 torr after 10 minutes?**
Common mixing lesions may not be excluded. Examples are total anomalous pulmonary venous return, tetralogy of Fallot with a predominant left-to-right shunt, and hypoplastic left heart syndrome.

Gessner IH, Victorica BE: Pediatric Cardiology: A Problem-Oriented Approach. Philadelphia, W.B. Saunders, 1993.

CONGESTIVE HEART FAILURE

32. **What are the major causes of heart failure in a fetus?**
Severe anemia, arrhythmia, infection, large systemic AV fistula (e.g., vein of Galen AV malformation), and severe atrioventricular valve insufficiency.

33. **What are signs and symptoms of heart failure in a newborn infant?**
Common signs and symptoms of heart failure in a neonate are tachypnea, tachycardia, cardiomegaly, pulmonary rales, hepatomegaly, weak peripheral pulses, and failure to thrive. Cyanosis may also occur in later stages of congestive heart failure, making diagnosis more difficult.

34. **What are some heart lesions that can present with heart failure in the first week of life?**
Ductal-dependent abnormalities
- Hypoplastic left heart syndrome with a large PDA
- Truncus arteriosus
- Interrupted aortic arch type B (i.e., interruption of the aorta between the left common carotid artery and the left subclavian artery)
- Coarctation of the aorta with a VSD
- Critical aortic stenosis
Non–ductal-dependent abnormalities
- Total anomalous pulmonary venous return
- Endocardial cushion defect

- Myocardial dysfunction (cardiomyopathy)
- Supraventricular tachycardia/arrhythmia
- Single ventricle complex
- Sepsis

35. **What are some heart lesions that can cause heart failure in an infant beyond the newborn period?**
Obstruction to systemic blood flow
  - Coarctation of the aorta
  - Severe aortic stenosis
  Left-to-right shunt
  - VSD
  - Endocardial cushion defect
  - PDA
  Mixing lesions
  - Total anomalous pulmonary venous return, without obstruction
  - Single ventricle, without pulmonic stenosis
  - D-transposition of the great arteries
  - Large VSD
  - Truncus arteriosus
  Myocardial dysfunction/pericardial disease
  - Anomalous left coronary artery
  - Myocarditis
  - Arrhythmia (supraventricular tachyarrhythmia [SVT])
  - Endocarditis/pericarditis

36. **Why does the newborn heart have a reduced ability to adapt to stress?**
The newborn heart has fewer myofilaments with which to generate the force of contraction. The newborn ventricle has decreased compliance compared with the older adult ventricle. Therefore, the newborn heart generates less augmentation in stroke volume for a given increase in diastolic volume. The oxygen consumption and cardiac output per meters squared are much higher in newborns, and there is very little systolic reserve. Tachycardia is therefore the usual neonatal response to stress, since increase in stroke volume is so limited.

37. **What three classes of medications are used for the treatment of congestive heart failure in the neonate?**
  - Inotropic agents
  - Diuretics
  - Afterload reduction agents

38. **What are compensatory mechanisms during heart failure?**
Increased heart rate, enhanced stroke volume (Frank-Starling mechanism), sympathetic nerve activation (increased sympathetic tone, renin-angiotensin system activation), increased 2,3-diphosphoglycerate, increased atrial natriuretic peptides, and myocardial hypertrophy.

Park MK: Pediatric Cardiology for the Practitioners, 3rd ed. St. Louis, Mosby, 1996.

TREATMENT OF HYPOTENSION ON THE NEONATE

39. **What is the most frequent primary cause of hypotension in the preterm neonate in the immediate postnatal period?**

Disturbance of peripheral vasomotor regulation is the most frequent primary cause of hypotension in preterm neonates. In cases of sepsis, the decrease in the peripheral vascular resistance is caused by the release of inflammatory mediators induced by infectious agents and/or endotoxins. However, in most cases of hypotension in a preterm neonate, there is no evidence of infection. In these patients, oxidant stress and other noninfectious stimuli initiate a nonspecific systemic inflammatory response resulting in a decrease in peripheral vascular resistance and systemic blood pressure. In addition, in over one third of hypotensive preterm neonates, impaired myocardial function may contribute to the cardiovascular compromise. Finally, unlike the hypovolemia observed in the pediatric patient population, absolute hypovolemia in a sick preterm neonate is infrequently the primary cause of hypotension during the immediate postnatal period.

40. **What are the mechanisms of action of the cardiovascular effects of dopamine in a preterm neonate?**

In a preterm neonate, dopamine increases systemic blood pressure by increasing total peripheral vascular resistance (i.e., afterload) and myocardial contractility. Dopamine increases the

---

KEY POINTS: TREATMENT OF HYPERTENSION IN NEONATES

1. Dopamine and dobutamine have different physiologic effects in a newborn.

2. Dopamine is a good inotrope to use (depending on the dose) if there is a risk of renal ischemia, low cardiac output, and/or hypotension with decreased systemic vascular resistance.

3. Dobutamine is a good inotrope to use for low cardiac output in patients at risk for myocardial ischemia, pulmonary hypertension, and left ventricular diastolic dysfunction.

---

effective circulating blood volume (i.e., preload) by decreasing venous capacitance, which may also contribute to the beneficial cardiovascular effects of the drug. Dopamine selectively increases total renal blood flow by inducing selective vasodilatation of the renal artery in the preterm neonate. Finally, dopamine has no direct effect on the cerebral and mesenteric circulation in this population.

41. **Why is dopamine superior to dobutamine in the treatment of hypotension in a preterm neonate?**

Dopamine is more effective than dobutamine in the treatment of systemic hypotension in a preterm neonate because the most frequent cause of hypotension in this patient population is abnormal regulation of the peripheral vascular tone with or without associated myocardial dysfunction. Because dopamine increases both total peripheral vascular resistance and myocardial contractility, it corrects the major underlying pathophysiologic abnormalities causing systemic hypotension in preterm neonates. Dobutamine effectively increases myocardial contractility. It can, however, cause peripheral vasodilatation. Thus, although the cardiac output is increased significantly with dobutamine, the blood pressure may not increase at all because of the dobutamine-induced decrease in the afterload. Furthermore, since cerebral blood flow in the neonatal period is determined primarily by the systemic blood pressure (and not the cardiac output), dobutamine administration alone may not result in an improvement of cerebral perfusion in a hypotensive preterm neonate unless blood pressure is normalized. Lastly, dobutamine lacks the beneficial renal vascular and tubular actions of dopamine, which may contribute to the recovery of the abnormal cardiovascular status and fluid homeostasis in a hypotensive preterm neonate.

Nichols DG, Cameron DE, Greeley WJ, et al: Critical Heart Disease in Infants and Children. St. Louis, Mosby, 1995.

CYANOTIC CONGENITAL HEART DISEASE

42. **What is the most common cyanotic lesion presenting in the newborn period?**
D-transposition of the great arteries is the most common form of cyanotic congenital heart disease in neonates and accounts for 6–10% of infants with congenital heart disease. In children "outside" the newborn period, tetralogy of Fallot is the most common, representing 7–9% of cardiac cases of cyanosis.

KEY POINTS: CYANOTIC CONGENITAL HEART DISEASE

1. An unrestrictive atrial communication is crucial in certain cyanotic congenital heart lesions to provide mixing and/or cardiac output.

2. The most common cyanotic lesion presenting in the newborn period is d-transposition of the great arteries.

3. A left axis in a cyanotic newborn baby is usually tricuspid atresia.

43. **What are the "five Ts" of cyanotic congenital heart disease?**
    - Transposition of the great arteries
    - Tetralogy of Fallot
    - Truncus arteriosus
    - Total anomalous pulmonary venous return
    - Tricuspid atresia

44. **What are other principal cyanotic heart lesions that do not begin with a *t*?**
    - Ebstein's anomaly of the tricuspid valve
    - Hypoplastic left heart syndrome
    - Pulmonary atresia

45. **How do infants with d-transposition of the great arteries present in the newborn period?**
In d-transposition of the great arteries, the aorta arises from the right ventricle, and the pulmonary artery arises from the left ventricle. Unless there is adequate mixing of the pulmonary and systemic circulation, the infant will become hypoxic and acidotic and will die in the first few days of life.

46. **How can other cardiac defects such as a VSD or a large atrial septal defect alter the clinical presentation of infants with d-transposition of the great vessels?**
The more mixing that occurs between the chambers of the heart, the later the clinical presentation of the infant. The majority of infants with d-transposition of the great arteries and an

intact ventricular septum have a patent foramen ovale. They commonly present in the first 6–24 hours of life with profound cyanosis, and depending on the size of the foramen ovale, they may require intervention (i.e., balloon atrial septostomy) before the surgical correction. Infants with a large atrial septal defect can present at 24–48 hours of life with moderate cyanosis and usually do not develop acidosis. Infants with d-transposition of the great arteries and a large VSD may present even later (2–6 weeks of life) and can demonstrate signs of congestive heart failure.

47. **How do prostaglandins work in d-transposition of the great arteries?**
Prostaglandins keep the ductus arteriosus patent and help assist with the mixing of the circulations.

48. **In infants with d-transposition of the great arteries, how does a balloon atrial septostomy improve systemic oxygen saturation?**
The balloon atrial septostomy permits unrestricted bidirectional mixing of fully saturated blood in the left atrium with desaturated blood in the right atrium to achieve a higher net saturation of blood in the systemic circulation. After this procedure, patency of the ductus is no longer essential. Variations in oxygen saturation can be expected, although mixing is excellent.

49. **What are the clinical manifestations of tetralogy of Fallot at birth?**
The most common clinical manifestation is a murmur secondary to obstruction across the right ventricular outflow tract. The murmur is not due to the VSD (large defect, equal pressures in both ventricles). Cyanosis depends on the severity of the right ventricular outflow tract obstruction along with the presence or absence of a PDA.

50. **What is total anomalous pulmonary venous return?**
In total anomalous pulmonary venous return, there is no direct communication between the pulmonary veins and the left atrium. The different types of total anomalous pulmonary venous return depend on their drainage sites. Total anomalous pulmonary venous return accounts for 1% of all congenital heart disease. There is a marked predominance of males for the infracardiac type.

51. **What are the different types of total anomalous pulmonary venous return?**
   - **Supracardiac:** Represents 50% of all total anomalous pulmonary venous return. The pulmonary veins usually drain into the right superior vena cava via a left vertical vein. They can be obstructed (the vertical vein is "pinched" between the left pulmonary artery and the left bronchus or at superior vena cava insertion) or unobstructed.
   - **Cardiac:** Represents 20% of all total anomalous pulmonary venous return. The pulmonary veins drain into the coronary sinus or directly into the right atrium. They can be obstructed (obstruction can occur at the site of the obligate right-to-left atrial shunt) or unobstructed.
   - **Infracardiac:** Represents 20% of all total anomalous pulmonary venous return. The common pulmonary vein drains below the diaphragm into the portal venous system, ductus venosus, inferior vena cava, or hepatic veins. These veins are usually obstructed.
   - **Mixed:** Represents 10% of all total anomalous pulmonary venous return. It is a combination of the other types.

52. **What accounts for the varying clinical manifestations of anomalous pulmonary venous return in a neonate?**
The different presentations of total anomalous pulmonary venous return depend on whether the pulmonary veins are obstructed.
   - With obstructed veins, infants present with cyanosis and respiratory distress.
   - With unobstructed veins, tachypnea develops gradually.

53. **Why is an atrial communication important in total anomalous pulmonary venous return?**
Without an atrial communication, there is no way that blood can get to the left atrium/left ventricle and out the aorta to provide any cardiac output. An atrial septal defect is necessary for survival with this lesion.

54. **What is scimitar syndrome?**
Scimitar syndrome has the following components: right lung hypoplasia, anomalous connection of the right pulmonary veins to the inferior vena cava, right pulmonary artery hypoplasia, anomalous systemic arterial supply to the right lung, bronchial anomalies, and dextroposition of the heart reflecting the hypoplastic right lung. The term *scimitar syndrome* derives from a feature on the chest x-ray: the right pulmonary veins cast a shadow like the handle of a scimitar in the right lower zone as they drain anomalously into the inferior vena cava.

55. **What are clinical manifestations of truncus arteriosus in a neonate?**
Cyanosis may or may not be seen immediately after birth. Signs of congestive heart failure develop days to several weeks after birth. Tachypnea or difficulty feeding can be a sign of congestive heart failure. With truncal stenosis there can be a systolic ejection murmur. There is a single second heart sound. The pulses are bounding, and the pulse pressure is wide.

56. **What syndrome can be associated with truncus arteriosus?**
DiGeorge syndrome with hypocalcemia is present in approximately one third of cases with truncus arteriosus.

57. **What are the clinical manifestations of a neonate with hypoplastic left heart syndrome?**
Infants with hypoplastic left heart syndrome can present within the first few hours to days of life. The more common clinical signs are tachypnea, hepatomegaly, pulmonary rales, weak peripheral pulses, vasoconstricted extremities, and a single second heart sound (S2). The patient may not appear cyanotic.

58. **Under what circumstances can information from an ECG in a cyanotic neonate rapidly indicate the presence of congenital heart disease?**
The key is an abnormal frontal plane axis:
   - A **leftward** axis for a newborn (i.e., left superior axis: –90 to 0 degrees or between 0 and 60 degrees) strongly implies a structural anomaly of the heart. Dominant left ventricular forces often accompany this anomaly. The differential diagnosis includes tricuspid atresia, pulmonary valve atresia with intact ventricular septum, critical pulmonary stenosis, or complex single left ventricle.
   - A **rightward** superior/northwest axis (i.e., –90 to –180 degrees) suggests an endocardial cushion defect.

59. **What are some common chest x-ray findings in infants with cyanotic congenital heart lesions?**
   - **D-transposition of the great arteries with an intact ventricular septum:** Cardiomegaly with increased pulmonary vascular markings. Egg-shaped cardiac silhouette, with a narrow, superior mediastinum.
   - **Tetralogy of Fallot:** Heart size normal or smaller than normal. Decreased pulmonary vascular markings, concave main pulmonary artery segment with an upturned apex (boot-shaped heart). May have a right aortic arch.
   - **Total anomalous pulmonary venous return:** Cardiomegaly with right atrial and ventricular enlargement and increased pulmonary vascular markings. "Snowman" heart can be seen with

supracardiac, unobstructed veins. Usually seen after several months. With pulmonary venous obstruction, there is radiographic evidence of pulmonary edema (diffuse reticular pattern).

- **Tricuspid atresia:** Normal size or mild cardiomegaly with straight right heart border and decreased pulmonary vascular markings.
- **Pulmonary atresia:** Normal size or mild cardiomegaly with right atrial enlargement and decreased pulmonary vascular markings.
- **Ebstein's anomaly of the tricuspid valve:** In severe cases, the heart is enormous, balloon-shaped, and occupies almost the entire cardiothoracic area.
- **Truncus arteriosus:** Cardiomegaly with increased pulmonary vascular markings. Right aortic arch may be seen.
- **Single ventricle:** Depends on the presence or absence of pulmonary stenosis. May have cardiomegaly with increased pulmonary vascular markings or a relatively normal-sized heart with decreased pulmonary vascular markings.

60. **What cardiac lesions should one consider when the radiologist says an infant has a right aortic arch?**
   - **Truncus arteriosus:** 36%
   - **Tetralogy of Fallot:** 13–34%
   - **Double-outlet right ventricle:** 20%
   - **Tricuspid atresia:** 5–8%
   - **Transposition of the great vessels:** 3%
   - **VSD:** 2–6%

   Emmanoulides GC, Allen HD, Riemenschneider TA, Gutgesell HP (eds): Moss and Adams' Heart Disease in Infants, Children and Adolescents Including the Fetus and Young Adult, 5th ed. Baltimore, Williams & Wilkins, 1994.

ACYANOTIC AND OBSTRUCTIVE CONGENITAL HEART LESIONS

61. **What are the common causes of left-to-right shunts in a newborn infant?**
   - VSD
   - PDA
   - Atrial septal defect
   - Endocardial cushion defect (AV canal)

KEY POINTS: ACYANOTIC AND OBSTRUCTIVE CONGENITAL HEART LESIONS

1. A PDA is needed in both severe right and left heart obstructive lesions.

2. Neonates with a large left-to-right shunt usually do not go into congestive heart failure until 3–6 weeks of age, when the pulmonary vascular resistance drops, and the left-to-right shunting increases with increased flow into the pulmonary arteries.

62. **What acyanotic heart defect is typically seen in children with Down syndrome?**
   Endocardial cushion defect (can be complete with ventricular and atrial components or incomplete with just a defect in the septum primum and VSD).

63. **Why do infants with large VSDs escape detection in the newborn period?**
   Infants with a VSD are usually identified after they leave the hospital because both the heart murmur of a VSD and the symptoms of heart failure do not appear during the first few days of

life. In the immediate postnatal period the pulmonary vascular resistance is still elevated, thereby limiting the shunting of blood from the left ventricle into the right ventricle and into the lungs. As the pulmonary vascular resistance falls, an increased volume flows through the defect, which increases the intensity of the murmur and the amount of pulmonary blood flow.

64. **Name three conditions associated with persistent patency of the ductus arteriosus.**
    - Prematurity
    - Hypoxia (pulmonary disease/high altitude)
    - Congenital rubella syndrome

65. **What are three common obstructive heart lesions that can present in the newborn period?**
    - Severe/critical pulmonary stenosis
    - Severe/critical aortic stenosis
    - Coarctation of the aorta

66. **What is critical pulmonary stenosis?**
    Pulmonary stenosis in a neonate severe enough to cause cyanosis and acidosis (rare) with signs of right heart failure (rare) is defined as *critical pulmonary stenosis*. Ductal patency is *essential* for maintaining pulmonary blood flow. Essential diagnostic features are limited or there is no forward flow through the stenotic pulmonary valve, absence of pulmonary atresia, and a right-to-left shunt across the foramen ovale. Pulmonary balloon valvuloplasty is undertaken to relieve the stenosis after stabilization of the infant.

67. **What is critical aortic stenosis?**
    Aortic stenosis in a neonate that results in congestive heart failure with circulatory shock is termed *critical aortic stenosis*. In affected infants, the systemic circulation is dependent on the patency of the ductus arteriosus with flow from the pulmonary artery into the descending aorta. *These infants are ductal dependent to provide cardiac output.* In some infants, inotropic support, ventilation, and correction of acidosis may be required. Most infants are palliated by an aortic balloon valvuloplasty. The aortic valve can be tricuspid, bicuspid, or unicuspid.

68. **What is a neonatal coarctation? How does it present?**
    Neonatal coarctation of the aorta is obstruction in the thoracic aorta or the transverse aortic arch and requires *patency of the ductus arteriosus* to maintain cardiac output. Typically, these infants become symptomatic when the ductus arteriosus closes. They have signs and symptoms of acute circulatory shock, with decreased or no pulses in the lower extremities, tachypnea, and acidosis, and they may or may not have a murmur. There is an obligate right-to-left ductal shunt, similar to that in critical aortic stenosis. After stabilization, all of these infants require surgery.

69. **If the apex of the heart is on the opposite side of the patient from the stomach, what is the likelihood that the patient has congenital heart disease?**
    The likelihood of congenital heart disease is between 90–95%. This condition is referred to as *dextrocardia*.

70. **What are the different types of interrupted aortic arch?**
    - **Type A:** Interruption is distal to the left subclavian artery.
    - **Type B:** Interruption is between the left carotid artery and the left subclavian artery. An aberrant right subclavian artery can also be seen in this condition (most common, occurring in approximately 40% of all cases).
    - **Type C:** Interruption is between the innominate artery and the left carotid artery.

71. **What other lesions are commonly seen with interrupted aortic arch?**
VSD and PDA.

72. **What genetic abnormality is associated with interrupted aortic arch?**
DiGeorge syndrome.

Freedom RM, Yoo SJ, Mikailian H, Williams W: The Natural and Modified History of Congenital Heart Disease. Elmsford, NY, Blackwell Publishing, 2004.

VASCULAR RINGS

73. **What is the difference between a complete and an incomplete vascular ring?**
A complete vascular ring is present when abnormal vascular structures form a ring around the trachea and the esophagus (e.g., double aortic arch or right aortic arch with a left ligamentum arteriosum). An incomplete vascular ring occurs when abnormal vascular structures surround but do not form a complete circle around the trachea and the esophagus.

KEY POINTS: VASCULAR RINGS

1. Vascular rings are suspected based on clinical symptoms.

2. Echocardiograms may not be the *best* imaging modality.

74. **What is the most common vascular ring?**
A double aortic arch is the most common type of vascular ring (40%).

75. **What are the different types of vascular rings? What are their radiographic findings, their symptoms, and treatment?**
See Fig. 5-3.

76. **What are the indications for surgical intervention?**
Respiratory distress, history of recurrent pulmonary infections, difficulty swallowing, and apneic spells are indications for surgical intervention.

77. **What imaging modalities are used for assessing vascular rings?**
Echocardiography can be used, but it does not always define the exact anatomy. Barium swallow and angiography can also be used; however, MRI has become the leading noninvasive imaging modality and is best in defining the anatomy.

78. **How does a surgeon repair some of the more common forms of vascular rings?**
- **Double aortic arch:** The smaller of the two arches is divided (usually the left) via a left thoracotomy.
- **Right aortic arch and left ligamentum arteriosum:** The ligamentum is divided via a left thoracotomy.
- **Anomalous left pulmonary artery:** The left pulmonary artery is divided and reimplanted.

Moes CAF, Freedom RM: Rings, slings and other things: Vascular structures contributing to a neonatal noose. In Freedom RM, Benson LN, Smallhorn JF (eds): Neonatal Heart Disease. New York, Springer-Verlag, 1992, pp 731–749.
Woods RK, Sharp RJ, Holcomb GW III, et al: Vascular anomalies and tracheoesophageal compression: A single institution's 25 year experience. Ann Thorac Surg 72:434–438; discussion, 438–439, 2001.

	Anatomy	Esophagogram	Other Radiographic Findings	Symptoms	Treatment
Double aortic arch	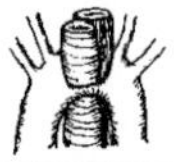	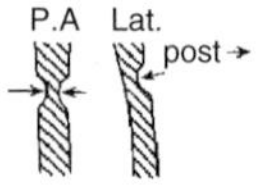 P.A Lat. post →	Anterior compression of trachea	Respiratory difficulty (onset <3 mos.) Swallowing dysfunction	Surgical division of a smaller arch
Right aortic arch with left ligamentum arteriosum	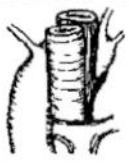	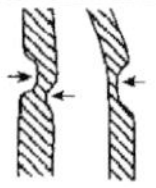		Mild respiratory difficulty (onset >1 year) Swallowing dysfunction	Surgical division of the ligamentum arteriosum
Anomalous innominate artery	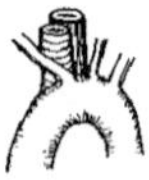	Normal	Anterior compression of trachea	Stridor and/or cough in infancy	Conservative management, or surgical suturing of the artery to the sternum
Aberrant right subclavian artery	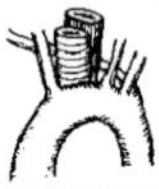	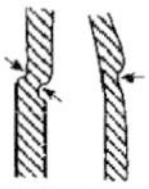		Occasional swallowing dysfunction	Usually no treatment is necessary
"Vascular sling"	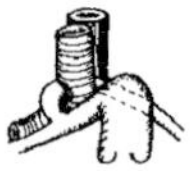	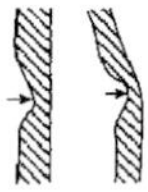	Right-sided emphysema or atelectasis. Posterior compression of trachea or right main stem bronchus	Wheezing and cyanotic episodes since birth	Surgical division of the anomalous LPA (from the RPA) and anastomosis to the MPA

Figure 5-3. Different types of vascular rings. LPA = left pulmonary artery, RPA = right pulmonary artery, MPA = main pulmonary artery. (From Park M: Pediatric Cardiology for Practitioners, 3rd ed. St. Louis, Mosby, 1996, p 246.)

SEGMENTAL CARDIAC AND CARDIAC MALPOSITION ANALYSIS

79. **How are segmental relationships expressed in congenital heart disease?**
    - **Visceroatrial relationship:** S (solitus), I (inversus), and A (ambiguous)
    - **Ventricular loop:** D loop, L loop, and X (uncertain or indeterminate loop)
    - **Great arteries:** S (solitus), I (inversus, or mirror image of normal), D (d-transposition), and L (l-transposition)

80. **How can an ECG localize where the anatomic right and left ventricles are located?**
    Because depolarization occurs in the left ventricle before the right ventricle, the presence/location of the Q waves over the precordium can assist in the anatomic location of the left ventricle and right ventricle. If Q waves are seen in V5, V6, and lead 1, the left ventricle is D-looped and on the left side. If Q waves are seen in V4R, V1, and V2, but not V5 and V6, it is likely that the ventricles are L-looped (Fig. 5-4).

81. **What are three noninvasive modalities used to assess atrial location?**
    The chest x-ray, the ECG, and the echocardiogram are three modalities that can help locate the position of the atria.

82. **How does the abdominal x-ray help to determine right atrial position?**
    - If the abdominal situs is solitus (liver on right and stomach on left), the right atrium is on the right side.

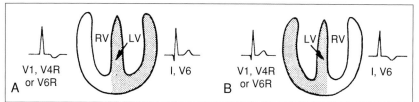

Figure 5-4. Locating the ventricles from the ECG. The left ventricle (LV) is usually located on the same side as the precordial leads that show Q waves. If V6 shows a Q wave, the LV is on the left side. If V4R and V1 show a Q wave, the LV is to the right of the anatomic right ventricle (RV). Note that SQ waves are also present in V1 in severe right ventricular hypertrophy (RVH). (From Park MK, Guntheroth WG: How to Read: Pediatric ECGs, 3rd ed. St. Louis, Mosby, 1992, p 253.)

- If the abdominal situs is inversus (liver on the left and stomach on the right), the right atrium is on the left side.
- If the liver is midline (situs ambiguous), there are either two right atria or two left atria. In this case, there are usually abnormalities of the spleen as well (e.g., polysplenia/asplenia).

83. **How does the ECG help determine atrial position?**
The sinoatrial node is located in the right atrium. The P wave axis, seen on the ECG, can determine where the sinoatrial node is originating from, and hence the locations of the right atrium (Fig. 5-5).

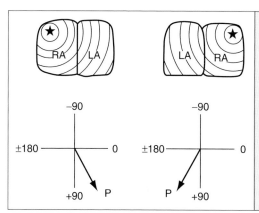

Figure 5-5. Locating the atria by the use of the P axis. When the right atrium (RA) is on the right side, the P axis is in the left lower quadrant (0 to +90 degrees). When the RA is on the left side, the P axis is in the right lower quadrant (+90 to −180 degrees). LA = left atrium. (From Park MK, Guntheroth WG: How to Read: Pediatric ECGs, 3rd ed. St. Louis, Mosby, 1992, p 252.)

84. **What determines the "right atrium" on echocardiogram?**
The drainage of the coronary sinus. The coronary sinus (there is almost always a coronary sinus) drains into the right atrium. In situs solitus with normal systemic and pulmonary venous connections, the pulmonary veins always drain into the left atrium, and the systemic veins (superior and inferior vena cava) drain into the right atrium. The coronary sinus, however, is the most reliable echocardiographic marker of the right atrium.

85. **What is dextrocardia?**
Dextrocardia is a condition in which the heart is located on the right side of the chest. Although it defines where the heart is located, it does not define segmental atrioventricular and ventricular-arterial relationships.

KEY POINTS: CARDIAC MALPOSITION

1. When evaluating a chest radiograph of a patient with suspected congenital heart disease, always locate the liver shadow and stomach bubble to help assess abdominal situs.

2. Dextrocardia is a condition in which the heart is located on the right side of the chest.

3. Mesocardia is designated when the heart is located in the midline of the thorax.

86. **What is mesocardia?**
Mesocardia is designated when the heart is located in the midline of the thorax.

> Park M: Pediatric Cardiology for Practitioners, 3rd ed. St. Louis, Mosby, 1996.
> Van Praagh R, Weinberg PM, Foran RB, et al: Malposition of the heart. In Adams FH, Emmanoulides GC, Reimenschneider TH (eds): Moss' Heart Disease in Infants, Children and Adolescents, 5th ed. Baltimore, Williams & Wilkins, 1994.

PREOPERATIVE STABILIZATION

87. **What are the principles of preoperative management in the neonate with critical congenital heart disease?**
In critical congenital heart lesions, the ultimate outcome depends on timely and accurate assessment of the structural anomaly and on evaluation and resuscitation of secondary organ damage. The principles of preoperative management are:
1. Initial stabilization airway management, vascular access, maintaining patency of a ductus arteriosus with prostaglandin E_1 (PGE_1) delineation of the anatomic defect by echocardiography
2. Evaluation and treatment of additional organ system dysfunction, particularly of the pulmonary, renal, hepatic, and central nervous system
3. Evaluation of other congenital heart defects
4. Genetic evaluation
5. Cardiac catheterization, if indicated
6. Surgical management, if indicated, when all other systems are optimized

88. **When does a neonate with critical congenital heart disease typically present, and what are the common presentations?**
The timing of the presentation with the accompanying symptoms depends on the nature and severity of the anatomic defect, in utero effects (if any), alterations in the systemic and pulmonary vascular resistance after birth, and timing of closure of the foramen ovale and the ductus arteriosus. Signs and symptoms may include cyanosis, congestive heart failure, shock, asymptomatic heart murmur, and arrhythmia.

89. **How should PGE_1 be administered?**
The starting dose of prostaglandin is 0.05–0.1 μg/kg/min. This should be administered using a continuous intravenous drip, preferentially through an umbilical venous line, or a well function-ing intravenous line. Once the effects of PGE_1 (e.g., improved oxygen saturations, decreased acidemia) are seen, the dose can be slowly reduced to 0.01 μg/kg/min.

90. **In which patients should PGE_1 be used?**
   - Neonates who fail a hyperoxia test; this procedure indicates an infant who is highly likely to have congenital heart disease that is ductal dependent

- Neonates with a confirmed congenital heart defect (by echocardiography) that is ductal dependent for pulmonary or systemic blood flow, or a lesion that requires a PDA for intercirculatory mixing
- Neonates who present with circulatory shock in the first or second week of life

KEY POINTS: PREOPERATIVE STABILIZATION

1. There are a variety of presentations in an infant with congenital heart disease.

2. The starting dose of PGE_1 is 0.05–0.10 µg/kg/min.

3. To maintain patency of the ductus arteriosus, PGE_1 is used in both right and left heart obstructive lesions.

91. **What are some of the side effects of PGE_1?**
    - **Cardiovascular:** Hypotension, peripheral vasodilatation; 16%
    - **Central nervous system:** Temperature elevation, seizure; 16%
    - **Respiratory:** Apnea, hypoventilation; 10%
    - **Metabolic:** Hypoglycemia, hypocalcemia; 3%
    - **Infectious:** Sepsis, wound infection; 3%
    - **Gastrointestinal:** Diarrhea, necrotizing enterocolitis; 4%
    - **Hematologic:** Disseminated intravascular coagulation, hemorrhage, thrombocytopenia; 3%
    - **Renal:** Renal failure and renal insufficiency; 1%
       These numbers reflect side effects for neonates weighing >2 kg. Side effects are increased in infants weighing <2 kg.

92. **In what lesions does keeping the ductus open help improve pulmonary blood flow? In what lesions does keeping the ductus open help improve cardiac output?**
    In lesions with right ventricular outflow obstruction, the ductus arteriosus helps to improve pulmonary blood flow by shunting blood into the pulmonary arteries (e.g., tetralogy of Fallot, tricuspid atresia, pulmonary atresia). In lesions with left ventricular outflow obstruction (e.g., hypoplastic left heart syndrome, critical aortic stenosis, neonatal coarctation of the aorta), the ductus arteriosus improves cardiac output by bypassing the obstruction.

93. **How is the hypoxemia resulting from d-transposition of the great arteries managed?**
    In a severely hypoxemic infant with transposition of the heart vessels, it is important to ensure adequate mixing between the two parallel circuits and maximize the mixed venous oxygen saturation. This is accomplished by:
    - Maintaining patency of the ductus arteriosus with PGE_1.
    - Providing mild hyperventilation and increased inspired oxygen to decrease pulmonary vascular resistance and increase pulmonary blood flow.
    - When these treatments do not work, an emergent balloon atrial septostomy is performed to enlarge the foramen ovale.

94. **What is a tet spell? How is it managed?**
    The classic tetralogy of Fallot spell includes the following symptoms: agitation/irritability, hyperpnea, profound cyanosis, and syncope. Auscultation during the spell frequently reveals an absent murmur due to minimal flow across the right ventricular outflow tract. If frequent or

inadequately managed, these spells can (in rare cases) result in death. Initial treatment typically consists of supplemental oxygen, sedation (subcutaneous morphine 0.1 mg/kg), and/or volume expansion. The knee/chest position for children can also be performed, which increases the systemic venous return and the systemic vascular resistance.

Lewis AB, Freed MD, Heyman MA, et al: Side effects of therapy with prostaglandin E1 in infants with critical congenital heart disease. Circulation 64:893–898, 1981.

POSTOPERATIVE MANAGEMENT

95. **What information is needed to care for a neonate with congenital heart disease after cardiothoracic surgery?**
    - The underlying anatomic defect
    - The clinical/physiologic status of the infant in the preoperative period
    - The anesthetic regimen used during surgery
    - The duration of the cardiopulmonary bypass, aortic cross clamp time, and circulatory arrest time
    - The details of the operative procedure and any concerns of the surgeon regarding the potential for residual defects
    - The data available from monitoring catheters, physical examination, radiographs, echocardiography, and ECG

96. **What are the most common noncardiac causes of respiratory compromise after cardiothoracic surgery?**
    See Table 5-3.

97. **What cardiac surgical procedures are associated with phrenic nerve palsy?**
    - **Arch reconstruction**
    - **Interrupted aortic arch repair or coarctation repair**
    - **Arterial switch operation**
    - **Tetralogy of Fallot/absent pulmonary valve repair:** Pulmonary artery placation
    - **Tetralogy of Fallot/pulmonary atresia: unifocalization**
    - **Truncus arteriosus repair**
    - **PDA ligation**
    - **Systemic-to-pulmonary shunt**

    Marino BS, Wernovsky G: Preoperative and postoperative care of the infant with critical congenital heart disease. In Avery GB, Fletcher MA, MacDonald MG (eds): Neonatology: Pathophysiology and Management of the Newborn. Philadelphia, Lippincott Williams & Wilkins, 1999.

    Newth CJL, Hammer J: Pulmonary issues. In Chang AC, Hanley FL, Wernovsky G, Wessel DL (eds): Pediatric Cardiac Intensive Care. Baltimore, Williams & Wilkins, 1998, p 352.

KEY POINTS: ASSESSMENTS AFTER CARDIAC CATHETERIZATION IN NEONATES

1. Vital signs

2. Femoral pulse

3. Dorsalis pedis pulse

4. Hematocrit

TABLE 5-3.   NONCARDIAC CAUSES OF RESPIRATORY COMPROMISE AFTER CARDIOTHORACIC SURGERY

Central Nervous System
1. General anesthesia
2. Administration of analgesics or sedative/hypnotics
3. Hypoxic-ischemic encephalopathy
4. Apnea of prematurity

Isolated Neuropathies
1. Hemidiaphragmatic paresis or paralysis—phrenic nerve injury
2. Vocal cord paralysis—recurrent laryngeal nerve injury

Airway Abnormalities Proximal to Alveoli
1. Tracheostomy or endotracheal tube obstruction
2. Postextubation subglottic edema
3. Laryngotracheomalacia
4. Left mainstem bronchomalacia from long-standing left atrial or left pulmonary artery enlargement

Neuromuscular Disorders
1. Residual neuromuscular blockade
2. Respiratory muscle weakness from disuse and/or malnutrition

Alveolar Disease
1. Acute lung injury from cardiopulmonary bypass
2. Increased lung fluid from left-to-right shunt lesions
3. Atelectasis
4. Pneumonia
5. Pulmonary hemorrhage
6. Pulmonary hypoplasia

Extrinsic Lung Compression
1. Pleural effusion (transudate versus exudate)
2. Pneumothorax, hemothorax, chylothorax

Chest Wall
1. Midsternal incisions
2. Thoracotomy incisions
3. "Clam shell" chest incisions

Adapted from Newth CJL, Hammer J: Pulmonary issues. In Chang AC, Hanley FL, Wernovsky G, Wessel DL (eds): Pediatric Cardiac Intensive Care. Baltimore, Williams & Wilkins, 1998, p 352.

INTERVENTIONAL CARDIOLOGY

98. **Which kinds of congenital heart disease may benefit from a cardiac catheterization interventional procedure?**
See Table 5-4.

99. **Which anomaly of the systemic veins prevents access to the right heart from the femoral veins?**
An interrupted inferior vena cava prevents access to the right heart from the femoral veins. This interruption, however, is usually below the level of the hepatic veins. Therefore, the umbilical vein remains an alternate way to access the right heart.

Freedom RM, Mawson JB, Yoo SJ, Benson LN: Congenital Heart Disease: Textbook of Angiography. Armonk, NY, Futura, 1997.

Lock JE, Keane JF, Fellows KE: Diagnostic and Interventional Catheterization in Congenital Heart Disease, 3rd ed. Boston, Martinus Nijhoff, 1987.

TABLE 5-4. CONGENITAL HEART DISEASES THAT MAY BENEFIT FROM CARDIAC CATHETERIZATION INTERVENTIONAL PROCEDURES

Congenital Heart Disease	Cardiac Interventional Procedure
Transposition of the great arteries/intact ventricular septum	Rashkind balloon atrial septostomy
Critical aortic stenosis	Aortic balloon valvuloplasty
Critical pulmonic stenosis	Pulmonary balloon valvuloplasty
Restrictive atrial septum (right heart lesions)	Balloon or blade atrial septostomy
Tricuspid atresia, pulmonary atresia with intact ventricular septum	
Restrictive atrial septum (left heart lesions)	
Total anomalous pulmonary venous return, mitral atresia with hypoplastic left heart syndrome	
Scimitar syndrome	Coil embolization of systemic-to-pulmonary collateral vessels

INTERPRETING NORMAL AND ABNORMAL ECGS IN THE NEWBORN PERIOD

100. **What is characteristic of a normal newborn ECG?**
Compared with the ECG of an older infant or child, the newborn ECG is remarkable for:
- Right axis deviation +90–180 degrees
- Right ventricular dominance, tall R wave in V1, and deep S wave in V6
- Positive T wave in the right precordial leads V3r, V4r, and V1
- Longer QTc interval up to 0.46 sec
Evidence of increased right ventricular forces decreases over the first 6 months of life (Fig. 5-6).

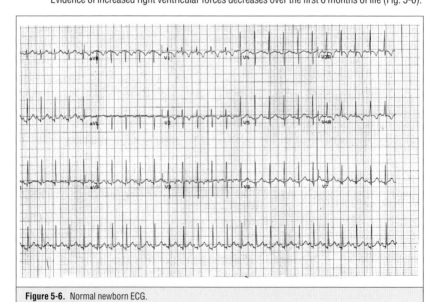

Figure 5-6. Normal newborn ECG.

KEY POINTS: ECGS IN THE NEWBORN PERIOD

1. Left axis deviation in a newborn ECG is abnormal.

2. T waves should be inverted in V1 by 3 days of age.

101. What ECG findings are always abnormal in a newborn?

The normal ECG in a newborn shows a preponderance of right ventricular forces because the right and left ventricles are of equal mass at birth. The mean QRS axis for a newborn is 110 degrees. Left axis deviation (<30 degrees) is always abnormal. Downward forces in the QRS in lead AVF and upward forces in lead 1 indicate a left axis deviation. Leads 1 and aVL may show a Q wave or negative deflection, which is known as left axis deviation with a counterclockwise loop. This finding is seen in infants with an endocardial cushion defect or infants who have an endocardial cushion type VSD.

102. What is the most common tachyarrhythmia in the newborn? How is it treated?

SVT (Fig. 5-7) is the most common tachycardia in term newborn infants and premature infants. It is usually a narrow complex tachycardia at rates of 250–300/minute. The mechanism is usually a reentrant type of tachycardia. It can be treated with adenosine (100–250 μg/kg) given as a rapid push. Adenosine blocks conduction through the AV node, resulting in a transient bradycardia and interruption of the reentrant circuit. Once converted to normal sinus rhythm, the infant should have a 12-lead ECG to rule out a delta wave and the presence of Wolff-Parkinson-White–type SVT.

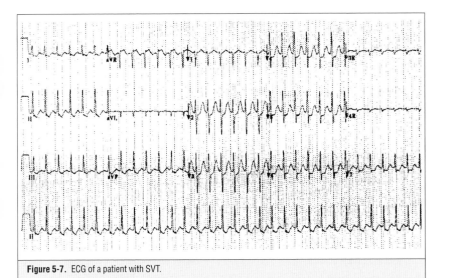

Figure 5-7. ECG of a patient with SVT.

103. What are ECG signs of abnormal right ventricular hypertrophy in a newborn?

- A Q wave in V1 (qR or qRs pattern) suggests right ventricular hypertrophy.
- An upright T wave in V1 after the third day of life also is consistent with right ventricular hypertrophy.

104. What are the ECG abnormalities observed in infants with hyperkalemia?
- The earliest change seen in a patient with hyperkalemia is the development of tall, peaked T waves in the precordial leads.
- With further elevation of the serum potassium concentration, there is a reduction in the R wave, a widening of the QRS complex, ST-segment elevation or depression, and PR prolongation.
- Ultimately, there is further widening of the QRS complex and cardiac arrest (Fig. 5-8).

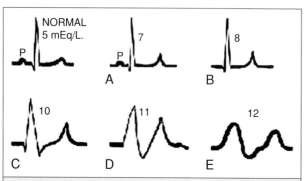

Figure 5-8. ECG changes of a patient with hyperkalemia. **A–E.** ECG changes seen with progressive increases in serum potassium levels as indicated by the numbers (mEq/L).

105. What are the ECG abnormalities observed in infants with hypokalemia?
- Depressions of the ST segment with flattening of the T wave
- Development of prominent U waves with QTU prolongation
- Development of ventricular arrhythmias

106. What other electrolyte disturbance mimics hypokalemia?
Hypomagnesemia.

107. What ECG disturbances are seen in infants with hypocalcemia?
Prolongation of the QT interval.

108. What are ECG changes associated with digitalis?
- **Digitalis effect:** Shortening of QTc, sagging of the ST segment, decreased T wave amplitude, and slowing of heart rate. Digitalis effects are usually seen during ventricular repolarization.
- **Digitalis toxicity:** Prolongation of PR interval, sinus bradycardia, heart block (second degree), and arrhythmias (supraventricular and ventricular). The toxic effects of digoxin are usually seen in the formation and conduction of the impulse.

109. What is a delta wave?
A delta wave is a slurring in the upstroke of the QRS complex; it generally occurs in association with a short PR interval. This is a sign of Wolff-Parkinson-White syndrome (Fig. 5-9). The delta wave signifies that atrial depolarization is proceeding down an abnormal bypass tract to the ventricle.

110. What is a bypass tract?
A bypass tract is a special group of cells that allows direct conduction from the atria to the ventricle. Normally, atrial depolarization goes down the AV node to the ventricle. Because conduction is slower through the AV node, the delta wave is that part of the QRS or ventricular depolariza-

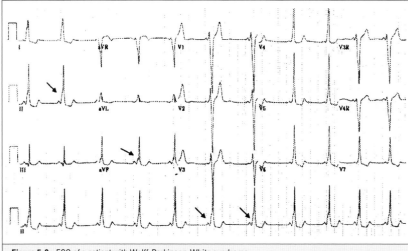

Figure 5-9. ECG of a patient with Wolff-Parkinson-White syndrome.

tion occurring first from the bypass tract. Once the depolarization gets through the AV node, the depolarization of the ventricles proceeds in a normal fashion. The short PR interval and the delta wave are indications of the presence of a bypass tract that can potentially place an infant at risk for supraventricular tachycardia.

111. What is a normal QTc interval in a newborn infant?
The normal QTc interval in a newborn is <0.46 sec. In children and adults, the upper limit of normal for QTc is 0.44 sec. Newborns with a prolonged QTc interval on the first day of life should have a repeat ECG in 1–2 days. Prolonged QTc interval has been associated with an increased risk of sudden infant death syndrome.

Gillette P, Garson A: Pediatric Arrhythmias: Electrophysiology and Pacing. Philadelphia, W.B. Saunders, 1990.

ARRHYTHMIAS

112. What are congenital anatomic and nonanatomic causes of congenital complete heart block in the fetus?
Complete congenital heart block in the fetus can occur secondary to structural congenital heart disease (levo-transposition of the great arteries [L-TGA], left atrial isomerism, or maternal collagen vascular disease). Heart block occurs in women with a variety of connective tissue diseases (e.g., systemic lupus erythematosus or Sjögren's syndrome). Anti-RO (SSA) and La (SSB) antibodies are found in many of these women, but only a minority of fetuses are affected. Most cases are identified between 18–24 weeks' gestation.

113. What are common benign arrhythmias seen in the fetus?
The most common benign arrhythmia in the fetus is a premature atrial contraction. This benign dysrhythmia is commonly detected during fetal monitoring. Blocked premature atrial contractions often cause what appears to be a pause on the monitoring strips, and they occur when the ventricle is refractory and not conducted.

KEY POINTS: ARRHYTHMIAS

1. Maternal connective tissue diseases (systemic lupus erythematosus and Sjögren's syndrome) can cause complete congenital heart block and/or dilated cardiomyopathy in a fetus or infant.

2. Atrial premature contractions are benign arrhythmias. On rare occasions, if frequent enough, they can trigger supraventricular tachycardia.

114. What type of arrhythmias can be diagnosed in the fetus?

All types of tachyarrhythmias and bradyarrhythmias can be detected. Premature beats account for 80–90% of fetal arrhythmias but are generally benign. Reentrant SVTs account for 5% of fetal arrhythmias, complete heart block 2.5%, and atrial flutter 1–2%. Ventricular arrhythmias are rare.

Friedman DM, Duncanson LJ, Glickstein JS, Buyon JP: A review of congenital heart block. Images Paediatr Cardiol 16:36–48, 2003.

Gillette P, Garson A: Pediatric Arrhythmias: Electrophysiology and Pacing. Philadelphia, W.B. Saunders, 1990.

Glickstein JS, Buyon J, Kim M, Friedman DM: The fetal Doppler mechanical PR interval: A validation study. Fetal Diagn Ther 19:31–34, 2004.

COR PULMONALE

115. What is cor pulmonale?

Cor pulmonale is a severe abnormality in right ventricular function that occurs as a result of lung pathology. The common denominator in all cases is a significantly elevated pulmonary vascular resistance and right ventricular hypertension. The right ventricular dysfunction is manifested as a combination of right ventricular hypertrophy with decreased right ventricular compliance, and right ventricular dilatation with decreased systolic function. By definition, cor pulmonale excludes all cases of right ventricular pathology due to congenital heart disease.

116. What are the causes of cor pulmonale in a newborn infant?

Cor pulmonale may be the result of any pathology that causes pulmonary vascular resistance to remain significantly elevated after birth. By far, the most common cause of cor pulmonale in infants is bronchopulmonary dysplasia. Other pulmonary causes include upper airway obstruction, neuromuscular disease, restrictive lung disease, thoracic cage abnormality, and parenchymal lung disease.

117. What are the signs and symptoms of cor pulmonale?

- **Poor feeding:** Inability to substantially increase cardiac output with exercise
- **Signs and symptoms of underlying pulmonary pathology:** Oxygen requirement
- **Tachypnea, retractions, rales, wheezing**
- **Heaving, right ventricular impulse, loud P2, tricuspid regurgitant murmur**
- **Hepatosplenomegaly**

Gewitz MH: Cor pulmonale—Pulmonary heart disease. In Emmanoulides GC, Allen HD, Riemenschneider TA, Gutgesell HP (eds): Moss and Adams' Heart Disease in Infants, Children and Adolescents, Including the Fetus and Young Adult, 5th ed. Baltimore, Williams & Wilkins, 1994.

ENDOCARDITIS

118. **Which neonates are at risk for developing endocarditis?**
    - Neonates with congenital heart disease
    - Neonates with structurally normal hearts who have an indwelling central venous catheter
    - Neonates with normal cardiac anatomy and PDA

119. **What are the pathogens that cause endocarditis in neonates?**
    Staphylococcus species, group B Streptococcus, *Escherichia coli,* Listeria monocytogenes, Candida species, and gram-negative organisms such as Acinetobacter species, Serratia species, Enterobacter species, and Klebsiella species.

120. **What are the signs of endocarditis in the neonate?**
    Heart murmurs, skin abscesses, and hepatomegaly are the most common signs found in neonatal patients. The findings in children with subacute bacterial endocarditis—splenomegaly, petechiae, and splinter hemorrhages—are not usually seen in newborn infants.

    Millar BC, Jugo J, Moore JE: Fungal endocarditis in neonates and children. Pediatr Cardiol 26:517–536, 2005.
    Pearlman SA, Higgins S, Eppes S, et al: Infective endocarditis in the premature infant. Clin Pediatr (Phila) 37:741–746, 1998.

CARDIOMYOPATHY IN THE NEONATE

121. **What are the echocardiographic findings in each of the three types of neonatal cardiomyopathy?**
    See Table 5-5.

TABLE 5-5. ECHOCARDIOGRAPHIC FINDINGS IN THE THREE TYPES OF NEONATAL CARDIOMYOPATHY		
Type of Cardiomyopathy	Function Seen on Echocardiography	Other Echographic Findings
Dilated cardiomyopathy	Globular left ventricle Globular and poorly contracting right ventricular size; contractility may be normal or similarly depressed	Endocardial fibroelastosis
Hypertrophic cardiomyopathy	Marked left or biventricular hypertrophy with normal or hyperdynamic systolic function	With or without presence of asymmetric septal hypertrophy (left ventricle) Left ventricular cavity is smaller than normal Ventricular filling is impaired by diastolic relaxation abnormalities
Restrictive cardiomyopathy	Normal ventricular size and contractility	Abnormal diastolic filling Markedly decreased ventricular compliance

122. **Which metabolic disease is associated with hypertrophic cardiomyopathy, short PR interval, and huge QRS voltage?**
Pompe's disease (glycogen storage disease type II or acid maltase deficiency).

123. **What common syndrome is associated with hypertrophic cardiomyopathy?**
Approximately 10–20% of patients with Noonan's syndrome have an associated hypertrophic cardiomyopathy.

> Keren A, Popp RL: Assignment of patients into the classification of cardiomyopathies. Circulation 86:1622–1633 1992.

KEY POINTS: CARDIOMYOPATHY IN NEONATES

1. The diagnosis of a cardiomyopathy in a neonate warrants a full genetic, metabolic, and infectious disease evaluation.

2. The three types of neonatal cardiomyopathy are dilated, hypertrophic, and restrictive.

CARDIAC TRANSPLANT

124. **What are the signs of rejection in a neonate who has undergone a cardiac transplant?**
Most rejection episodes in the era of cyclosporine immunosuppression are relatively asymptomatic, especially in older children. The neonatal recipient, however, can often have the nonspecific findings of fever, irritability, tachycardia, loss of appetite, and an S3 gallop on physical examination.

125. **What are major long-term complications that can occur following heart transplantation?**
Rejection, infection, coronary artery disease, hypertension, renal dysfunction, and tumors.

126. **Can a heart that is rejecting have preserved systolic function on echocardiogram?**
Yes.

127. **What are the important hemodynamic considerations in a transplanted heart?**
During cardiac transplantation, all nerves to the heart are severed so that there is no direct sympathetic or parasympathetic control of heart rate. Concomitantly, during the first few postoperative days the stroke volume of the transplanted heart is relatively fixed, and the contractility of the heart is diminished because of ischemia that occurred during harvest and implantation. Cardiac output is directly proportional to changes in the heart rate in the early postoperative period. Therefore, many surgeons try to maintain cardiac output by pacing the heart with temporary pacing wires.

> Addonizio LJ: Late complications of pediatric cardiac transplantation. Am Coll Cardiol Curr J Rev 3:23–25, 1994.

CARDIAC TUMORS

128. What are the most frequent histologic types of primary cardiac tumors in infants and newborns?

- **Rhabdomyoma:** Most common cardiac tumor in newborns and infants (~ 50%). Tumors involve the myocardium, usually the interventricular septum; they may be single or multiple as well as intramural. Rhabdomyomas seldom cause obstruction and usually regress.
- **Fibroma:** Second most common primary cardiac tumor in infants and young children, accounting for ~25% of such tumors. They are usually single and intramural; they may involve the left ventricular posterior wall and interventricular septum. Fibromas are often located at the left ventricular apex.

128. What are other types of cardiac tumors?

- **Intrapericardial teratomas**
- **Atrial myxomas:** More frequent in older children and adolescents
- **Mesothelioma localized to the AV node:** Can produce heart block or sudden death in adolescents)
- **Sarcoma/angiosarcoma:** Seen primarily in right atrium; metastases to lung, lymph nodes, mediastinum, liver, kidneys, and adrenal glands

129. What is the most frequent disease associated with primary rhabdomyoma?
Approximately 50% of patients with cardiac rhabdomyomas have tuberous sclerosis. Multiple rhabdomyomas are more consistent with the diagnosis of tuberous sclerosis than a solitary tumor. Neonates with this syndrome may have no clinical manifestation other than cardiac tumors or cutaneous and neurological findings.

130. How do intracardiac tumors cause perinatal or neonatal death?
Depending on size and location, cardiac tumors have been demonstrated to cause death from:

- Severe intractable dysrhythmia
- Nonimmune hydrops
- Decreased cardiac output secondary to inflow or outflow obstruction

Bharati S, Lev M: Cardiac tumors. In Emmanoulides GC, Allen HD, Riemenschneider TA, Gutgesell HP (eds): Moss and Adams' Heart Disease in Infants, Children and Adolescents, Including the Fetus and Young Adult, 5th ed. Baltimore, Williams & Wilkins, 1994.

CARDIAC SURGERY

131. What congenital heart lesions are treated with the placement of a shunt in the newborn period?
The modified Blalock-Taussig shunt is a Gore-Tex interposition shunt placed between the subclavian artery (right or left) and the right or left pulmonary artery. It is used for congenital heart lesions that require increased pulmonary blood flow in the neonatal/infant period. Examples include lesions with a hypoplastic pulmonary annulus, atretic pulmonary valve annulus, or severely hypoplastic main and branch pulmonary arteries. The cardiac malformations in such instances would include severe tetralogy of Fallot, tetralogy of Fallot with pulmonary atresia, tricuspid atresia, pulmonary atresia/VSD, and pulmonary atresia with intact ventricular septum. A modified Blalock-Taussig shunt is used in the first stage of a hypoplastic left heart syndrome repair (modified Norwood operation).

132. What are the major shunts used in heart surgery?

The modified Blalock-Taussig shunt, the bidirectional Glenn procedure (shunt), and the Sano modification of the Norwood operation are the most common types of shunts used today. Shunts that were used in the past to increase pulmonary blood flow include the Waterston shunt (anastomosis from the ascending aorta to the right pulmonary artery) and the Potts shunt (anastomosis from the descending aorta to the left pulmonary artery). These two shunts are not used any more (Fig. 5-10).

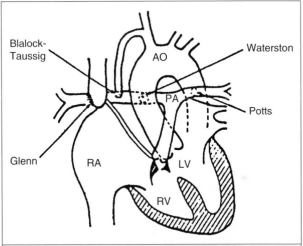

Figure 5-10. Major shunt operations for congenital heart disease. AO = aorta, PA = pulmonary artery, RA = right atrium, LV = left ventricle, RV = right ventricle. (From Park M: Pediatric Cardiology for Practitioners, 3rd ed. St. Louis, Mosby, 1996.)

133. What is a Glenn procedure? In what kinds of congenital heart disease is it used?

A bidirectional Glenn anastomosis is a connection from the right superior vena cava to the right pulmonary artery, or the left superior vena cava to the left pulmonary artery, or both (i.e., bicaval bidirectional Glenn anastomosis). The pulmonary arteries are in continuity, so a right bidirectional Glenn anastomosis connection will send blood flow into the right and the left pulmonary arteries. This anastomosis is usually the intermediate step to a Fontan procedure. Lesions for which a bidirectional Glenn procedure is used include those with single ventricle anatomy (e.g., hypoplastic left heart syndrome, hypoplastic right heart syndrome, tricuspid atresia, and pulmonary atresia).

134. What is the Jatene operation (switch procedure)?

The Jatene procedure (arterial switch) is performed for d-transposition of the great arteries. The coronary arteries are removed from the aorta and reimplanted into the pulmonary artery, which becomes the new aorta.

135. What is the Mustard or Senning procedure?

The Mustard or Senning (atrial switch) procedure is used in d-transposition of the great arteries to baffle systemic and pulmonary venous drainage. In this procedure, the systemic venous drainage returning to the right atrium is baffled through the mitral valve, where it enters the left ventricle, and then the pulmonary artery. The pulmonary venous drainage returning to the left atrium is baffled through the tricuspid valve, into the right ventricle, and then out the aorta. This procedure is not as commonly performed today, and the Jatene Procedure is more commonly used in d-transposition of the great vessels.

136. **What are the stages of the modified Norwood procedure?**
  - **Stage 1:** Anastomosis of the proximal main pulmonary artery to the aorta, with aortic arch reconstruction and transection and patch closure of the distal main pulmonary artery; a modified right Blalock-Taussig shunt (right subclavian artery to right pulmonary artery) to provide pulmonary blood flow; and lastly, atrial septectomy to allow for adequate left-to-right atrial communication.
  - **Stage 1 (alternate approach):** In some centers, a Norwood-Sano operation is performed as a first stage. In this operation, the modified Blalock-Taussig shunt is replaced with a right ventricle to the main pulmonary artery connection (Sano modification) to provide pulmonary blood flow.
  - **Stage 2:** Bidirectional Glenn anastomosis (*see* question 133).
  - **Stage 3:** Completion of a Fontan operation (*see* question 137).

137. **What is the modified Fontan procedure?**
  The modified Fontan procedure is a two-step operation that, when completed, entails the end-to-side anastomosis of the superior vena cava into the right pulmonary artery (i.e. the bidirectional Glenn operation) and the construction of a baffle or lateral tunnel from the inferior vena cava orifice to the orifice of the SVC, where it enters into the right pulmonary artery (Fig. 5-11). The bidirectional Glen operation is the first step to completing the Fontan circuit. Another technique used to connect the SVC flow into the right pulmonary artery is called the hemiFontan. The creation of the lateral tunnel (with or without a fenestration) is the second and final step to completing the Fontan circuit.

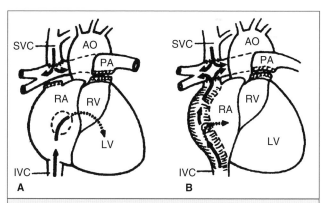

Figure 5-11. Modified Fontan operation. *A,* Bidirectional Glenn operation or SVC to RPA anastamosis. *B,* Cavocaval baffle to PA connection, with or without fenestration. AO = aorta, PA = pulmonary artery, SVC = superior vena cava, RA = right atrium, RV = right ventricle, LV = left ventricle, IVC = inferior vena cava. (From Park M: Pediatric Cardiology for Practitioners, 3rd ed. St. Louis, Mosby, 1995, p 213.)

138. **What congenital heart lesions are considered inoperable?**
  Newborn infants in whom important anatomic structures are not present can be considered inoperable. Some of the involved conditions might include tetralogy of Fallot with multiple aor-

topulmonary collaterals and no main or branch pulmonary arteries, neonates with absence of pulmonary veins or severe pulmonary venous stenosis, or infants with tracheal agenesis. In infants with multiple anatomic or severe chromosomal abnormalities, the heart lesions might be repairable, but the overall prognosis for the baby may be so bleak that operating on the heart may not improve the quality of life or even extend the life of the baby.

139. What are some of the initial treatment objectives for a neonate after corrective cardiac surgery?

1. Minimize stress response with continuous narcotic administration.
2. Minimize oxygen consumption and regulate ventilation with neuromuscular blockade.
3. Support cardiac performance, including:
   - Preload (monitoring and maintenance of filling pressures)
   - Afterload (initiation of afterload reduction, as tolerated)
   - Contractility (anticipation of the need for inotropic support)
   - Heart rate (monitoring and maintenance of optimal heart rate and rhythm)
4. Maintain metabolic homeostasis, including:
   - Monitoring and maintenance of core temperature and optimal pH
   - Monitoring and correction of electrolyte imbalances and coagulopathy
   - Monitoring and regulation of serum glucose
   - Monitoring and avoidance of fluid overload

Feltes T: Postoperative recovery from congenital heart disease. In Garson A, Bricker JT, Fisher DJ, Neish SR (eds): The Science and Practice of Pediatric Cardiology. Baltimore, Williams & Wilkins, 1990.

140. What are some of the warning signs of cardiac tamponade?

The signs of tamponade can occur quickly. They include tachycardia, decrease in oxygen saturation, increase in cardiac filling pressures, abrupt decrease in chest tube drainage, increasing cardiac size on chest x-ray, and poor perfusion. Pulsus paradoxus may not be evident in a mechanically ventilated patient unless he or she is spontaneously breathing.

141. What are some of the concerns in a neonate with an "open chest" after heart surgery?

The infant should be kept deeply sedated and paralyzed. The wound should be covered. Lung tidal volume should be adjusted appropriately so the lung does not herniate. Monitored cardiac pressures are usually low. These patients require broad-spectrum antibiotic coverage. Before closing the chest, vigorous diuresis is usually required. When the chest is eventually closed, all of the intravascular pressures will increase, airway compliance will increase, and tidal volume should be adjusted downward.

142. If the infant cannot be taken off cardiopulmonary bypass after surgery, what are the options?

Extracorporeal membrane oxygenation (ECMO) can provide a means to assist the heart and/or lungs for a temporary amount of time. Venoarterial ECMO is used in neonatal patients with either life-threatening pulmonary disease (e.g., congenital diaphragmatic hernia or persistent fetal circulation) or neonates with postoperative ventricular failure. The survival rate in postoperative cardiac patients is about 42%.

Castaneda A, Jonas R, Mayer J, Hanley F: Cardiac Surgery of the Neonate and Infant. Philadelphia, W.B. Saunders, 1994.

Feltes T: Postoperative recovery from congenital heart disease. In Garson A, Bricker JT, Fisher DJ, Neish SR (eds): The Science and Practice of Pediatric Cardiology. Baltimore, Williams & Wilkins, 1990.

Klein MD, Shaheen KW, Whittlesey GC, et al: Extracorporeal membrane oxygenation for the circulatory support after repair of congenital heart disease. J Thorac Cardiovasc Surg 100:498, 1990.

CHAPTER 6

DERMATOLOGY

Kimberly D. Morel, MD, Elizabeth Alvarez Connelly, MD, and Lawrence F. Eichenfield, MD

1. **Name three forms of epidermal inclusion cysts that are commonly found in neonates.**
   1. **Milia:** Tiny cysts, usually found on the face, occurring in up to 40% of newborns
   2. **Epstein pearls (Fig. 6-1):** Cysts found on the palate of approximately 64% of newborns
   3. **Bohn nodules:** Alveolar cysts

   All three forms represent cystic retention of keratin, appear and resolve in the first month, and can be present at birth. They are white, 1- to 2-mm papules that can be found singularly or in clusters.

2. **What are neonatal acne and transient cephalic neonatal pustulosis (TCNP)? How do these entities differ from infantile acne?**
   There is some degree of controversy regarding the cause and nomenclature of these conditions. Some neonatal outbreaks, while commonly called *neonatal acne,* are not composed of distinct pimples (i.e., comedones), but superficial pustules.
   - **Neonatal acne:** Usually begins at a few weeks of life and resolves over several months. Affected infants exhibit multiple inflammatory erythematous papules and pustules. Treatment is rarely needed.
   - **TCNP:** Has been proposed as a subset of what has been called neonatal acne, which is caused by *Malassezia* species rather than by an elevation in androgen levels (which occurs in infantile or classic acne). Others have proposed that there is no true neonatal acne and that the term

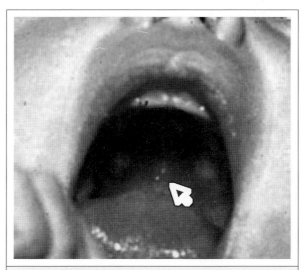

Figure 6-1. Epstein pearls.

TCNP (or neonatal cephalic pustulosis) should be used as a substitute. Like neonatal acne, TCNP usually begins at a few weeks of life and resolves in several months. Affected infants demonstrate multiple inflammatory erythematous papules and pustules. Comedonal lesions are rare, and treatment is rarely needed, although some experts believe that topical anti-yeast agents speed resolution.

- **Infantile acne:** Truly an acneiform condition, with open and closed comedones as well as papules and pustules. It usually presents later, usually beyond the age of 2–3 months, and generally resolves between the ages of 6 and 12 months. That time sequence parallels decreases in fetal adrenal pubertal androgen levels and male testosterone levels (one possible reason males are more commonly affected). Unlike neonatal acne or TCNP, infantile acne may persist and cause scarring. For this reason, like adolescent acne, it is treated with topical antibiotics and occasionally with retinoids or systemic agents.

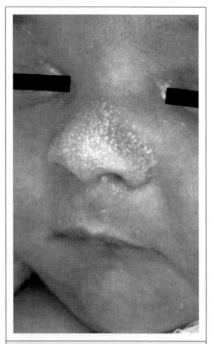

Figure 6-2. An infant with sebaceous hyperplasia.

3. **What is the standard treatment for milia, sebaceous gland hyperplasia (Fig. 6-2), transient neonatal pustular melanosis, erythema toxicum, and sucking blisters?**
   The treatment is the same for all—that is, no treatment other than reassuring the family that the condition will resolve with time (Table 6-1).

4. **What is prickly heat? Which bacteria are believed to contribute to its cause?**
   Prickly heat is the term for *miliaria rubra*, which is caused by obstruction of the eccrine ducts. The extracellular polysaccharide substance from *Staphylococcus epidermidis* has been implicated in its pathogenesis.

TABLE 6-1. NEONATAL SKIN LESIONS			
Condition	**Onset**	**Resolution**	**Treatment**
Milia	Can be at birth, <1 month old	Usually <1 month	None
Sebaceous gland hyperplasia	Can be at birth, <1 month old	Usually <1 month	None
Transient neonatal pustular melanosis	Usually present at birth	Vesicopustules <5 days; pigment macules <3 month	None
Erythema toxicum	24–48 h, new lesions <10 days old	Each lesion, <5 days; all lesions, <2 weeks	None
Sucking blisters	Present at birth	Days	None

5. **How are miliaria crystallina and miliaria rubra differentiated? How are they treated?**
Miliaria is found in up to 15% of newborns. Both forms are caused by eccrine duct obstruction and resultant sweat leakage to different levels of skin (crystallina if the leakage occurs under the stratum corneum, and rubra if it takes place at the upper dermis). Miliaria is more common in hot, humid environments and is distributed to the forehead, upper trunk, or other covered surfaces. Don't sweat about the treatment—just keep the baby from being overheated. The removal of excess layers of clothing (or moving the infant to Alaska) is helpful. Air conditioning may also be helpful.

6. **Is erythema toxicum toxic? In which kind of infant is it rarely seen?**
Erythema toxicum is a benign condition (Fig. 6-3). Erythema toxicum is no alien to the nursery; it is present in 50% of term newborns. It is much less prevalent in premature infants, however, occurring in only approximately 5%.

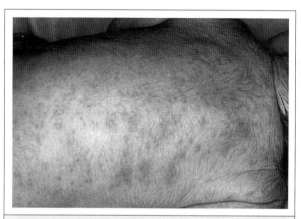

Figure 6-3. Erythema toxicum. White papules on an erythematous base are seen.

7. **When do the lesions of erythema toxicum occur? What do they look like?**
Erythema toxicum usually begins between 24 and 48 hours of life and spontaneously resolves in 4–5 days; however, new lesions can occur up to day 10 of life. All lesions should resolve by 2 weeks. Erythema toxicum lesions are irregularly bordered, erythematous macules, 2–3 cm in diameter, with central yellowish vesicopustules. They are mostly discrete, but some erythematous macules become confluent. Lesions do not involve the palms or soles.

8. **Which type of cells is seen on microscopic examination of pustules scraped from erythema toxicum lesions?**
Wright-Giemsa stains of pustule scrapings show mostly eosinophils. Up to 15% of affected infants demonstrate peripheral eosinophilia as well.

9. **What is harlequin color change?**
Harlequin color change is a demarcated erythema forming on the dependent half of the body of newborns. In some cases, the baby appears as if a line were drawn right down the midline. The more superior half of the body appears pale. This appearance can occur in any position and commonly lasts from seconds up to 20 minutes. It is rarely seen after 10 days of life. Harlequin color change is explained by immature autonomic vasomotor control because it is more common in premature infants and is reversible. If the baby is flipped over during an episode, the newly dependent portion will become erythematous.

10. **What are the modes of inheritance of neurofibromatosis types 1 and 2? What protein mutations are involved in these genetic diseases?**
Both diseases are autosomal dominant, but spontaneous mutations account for approximately half of cases. The incidence of neurofibromatosis type 1 is 1 in 2500; the mutated gene product is neurofibromin, a protein involved in tumor suppression. Neurofibromatosis type 2 has a reported incidence of 1 in 33,000; the involved gene product is Merlin, which mediates cytoskeleton and extracellular movement.

11. **When should neurofibromatosis type 1 be suspected in a newborn?**
Neurofibromatosis type 1 should be suspected in any infant with multiple café-au-lait spots, congenital glaucoma, a plexiform neurofibroma, or pseudoarthrosis. Without a positive family history, it can be difficult to diagnose neurofibromatosis in the first months of life. The diagnosis requires two or more of the following criteria: ≥6 café-au-lait macules of 0.5 cm before puberty (1.5 cm postpuberty), ≥2 neurofibromas, one plexiform neurofibroma, axillary freckles or inguinal freckles, ≥2 Lisch nodules (iris hamartomas), osseous lesions, or a first-degree relative with neurofibromatosis type 1. Other features that are associated with neurofibromatosis in older children include learning disability, macrocephaly, short stature, juvenile xanthogranulomas, angiomas, mental retardation, impaired coordination, seizures, cerebral tumors (i.e., optic gliomas), increased risk of malignancy, and hypertension.

KEY POINTS: DIFFERENTIAL DIAGNOSIS OF CONGENITAL VASCULAR-APPEARING NODULE

1. Vascular tumor (e.g., congenital hemangioma)

2. Vascular malformation (e.g., arterial, venous, lymphatic, capillary malformation)

3. Congenital malignancy (e.g., neuroblastoma, rhabdomyosarcoma, fibrosarcoma, primitive neuroectodermal tumor, lipoblastoma, liposarcoma)

12. **What is the most common cutaneous finding in neonates with tuberous sclerosis?**
Hypopigmented macules, known as ash-leaf spots, are the most common skin findings of tuberous sclerosis in infants. Connective tissue nevi, known as *shagreen patches,* may also be present at birth. Adenoma sebaceum (facial angiofibromas) generally appear at age 3 years and older; periungual or gum fibromas appear in early adulthood. During the first months of life, hypopigmented macules may be recognizable only with a Wood's lamp because of the general lack of pigmentation in the skin. Another manifestation of tuberous sclerosis during the neonatal period that is of great concern is a rhabdomyoma within the heart. Children diagnosed with tuberous sclerosis should have a cardiac echocardiography examination performed.

13. **Are hypopigmented macules always a sign of tuberous sclerosis?**
No! Most hypopigmented macules are a variant of normal conditions. However, multiple ash-leaf–like macules, a family history of tuberous sclerosis, neonatal seizures, cardiac rhabdomyomas, or renal cysts may alert you to the diagnosis of tuberous sclerosis.

14. **Tuberous sclerosis is inherited in an autosomal dominant fashion. What is peculiar about the genetic abnormalities associated with the tuberous sclerosis phenotype?**
Two distinct chromosomal complexes on two different chromosomes are implicated as areas of mutation that result in tuberous sclerosis. Tuberous sclerosis complex 1 is due to mutations in

the gene hamartin on chromosome 9, located at 9q34.3. Tuberous sclerosis complex 2 is caused by mutations in the tuberin gene on chromosome 16 at 16p13.3.

15. **What is a collodion baby?**
   Collodion baby is a term used to describe a neonate born with a yellow, shiny membrane that resembles collodion.

16. **Which type of ichthyosis is most commonly associated with a collodion baby?**
   Of newborns with collodion membrane, the most common ichthyosis that develops is nonbullous ichthyosiform erythroderma, also called *congenital ichthyosiform erythroderma*. Lamellar ichthyosis is another rare form of ichthyosis that may present initially with collodion membrane. Approximately 5% of babies with collodion membrane do not go on to have clinically significant skin disease. Furthermore, not all patients with ichthyotic skin disease have a collodion membrane at birth.

17. **How should one care for a baby with collodion membrane?**
   Supportive care is important until the collodion membrane sheds. Affected newborns have difficulty with temperature regulation, are prone to sepsis, and have increased fluid and nutritional requirements. Therefore, temperature should be controlled in an incubator, and any signs of infection should be promptly investigated and treated. Ectropion occurs as a result of taut skin everting eyelid margins, which leaves patients at risk for corneal ulceration. Topical ocular lubricants should be instituted early. Eclabium occurs by a similar mechanism of taut skin everting the lips. Nasogastric tube feedings may be required for poor suck and feeding difficulties.

18. **What is a harlequin baby?**
   The term *harlequin baby* is used to describe neonates born with massive shiny plates of stratum corneum with deep, red fissures that form geometric patterns resembling a harlequin costume. This entity is quite different from a harlequin color change, which is benign in nature. As in neonates with collodion membrane, temperature regulation is defective, fluid requirements are increased, and there is a high risk of infection. The skin defect is usually restrictive, and respiratory insufficiency results. Harlequin babies rarely survive beyond the neonatal period.

19. **What is KID syndrome? How does it present in kids?**
   KID syndrome is a rare disorder characterized by keratitis, ichthyosis, and congenital neurosensory deafness. Newborns have erythematous, thickened skin that eventually peels. The face and extremities then become ichthyotic; scaly keratoconjunctivitis usually develops during infancy.

20. **Are newborns with epidermolytic hyperkeratosis hyperkeratotic?**
   Epidermolytic hyperkeratosis is also called *bullous congenital ichthyosiform erythroderma*. Newborns most often have blisters or bullae along with denuded skin. Although subtle hyperkeratosis appears in some newborns, it usually develops over time as the blistering subsides.

21. **What is subcutaneous fat necrosis of the newborn?**
   Subcutaneous fat necrosis of the newborn usually presents within the first month of life with red to violaceous mobile plaques, especially on the back, thighs, and cheeks. The cause of subcutaneous fat necrosis is not definitively known.

22. **In which clinical situations may subcutaneous fat necrosis of the newborn occur?**
   Subcutaneous fat necrosis may occur in cases of prematurity, fetal distress, birth trauma, infection, or cold stress.

23. **How should newborns with subcutaneous fat necrosis be monitored?**
    Although the disorder is most often benign and self-limited, in some cases subcutaneous fat necrosis of the newborn may be associated with hypercalcemia and death. Therefore, serum calcium levels must be monitored, and caregivers must be vigilant for clinical signs and symptoms of hypercalcemia.

24. **What is a blueberry muffin baby?**
    Blueberry muffin baby is a term used to describe neonates whose skin resembles a blueberry muffin (i.e., the skin shows diffuse, dark blue to violaceous purpuric macules and papules). The spots represent dermal hematopoiesis and are a sign of serious systemic disease, most often congenital infection. The congenital infection most commonly associated with this appearance is congenital rubella, although it may have other causes.

25. **Which diseases may cause blueberry muffin syndrome?**
    - Congenital infections
    - Hemolytic disease of the newborn
    - Toxoplasmosis
    - Neoplastic disease
    - Rubella
    - Leukemia
    - Cytomegalovirus
    - Neuroblastoma
    - Herpes
    - Langerhans' cell histiocytosis
    - Coxsackie B2
    - Congenital rhabdomyosarcoma with cutaneous metastases
    - Parvovirus B19

26. **What is the clinical presentation of sclerema neonatorum?**
    Findings usually appear in the first 2 weeks of life but can begin as late as 4 months. Infants who are poorly nourished, dehydrated, hypothermic, or septic are most commonly affected. Sclerema neonatorum begins in the lower extremities with the appearance of hard, cool skin and decreased mobility and subsequently involves the trunk and face. Palms, soles, and genitalia are not involved. Joints become immobile, and the face appears mask-like. Sclerema may be associated with necrotizing enterocolitis, pneumonia, intracranial hemorrhage, hypoglycemia, and electrolyte disturbances.

27. **What is the cause of sclerema? Why is it more common in infants with infection, hypothermia, or other stressors?**
    Sclerema is likely a result of lipoenzyme dysfunction and occurs in infants who are stressed with severe illnesses. More specifically, dysfunction of enzymes regulating the conversion of saturated fatty acids to unsaturated fatty acids results in excess saturated fatty acids. This dysfunction promotes fat solidification. The incidence of sclerema has decreased significantly because events such as malnutrition, dehydration, and hypothermia occur less commonly in modern nurseries. Treating the underlying condition can result in resolution of sclerema. Some authors also propose systemic steroids or therapy with exchange transfusions.

28. **Why is presence of pruritus a poor way to differentiate atopic dermatitis from seborrheic dermatitis in infants?**
    Hope you are itching for the answer! Although atopic dermatitis classically includes pruritus, infants and especially newborns may not have the coordination to scratch. However, occipital alopecia can occur as a result of excessive rubbing of the back of the head against the bed sheets. In this situation, hair may fall out or break off due to friction.

29. **Describe the usual distributions of the rash caused by atopic dermatitis and that caused by seborrheic dermatitis in neonates.**

    If dermatitis involves the axillae or groin, it is more likely to be seborrheic dermatitis. If extensor surfaces such as forearms and shins are involved, atopic dermatitis is more likely. Both atopic dermatitis and seborrheic dermatitis involve scalp and posterior auricular areas, although seborrheic dermatitis has large, yellowish scale and, when severe, characteristically extends down to the forehead and eyebrow areas.

30. **What is scalded skin syndrome?**

    Staphylococcal scalded skin syndrome (SSSS) is caused by toxins released by *Staphylococcus aureus* that lead to blistering and desquamation of the skin. The Nikolsky's sign is positive; simply rubbing the skin causes a blister to form. Outbreaks of such blistering have been reported in newborn nurseries. Remember, however, that scalding thermal burns have been reported in neonates bathed in overly hot water—another "scalding skin syndrome."

31. **What is aplasia cutis congenita?**

    Aplasia cutis congenita occurs as a result of failure of development of the normal layers of skin. It occurs most often on the scalp and may present clinically as an ulcer, healed erosion, or well-formed scar. Therefore, it is often mistaken for trauma due to a scalp pH probe. In cases of large lesions or lesions overlying the midline neurocranial axis, imaging should be considered because aplasia cutis congenita may be associated with underlying malformations of bone or may extend deeply to the meninges.

32. **What is the significance of preauricular skin tags?**

    Preauricular skin tags, also called *accessory tragi,* are embryonic remnants of the first branchial arch (Fig. 6-4). The formation of the first branchial arch occurs during the fourth week of fetal development. The kidneys and heart also develop during this time. Renal ultrasound has been recommended in patients with preauricular skin tags because they can be associated with urinary tract abnormalities (8.6% of cases according to one prospective study).

33. **What are accessory nipples? Where are they located?**

    Accessory nipples, also called *supernumerary nipples* (Fig. 6-5), are embryonic remnants of the mammary line that extend from the axilla to the inner thigh. They appear as pink or brown

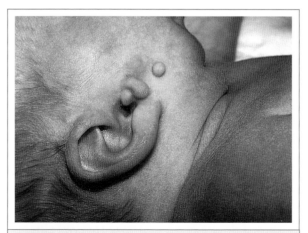

Figure 6-4. Preauricular skin tags.

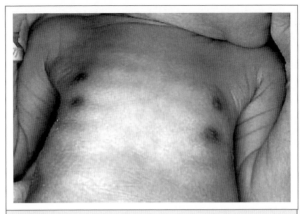

Figure 6-5. Supernumerary nipples.

papules, with or without surrounding areola, anywhere along the mammary line. There have been conflicting reports about an association with urinary tract abnormalities.

34. **What are the risk factors for development of hemangiomas?**
Infantile hemangiomas are common vascular tumors that arise during the neonatal period. One study found that 10% of Caucasian children had hemangiomas when examined at 1 year of age. Hemangiomas occur more frequently in female children, with a female/male incidence of 2–5:1. In addition, they arise more commonly in premature infants and in infants whose mothers underwent chorionic villus sampling.

35. **What do strawberries and caverns have to do with hemangiomas?**
In the older and lay literature, superficial hemangiomas were called *strawberry birthmarks* because the color and texture of the skin is somewhat reminiscent of a strawberry. Deep hemangiomas have been called *cavernous hemangiomas,* but the term is particularly confusing because it has also been used to describe venous malformations, which are a completely different kind of vascular birthmark. So it is prudent to avoid both terms and to use the terms *superficial, deep,* or *mixed hemangiomas* to describe a particular type of hemangioma.

36. **What are the differences between hemangiomas and vascular malformations?**
The classification of vascular birthmarks has historically been a problematic issue. The most commonly accepted classification was introduced almost 20 years ago and has been modified slightly. It divides vascular birthmarks into two broad categories:
   - **Vascular tumors:** These include the most common birthmark, the hemangioma of infancy, and other rare childhood-onset vascular tumors. The lesions are proliferating lesions composed of blood vessels. Hemangiomas have a characteristic natural history. They are usually noted in the first few weeks of life, undergo rapid proliferation that may last for several months, and then slowly regress over several years. At the end of the period of spontaneous regression, they may be undetectable or leave a residual mass or textural changes. Hemangiomas are distinct histologically and show increased endothelial turnover.
   - **Vascular malformations:** These include various lesions (e.g., capillary malformations [port-wine stains]). They are classified according to the type of vessels that compose them. They are often noted in the immediate newborn period. Vascular malformations grow with the child, although they may become more prominent as the child matures. They do not show a marked increase in proliferation and differ histologically from tumors.

Most importantly, they do not regress spontaneously, and they persist throughout the patient's lifetime. Therefore, management is significantly different from that undertaken for a hemangioma.

37. **In which situations should you worry about coexistent internal hemangiomas?**
Infants who present with multiple cutaneous hemangiomas or large hemangiomas may have underlying internal hemangiomas. The liver, gastrointestinal tract, central nervous system, eyes, and lungs are the most common sites of extracutaneous involvement. Not all children with multiple skin hemangiomas have underlying systemic involvement; conversely, children with visceral hemangiomas may have no skin lesions. Children with hemangiomas located on the lower face in a "beard" pattern often have laryngeal hemangiomas that may not become detectable until they compromise breathing. Therefore, a pediatric otolaryngologist should evaluate these children early in life.

38. **In newborns with multiple cutaneous hemangiomas, what is the most common location of internal organ hemangiomas?**
The gastrointestinal tract, especially the liver. Hepatomegaly or signs of high-output cardiac failure are clinical clues to hepatic hemangiomatosis. It is important to remember that normal liver sonogram results in the neonatal period do not rule out subsequent hepatic hemangiomatosis because symptoms may develop during the proliferative phase of the hemangioma.

39. **In addition to multiple cutaneous hemangiomas, what is a risk factor for hepatic hemangiomatosis?**
Large hemangioma size, especially segmental.

40. **What are some of the complications that can occur with a large hemangioma?**
Large hemangiomas may impair vital functions. Even smaller lesions in problematic locations can lead to complications. Hemangiomas located around the eye may obstruct the visual axis or lead to astigmatism by deforming the shape of the globe, which leads to visual impairment. Large lesions with high flow may cause congestive heart failure. Large facial hemangiomas have been seen in association with underlying congenital anomalies, including cardiac and central nervous system malformations. Finally, large hemangiomas may lead to significant disfigurement even as they regress spontaneously. Ulceration may complicate large or small hemangiomas.

41. **What endocrine study should be considered in an infant with a large hemangioma?**
Thyroid function testing. Hemangioma tissue may exhibit enzyme activity (type 3 iodothyronine deiodinase), which inactivates thyroid hormone. Infants with large, proliferating hemangiomas, especially hepatic hemangiomas, should be monitored for symptoms of hypothyroidism. Laboratory testing should be performed even if the newborn screen results were within normal limits because enzyme activity can increase during the proliferative phase of the hemangioma.

42. **What is a RICH?**
RICH is an acronym for a rapidly involuting congenital hemangioma.

43. **What is the difference between hemangioma of infancy and RICH?**
Hemangiomas of infancy can have precursor lesions present at birth but usually do not begin to proliferate until after 2 weeks of age. They proliferate for several months and slowly involute over years. Congenital hemangiomas are present more fully formed at birth. They undergo rapid involution, usually within 1–2 years, and are thus named *rapidly* involuting congenital

hemangiomas. There is also a subtype of congenital hemangiomas that do not involute and are therefore named non-involuting congenital hemangiomas (NICH).

44. **Which malignancies can mimic the appearance of a congenital hemangioma?**
Neuroblastoma, rhabdomyosarcoma, fibrosarcoma, primitive neuroectodermal tumor, liposarcoma, and lipoblastoma may all mimic the appearance of a hemangioma.

45. **What treatments have been used for problematic hemangiomas?**
Problematic hemangiomas include those that compromise vital functions, cause significant distortion or disfigurement of normal underlying structures, and have ulcerated or become infected. Treatment strategy varies depending on the clinical situation. Oral prednisone or prednisolone is the most commonly used treatment for problematic hemangiomas; the duration of treatment varies according to the age of the patient and the lesion. Intralesional injection of other types of corticosteroids may also be indicated. Vincristine or interferon-alpha have also been used to treat some patients with life-threatening hemangiomas. The use of interferon-alpha has been complicated by neurotoxicity (spastic diplegia). Other treatments for problematic hemangiomas include laser therapy, surgery, embolization, and cryotherapy.

46. **How should a child with a hemangioma located over the lumbosacral spine be evaluated?**
Hemangiomas in this location may be associated with underlying spinal cord anomalies (such as a tethered spinal cord), underlying bony defects, and anomalies of the genitourinary and gastrointestinal systems. For detection of a tethered cord, magnetic resonance imaging is the study of choice. See "Key Points" box to follow for additional cutaneous clues to underlying spinal cord abnormalities, and see Fig. 6-6 for a striking example of multiple congenital anomalies overlying the midline lumbrosacral spine.

KEY POINTS: MIDLINE LUMBOSACRAL CUTANEOUS CLUES TO AN UNDERLYING TETHERED CORD OR OCCULT SPINA BIFIDA

1. Sacral pits (particularly with lateral deviation of the gluteal cleft)

2. Hairy patches

3. Appendages (skin tag or tail)

4. Sacral lipoma

5. Vascular lesions (hemangioma, port-wine stain, telangiectases)

6. Pigmentation variants (hyperpigmentation, including lentigo and melanocytic nevus, and hypopigmentation)

7. Aplasia cutis congenita

47. **What is Kasabach-Merritt phenomenon? With which tumors is it associated?**
Kasabach-Merritt phenomenon/syndrome is a rare complication that occurs in infants with large vascular tumors. Patients usually present in the first few months of life with a rapidly enlarging vascular mass associated with profound thrombocytopenia and coagulopathy. It is a life-threat-

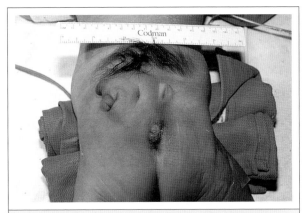

Figure 6-6. Multiple congenital anomalies located over the lumbosacral spine.

ening condition. In the past, this phenomenon was thought to be a complication of "garden variety" hemangiomas, but recent evidence indicates an association with rare vascular tumors such as the kaposiform hemangioendothelioma and the congenital tufted angioma.

48. **What is a lymphangioma?**

A lymphangioma is a vascular malformation composed of lymphatic tissue. These lesions are sometimes noted in the immediate newborn period or may become more prominent as a child grows. They do not regress spontaneously. A cystic hygroma is one type of lymphatic malformation that is composed of larger cystic spaces. It usually is apparent in the immediate newborn period and is located on the head and neck. Some patients with cystic hygroma have underlying genetic abnormalities such as Turner's syndrome.

49. **How is a port-wine stain capillary malformation treated?**

A port-wine stain is a malformation composed of small capillary and venular-sized vessels. As a child matures, the lesion may darken, thicken, and develop blebs. Pulsed dye laser therapy is the preferred method of treatment and may lead to significant lightening in many patients. Multiple treatments are usually required.

50. **When should Sturge-Weber syndrome be considered in a child with facial port-wine stain? What are the characteristic findings in Sturge-Weber syndrome?**

Approximately 10% of children with a port-wine stain in the distribution of the ophthalmic branch of the trigeminal nerve have findings of Sturge-Weber syndrome. Sturge-Weber syndrome is characterized by seizures (onset usually occurs in patients younger than 2 years old), hemiplegia, mental retardation, and glaucoma. However, in infancy many of these findings may not be present or may be difficult to discern. Similarly, a computed tomography or magnetic resonance imaging scan in infancy may not show the characteristic calcification, cerebral atrophy, or abnormalities of the cortex and white matter. However, an enlarged choroid plexus or increased myelination may be present early in the course of Sturge-Weber syndrome. Neonates with a port-wine stain in that distribution should have an urgent eye examination to assess for possible glaucoma.

51. **What is epidermolysis bullosa?**

Epidermolysis bullosa is a heterogeneous group of inherited disorders characterized by skin fragility and blistering (Fig. 6-7). The majority of patients develop symptoms in the newborn period. The most common types are epidermolysis bullosa simplex, junctional epidermolysis

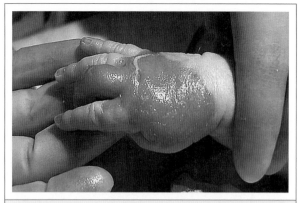

Figure 6-7. Epidermolysis bullosa.

bullosa, and dystrophic epidermolysis bullosa. Within each subset there are different clinical phenotypes. It is now understood that these diseases are caused by an inability to synthesize proteins that play an important role in maintaining the skin's integrity. Epidermolysis bullosa simplex is caused by mutations in keratins located in the basal layer of the epidermis; junctional epidermolysis bullosa is caused by defects in the protein laminin 5 and other proteins at the dermal-epidermal junction, and dystrophic epidermolysis bullosa is caused by a defect in collagen VII. There is no cure for these conditions, and treatment is supportive.

52. **What are the basic principles of skin care for children with epidermolysis bullosa?**
Skin trauma (rubbing, chafing) should be avoided, because the skin will likely blister at the site. Tape should not be applied directly to the skin. New skin blisters should be ruptured with a sterile needle or lancet (to prevent them from enlarging) and dressed with a topical antibiotic and nonadherent dressing such as plain petrolatum gauze. The blisters need to be monitored closely because superinfection may be a complication. Infants with severe forms of epidermolysis bullosa are at risk for nutritional deficiencies, poor weight gain, and anemia.

53. **Define congenital melanocytic nevus.**
A congenital melanocytic nevus is usually defined as a melanocytic lesion that is present at birth. The incidence is reported to be 0.5–2%.

54. **What are some complications of congenital melanocytic nevi?**
Congenital melanocytic nevi are often subdivided according to their size. Melanoma has been reported to arise within congenital lesions, but the exact risk for this complication is controversial. It is known that large lesions carry the greatest risk and that melanoma, when it occurs, does so earlier in life. In large congenital melanocytic nevi, the incidence is reported to be between 4.6% and 14%. One prospective study reported a 5-year cumulative risk of 4.5% compared with that in the general population. Leptomeningeal melanosis is a rare complication that may occur in association with a giant congenital nevus located over the head, neck, or spine or multiple (>3) congenital nevi.

55. **An infant is born at 29 weeks' gestation. Name five clinical problems that may be related to immature skin barrier function in this baby.**
The skin of premature infants is immature and has compromised barrier function (Fig. 6-8). Clinical consequences include increased transepidermal water loss, fluid and electrolyte

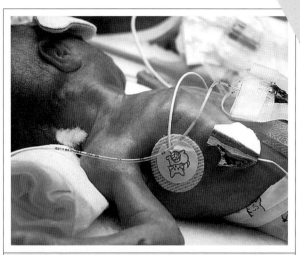

Figure 6-8. Premature infant skin. The skin is very translucent-appearing, and blood vessels are readily apparent.

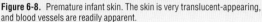

disturbances, temperature instability, infection (cutaneous and systemic), absorption of substances applied to the skin, and susceptibility to mechanical, chemical, and thermal stresses.

56. **Approximately when will an infant born at 30 weeks' gestation have skin barrier function equivalent to that of an adult?**
Most premature infants exhibit rapid maturation of skin barrier function over the first 2–3 weeks of life. In infants of <25 weeks' gestation, skin barrier function may require 8 weeks or longer after birth to mature.

57. **Methemoglobinemia is a potential toxic side effect of topical application of which preparations?**
Prilocaine, resorcinol, aniline dyes, and methylene blue.

58. **Which endocrine side effect has been reported after topical application of povidone-iodine on newborn, especially preterm, skin?**
Hypothyroxinemia and goiter.

59. **What are the toxic side effects of topical alcohol in the neonate?**
Hemorrhagic necrosis, especially on occluded skin, and neurotoxicity.

60. **What side effect can be caused by topical application of moisturizer containing lactic acid to infant skin?**
Metabolic acidosis.

61. **Two weeks into a neonatal intensive care unit course, an infant born at 27 weeks' gestation develops two superficial erosions on the anterior trunk. Subsequently, these heal with a brownish, wrinkled appearance. What is the diagnosis? What is the cause?**
Skin injury may accompany routine care of very premature infants. *Anetoderma of prematurity* is the term for focal depressions or outpouchings, which are presumed to be a response to mechanical or thermal injury to the skin.

62. **What infection should be considered in a premature infant developing pustules around a tape site (as used around an armboard for stabilization of an intravenous tube)?**
Although bacteria, especially *Staphylococcus* and *Streptococcus* species, should always be considered as a cause of cutaneous pustules, tape sites have been associated with opportunistic fungal infections of the skin, especially involving *Aspergillus* species. Other fungi and yeast, including *Rhizopus* and *Candida* organisms, should also be considered. Performing a biopsy and culture is a standard approach to diagnosis.

WEBSITES

Online Mendelian Inheritance in Man (OMIM)

http://www.ncbi.nlm.nih.gov/entrez/query.fcgi?db=OMIM

Dermatology Atlas

http://dermatlas.med.jhmi.edu/derm

Society for Pediatric Dermatology

http://www.pedsderm.net

Foundation for Ichthyosis and Related Skin Types (FIRST)

http://www.scalyskin.org

BIBLIOGRAPHY

1. Eichenfield LF, Frieden IJ, Esterly NB: Textbook of Neonatal Dermatology. Philadelphia, W.B. Saunders, 2001.
2. Fine J, Eady RAJ, Bauer EA, et al: Revised classification system for inherited epidermolysis bullosa: Report of the second international consensus meeting on diagnosis and classification of epidermolysis bullosa. J Am Acad Dermatol 42:1051–1066, 2000.
3. Harper J, Oranje A, Prose N (eds): Textbook of Pediatric Dermatology. Oxford, Blackwell Science, 2000.

4. Huang SA, Tu HM, Harney JW, et al: Severe hypothyroidism caused by type 3 iodothyronine deiodinase in infantile hemangiomas. N Engl J Med 343:185–189, 2000.

5. Mancini AJ: Skin. Pediatrics 113:1114–1119, 2004.

6. Metry DW, Hawrot A, Altman C, Frieden IJ: Association of solitary, segmental hemangiomas of the skin with visceral hemangiomatosis. Arch Dermatol 140:591–596, 2004.

7. Niamba P, Weill FX, Sarlangue J, et al: Is neonatal cephalic pustulosis (neonatal acne) triggered by *Malassezia sympodialis*? Arch Dermatol 134:995–998, 1998.

8. Resnick SD: Staphylococcal and streptococcal skin infections: Pyodermas and toxin-mediated syndromes. In Harper J, Oranje A, Prose N (eds): Textbook of Pediatric Dermatology. Oxford, Blackwell Science, 2000, pp 369–383.

9. Schachner LA, Hansen RC. Pediatric Dermatology, 3rd ed. New York, Mosby, 2003.

CHAPTER 7

ENDOCRINOLOGY AND METABOLISM

Mary Pat Gallagher, MD, Wendy K. Chung, MD, PhD, and Sharon E. Oberfield, MD

HYPOCALCEMIA

1. **What perinatal factors are associated with hypocalcemia in the immediate newborn period?**
   - Prematurity
   - Asphyxia
   - Maternal diabetes
   - Maternal hyperparathyroidism
   - Transient congenital hypoparathyroidism
   - Congenital absence or hypoplasia of the parathyroid glands (sporadic or as part of DiGeorge syndrome)

2. **How are calcium levels expected to change in premature infants during the first few days of life?**
   In newborn infants, there is a physiologic decline in serum total and ionized calcium during the first 48 hours of life. This decline is exaggerated in preterm infants compared with term infants, with a direct correlation between serum calcium and gestational age (Fig. 7-1). Because no symptoms are specific for early hypocalcemia in preterm infants, the diagnosis is made by demonstrating a serum calcium level <17.0 mg/dL (1.75 mmol/L).

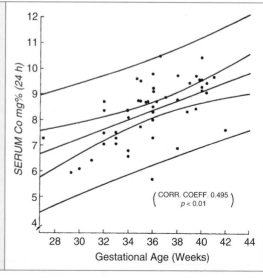

Figure 7-1. Serum calcium in relation to gestational age at 24 hours of age. (From Tsang RC, Light IJ, Sutherland JM, Kleinman LI. Possible pathogenetic factors in neonatal hypocalcemia of prematurity. J Pediatr 82:423–429, 1973.)

3. **Is treatment of hypocalcemia necessary in premature infants?**
   Arguing against the need for the treatment of incidentally noted hypocalcemia in the preterm infant are the following:
   - Hypocalcemia of prematurity is usually asymptomatic.
   - It resolves spontaneously.
   - Long-term follow-up studies have shown no benefit with treatment.
   - Total serum calcium level is a poor predictor of ionized serum calcium in premature infants.
   - IV calcium is associated with complications such as cardiac arrhythmias and ulcerations due to soft tissue infiltration of the infusate.

   In addition, calcium therapy may block the normal physiologic adaptation to hypocalcemia in premature infants, which includes increasing serum levels of parathyroid hormone (PTH) and $1,25(OH)_2$ vitamin D in the first few days of life.

   Loughead JL, Tsang RC: Neonatal calcium and phosphorus metabolism. In Cowett RM (ed): Principles of Perinatal-Neonatal Medicine. New York, Springer-Verlag, 1998, pp 879–908.

4. **When is treatment of hypocalcemia recommended in premature infants?**
   In the absence of additional data, it is conventional to treat all serum calcium levels < 6.0 mg/dL, even in asymptomatic neonates. The addition of 200 mg/kg/day of 10% calcium gluconate to standard intravenous (IV) solutions provides 20 mg/kg/day of elemental calcium. If symptoms are present (especially cardiac arrhythmia or seizures), a bolus of 100 mg/kg of 10% calcium gluconate (10 mg/kg elemental calcium) may be given intravenously over 10 minutes with careful cardiac monitoring.

KEY POINTS: HYPOCALCEMIA

1. Neonatal hypocalcemia is associated with prematurity, asphyxia, maternal diabetes, transient hypoparathyroidism, permanent congenital hypothyroidism, and rarely, maternal hyperparathyroidism.

2. The most common reason for hypocalcemia in the newborn period is prematurity.

3. Breast milk rickets is seen in premature infants due to the relatively low mineral (e.g., calcium and phosphorus) content of breast milk.

4. Serum calcium levels are frequently elevated in patients with Williams syndrome.

5. Normal magnesium levels are needed for optimal functioning of the parathyroid glands.

5. **How can the calcium requirements for premature infants be met by oral feedings?**
   Recent studies in premature infants using stable isotopes of calcium showed a true calcium absorption rate of 50–90%. Thus, to meet an accretion rate of 100 mg/kg/day with an absorption rate of 75% and an assumed retention rate of 75% (which may be on the high side), oral intake of calcium for growing premature infants should be about 200 mg/kg/day. This large intake in infants with very low birth weight can be achieved only with special formulas for low-birth-weight infants or mineral fortifiers for breast milk–fed preterm infants.

   Tsang RC, Lucas A, Uauy R, et al (eds): Nutritional Needs of the Preterm Infant. Baltimore, Williams & Wilkins, 1993.

6. **How can the calcium requirements for premature infants be met by hyperalimentation solutions?**
   This problem is much more difficult to address, although intestinal absorption is not a factor. In the early weeks of life with fluid intakes of 150 mg/kg/day, it is difficult to exceed an IV calcium

intake of 60 mg/kg/day in the smallest premature infants (weight < 1000 gm) with standard total parenteral nutrition (TPN) solutions. When the concentration of calcium exceeds 60 mg/dL (3 mEq/dL) in TPN solutions, precipitation with phosphate may occur, depending on variables such as temperature, pH, amino acid content, and even how the nutrients are added to the solution.

7. **What is the pathophysiology of "breast milk rickets" in premature infants?**
Clinical rickets develops in preterm infants with very low birth weight who are fed human milk not fortified with minerals and vitamins. Typically, the disease presents after 8 weeks of life with severe hypophosphatemia, "relative hypercalcemia," and hypercalciuria. The x-ray findings mimic those of rickets due to vitamin D deficiency. The biochemical findings are the result of low mineral intake. Because human milk is low in both calcium and phosphorus, the very low phosphorus intake (about 50% of calcium intake) severely limits deposition of calcium in bone.
   Caution: Because treatment with phosphorus alone can result in severe hypocalcemia, supplements of both minerals are imperative.

8. **What is the differential diagnosis of the etiology of a hypocalcemic seizure in a 14-day-old, term infant?**
Seizures secondary to hypocalcemia are very unlikely in a previously healthy, term infant at 2 weeks of age. The differential diagnosis includes congenital hypomagnesemia (rare), late infantile tetany associated with high phosphate load (e.g., feedings with cow milk), and acid-base disturbances caused by diarrhea treated with alkali therapy.

9. **What is the appropriate therapy for a hypocalcemic seizure in a 14-day-old, term infant?**
Treatment of hypocalcemic seizures is the same for both premature and term infants. In general, 10% calcium gluconate containing 9.4 mg/mL of elemental calcium is the drug of choice. The usual dose of 2 mL/kg body weight (18 mg/kg of elemental calcium) should be given in a peripheral vein over the course of 10 minutes with heart rate monitoring. Make sure the venous line is patent before infusing calcium.

HYPERCALCEMIA

10. **How many fractions of calcium are found in the serum? Which can be measured in the clinical laboratory?**
There are three fractions of calcium in serum: ionized calcium (50%), calcium bound to serum proteins (40%), and calcium complexed to serum anions (10%). Ionized calcium and total calcium can be measured in most hospital laboratories.

11. **What are the normal serum calcium values in term infants?**
Normal values (in milligrams per deciliter, expressed as mean and range) depend on chronologic age and laboratory variation (to a lesser degree):
   - **Cord:** 9.34 (8.2–11.1)
   - **5 hours:** 8.38 (7.3–9.2)
   - **11 hours:** 8.22 (6.9–10.2)
   - **24 hours:** 7.7 (6.2–9.0)
   - **48 hours:** 7.94 (5.9–9.7)

12. **What are the normal serum values in preterm infants?**
As in term infants, normal values (in milligrams per deciliter, expressed as mean ± standard deviation and range) depend on chronologic age:
   - **1 week:** 9.2 ± 1.1 (6.1–11.6)
   - **3 weeks:** 9.6 ± 0.5 (8.1–11.0)
   - **5 weeks:** 9.4 ± 0.5 (8.6–10.5)
   - **7 weeks:** 9.5 ± 0.7 (8.6–10.8)

13. **List the manifestations of hypercalcemia in neonates.**
    - Lethargy
    - Irritability
    - Polyuria
    - Vomiting
    - Constipation
    - Failure to thrive

14. **What values "define" hypercalcemia in newborn infants?**
    Total serum calcium > 10.8 mg/dL or ionized serum calcium > 5.4 mg/dL.

15. **What are some of the causes of hypercalcemia in neonates?**
    - Iatrogenic hypercalcemia
    - Subcutaneous fat necrosis
    - Idiopathic infantile hypercalcemia
    - Williams syndrome
    - Hyperparathyroidism (primary and secondary)
    - PTH-related peptide tumor
    - Hyperprostaglandin E syndrome
    - Hypophosphatasia
    - Familial hypercalciuric hypercalcemia
    - Blue diaper syndrome
    - Thyrotoxicosis
    - Vitamin A intoxication
    - Chronic thiazide toxicity
    - Excessive maternal intake of vitamin D

16. **How is acute hypercalcemia managed in newborn infants?**
    - Promote diuresis by administering IV fluids (normal saline).
    - Administer furosemide, and monitor serum electrolytes carefully.
    - Hydrocortisone (1 mg/kg every 6 hours) is of value only in chronic situations to reduce intestinal absorption of calcium.
    - In severe cases, dialysis may be required to lower calcium levels while the patient is awaiting definitive treatment of the underlying cause.
      Calcitonin cannot be recommended because of insufficient data. There are rare case reports of the successful use of bisphosphonate therapy in the neonatal period.

    Bachrach LK, Lum CK: Etidronate in subcutaneous fat necrosis of the newborn. J Pediatr 135:530–531, 1999.

17. **A 3-day-old infant born small for gestational age at term has a total serum calcium level of 13.2 mg/dL. She was delivered by emergency cesarean section and was diagnosed with supravalvular aortic stenosis. What is the likely diagnosis?**
    Williams syndrome is the likely diagnosis in an infant with hypercalcemia and supravalvular stenosis who was born small for gestational age. Affected infants are often described as having "elfin" facies.

18. **A term infant is incidentally noted to have a calcium level of 12.2 mg/dL at 4 days of age. Family history reveals that the father has also been evaluated for elevated calcium levels. What would you expect to find on measurement of the infant's urinary calcium level? What is the most likely diagnosis? What is the appropriate therapy?**
    The most likely diagnosis is an autosomal-dominant mutation of the calcium sensing receptor, or "hypocalciuric hypercalcemia." The infant's urinary calcium level will be inappropriately low for the serum calcium. In the heterozygous state, this is generally thought to be a benign

condition, and treatment is not indicated. Rare cases of homozygous mutations result in severe neonatal hyperparathyroidism, which is a life-threatening disorder.

Hsu SC, Levine MA: Perinatal calcium metabolism: Physiology and pathophysiology. Semin Neonatol 9:23–36, 2004.

19. **Why is the diaper blue in blue diaper syndrome?**
A defect in the intestinal transport of tryptophan causes excretion of blue, water-insoluble tryptophan metabolites. It is not well understood why these children have high calcium levels.

HYPOMAGNESEMIA AND HYPERMAGNESEMIA

20. **How are millimoles (mmol) of magnesium converted to milliequivalents (mEq) and milligrams (mg)?**

$$1 \text{ mmol} = 2 \text{ mEq} = 24 \text{ mg. Therefore, } 1 \text{ mEq of magnesium} = 12 \text{ mg.}$$

21. **What two types of magnesium reactions are important in human physiology?**
Intracellular and extracellular.

22. **What are the important intracellular reactions?**
Magnesium is the second most abundant intracellular cation after potassium and helps to regulate cellular metabolism. As part of the magnesium-adenosine triphosphate complex, it is essential for all biosynthetic processes, including glycolysis, formation of cyclic adenosine monophosphate, and transmission of the genetic code. In addition, any reaction that uses or produces energy requires magnesium.

23. **What are the important extracellular reactions?**
Only 1% of magnesium is contained in extracellular fluid. However, extracellular concentrations are critical for maintenance of electric potentials of nerve and muscle membranes and for the transmission of impulses across the neuromuscular junction. Magnesium and calcium may act synergistically or antagonistically in many of these processes.

24. **What causes magnesium depletion in neonates?**
- Maternal diabetes
- Maternal magnesium deficiency
- Renal losses of magnesium in acidotic states
- Use of nutrient solutions containing insufficient amounts of magnesium
- Renal tubular defects
- Intestinal wasting of magnesium (rare X-linked condition)
- Gastrointestinal losses (through emesis, nasogastric suctioning, and diarrhea)
- Prematurity, which increases the risk for magnesium deficiency
- Intrauterine growth retardation

Rubin LP: Neonatal disorders of serum magnesium. In Taeusch HW, Ballard RA (eds): Avery's Diseases of the Newborn, 7th ed. Philadelphia, W.B. Saunders, 1998, pp 1189–1206.

25. **Discuss the signs and symptoms of magnesium deficiency in neonates.**
Most infants are asymptomatic. On rare occasions, the following signs and symptoms may be seen:
- **Color:** Pallor, cyanosis, or duskiness
- **Affect:** Out of touch with surroundings, apathetic, irritable when disturbed, restless
- **Eyes:** Staring with infrequent blinking, oculogyric crises
- **Heart:** Tachycardia (bradycardia during apneic episodes)

- **Respiration:** Brief apnea, sometimes followed by tachypnea
- **Neuromuscular system:** Motor weakness, transient spasticity, abnormal reflexes; if hypocalcemia develops (see below), the infant may show signs associated with calcium deficiency, including seizures

26. **Describe the effects of hypomagnesemia on calcium homeostasis.**
Hypomagnesemia usually increases the secretion of PTH, thereby increasing calcium levels. In chronic magnesium-deficient states, however, secretion of PTH is reduced. In such circumstances, hypomagnesemia may induce hypocalcemia.

27. **What causes hypermagnesemia in neonates?**
   - Maternal treatment with magnesium (for preeclampsia or tocolysis)
   - Excessive magnesium administration to neonate (e.g., TPN, antacids, treatment of pulmonary hypertension)

28. **How should hypomagnesemia be treated parenterally?**
   - Hypomagnesemia usually is treated intravenously or intramuscularly with a 50% solution of magnesium sulfate.
   - One milliliter of a 50% solution contains 4 mEq of elemental magnesium. The usual dose is 0.1–0.25 mL/kg/day.
   - Serum magnesium levels should be monitored every 12 hours.

29. **List the signs of hypermagnesemia in neonates.**
   - Flaccidity
   - Unresponsiveness
   - Respiratory insufficiency
   - Apnea
   - Ileus
   - Delayed passage of meconium
   In extreme cases, cardiorespiratory function ceases and death ensues.

30. **How is hypermagnesemia treated?**
   - Stop the administration of magnesium.
   - Make sure the infant is well hydrated.
   - Consider diuretic therapy.
   - In severe cases, exchange transfusion (with acid-citrate-dextrose solution) is effective.
   - The effects of calcium salts are equivocal.

THYROID DISORDERS

31. **What is the incidence of congenital hypothyroidism?**
One in 4000 liveborn infants.

32. **What are the embryonic stages of development of the fetal hypothalamic-pituitary-thyroid axis?**
   - Thyroid tissue is first identified at the base of the tongue 16–17 days after conception.
   - By 7 weeks' gestation, the gland has migrated to its final position in the anterior neck and has developed its characteristic bilobed structure.
   - By 10 weeks' gestation, the fetal thyroid gland is trapping iodine and synthesizing thyroxine (T_4).
   - By 10 weeks' gestation, the fetal hypothalamus is synthesizing thyrotropin-releasing hormone (TRH). Most fetal TRH, however, is made in extrahypothalamic tissues (e.g., placenta, pancreas). Hypothalamic TRH production does not mature fully until the perinatal period.

- By 10–12 weeks' gestation, the fetal pituitary gland is synthesizing thyroid-stimulating hormone (TSH).

Fisher DA, Dussault JH, Sack J, Chopra IJ: Ontogenesis of hypothalamic-pituitary-thyroid function and metabolism in man, sheep and rat. Rec Prog Hormone Res 33:59–116, 1977.

33. **When does the fetal hypothalamic-pituitary-thyroid axis begin to function?**
The hypothalamic-pituitary-thyroid axis is in place by the end of the first trimester. The thyroid and pituitary glands reach mature secretory capacity by 30–35 weeks of gestation. The feedback interrelationship among the units is fully established when hypothalamic TRH maturation is completed by 1–2 months after birth.

Fisher DA, Klein AH: Thyroid development and disorders of thyroid function in the newborn. N Engl J Med 304:706, 1981.

34. **Describe the pattern of secretion of T_4 during gestation.**
The amount of T_4 secreted by the fetal thyroid gland increases slowly until midgestation (20–24 weeks) when, stimulated by increasing amounts of TSH from the fetal pituitary, T_4 levels begin to increase more rapidly, reaching a normal adult level by about 30 weeks' gestation. Thereafter, T_4 increases slowly to high normal levels at term.

Fisher DA: Fetal thyroid function: Diagnosis and management of fetal thyroid disorders. Clin Obstet Gynecol 40:16–31, 1997.

35. **Describe the pattern of TSH secretion during gestation.**
The amount of circulating TSH begins to increase in midgestation (20 weeks) and reaches a peak level of approximately 15 µU/mL by 30 weeks' gestation. The TSH level then declines gradually to about 10 µU/mL at term.

36. **Do maternal TSH and maternal iodine cross the placenta?**
Maternal TSH does not cross the placenta, but maternal iodine crosses the placenta freely and is essential for the synthesis of thyroid hormones by the fetus.

37. **Do maternal T_3 and T_4 levels have any effect on the fetus?**
The placenta is a barrier to the passages of thyroid hormones and contains enzymes that break down maternal T_4 and T_3 into inactive metabolites. Only a small percentage of circulating maternal T_4 and very little (if any) T_3 reach the fetus. However, the amount of maternal T_4 that does cross the placenta is significant. During the first 10–12 weeks of gestation, all of the circulating T_4 in the fetus is from maternal sources; thus, early brain development depends on maternal hormone. Even after the fetus synthesizes its own T_4 in the second and third trimesters, maternal T_4 is essential for normal neurologic development, including neuronal proliferation and maturation, dendritic arborization, and synapse formation. It accounts for about 30% of fetal T_4 levels at term.

38. **What happens to TSH levels at parturition?**
Within 15–20 minutes after birth, the fetal pituitary releases a surge of TSH, probably in response to cooling. TSH reaches a peak of about 80 µU/mL in about 30 minutes, decreases rapidly over the first 24 hours of life, and then drops more gradually to levels comparable to normal adult levels by the end of the first 1–2 weeks of life.

39. **How does the TSH surge affect T_4 levels?**
Serum T_4 levels increase rapidly, reaching a peak level of about 17 µg/dL at 24 hours. T_4 then gradually decreases to levels at the upper limit of normal adult values over the first 4–5 weeks of life. Free T_4 levels follow the same pattern, reaching a peak of 3.5 ng/dL at 24–36 hours.

40. **How do levels of thyroid hormone differ in premature and term infants?**
    The levels of TRH, TSH, T4, free T_4, and T_3 are lower in premature infants than in term infants, and the postnatal surges of TSH and T_4, although qualitatively similar, are blunted. These differences are related directly to gestational age: the lower the gestational age, the lower the levels and responses of thyroid-related hormones (Table 7-1).

41. **What is hypothyroxinemia of prematurity?**
    The term refers to infants with low birth weight (30–35 weeks' gestation) or very low birth weight (<30 weeks' gestation), who have an even more attenuated rise in T_4, after which T_4 levels drop below cord levels in the first week of life. Then they rise gradually over 3–6 weeks to approach levels of term infants (Table 7-2).

42. **Should hypothyroxinemia of prematurity be treated?**
    The premature infant with low T_4 and *persistently elevated* TSH has either transient or permanent hypothyroidism and should be treated with T_4 until the nature of the condition becomes clear. However, whether premature infants with low T_4 and normal TSH should be treated remains controversial.

    Fisher DA: Hypothyroxinemia in premature infants: Is thyroxine treatment necessary? Thyroid 9:715–720, 1999.
    Fisher DA: Thyroid function in premature infants: The hypothyroxinemia of prematurity. Emerg Concepts Perinat Med 25:999–1014, 1998.

TABLE 7-1. SERUM THYROXINE (μg/dL) AT DIFFERENT GESTATIONAL AGES*

Time	30–31	31–33	34–35	36–37	Term
Cord	6.5 (1.0)	7.5 (2.1)	6.7 (1.2)	7.5 (2.8)	8.2 (1.8)
3–10 days	7.7 (1.8)	8.5 (1.9)	10.0 (2.4)	12.7 (2.5)	15.9 (3.0)
11–20 days	7.5 (1.8)	8.3 (1.6)	10.5 (1.8)	11.2 (2.9)	12.2 (2.0)

*Mean (standard deviation).
Adapted from Cuestas RA: Thyroid function in healthy premature infants. J Pediatr 92:963–967, 1978.

TABLE 7-2. THYROID FUNCTION IN INFANTS = 28 WEEKS' GESTATION*

Postnatal Age	T_4 (μg/dL)	T_3 (ng/dL)	TSH (μU/mL)
Birth	3.8 (1.5)	58.6 (26)	16 (8)
24 hours	3.1 (1.6)	71.6 (26)	16 (8)
72 hours	2.7 (1.5)	65.1 (39.1)	11 (5)
1 week	2.3 (1.2)	58.6 (19.5)	12 (7)
3 weeks	3.9 (1.8)	71.6 (26)	11 (4)
4 weeks	4.0 (1.8)	71.6 (26)	11 (6)
6 weeks	4.7 (2.2)	78.1 (13)	12 (6)

T_4 = thyroxine, T_3 = triiodothyronine, TSH = thyroid-stimulating hormone.
*Mean (standard deviation).
Adapted from Mercado M, Yu VYH, Francis I, et al: Thyroid function in very preterm infants. Early Hum Devel 16:134–141, 1988.

43. **Does breast-feeding provide needed T_4 to premature infants with an immature hypothalamic-pituitary-thyroid axis?**
   This question has not yet been answered. There are some case reports in the literature that suggest that breast-feeding delays the onset of hypothyroidism, but others argue against that finding.

44. **Why do we screen for congenital hypothyroidism?**
   Signs and symptoms of hypothyroidism are subtle at birth, and the characteristic appearance of cretinism may not be apparent for 3–4 months. The brain requires thyroid hormone for normal development until about 2–3 years of age, and deficiency of thyroid hormone during this period causes irreversible brain damage to an extent related directly to the length of time of the hypothyroidism. Thus, it is of vital importance to identify a hypothyroid infant as quickly as possible, even before clinical signs appear.

45. **When and how is thyroid screening done?**
   A heel-stick blood sample is taken at discharge or 3 days of life, whichever is earlier. In North America, T_4 is measured first; then TSH is measured in samples with the lowest 10–29% of T_4 results.
   American Academy of Pediatrics: Newborn screening for congenital hypothyroidism: Recommended guidelines. Pediatrics 91:1203–1209, 1993.

46. **List the causes of congenital hypothyroidism and give the incidence of each.**
   See Table 7-3.

47. **How does maternal Graves' disease affect the fetus and neonate?**
   The thyroid-stimulating immunoglobulins (TSIs) cross the placenta and may cause fetal thyrotoxicosis, resulting in goiter, tachycardia, rapid skeletal maturation, premature birth, and congestive heart failure. Long-term neurologic deficits may result because excessive T_4 reduces the neuronal proliferation.
   Only about 1 in 70 neonates born to thyrotoxic mothers exhibit clinical thyrotoxicosis. Such infants may show a phase of transient hypothyroidism due to antithyroid drugs (half-life, 2–3 days), then thyrotoxicosis resulting from maternal TSIs.

TABLE 7-3. CAUSES OF CONGENITAL HYPOTHYROIDISM AND INCIDENCE OF EACH

Cause	Incidence	Percent of Cases
Thyroid dysgenesis (aplasia, hypoplasia, ectopy)	1:4000	75
Thyroid dyshormonogenesis	1:30,000	10
Hypothalamic-pituitary hypothyroidism	1:100,000	5
Transient hypothyroidism (secondary to drugs or maternal antibodies, idiopathic)	1:40,000	10

From Fisher FA: Disorders of the thyroid in the newborn and infant. In Sperling MA (ed): Pediatric Endocrinology. Philadelphia, W.B. Saunders, 1996, p 57.

48. **How may treatment of maternal Graves' disease affect the fetus and neonate?**
    - Antithyroid drugs (e.g., propylthiouracil [PTU], methimazole) cross the placenta and may block the fetal thyroid, leading to fetal hypothyroidism.
    - Radioactive iodine crosses the placenta and ablates the fetal thyroid.
    - Beta-adrenergic agents (e.g., propranolol) cross the placenta and have been associated with intrauterine growth retardation, bradycardia, respiratory distress, and hypoglycemia.

49. **Is breast-feeding contraindicated in mothers with Graves' disease?**
    Methimazole and carbamazole are excreted into breast milk in quantities that may affect the infant adversely. If breast-feeding cannot be avoided, the infant should undergo thyroid function tests at weekly intervals to avoid potential hypothyroidism. PTU is not a contraindication to breast-feeding because only about 0.1% is excreted in breast milk.

50. **What are the signs of neonatal thyrotoxicosis?**
    - Goiter
    - Low birth weight with normal length
    - Proptosis
    - Periorbital edema
    - Hyperactivity, hyperirritability
    - Poor weight gain despite ravenous feeding
    - Frequent stooling

KEY POINTS: THYROID-RELATED DISORDERS

1. Hypothyroxinemia of prematurity is associated with a developmental immaturity of the hypothalamic-pituitary-thyroid axis and therefore should never be used as an explanation for low thyroid levels in the presence of an elevated TSH level.

2. Hypopituitarism in a neonate most often presents with hypoglycemia and may also cause hyponatremia, jaundice, micropenis, and undescended testes.

3. The most common cause of virilized external genitalia in a 46,XX infant is 21-hydroxylase deficiency.

4. The fetal hypothalamic-pituitary-thyroid axis is in place by the end of the first trimester but is not fully mature until 2 months postpartum (term).

5. Maternal T_4 does cross the placenta and is essential for the normal neurologic development of the fetus.

6. TSH and T_4 levels rise in both premature and term infants immediately after birth; however, the rise in premature infants is blunted.

7. Infants with neonatal thyrotoxicosis are at an increased risk for congestive heart failure and learning disorders.

51. **Does neonatal thyrotoxicosis require treatment?**
    Neonatal thyrotoxicosis normally is a self-limited disease that subsides by about 3 months of age when maternal TSIs are metabolized. However, tachycardia, irritability, and poor weight gain require treatment with low-dose PTU with or without propranolol. The danger of treatment is oversuppression of the neonatal thyroid and consequent hypothyroidism.

52. **How do iodide-containing medicines affect the fetal thyroid state?**
The mature thyroid stops synthesis of T_4 in the presence of excessive iodine (i.e., Wolff-Chaikoff effect) but escapes from this inhibition when intrathyroidal iodine pools are depleted. The fetal thyroid cannot "escape" the inhibition and develops into a goiter that can be large enough to require emergency transection at birth. In addition, the continued blockade of T_4 production by iodine leads to fetal hypothyroidism.

    Note: Premature infants are also unable to escape from the inhibitory effect of iodine and may become hypothyroid when subjected to multiple povidone-iodine washings or iodinated contrast agents. This is particularly important in infants who have required repeated procedures.

    Allemand D, Grüters A, Beyer P, Weber B: Iodine in contrast agents and skin disinfectants is the major cause for hypothyroidism in premature infants during intensive care. Hormone Res 28:42–49, 1987.

ADRENAL DISORDERS

53. **Which disorders of adrenal steroidogenesis should be suspected as a possible cause for virilization of a 46,XX fetus?**
    - **21-hydroxylase deficiency:** Manifestations depend on whether the deficiency is partial or complete. Partial deficiency results in virilization in females, and complete deficiency results in salt wasting and signs of cortisol deficiency (e.g., hypoglycemia, shock).
    - **11-hydroxylase deficiency:** Salt retention and hypertension are seen in 50–80% of cases, and virilization is seen in females.

54. **Which disorders of adrenal steroidogenesis should be suspected as a possible cause for undervirilization of a 46,XY fetus?**
    - Steroidogenic acute regulatory (StAR) protein deficiency (i.e., congenital adrenal lipid hyperplasia) leads to salt wasting and ambiguous genitalia in males.
    - 3-β-hydroxysteroid dehydrogenase deficiency results in salt wasting, mild virilization in females, and ambiguous genitalia in males.
    - 17-α-hydroxylase deficiency results in hypertension and ambiguous genitalia in males.

55. **In infants with congenital adrenal hyperplasia (CAH) due to 21-hydroxylase deficiency, which of the following is abnormal: (1) genetic sex, (2) gonadal differentiation, (3) internal genital formation and structure, or (4) external genitalia in females?**
The answer is (4). In females with CAH, the karyotype (genetic sex) is normal (46XX). The müllerian ducts develop normally into a uterus and fallopian tubes without secretion of antimüllerian hormone. No wolffian duct derivatives are formed because no fetal testis is present. The elevated adrenal androgen levels cause virilization of the external genitalia.

    http://www.sickkids.ca/childphysiology/cpwp/Genital/genitaldevelopment.htm

56. **List the sources of maternal androgens that cause masculinization.**
    - Androgen-secreting tumors
    - Ingestion of synthetic progestins, androgens, or danazol (a derivative of testosterone)

57. **A male fetus is exposed to maternal progestin at 10 weeks of gestation. What is the possible manifestation?**
Exposure of male fetuses to progestin at 8–14 weeks of gestation may result in hypospadias.

58. **What causes adrenal hemorrhage in neonates?**
Adrenal hemorrhage occurs more frequently after breech delivery, with eventual calcification in some cases. Hypoxia, fetal distress, maternal diabetes, and congenital syphilis also have been associated with adrenal hemorrhage.

59. **What are the manifestations of adrenal hemorrhage?**
Even with bilateral adrenal hemorrhage, most infants are asymptomatic. On occasion, however, severe abnormalities of glucose, sodium, and potassium may be noted, with signs of shock.

60. **Describe the evaluation of adrenal hemorrhage.**
The evaluation should include a 60-minute adrenocorticotropic hormone stimulation test with measurement of baseline and 60-minute cortisols. The normal peak is >20 μg/dL.

61. **A pregnant woman has a low urinary estriol level. At delivery, her male infant develops hyponatremia, hyperkalemia, and hypoglycemia. What diagnosis should you consider?**
Congenital adrenal hypoplasia. A low maternal estriol level occurs because the fetus contributes to the precursors for placental formation of maternal estriols.

62. **How common is congenital adrenal hypoplasia?**
Congenital adrenal hypoplasia is an X-linked disorder affecting 1 in 12,500 live births.
   http://www.ncbi.nlm.nih.gov/entrez/dispomim.cgi?id=300200

63. **With what other disorders may it be associated?**
   - Anencephaly
   - Pituitary hypoplasia
   - Gonadotropin deficiency

   Bassett JH, O'Halloran DJ, Williams GR, et al: Novel DAX1 mutations in X-linked adrenal hypoplasia congenita and hypogonadotrophic hypogonadism. Clin Endocrinol (Oxf) 50:69–75, 1999.

64. **What is StAR protein?**
StAR protein is necessary for proper reduction of aldosterone, cortisone, and sex hormones. Its absence leads to feminization of males as part of congenital lipoid adrenal hyperplasia. In a subset of patients with congenital lipoid adrenal hyperplasia, mutations in StAR protein result in severe impairment of steroid biosynthesis in the adrenal glands and gonads.

65. **What is the best time to obtain a cortisol level in premature neonates?**
Collect the blood specimen at any time. Circadian rhythms do not affect the level of cortisol in very premature infants. Infants with extremely low birth weight may have quite low cortisol levels (9.2 ± 9.8 μg/mL) and lack the typical early-morning rise in cortisol. Whether such low corticosteroid levels in premature infants with very low birth weight indicate adrenal insufficiency is not fully known.

   Metzger DL, Wright NM, Veldhuis JD, et al: Characterization of pulsatile secretion and clearance of plasma cortisol in premature and term neonates using deconvolution analysis. J Clin Endocrinol Metab 77:458–463, 1993.

66. **What is pseudohypoaldosteronism?**
Pseudohypoaldosteronism is an inherited disease (autosomal recessive or dominant pattern) characterized by renal tubular unresponsiveness to the kaliuretic and sodium and chloride reabsorptive effects of aldosterone. In contrast to CAH or adrenal insufficiency, it is accompanied by excessive levels of renin and aldosterone. Unresponsiveness to aldosterone may be generalized, in which case sodium excretion is increased in sweat, saliva, stool, and urine, or limited to the renal tubule, in which case sodium excretion is increased in urine only.

67. **How is pseudohypoaldosteronism treated?**
With salt supplementation and potassium-lowering agents such as Kayexalate (sodium polystyrene sulfonate).

KEY POINTS: ADRENAL DISORDERS

1. CAH due to 21-hydroxylase deficiency is the most common cause of ambiguous genitalia in a 46,XX newborn.

2. Even with bilateral adrenal hemorrhage, adrenal function is usually preserved.

3. Newborn infants lack established circadian rhythms for cortisol secretion.

PITUITARY DISORDERS

68. **When does growth hormone first appear in fetal plasma?**
At 10 weeks' gestation. Levels increase in midgestation and decrease toward term.

69. **Does placental growth hormone contribute to fetal levels?**
No. Placental growth hormone is secreted only into the maternal circulation.

70. **When does the hypothalamic-pituitary-gonadal axis develop in the fetus?**
Gonadotropin-releasing hormone is detectable in the hypothalamus at 8 weeks' gestation. Luteinizing hormone and follicle-stimulating hormone are present in the pituitary gland by 11–12 weeks' gestation, and at term are found in low levels in cord blood. The fetal testis responds to human chorionic gonadotropin (hCG), but the fetal ovary does not respond because it lacks hCG receptors.

71. **What manifestations of adrenocorticotropic hormone insufficiency are seen in neonates?**
   - Hypoglycemia
   - Hyponatremia (without hyperkalemia)
   - Direct hyperbilirubinemia

72. **What are the symptoms of growth hormone deficiency in neonates?**
The most common presenting symptom is hypoglycemia. Micropenis is also common in male neonates. Jaundice may be present for a prolonged period. Because growth hormone is not necessary for intrauterine linear growth, intrauterine growth retardation is not a feature of growth hormone deficiency.
   Palma Sisto PA: Endocrine disorders in the neonate. Pediatr Clin North Am 51:1141–1168, 2004.

KEY POINTS: PITUITARY DISORDERS

1. Hypoglycemia and microphallus are commonly presenting symptoms and signs of neonatal hypopituitarism.

2. Midline facial defects are associated with pituitary hormone deficiencies.

3. Placental growth hormone is secreted only into the maternal circulation.

73. **What are the typical findings in neonates with hypogonadotropic hypogonadism (HHG)?**
In male neonates, HHG is associated with micropenis (stretched penile length < 2.5 cm). Undescended testes also may be present. In female neonates, there are no clinical findings of HHG.

74. **What major malformations may be associated with disorders of the hypothalamic-pituitary axis in neonates?**
Cleft lip and palate, optic nerve atrophy, septo-optic dysplasia, and holoprosencephaly.

Traggiai C, Stanhope R: Endocrinopathies associated with midline cerebral and cranial malformations. J Pediatr 140:252–255, 2002.

INTERSEX DISORDERS

75. **What is the initial gene thought to be responsible for differentiation of the bipotential gonad into the testis?**
Sex-determining region of Y-chromosome (SRY) is thought to be the first in a cascade of transcription factors that initiate the process of testicular development. SRY is located on the short arm of the Y chromosome, and the gonad loses bipotentiality at approximately 6–8 weeks' gestation. In the absence of SRY expression, the bipotential gonad will develop into an ovary.

76. **What two hormones, produced by the testes in utero, result in a phenotypic male?**
Testosterone is produced by Leydig cells within the fetal testes by 6 weeks of gestation. In addition, the testes produce the peptide hormone, *müllerian inhibitory substance* (MIS), which eliminates all müllerian structures in the male. An isolated deficiency in MIS produces a normal external male phenotype, but the internal phenotype is characterized by a fallopian tube running parallel to the vas deferens.

77. **What causes the XX male sex reversal syndrome?**
There are a number of cases of 46,XX sex reversal in the literature. Only a minority of these cases have been shown to have been caused by translocation of SRY. At least one case of SOX9 duplication (a transcription factor downstream of SRY) has been reported. The majority of cases are unexplained at this time.

Huang B, Wang S, Ning Y, et al: Autosomal XX sex reversal caused by duplication of SOX9. Am J Med Genet 87:349–353, 1999.

78. **You are asked to assess a neonate with nonpalpable gonads and genital ambiguity (i.e., severe hypospadias and an intermediate-sized phallic structure). What is the most likely diagnosis? Why?**
The most likely diagnosis is CAH because it is the most common intersex diagnosis and because no gonadal tissue is palpable. Other diagnoses, such as mixed gonadal dysgenesis or hermaphroditism, generally present with one palpable gonad.

79. **Which *one* serum test has the greatest chance of confirming the correct diagnosis?**
Several steps leading to cortisol synthesis may be affected and produce the virilized female phenotype. The most likely missing enzyme is 21-hydroxylase, and the result is a major accumulation of its immediate precursor, 17-hydroxyprogesterone. A serum radioimmunoassay for 17-hydroxyprogesterone should be diagnostic in approximately 90% of cases. In the remaining 8–9%, a serum radioimmunoassay for deoxycortisone establishes the missing 11-hydroxylase activity. It is reasonable to send serum for both radioimmunoassays. If both assays yield negative results, further studies may be ordered.

80. **A neonate presents with severe penoscrotal hypospadias and a palpable gonad in the left hemiscrotum; the right hemiscrotum is empty. Amniocentesis shows a classic 46,XX karyotype, and ultrasound shows a cystic structure behind the bladder but no uterus. The genitogram shows**

a vagina with low insertion and a tiny atretic uterine cavity. What is the differential diagnosis?

The two most likely diagnoses are mixed gonadal dysgenesis and true hermaphroditism. The combination of a descended gonad and virilization indicates the presence of some functional testicular tissue. An ovary usually does not descend into the scrotum, and an ovotestis does so only in rare cases. In mixed gonadal dysgenesis, one gonad is a streak found within the abdomen, and one testis descends into an inguinal or scrotal position. True hermaphroditism is characterized by a combination of both ovarian-follicular and testicular tissue, which may be combined within one testis (ovotestis). The rudimentary vagina and uterus reflect inadequate production of MIS despite the presence of some testicular tissue. Because the action of MIS is also paracrine, the vaginal and uterine structures are lateralized primarily to the side opposite the testis.

81. **A neonate presents with genital ambiguity, including significant clitoromegaly and a palpable gonad on the left side in a labioscrotal fold. The right gonad is palpable in the right inguinal canal. The infant's family recently migrated from the Dominican Republic. What is the most likely diagnosis?**

The most likely diagnosis is 5-alpha reductase deficiency, which was first characterized by its striking clinical presentation. Cases are clustered in the Dominican Republic, where the culture is extremely supportive.

82. **You are asked to evaluate a neonate in the delivery room. Amniocentesis during pregnancy revealed a 46,XY karyotype, but the infant has a perfectly normal female phenotypic appearance. What is the most likely diagnosis?**

Androgen insensitivity syndrome (AIS). Patients with AIS have a normal XY karyotype. The testes are fully developed but never descend, and the external genitalia are those of a normal female. Serum testosterone levels are markedly elevated, but no virilization takes place. Because of a mutation in the androgen receptor, androgen has no effect on its target tissues. AIS, in effect, is end-organ failure based on molecular mutation; it is a syndrome in the sense that several point mutations have been identified.

83. **What are the likely findings on pelvic examination?**

Absence of the uterus and upper two thirds of the vagina. These structures originate from the müllerian ducts, which involute in response to secretion of MIS. The testes are normal and produce normal amounts of testosterone and MIS.

84. **A male neonate in the intensive care unit has a right hernia and a left undescended testis. When the bulging hernia enlarges, intervention is recommended. The surgeon reports that a fallopian tube has been found in the hernia sac. What is the diagnosis?**

Hernia uteri inguinalis.

KEY POINTS: INTERSEX DISORDERS

1. Informative findings in narrowing the differential diagnosis in an infant with ambiguous genitalia are the presence or absence of palpable gonads and/or the presence or absence of a uterus.

2. MIS levels may be useful in documenting the presence of testicular tissue (Sertoli cells).

3. Complete androgen insensitivity is rarely diagnosed in infancy but may present in the newborn period when a phenotypically normal female infant is born after a prenatal karyotype of 46,XY has been documented on amniocentesis.

85. **What causes hernia uteri inguinalis?**

Absence of MIS, which is produced by the testis and results in involution of müllerian ducts during the course of normal male sexual differentiation. A normal-appearing testis that produces testosterone may lack the capacity to synthesize or secrete MIS. The result is a normal external prominent utricle.

http://www.ncbi.nlm.nih.gov/entrez/dispomim.cgi?id=261550

HYPOGLYCEMIA

86. **How is neonatal hypoglycemia defined?**

In adults, *hypoglycemia* is defined as a condition involving a plasma glucose level <40 mg/dL. A plasma glucose concentration of 70–100 mg/dL is considered normal, and the therapeutic target range for adults with hypoglycemia is >60 mg/dL. The definition in neonates is controversial. Some physicians accept significantly lower plasma glucose concentrations as normal for neonates. However, in the absence of scientific evidence that neonates tolerate lower concentrations than adults, many clinicians now believe that values <50 mg/dL are abnormal. This definition is supported by Koh et al., who demonstrated electrophysiologic changes in the brains of infants when glucose reaches 50 mg/dL.

87. **Why is glucose important?**

Glucose is the primary fuel for the brain and accounts for over 90% of total body oxygen consumption early in fasting. Because of their larger brain-to-body size ratio, infants have greater glucose requirements than adults. Hepatic glucose production rates in infants are approximately 6 mg/kg/min (3–6 times greater than those of adults).

88. **What causes hypoglycemia in neonates?**

Hypoglycemia results from either abnormal control of fasting adaptations or failure of a particular fasting metabolic system. In the first 12–24 hours of life, normal newborns are at increased risk for hypoglycemia because gluconeogenesis and especially ketogenesis are incompletely developed. Hypoglycemia occurring or persisting after the first 24 hours of life is abnormal and implies failure of one of the fasting systems.

89. **What physical features suggest the cause of hypoglycemia in neonates?**

- **Macrosomia:** Because insulin is a growth factor, hyperinsulinism leads to macrosomia. Infants of diabetic mothers and infants with severe forms of congenital hyperinsulinism typically are large for gestational age. In addition, neonates with Beckwith-Wiedemann syndrome are macrosomic and may have hyperinsulinism.
- **Midline defects:** Congenital pituitary deficiency may be associated with midline defects such as cleft lip, cleft palate, single central incisor, and micro-ophthalmia.
- **Micropenis:** Congenital gonadotropin deficiency can cause micropenis.
- **Hepatomegaly:** Glycogen storage diseases (GSDs) and fatty acid oxidation disorders may be associated with hepatomegaly.

90. **Which hormonal abnormalities cause hypoglycemia in neonates?**

- **Hyperinsulinism:** The most common cause of recurrent hypoglycemia in neonates
- **Hypopituitarism:** Combination of growth hormone, thyroid hormone, and cortisol deficiencies

91. **How is hypoglycemia treated acutely?**

Hypoglycemia can be treated emergently with oral or nasogastric tube feeding of dextrose or formula. If symptoms are severe, 200 mg/kg of dextrose (2 mL/kg of 10% dextrose) can be administered intravenously. Blood glucose should be checked within 15 minutes of intervention and subsequently monitored to ensure adequate treatment (plasma glucose > 60 mg/dL) and to prevent hypoglycemic episodes. If necessary, continuous IV dextrose is initiated (6–12 mg/kg/min).

92. **Which defects in fasting metabolic systems cause hypoglycemia in neonates?**
    - Defects of glycogenolysis (i.e., GSDs) are associated with hepatomegaly. Examples include deficiencies of debranching enzyme (GSD type 3), liver phosphorylase (GSD type 6), and phosphorylase kinase (GSD type 9).
    - Defects of gluconeogenesis include deficiencies of glucose-6-phosphatase (i.e., GSD type 1) and fructose-1,6-diphosphastase. Defects of gluconeogenesis and glycogenolysis rarely present in early infancy because neonates are not exposed to fasting for more than 4 hours at a time.
    - Fatty acid oxidation disorders include medium-chain acyl dehydrogenase deficiency. Unless a neonate is breast-feeding poorly or experiences an illness that limits oral intake, a fatty acid oxidation disorder is unlikely to present in infancy. This disorder, however, can cause serious problems during fasting later in life and should be tested for as part of neonatal screening.

93. **List and explain the hormonal controls necessary for fasting adaptation.**
    - **Insulin:** Inhibits fasting metabolic systems
    - **Epinephrine:** Stimulates hepatic glycogenolysis, hepatic gluconeogenesis, and hepatic keto-genesis
    - **Glucagon:** Stimulates hepatic glycogenolysis
    - **Cortisol:** Stimulates hepatic gluconeogenesis
    - **Growth hormone:** Stimulates lipolysis

94. **What tests should be included in the "critical sample" during a hypoglycemic episode?**
    Once hypoglycemia is confirmed (i.e., glucose ≤ 50 mg/dL), blood should be analyzed for the following:
    - Insulin
    - Free fatty acids
    - Growth hormone
    - Lactate/pyruvate
    - Bicarbonate
    - Ammonia
    - Ketones
    - Cortisol

95. **What causes transient hyperinsulinism?**
    Transient hyperinsulinism occurs in infants of diabetic mothers whose up-regulated insulin secretion in response to a hyperglycemic fetal environment persists in the immediate postnatal period. In perinatally stressed neonates (e.g., infants who are small for gestational age or have birth asphyxia or toxemia), hyperinsulinism due to dysregulated insulin secretion may persist for up to several months after birth.

96. **How is transient hyperinsulinism treated?**
    Initial management consists of IV dextrose and frequent or continuous feeds. In persistent cases, diazoxide (5–15 mg/kg/day) may be effective in controlling insulin secretion.

97. **What causes congenital hyperinsulinism?**
    Genetic defects of insulin secretion include recessive mutations of the β-cell sulfonylurea recep-tor/potassium channel genes and dominant gain of functional mutations of glucokinase and

glutamate dehydrogenase. Dominant functional mutations are milder and usually present later in infancy.

98. **What is the treatment for congenital hyperinsulinism?**
Congenital hyperinsulinism due to severe sulfonylurea receptor/potassium channel mutation is often resistant to diazoxide. Octreotide (a somatostatin analog) tempers excessive insulin secretion but rarely prevents hypoglycemia completely or normalizes fasting tolerance. Continuous glucagon infusion can stabilize blood glucose until surgery is performed, but experience with long-term use is limited. If the combination of octreotide and frequent feeds fails, pancreatectomy is necessary. Surgery may be curative if a focal lesion is present and completely resected.

Glaser B, Thornton P, Otonkoski T, Junien C: Genetics of neonatal hyperinsulinism. Arch Dis Child Fetal Neonatal Ed 82:79–86, 2000.

99. **What is the cornerstone of treatment for defects of glycogenolysis and gluconeogenesis?**
Frequent feedings.

KEY POINTS: HYPOGLYCEMIA

1. A work-up for hypoglycemia should be considered in any newborn who is documented to have a blood sugar level persistently less than 50 mg/dL.

2. The three common etiologies for hypoglycemia in a neonate are decreased production due to an inborn error of metabolism, increased utilization, and altered hormonal regulation.

3. An infant with hypoglycemia should be carefully examined for hepatomegaly, macroglossia, macrosomia, and midline abnormalities, including clefting defects.

4. The etiology of hypoglycemia is most readily identified by measuring metabolites and hormones at the time of hypoglycemia and should include measures of glucose, free fatty acids, ketones, lactate, pyruvate, ammonia, insulin, cortisol, and growth hormone. Abnormalities in any of these studies may then suggest definitive diagnostic studies.

5. Treatment of hypoglycemia depends on the etiology but may include avoidance of fasting, a diet altered to circumvent a metabolic block, insulin suppression with diazoxide or pancreatic resection, or replacing deficiency growth hormone or cortisol.

6. Abnormalities of both the β-cell sulfonylurea receptor and the potassium channel have been documented to cause congenital hyperinsulinism.

100. **How are fatty acid oxidation disorders treated?**
By instituting a high-carbohydrate diet (and for certain long-chain fatty acid oxidation disorders, metabolic diets high in medium-chain triglyceride) and by ensuring that fasting is limited to 12 hours. If an affected infant is feeding poorly or experiences vomiting, IV dextrose must be initiated emergently. The finding of euglycemia in the setting of a concurrent illness should not deter the clinician from initiating IV dextrose. By the time hypoglycemia is detected in fatty oxidation disorders, liver failure, cerebral edema, and cardiac toxicity are already present or developing. The mortality rate of >25% during a first episode dramatizes the need for prompt intervention.

NEONATAL SCREENING

101. **Routine neonatal screening commonly tests for which diseases?**
    - Hypothyroidism
    - Phenylketonuria (PKU)
    - Glucose-6-phosphate dehydrogenase (G6PD) deficiency
    - Galactosemia
    - Maple syrup urine disease (MSUD) (G6PD deficiency)
    - Biotinidase deficiency
    - Medium-chain acyl–coenzyme A (CoA) dehydrogenase
    - Homocystinuria
    - Sickle cell disease
    - CAH
    - Cystic fibrosis

    In an expanded neonatal screening, as many as 55 disorders can be tested for. Recent protocols from the American College of Medical Genetics recommends 29 disorders for which clinicians should screen during the neonatal period.

102. **Which of these groups of diseases is likely to be life-threatening in the neonatal period: (1) galactosemia, MSUD, and CAH; or (2) sickle cell disease, G6PD deficiency, and biotinidase deficiency?**
    The answer is (1). Galactosemia can cause acute liver failure promptly after institution of milk feedings. It also predisposes neonates to *Escherichia coli* septicemia. MSUD causes lethal depression of the function of the central nervous system in the neonatal period. Salt-losing CAH, caused by 21-hydroxylase deficiency, can cause addisonian crisis with hypovolemic/hyponatremic shock, hypoglycemia, and (most dangerous of all) severe hyperkalemia.

103. **In which of these groups of diseases is delayed or impaired development of the central nervous system expected if effective treatment is begun at 3 months of age: (1) PKU, hypothyroidism, MSUD, and galactosemia; or (2) PKU, hypothyroidism, and homocystinuria?**
    The answer is (1). Effective treatment of PKU, hypothyroidism, and MSUD must begin within the first few weeks of life to avoid significant problems in development. In infants with galactosemia, learning disabilities are quite prominent even if treatment is begun expectantly. Developmental disabilities are found in 50% of untreated homocystinuric patients, but the age by which treatment must begin is not known.

104. **In which of these groups of diseases may physical signs be present at or shortly after birth: (1) sickle cell disease, G6PD deficiency, and homocystinuria; (2) galactosemia and CAH; or (3) galactosemia, CAH, and PKU?**
    The answer is (2). Some infants affected by galactosemia have cataracts shortly after birth. The female infant with CAH due to 21-hydroxylase deficiency often has ambiguous genitalia (i.e., enlarged clitoris, labial fusion) at birth.

105. **What are the benefits of detecting sickle cell disease by neonatal screening?**
    Sickle cell disease presents at various ages and in various ways, but the major threat to life for small infants is bacterial sepsis, with *Streptococcus pneumoniae* high on the list of causative organisms. Preclinical detection of sickle cell disease allows prophylaxis against pneumococcal infection.

106. **A 5-day-old breast-fed infant has a strongly positive test result for urinary-reducing substance but a negative test result for urinary glucose. What action should be taken?**
    In breast-fed infants, the dietary carbohydrate is lactose, which is hydrolyzed during absorption to glucose and galactose, both reducing sugars. Therefore, a non–glucose-reducing substance

in the urine is almost certainly galactose, and its presence strongly suggests the diagnosis of galactosemia. Intake of lactose should be stopped immediately and not reinstituted until galactosemia has been ruled out by assay for red blood cell galactose-1-phosphate uridylyltransferase. Because galactosemia can be rapidly lethal, do not delay this decision until the result of the screening test is known.

107. How is newborn screening for cystic fibrosis performed?
It is a two-tiered test in which immunoreactive trypsinogen is first measured. Babies with the highest immunoreactive trypsinogen levels are then genetically tested for the most common mutations in cystic fibrosis transmembrane conductance regulator, including the most common ΔF508 mutation.

108. How is genetic testing used in newborn screening?
To increase the specificity of newborn screening for diseases with a common genetic etiology, a two-tiered test can be developed to screen for the disorder based on a metabolite or protein in the blood. The subset of newborns with the highest levels can then go on to genetic testing for the most common mutations to confirm the diagnosis genetically. This strategy has been commonly used for cystic fibrosis and medium-chain acyl-CoA dehydrogenase for which there are common mutations in the population.

KEY POINTS: NEONATAL SCREENING

1. New technologic advances in tandem mass spectrometry have revolutionized newborn screening and allow for detection of dozens of inborn errors of metabolism from blood spots.

2. Specimens should be collected after 24 hours of life and, with the exception of sickle cell disease and G6PD deficiency, should not be affected by transfusions.

3. DNA diagnostic tests are also being added to newborn screening regimens to increase the specificity of testing and reduce the number of false-positive results.

4. The majority of positive results from newborn screening are false positives, and repeat and/or additional diagnostic testing is required to distinguish true positives from false-positive results.

5. Treatment should be initiated as soon as the diagnosis is made and, for some conditions such as congenital hypothyroidism, PKU, and MSUD, permanent neurologic damage can result if treatment is delayed.

109. What new diagnostic method is being used in newborn screening to increase testing sensitivity and specificity, to decrease cost, and to increase the number of inborn errors of metabolism that can be effectively screened?
Tandem mass spectrometry (MS-MS) can be performed on dried blood spots and can measure hundreds of metabolites to facilitate screening of dozens of inborn errors of metabolism while more precisely quantitating the levels of the metabolites to improve screening sensitivity and specificity.

INBORN ERRORS OF METABOLISM

110. What clinical signs suggest metabolic disease in neonates?
- Lethargy and coma
- Recurrent vomiting

- Jaundice
- Dysmorphism
- Ocular abnormalities
- Marked hypotonia
- Seizures
- Unusual odors
- Visceromegaly
- Abnormalities of skin or hair
- Unstable body temperature
- Bleeding
- Tachypnea unrelated to pulmonary disease
  Note: The signs of metabolic disease are nonspecific. More common diseases such as sepsis must be considered in the differential diagnosis.

111. **If a neonate misses one or two feedings, is large ketonuria likely to develop?**
No. Large ketones usually are not detectable in the urine of normal newborn infants with fasting, including those with fasting-induced hypoglycemia. Conversely, ketonuria often is present in neonates with defects in gluconeogenesis and amino acid or organic acid metabolism. The rate of use of ketones as a fuel is greater in infants compared with children. Experimental data suggest that some inborn errors of metabolism may be associated with a secondary defect in ketone body use. Severe acidemia also may perturb the use of ketones.

112. **Which metabolic disorders are associated with a distinctive odor?**
- PKU
- Multiple CoA carboxylase deficiency
- MSUD
- b-Methylcrotonyl-CoA carboxylase deficiency
- Isovaleric acidemia
- Type II glutaric aciduria
- Type I tyrosinemia

113. **Which metabolic disorders are commonly associated with acidosis?**
- Methylmalonic acidemia
- Holocarboxylase synthetase deficiency
- Propionic acidemia
- Fructose 1,6-diphosphatase deficiency
- Isovaleric acidemia
- Succinyl CoA acetoacetate CoA transferase deficiency
- MSUD
- Primary lactic acidosis due to mitochondrial disorders
- Ketothiolase deficiency, pyruvate dehydrogenase complex deficiency, citric acid cycle deficiencies, and respiratory chain deficiencies
- Type II glutaric aciduria

114. **What are the first items the neonatal transport team must address in an infant with a suspected inborn error of metabolism?**
- ABCs: airway, breathing, circulation
- Hypoglycemia, metabolic acidosis

115. **What complications may the transport team encounter in infants with an inborn error?**
- Coma
- Seizures

- Brain swelling
- Intracranial hemorrhage
- *E. coli* sepsis in infants with galactosemia
- Bleeding

116. **What congenital abnormalities are more common in infants born to women with PKU?**
Microencephaly (mental retardation) and congenital heart defects, which are thought to result from high levels of phenylalanine.

117. **Which inborn errors of metabolism are commonly associated with neonatal seizures?**
- Nonketotic hyperglycemia
- Pyridoxine-responsive seizure disorders
- Peroxisomal disorders (e.g., neonatal adrenoleukodystrophy)
- Sulfite oxidase deficiency
- Glucose transporter (e.g., GLUT 1) deficiency with hypoglycorrhachia
- Disorders of ammonia metabolism (e.g., ornithine transcarbamylase deficiency)
- Disorders causing hypoglycemia (e.g., fatty acid oxidation disorders, GSDs, hyper-insulinemia)

118. **What common metabolic diseases can cause Fanconi syndrome?**
- Hereditary tyrosinemia
- Galactosemia
- Hereditary fructose intolerance
- Cytochrome C oxidase deficiency
- Pyroglutamic aciduria
- GSD type I

119. **What should the initial diagnostic assessment of an infant with suspected metabolic disease include?**
- Serum electrolytes
- Blood amino acid quantitation
- Blood pH and partial pressure of carbon dioxide
- Liver function tests
- Ophthalmologic examination
- Blood lactate and pyruvate
- Urine Clinitest reaction (while the infant is ingesting a lactose-containing formula)
- Urine organic acid quantitation
- Blood ammonia (urine orotic acid, if elevated)

120. **How can the five major kinds of metabolic diseases be distinguished?**
See Table 7-4.

121. **If an inborn error of metabolism is strongly suspected, what should the baby be fed?**
Nothing. The baby should be made NPO and given IV fluids containing only dextrose and electrolytes with enough dextrose to keep the baby anabolic.

122. **If an inborn error of metabolism is suspected, when is the best time to obtain samples for diagnostic testing?**
At the time the baby is most severely clinically affected, the diagnostic yield is highest.

TABLE 7-4. SUMMARY OF MAJOR FINDINGS IN THE FIVE MAJOR KINDS OF METABOLIC DISEASE

Finding	Organic Acidurias	Primary Lactic Acidoses	Urea Cycle Defects	Classic Galactosemia	Nonketotic Hyperglycemia	Fatty Acid Oxidation Defects
Metabolic acidosis	Frequent	Frequent	No	No	No	Variable
Ketoaciduria	Frequent	Variable	No	No	No	No
Urine organic acids	Abnormal	Increased lactate	Normal	Nondiagnostic	Normal	Increased dicarboxylics
Lactic acidosis	No	Frequent	No	No	No	Not initially
Hyperammonemia	Usually <500 μmol/L	Usually <500 μmol/L	Usually >500 μmol/L	No	No	Possible
Blood amniogram	Nondiagnostic	Increased alanine	Very abnormal	Nondiagnostic	Marked glycine	Nondiagnostic
CSF amniogram	Nondiagnostic	Increased alanine	Very abnormal	Nondiagnostic	Marked glycine	Nondiagnostic
Urine orotic acid	Usually normal	Normal	Very high	Normal	Normal	Normal
Neutropenia	Frequent	Variable	Unusual	No	No	No
Thrombocytopenia	Frequent	Variable	Unusual	No	No	No
Urine Clinitest	Negative	Negative	Negative	Positive	Negative	Negative
Hepatic failure	No	Uncommon	No	Frequent	No	Frequent
Cataracts	No	No	No	Frequent	No	No
Cardiac disease	No	Variable	No	No	No	Frequent
Rhabdomyolysis	No	Variable	No	No	No	Frequent
Congenital malformation	Not usually	Variable	No	No	No	Variable

From Spitzer A: Intensive Care of the Neonate. St. Louis, Mosby, 2005, p 1209.

KEY POINTS: INBORN ERRORS OF METABOLISM

1. Common presentations for inborn errors of metabolism include lethargy and coma, dysmorphism, recurrent vomiting, ocular abnormalities, tachypnea unrelated to pulmonary disease, visceromegaly, unusual odors, marked hypotonia, skin or hair abnormalities, seizures, unstable body temperature, bleeding, and jaundice.

2. Common strategies for treating inborn errors of metabolism include avoidance of fasting, dietary manipulation to avoid substrates that cannot be metabolized, medications to clear toxic byproduct, supplementation with high doses of cofactors and vitamins used by the deficient enzyme, and, when appropriate, enzyme replacement therapy or organ transplants such as liver or bone marrow transplant.

3. Infants with inborn errors of metabolism may not be symptomatic until metabolically stressed by an intercurrent illness or fasting.

4. Fetal development for inborn errors of metabolism may be normal if the metabolites are able to cross the placenta and may be metabolized by the mother for the fetus.

5. Sudden infant death syndrome can be caused by inborn errors of metabolism, and a family history of a death in infancy of unknown etiology should suggest screening for inborn errors of metabolism.

123. **What general treatment strategies can be used for inborn errors of metabolism?**
   - Avoiding nonmetabolizable substrate (e.g., avoiding lactose in galactosemia and fructose in hereditary fructose intolerance)
   - Supplementation with essential metabolites that are not synthesized (e.g., arginine in argininosuccinic aciduria and biotin in biotinidase deficiency)
   - Supplementation with vitamins or cofactors (e.g., carnitine and riboflavin in fatty acid oxidation disorders)
   - Inhibition of toxic byproduct accumulation (e.g., NTBC in type I tyrosinemia)
   - Enzyme replacement (e.g., Gaucher's disease)
   - Liver transplant (e.g., urea cycle defects)

CHAPTER 8

FLUID, ELECTROLYTES, AND RENAL DISORDERS

John M. Lorenz, MD

1. **How does the principal function of the kidney differ in fetal and neonatal life?**
   The principal and unique function of the fetal kidney is the continuous provision of fluid and electrolytes into the amniotic cavity, which is essential for maintenance of amniotic fluid volume. It also appears that the amniotic fluid intrauterine pressure is essential for normal lung development. Consequently, the interplay between kidney and lung during gestation is unique and notable. In neonatal life, the kidney is responsible for maintenance of an appropriate fluid and electrolyte milieu.

2. **Name the factors that contribute to the decline in postnatal renal vascular resistance.**
   - A fall in circulating catecholamine and renin levels
   - A rise in vasodilating prostaglandins

3. **What percentage of cardiac output do the kidneys receive in fetal life?**
   The kidneys receive 2–3% of cardiac output in fetal life (versus 15–18% in adults).

4. **When is nephrogenesis complete?**
   Nephrogenesis is complete at 36 weeks. Adequate renal function to sustain life, however, occurs much earlier in utero, at approximately 22–23 weeks' gestation.

5. **What are the changes in glomerular filtration rate (GFR) that occur prenatally?**
   Before 36 weeks' gestation, there is a gradual increase in GFR through the period of nephrogenesis. Between 36 weeks' and term gestation, the GFR remains stable and then increases dramatically at the time of birth. By 2 weeks of age, it has already doubled. In preterm infants born before the 34th week of gestation, the increase in GFR occurs more gradually.

6. **Why is the fractional excretion of sodium higher in newborn infants?**
   - Glomerular-tubular imbalance
   - Intravascular volume expansion

7. **How does sodium balance differ in term and preterm infants?**
   Term infants conserve sodium effectively after the first few hours of life (following intravascular volume contraction). Preterm infants conserve sodium less effectively because of the following:
   - Decreased proximal tubular reabsorption
   - Decreased distal response to aldosterone
   - Different set point for glomerular-tubular balance

8. **What are normal values for GFR in a newborn infant?**
   See Table 8-1.

TABLE 8-1.   GLOMERULAR FILTRATION RATE (GFR [mL/min/1.73 m^2])

Gestational Age	Postnatal Age		
	1 Week	2–8 Weeks	>8 Weeks
25–28 weeks	11.0 ± 5.4	15.5 ± 6.2	47.4 ± 21.5
29–34 weeks	15.3 ± 5.6	28.7 ± 13.9	51.4 ± 20.7
38–42 weeks	40.6 ± 14.8	65.8 ± 24.8	95.7 ± 21.7

9. **What are normal values for creatinine in a newborn infant?**
    See Table 8-2.

10. **What are the developmental differences in acidification mechanisms in a newborn infant?**
    - H$^+$ excretion in preterm infants is decreased.
    - Both term and preterm infants exhibit an altered threshold for bicarbonate reabsorption at birth.
    - In term infants, the bicarbonate wastage disappears by 1–2 weeks of life; however, in preterm infants it may persist.

11. **What are the developmental differences in water conservation and excretion in a newborn infant?**
    Although the capacity to dilute urine is normal, concentrating ability is limited in the immediate newborn period because of: (1) diminished tonicity of the renal medullary interstitium and (2) diminished response to arginine vasopressin.

12. **Why do preterm infants have difficulty excreting a potassium load?**
    Preterm infants have difficulty excreting potassium for the following reasons:
    - Distal immaturity of sodium-potassium-adenosine triphosphatase (Na$^+$-K$^+$-ATPase)
    - Reduced permeability of peritubular cells
    - Diminished tubular surface area
    - Diminished GFR

13. **When should the time of first voiding be considered delayed?**
    Ninety-seven percent of infants pass urine in the first 24 hours of life and 100% by 48 hours. During the first 2 days of life, infants urinate two to six times per day (Table 8-3).

TABLE 8-2.   NORMAL CREATININE VALUES

Gestational Age	Postnatal Age		
	1 Week	2–8 Weeks	>8 Weeks
25–28 weeks	1.4 ± 0.8	0.9 ± 0.5	0.4 ± 0.2
29–34 weeks	0.9 ± 0.3	0.7 ± 0.3	0.3 ± 0.2
38–42 weeks	0.5 ± 0.1	0.4 ± 0.1	0.4 ± 0.1

TABLE 8-3.   TIME OF FIRST VOID IN 500 INFANTS*

Hours	No. of Cumulative Infants (Term)	%	No. of Cumulative Infants (Preterm)	%	No. of Cumulative Infants (Postterm)	%
In delivery room	51	12.9	17	21.2	3	12
1–8	151	51.1	50	83.7	4	38
9–16	158	91.1	12	98.7	14	84
17–24	35	100	1	100	4	100
>24	0	—	0	—	0	—

*395 term infants, 80 preterm infants, 25 postterm infants.
Adapted from Clark DA: Time of first void and first stool in 500 newborns. Pediatrics 60:457, 1977.

MAINTENANCE FLUID REQUIREMENTS

14. **Why do premature infants lose weight after birth?**
     This decrease in weight is the result of catabolism secondary to low caloric intake and a
     decrease in extracellular volume that is independent of caloric intake. Most premature babies
     manifest diuresis and natriuresis in the first few days of life that results in negative net total body
     water and sodium balance and, thereby, a decrease in extracellular water volume, as shown in
     Fig. 8-1. Although we do not understand why this decrease in extracellular volume occurs, it is
     generally accepted that it is physiologically appropriate.

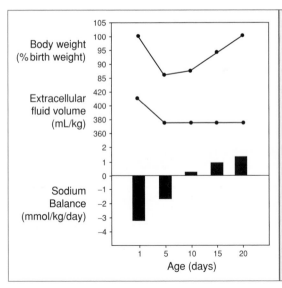

Figure 8-1. Postnatal changes in body weight, extracellular fluid volume, and sodium balance. (From Schaffer SC, Weisman DN: Fluid requirements in the preterm infant. Clin Perinatol 19:233–250, 1992.)

15. **Why is the reduction in extracellular volume considered physiologic?**
    - First, relatively large differences in water and sodium intake are required to moderate this weight loss. Furthermore, higher caloric intake has been correlated with less postnatal weight loss but no difference in the magnitude of decrease in extracellular volume.
    - Second, extracellular volume *per kilogram of body weight* remains stable with subsequent weight gain, suggesting that the relative decrease in extracellular volume shortly after birth is not a transient phenomenon.
    - Third, fluid and sodium intakes high enough to prevent this decrease in extracellular volume have been associated with increased morbidity in premature newborns (e.g., patent ductus arteriosus, necrotizing enterocolitis, chronic lung disease). It is not clear whether this same phenomenon occurs in growth-retarded or term babies.

16. **What are the main variables to consider when estimating insensible water loss (IWL)?**
    The most important determinants of IWL are gestational age, postnatal age, and environment. IWL decreases with increasing gestational and postnatal age (Fig. 8-2). IWL also decreases with increasing ambient humidity. Therefore, IWL will be lower in a humidified incubator than under a radiant warmer with ambient humidity.

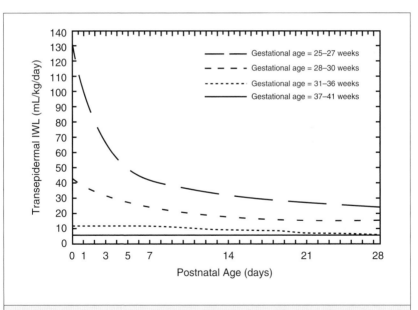

Figure 8-2. Transdermal loss as a function of gestational and postnatal age in naked, appropriate-for-gestational-age infants in a neutral thermal environment in incubators with 50% ambient humidity. (From Hammarlund K, Sedin G, Strömberg B: Transepidermal water loss in newborn infants. Part VIII: Relation to gestational and post-natal age in appropriate and small-for-gestational-age infants. Acta Pediatr Scand 72:721–728, 1983.)

17. **What concentration of dextrose is ordered for infants who must avoid oral ingestion?**

The relevant variable is the dextrose administration rate. Neonates normally produce 4–8 mg/kg/min of glucose endogenously. Administration at this rate usually maintains serum glucose concentration in the normal range and conserves glycogen stores. Once the rate of water administration is determined, a dextrose concentration is selected that provides somewhere between 4 and 8 mg/kg/min. In some infants, higher glucose infusion rates may be necessary, occasionally exceeding even 12–14 mg/kg/min in some circumstances to maintain appropriate blood glucose levels.

18. **How can the dextrose concentration necessary to provide a target dextrose administration rate be calculated once the fluid administration rate is determined?**

$$\text{Dextrose concentration (\%)} =$$
$$\text{target dextrose administration rate (mg/kg/min)} \div \text{infusion rate (mL/kg/day)} \times 170$$

19. **Is there a simple way to calculate the dextrose administration rate that will be provided with a given dextrose concentration and administration rate of the intravenous fluid?**

Yes.

$$\text{Dextrose administration rate (mg/kg/min)} =$$
$$\text{dextrose concentration (\%)} \times \text{infusion rate (mL/kg/day)} \times 0.006$$

20. **The specimen used for bedside glucose measurement with dry reagent strips uses whole blood. Is it necessary to "correct" glucose concentration determined with these reagent strips for the measurement to reflect plasma concentration?**

No. Glucose dry reagent strips measure plasma glucose concentration. Although whole blood is applied to the reagent, plasma diffuses out of the sample into the reaction zone of the strip, with membrane porosity metering sample flow. This is why reading the strip at the exact time designated by the manufacturer is so important. It is the glucose in this plasma that is measured.

21. **How much sodium should be given on the first day of life?**

In the absence of unusual sodium losses (i.e., loss of gastrointestinal or cerebrospinal fluid), no sodium should be given. During the first day of life, urine excretion is low (0.5–2 mEq/kg/day), and, in the absence of abnormal sodium losses, the kidney is the principal route of sodium loss. Therefore, sodium losses will be low so long as urinary output is low. Moreover, if IWL is unexpectedly high or with the onset of the postnatal diuresis (when water loss often exceeds sodium loss), the serum sodium (Na^+) level often rises. Therefore, it is usually best to withhold sodium initially, especially in extremely premature infants who are particularly at risk for developing significant hypernatremia in the first few days of life.

22. **When should maintenance potassium be started in an extremely premature infant?**

The main route of potassium loss is in the urine. Urine potassium losses are low initially because GFR and urine output are relatively low after birth. Moreover, serum potassium (K^+) levels may rise in extremely premature infants even in the absence of exogenous potassium. Therefore, potassium should be withheld until it can be ascertained that renal function is normal and, in extremely premature babies, the serum K^+ level is normal and not increasing.

23. **What are the maintenance fluid and electrolyte (Na+, K+, Cl−) requirements for preterm infants in the first month of life?**
See Table 8-4.

24. **Baby R is a 22-hour-old, 25-weeks'-gestation male in a humidified incubator who has received 150 mL/kg/day of fluid during the first day of life. Serum sodium is 128 mmol/L. Should sodium intake be increased?**
Not necessarily. Serum Na+ is the *concentration*, not the amount, of sodium in the extracellular fluid (ECF) space. If it is abnormal, the amount of sodium in the ECF space is abnormal *for the amount of water* in the ECF space. Thus, serum Na+ may be low because there is too little extracellular sodium and/or too much extracellular water. Total body water and sodium balance over the interval in which the serum Na+ fell must be estimated to distinguish between these two possibilities. The most common cause of hyponatremia in neonates in the first 1–2 days of life is excess fluid administration. In such situations, the serum Na+ will rise with fluid restriction.

TABLE 8-4.   FLUID RECOMMENDATIONS FOR PRETERM INFANTS

Transitional Phase (First 3–5 days)

Weight (gm)	Weight Loss (%)	Water* (mL/kg/day)	Na+ (mEq/kg/day)	Cl− (mEq/kg/day)	K+ (mEq/kg/day)
<1000	15–20	90–140	0–1	0–1	0
1001–1500	10–15	80–120	0–1	0–1	0–1
1501–2000	5–10	70–100	0–1	0–1	0–1
<2000	5–10	60–80	0–1	0–1	0–1

Stabilization Phase (<14 days)

Weight (gm)	Weight Loss (%)	Water (mL/kg/day)	Na+ (mEq/kg/day)	Cl− (mEq/kg/day)	K+ (mEq/kg/day)
<1000	0	80–120	2–3	2–3	1–2
1001–1500	0	80–120	2–3	2–3	1–2
1501–2000	0	80–120	2–3	2–3	1–2
<2000	0	80–120	2–3	2–3	1–2

Growth Phase (>14 days)

Weight (gm)	Weight gain (gm/day)	Feedings (mL/kg/day)	Na+ (mEq/kg/day)	Cl− (mEq/kg/day)	K+ (mEq/kg/day)
<1000	15–20	150–200	3–5	3–5	2–3
1001–1500	15–20	150–200	3–5	3–5	2–3

*Requirements are 10–20% less with a humidified Isolette or plastic shield.

25. The central laboratory calls with a critical serum (Na⁺) value of 122 mEq/L for baby boy Z, who is receiving total parenteral nutrition. Should you:

A. Send a sample of the parenteral fluid stat for Na⁺ analysis?

B. Give hypertonic saline to correct the serum (Na⁺)?

C. Call the lab to see whether the serum sample was lipemic?

D. Recheck the serum (Na⁺) using a point of contact instrument?

C or D. Hyperlipemia may occur in infants receiving intravenous lipid infusion as part of parenteral nutrition. This may result in fictitious hyponatremia. However, whether it does depends on the analytic method used to measure serum (Na⁺). *Indirect* ion-specific electrode analysis is typically used in large automated chemistry analyzers. It involves dilution of the serum sample with a large volume of diluents and, therefore, measures the concentration of sodium in the total serum sample (serum water and serum solids [i.e., lipids and protein]. Hyperlipemia will result in relatively less water (and thereby sodium) in a given volume of serum, causing the reported serum sodium concentration to be spuriously low. This is also the case when serum sodium concentration is measured using flame photometry, which also requires sample dilution. The same measurement error will occur with any electrolyte analyzed in diluted serum, but it is clinically significant only for sodium and chloride. Hyperlipemia can be avoided by discontinuing the intravenous lip infusion for several hours before obtaining the serum sample for analysis, but this is often impractical. *Direct* ion-specific electrode analysis, which is typically used in blood gas analyzers and point-of-contact instruments, measures electrical activity in plasma water (which is the physiologically relevant measure) in undiluted whole blood or plasma samples. Plasma electrical activity is then converted to plasma concentration by a fixed ion-specific multiplier, which is independent of plasma solids. The result, therefore, is unaffected by variations in the amount of solids in plasma.

26. Which should be used—birth weight or daily weight—to calculate water and sodium requirements during the first week of life?

You should use what the attending tells you to use! After the first day of life, however, it is the absolute fluid and electrolyte intake (milliliters or millimoles per day) *relative to the previous 12–24 hours* that one should be thinking about. In other words, should the absolute fluid or electrolyte intake be more or less than it was previously? The answer depends on what fluid and electrolyte balances resulted from the previous intakes and on what water and electrolyte losses are anticipated. There is no magic amount of water per kg/day that is appropriate for all infants, even at the same weight, gestational age, and postnatal age, and in the same environment. If the infant loses more water (and therefore weight) than you judge to be appropriate and you anticipate that water losses will remain approximately the same, the absolute amount of water (milliliters per day) given should be increased. However, if the current weight is used to calculate fluid

KEY POINTS: FLUIDS AND ELECTROLYTES

1. Like the lung, the premature kidney is very immature in its function for some period of time, with reduced glomerular filtration, an inability to handle electrolytes, and a diminished capacity for acidification of urine.

2. All premature neonates lose weight after birth. This is a normal process of constricting ECF volumes. Only when more than 10–15% of body weight has been lost should one consider the process as possibly pathophysiologic and investigate further.

3. Sodium and potassium do not usually need to be given on the first day of life, but glucose and calcium are necessary.

requirements, the absolute amount of water administered may be only slightly more or even less than the amount given the day before. For example, an 860-gm infant loses 110 gm (~13% of birth weight) in the first day of life after receiving 100 mL/kg/day (86 mL/day). You decide this rate of weight loss is too great and increase water intake by 25% to 125 mL/kg/day. Based on the current weight of 750 gm, however, this is only 94 mL/day, which is less than that given the previous day. If water losses remain the same, weight loss will be even greater over the next 24 hours despite an increase in water intake.

USING YOUR HEAD: SOME QUICK METHODS IN FLUIDS AND ELECTROLYTE THERAPY

It pays to know a few quickie math tricks so you are not fumbling for your calculator and then coming up with a ridiculous answer that is due to random finger error or is three orders of magnitude too large or small. You can perform many simple calculations in your head by rounding off weights, times, and fluid requirements. The answers you get won't be exact, but they will probably be close enough and are unlikely to be hugely divergent like the errors made with calculators. The following are examples of calculations you can do in your head. They involve issues that arise repeatedly.

27. **If you switch the umbilical artery line infusion from 5% dextrose in water (D5W) to normal saline, how much additional sodium will you be giving the baby?**
Usually the scenario goes something like this: the tiny baby is hyponatremic, and it is too late in the day to change his total parenteral nutritional constituents. But he is receiving 1.5 mL/h of D5W via his umbilical artery catheter (UAC). Someone suggests that the UAC infusate could be changed to normal saline to provide additional sodium. Is such a change likely to help the baby? The answer is that each milliliter per hour of normal saline provides about 4 mEq Na. The quick in-your-head calculation goes like this:

$$(24/1000) \times 154 \sim (25/1000) \times 160 = 160/40 = 4 \text{ (actual value} = 3.7)$$

So, for a 1-kg baby, a 1.5-mL/h infusion provides approximately an additional 6 (actual, 5.5) mEq Na over 24 hours. Not enough to make a dent in hyponatremia if the baby is a 3.5-kg term giant, but if he (or more likely *she,* if she has survived) is a 500-gm peanut, then you have added about 12 mEq/kg/day additional Na (actual 11). And that's a lot of extra sodium!

28. **How do I quickly estimate the correct infusion rate for an intravenous line?**
Here's a quickie that is certain to "win friends and influence your uncle." Suppose you want your 3.2-kg baby to receive 125 mL/kg/day of fluid. At what rate should the intravenous pump be set?
The first step is to quickly estimate the total daily fluid volume. An easy way to do this is break the calculation into pieces: 100 mL/kg/day is 320 mL/day. An extra quarter of that is 80 mL/day. So the baby should receive 400 mL/day. Next, instead of dividing by 24, multiply this number by 0.04, which is the same as dividing by 25. The answer is 16 mL/h. It is a little shy of the actual desired rate (16.7 mL/h), but it is close enough. At least it is in the right ballpark, unlike the number generated by your finger-fumbling friend with the calculator.

29. **I look on the intravenous bag and see a bewildering set of numbers: NaCl 12.5 mEq; KCl 8.3 mEq; Ca gluconate 6.25 mEq. How can I quickly tell how many mEq/kg/day of these constituents my baby is receiving?**
The first step to knowing what these numbers mean is to understand that when intravenous solutions are prepared, the weight of the baby is irrelevant. Only the rate of infusion is important. One reliable way to calculate the amount of intravenous constituents is to use something called a *"P" factor.* The P factor is merely the bag volume divided by the number of mL/kg/day the baby

is supposed to receive from this particular intravenous line. Suppose you want your baby to receive 120 mL/kg/day. For a 1-L bag of fluid, P = 1000/120 = 8.33. For a rate of 100 mL/kg/day, P = 10, and so on.

The next thing you need to know is how many mEq/kg/day of each constituent is needed. Suppose you want your baby to receive 3 mEq/kg/day Na, 2 mEq/kg/day K, and 1.5 mEq/kg/day Ca. The amount added to the 1-L bag is merely "P" times the quantity of each of these constituents:

$$Na \ (as \ NaCl) = 3 \times 8.33 = 25 \ mEq$$
$$K \ (as \ KCl) = 2 \times 8.33 = 16.67 \ mEq$$
$$Ca \ (as \ gluconate) = 1.5 \times 8.33 = 12.5 \ mEq$$

If the infusion bag contains only 500 mL instead of 1 L, these numbers are halved, giving us the numbers in the question. With a little practice you will recognize the P factors as old friends, and the numbers on the intravenous bags will not seem so intimidating.

30. **What's the point anyway? These calculations will all be automated soon by safety committees, and these in-your-head methods will become outmoded.** Things have not quite been automated yet. Just look around your hospital. And it is in an emergency, especially, that errors are made because everyone assumes that the amount and rate of dopamine, or PG, or epi, must be correct; after all, old reliable so-and-so did the calculations. But that is not always true. And wouldn't it be nice, for the sake of good care, if you could glance at the intravenous rate and say, "Wait a minute, this can't be right." So, *use your head! After all, that's what it's there for!*

ACID–BASE BALANCE

31. **How are acid-base measurements made?**
    Arterial oxygen activity is measured amperometrically by the Clark electrode. The reduction reaction of interest is as follows: $4e^- + O_2 + 2H_2O = 4OH^-$. Current flows in linear proportion to the activity of dissolved oxygen.

    Hydrogen ion concentration (pH) is measured potentiometrically using a complicated system that employs two electrodes (usually Ag/AgCl) designed such that the potential between them is sensitive to the concentration of H^+ ions in the intervening medium.

    Carbon dioxide (CO_2) activity is measured using an electrode with a semipermeable membrane that allows only CO_2 to diffuse into the electrode compartment, where it is converted to carbonic acid. The hydrogen ions produced by this reaction are then measured as above. The semipermeable membrane ensures that this measurement is completely independent of blood pH.

    Bicarbonate is not measured but is calculated from the Henderson-Hasselbalch equation:

    $$pH = \frac{pK' + \log(HCO_3^-)}{(0.0307 \times pCO_2)}$$

    where 0.0307 = solubility coefficient of CO_2 at 37°C. The equation uses pK', not just pK, because the pK is a composite of two reaction constants and only an "apparent" pK for H_2CO_3 dissociation.

32. **What is base excess? How is it measured?**
    The total blood buffers of human adults are composed of the buffers listed at the end of the paragraph. Values for infants are 3–4 mEq/L blood lower, so infants tend to have a persistent base deficit in that range. The effect of these buffers is to establish and stabilize a pH of roughly 7.40 in the blood.
    - Plasma HCO_3^-: 24 mEq/L blood
    - Plasma protein: 13 mEq/L blood

- Red cell HCO_3^-:14 mEq/L blood
- Red cell hemoglobin: 6 mEq/L blood

Base deficit or excess is the difference between the sum of these values and what actually is measured (or calculated) in the test sample. Thus, base excess is defined as the number of millimoles of strong base or strong acid needed to titrate 1 L of blood (Hgb = 15.0 gm/dL) to pH = 7.40 at 37°C while pCO_2 is held at 40 mmHg (at which point the buffers have been restored to normal values). It may be calculated from the following equation:

$$BE = [1 - 0.014(Hgb)] \{(HCO_3^-) - 24 + [1.43(Hgb) + 7.7](pH - 7.4)\}$$

33. **In acid-base disorders in human biology, in which body compartment is the measurement made?**
Acid-base measurements are made of the ECF, which includes the intravascular and the interstitial fluid compartments. Intracellular acid-base status, which likely influences cell function significantly, is difficult to assess and not routinely measured. Because CO_2 exchanges with the intracellular fluids much more rapidly than HCO_3^-, it is possible for rapid changes in pCO_2 to change the acid-base profile of the two compartments in different directions and at different rates. When attempting to treat acid-base disorders, pediatricians must consider the possible consequences: worsening intracellular acidosis in the face of alkalinization of the ECF with infusions of bicarbonate.

34. **What are the principal mechanisms whereby infants compensate for abnormal acid-base profiles?**
- **Metabolic alkalosis compensation:** Hypoventilation
- **Metabolic acidosis compensation:** Hyperventilation
- **Respiratory acidosis compensation:** Increased renal absorption of bicarbonate
- **Respiratory alkalosis compensation:** Diminished renal retention of bicarbonate

35. **Explain the importance of the volume of distribution in correcting acid-base derangements.**
After a known amount of solute is introduced into a solution, the concentration is measured, and the apparent volume in which the solute is distributed is calculated. This volume is called the *volume of distribution*, and it is used to estimate how much solute is needed to change the measured concentration of that solute. For simple, single compartments and inert solutes, the calculation measures the true volume. For multicompartment systems and unstable solutes, the solute may be distributed unevenly (i.e., either concentrated in or excluded from various compartments), metabolized, or otherwise eliminated. In these systems, the calculated volume is different from the true volume in which the solute is distributed. Because of its interaction with a number of buffer systems, both intracellular and extracellular, and its elimination as CO_2 through the lungs, the volume of distribution of bicarbonate is variable and difficult to predict. A good guess for use in dosing is 30% of body weight.

36. **What do we know for sure about the indications for the therapeutic use of sodium bicarbonate in pediatrics?**
Much less than you think. As a general rule, replacement of bicarbonate when body losses of bicarbonate are excessive (e.g., through the stool or urine) is appropriate. On the other hand, evidence documenting the value of sodium bicarbonate infusions to correct acidosis from many, if not most, other causes is very sketchy; therefore, sodium bicarbonate–replacement treatment should be used cautiously, if at all. Although it is relatively easy to make the numbers in the ECF change in the desired direction, it is much more difficult to be certain that the patient will improve or that this therapy is beneficial in any way. Review the literature thoroughly before reaching for the alkali.

KEY POINTS: ACID-BASE BALANCE

1. A primary acid-base disturbance is always defined by the pH. A pH less than 7.3 indicates a primary academia, whereas a pH greater than 7.5 indicates a primary alkalemia.

2. One must then turn to the underlying clinical situation to define the cause of the primary disturbance.

3. Sodium bicarbonate should be used sparingly to treat acidemia. One also should never give bicarbonate until the ability to excrete carbon dioxide is ensured; otherwise the clinical acid-base disturbance may be made worse.

4. When giving bicarbonate, a half-correction is usually appropriate, since the simultaneous treatment of the underlying disorder will often assist in aiding the correction.

---

37. **Is an infant able to make more or less acid when the pH is out of the normal range, thereby helping in the correction of systemic acidosis?**
Yes. According to Hood and Tannen, "There is convincing evidence that small changes in systemic pH modify the rate of endogenous acid production in a direction and amount that can attenuate the effect of an acid challenge in a variety of physiologic and pathologic situations."

> Hood VL, Tannen RL: Protection of acid–base balance by pH regulation of acid production. N Engl J Med 339:819–826, 1998.

38. **What mechanism underlies dilution acidosis and contraction alkalosis?**
When the concentration of HCO_3^- is changed by increasing or decreasing the volume in which it is distributed and the pCO_2 remains constant, the pH changes in the direction dictated by the Henderson-Hasselbalch equation.

39. **What is the difference between the units torr and mmHg?**
There is no difference.

DIURETICS

40. **Furosemide and bumetanide are loop diuretics that clinicians commonly prescribe for infants who have one of various diseases including respiratory distress syndrome, bronchopulmonary dysplasia, posthemorrhagic hydrocephalus, and congenital heart disease. What damage can chronic administrative loop diuretics inflict on the kidney and/or urinary tract?**
Loop diuretics induce hypercalciuria by inhibiting renal tubular calcium reabsorption. Therefore, chronic administration of these agents can cause nephrocalcinosis and/or calcium nephrolithiasis.

41. **How does one know whether a patient is at risk for developing furosemide-induced renal and/or genitourinary disease?**
Hypercalciuria induced by loop diuretics is a risk factor for nephrolithiasis and/or nephrocalci-nosis. Urinary calcium excretion can be evaluated by calculating the urinary calcium concentra-tion–to–urinary creatinine (Uca/Ucreat) concentration ratio from a random urine specimen or in an aliquot of a timed urine collection. Hypercalciuria in the newborn is identified when the Uca/Ucreat concentration ratio is significantly greater than 0.8.

42. **Explain the means by which furosemide-induced hypercalciuria and the consequent risk of nephrocalcinosis/nephrolithiasis can be reversed.**
Obviously, the best way to treat hypercalciuria that is induced by loop diuretics is to discontinue treatment. However, discontinuation of diuretics is not always possible. In contrast to loop diuretics, thiazide diuretics have an anticalciuric effect. Thus, changing an infant's diuretic regimen from furosemide/bumetanide to a thiazide may reduce urinary calcium excretion. If it is not feasible to discontinue treatment with a loop diuretic, adding a thiazide may effectively reverse hypercalciuria, thereby reducing the risk of nephrocalcinosis and/or nephrolithiasis. An alternative is to reduce the frequency of loop diuretic therapy and treat on an every-other-day or every-third-day basis to minimize the calciuria.

43. **What is the most rational treatment for the hypokalemic, hypochloremic metabolic alkalosis that may occur in newborns who receive intensive diuretic therapy?**
The rational treatment is spironolactone and potassium chloride supplementation. Diuretic therapy induces a reduction in effective intra-arterial volume and thereby activates the renin-angiotensin-aldosterone system, which, in turn, stimulates secretion of potassium in the distal tubule. Blocking the effect of aldosterone on the distal tubule, therefore, should counteract the metabolic consequences of pharmacologic diuresis. Accordingly, adding spironolactone, a competitive inhibitor of aldosterone, to the diuretic regimen improves the derangements in serum bicarbonate and potassium concentrations. Recent data also suggest that spironolactone therapy may improve cardiac function by a mechanism that is independent of its effect on the kidney.
   In general, it is helpful to initiate potassium chloride supplementation as soon as diuretics are considered to minimize the hypokalemic, hypochloremic effects of diuretic therapy.

KEY POINTS: DIURETICS

1. When initiating diuretic therapy in neonates, chloride usually needs to be given as well, typically in the form of potassium chloride, else metabolic alkalosis may be aggravated.

2. Loop diuretics tend to be more effective in neonates but may provoke calciuresis and renal stone formation.

3. Diuretic therapy has not been shown to significantly alter the course of bronchopulmonary dysplasia, although it may provide some immediate assistance in improving ventilation. The benefits should be carefully weighed against the risks of metabolic and bone disturbances.

44. **How can the addition of acetazolamide be detrimental to infants who are being treated with other diuretics?**
Some neonatologists and cardiologists prescribe acetazolamide, an inhibitor of carbonic anhydrase, to treat the alkalosis that is caused by diuretic therapy. Although acetazolamide may lower the blood bicarbonate concentration by virtue of its ability to block reabsorption of bicarbonate in the proximal tubule, it also increases renal potassium excretion. Therefore, treatment with acetazolamide may cause an undesirable decrease in the patient's already low serum potassium concentration.

DIFFERENTIAL DIAGNOSIS AND EVALUATION OF OLIGURIA

45. **Does the fetus make urine? If so, where does it go?**
Urine is made by the fetus in increasing amounts as gestation advances. Fetal urine, along with tracheobronchial secretions, is an important contributor to amniotic fluid. The process is

dynamic, with amniotic fluid being secreted continuously, then swallowed and reabsorbed from the gastrointestinal tract. Fetal oliguria may produce oligohydramnios, and swallowing difficulty or obstruction in the gastrointestinal tract may produce polyhydramnios.

46. **What determines urine output in the postnatal period?**
The volume of urine in the postnatal period is determined by water intake, GFR, the concentration gradient in the renal medullary interstitium, and the presence or absence of antidiuretic hormone (ADH).

47. **Is the urinary concentrating ability of an infant the same as that for older children? If not, why is it different?**
Children and adults can concentrate the urine maximally to 1200 mOsm/L. Neonates can concentrate only to 700 mOsm/L or less. Concentrating ability is limited in infants for several reasons. Protein intake by the infant is used to make new cells during this period of rapid growth, and relatively little nitrogen is diverted to urea. Urea is an important component of the tonicity of the medullary interstitium and the osmolality of urine. Additional factors include (1) the relatively short loops of Henle in the neonatal nephrons that limit the surface area available for equilibration with the interstitium and (2) a high level of prostaglandins that could increase medullary blood flow, "wash out" the medullary concentration gradient, and blunt the ability of ADH to increase water reabsorption. There may also be decreased production of cyclic adenosine monophosphate in response to ADH, decreasing the insertion of water channels into the collecting duct.

48. **The nurse says a 3-day-old infant is oliguric. You wonder, "How do I know whether there really is oliguria in this infant?" What qualifies as oliguria?**
Your question is not so naïve, given the wide range of urine volumes from the most dilute to the most concentrated. The nurse likely responds on the basis of physical evidence; for example, he or she may say that the infant had only three wet diapers over the past 24 hours. If the baby is in an intensive care unit and the urine volume is being quantified, a rate of urine flow can be calculated. Within the first 48 hours after delivery the volume may be as low as 0.5–0.7 mL/kg/h, but beyond this period it is greater than 1 mL/kg/h. Values less than 1 mL/kg/h, if persistent, qualify for oliguria.

49. **If an infant is found to be oliguric, what are the possible causes?**
It is most useful to approach the differential diagnosis in terms of the factors that determine urine output (*see* question 46). First, one should evaluate the intake, look for signs of dehydration, and reexamine fluid requirements, taking into account gestational age and the use of lights and warmers, which increase fluid requirements. A decrease in GFR is manifested by a rising serum creatinine concentration. This acute renal failure (ARF) should be analyzed for prerenal causes (e.g., congestive heart failure, increased IWL, intrarenal causes (e.g., acute tubular necrosis after perinatal asphyxia, renal malformations), and postrenal causes (e.g., obstruction, often posterior urethral valves [PUVs]). An increase in ADH leading to increased water reabsorption and oliguria occurs in heart failure. The syndrome of inappropriate secretion of ADH occurs only rarely in the neonatal period.

50. **An oliguric infant had a serum creatinine of 0.7 mg/dL at birth and 1.0 mg/dL at 48 hours of life. How do you interpret these levels?**
The serum creatinine of the infant at birth reflects that of his or her mother. Thereafter, the level in a term infant should decline to the normal value of 0.3–0.4 mg/dL. The rate of decline varies depending on the initial GFR, rate of increase in GFR, and gestational age. The important point is that the serum creatinine level should decline. In this case, it is rising and therefore is abnormal.

51. **How can the urine sodium concentration be helpful in evaluating oliguria?**
Urinary indices to separate prerenal ARF from intrarenal ARF are not as useful in neonates as in older children and adults. The best index is the fractional excretion of sodium (FE_{Na}), which is calculated as follows:

$$FE_{Na} = (U_{Na})(Screat) \times 100/(S_{Na})(Ucreat)$$

Prerenal failure is associated with $FE_{Na} = 2.5\%$, whereas intrarenal ARF is associated with $FE_{Na} = 3\%$. However, because of overlap between the two groups, specificity is limited. Premature infants with gestations <32 weeks have a high rate of sodium excretion; therefore, a high FE_{Na} is not useful as an index. However, if FE_{Na} is low, prerenal ARF is suggested.

52. **The nurse says a 2-day-old infant is oliguric. the baby has respiratory distress and is on a respirator. In reviewing his chart, you note that his mother had oligohydramnios. several people have noted that the baby looks "funny." Can you hazard an armchair differential diagnosis before going to see the baby?**
Oligohydramnios may be associated with severe renal anomalies that produce fetal oliguria. The lack of amniotic fluid can produce a fetal compression syndrome characterized by positional abnormalities of the extremities, a characteristic facial appearance, and pulmonary hypoplasia. The classic renal anomaly is renal agenesis, and the facial appearance in this condition is known as *Potter's facies*. A similar syndrome can be produced by autosomal recessive (infantile) poly-cystic kidney disease (ARPKD) or severe obstructive uropathy involving both kidneys, the blad-der neck, or the urethra. If the nurse adds that the baby's abdomen is very distended, the most likely suspicion is ARPKD, and severe obstruction is less likely.

53. **In the case of the 2-day-old infant in question 52, what diagnostic findings might the physical examination show?**
The physical examination might show large abdominal masses, in ARPKD or obstruction, that produce hydronephrosis but no masses in renal agenesis.

54. **Which initial test would help in the evaluation?**
The most helpful initial test would be abdominal sonography concentrating on the kidneys, ureters, and bladder.

DIFFERENTIAL DIAGNOSIS AND EVALUATION OF POLYURIA

55. **A newborn male infant is found to have renal failure due to obstructive uropathy from PUVs. A catheter is inserted into the bladder through the urethra. There is a large diuresis, and the ARF gradually subsides with normalization of the serum creatinine. Months later, the mother complains that her infant requires many more changes of diapers than did her other children. What is the likely explanation?**
Severe obstruction of the urinary tract during nephrogenesis may lead to renal maldevelopment and can result in renal dysplasia. An early sign of dysplasia is a renal concentrating defect that manifests as polyuria and polydipsia. Some affected children maintain a normal GFR throughout life, but others have a slowly progressive decline in renal function resulting in end-stage renal disease, often during the teenage years.

56. **What constitutes polyuria in the newborn period?**
Infants with polyuria have a rate of excretion of urine that is 4–5 mL/kg/h or greater.

57. **The mother of a 2-month-old infant complains about the baby's large urine output, which she believes is due to his drinking too much water. She is trying to control it by limiting fluid intake. What is wrong with her reasoning?**
Psychogenic water drinking does not occur in infants. The infant may be drinking excessive amounts of water to compensate for a urinary concentrating defect and to maintain water balance. In such cases, limiting oral intake results in dehydration. This infant needs further evaluation.

KEY POINTS: OLIGURIA AND POLYURIA

1. Oliguria is common in neonates during the first day of life because glomerular filtration is reduced. Nearly all babies will void, however, by 24 hours of life.

2. The creatinine measurement on the first day of life reflects the mother's creatinine level, whereas the 48-hour creatinine level is much more a reflection of neonatal renal function.

3. Normal urine output should exceed about 1 mL/kg/day in the neonatal period. Below that level can be considered oliguria after the first day of life. Polyuria can be considered when urine output exceeds 4–5 mL/kg/day.

4. Neonates cannot induce water intoxication through excessive water intake.

58. **If the infant in question 57 is fluid restricted, what would you expect his serum electrolyte measurements to show?**
The serum electrolytes most likely would show hypernatremia because of a negative water balance. The sodium balance probably is normal.

59. **An infant born prematurely to a mother who had polyhydramnios required mechanical ventilation for 1 week. At 6 days of life he had a rising serum creatinine level, hypotension with cool extremities, hyponatremia, and mild hypokalemia. Despite the appearance of ARF and hypovolemia, the infant had a large urine output with a high urinary concentration of sodium. What might be the cause? Is treatment available?**
Neither central nor nephrogenic diabetes insipidus commonly presents with polyuria in the newborn period, but the neonatal form of Bartter syndrome, also known as *hyperprostaglandin syndrome,* may present this way. In such cases, the mother has polyhydramnios due to increased fetal urine excretion, and the infant is often born prematurely. Postnatally, polyuria and renal sodium wasting continue, resulting in hypovolemia and prerenal ARF. Infants with Bartter syndrome also have hypercalciuria and increased excretion of prostaglandin E_2. Findings may include hypokalemia and an elevated serum bicarbonate level, but not as frequently in infants as in older children with Bartter syndrome.

The defect appears to be in the ascending limb of the loop of Henle involving the NaCl, KCl cotransporter, and the potassium channel. There are two genetic forms of neonatal Bartter syndrome, one involving the gene that codes for the cotransporter (locus *SLC12A1* on chromosome bands 15q–21) and one that results from mutation in the ROMK gene (locus *KCNJ1* on chromosome bands 11q24–25), which controls the potassium channel. Treatment with a prostaglandin synthetase inhibitor (e.g., indomethacin, ibuprofen) reverses many of the abnormalities. Salt-losing adrenal insufficiency must be excluded, but it is usually associated with hyperkalemia and acidosis.

POTTER SYNDROME AND OLIGOHYDRAMNIOS SEQUENCE

60. **What are the features of the oligohydramnios sequence (i.e., Potter's syndrome)?**
Typical signs of the oligohydramnios sequence include deformation of the limbs; pulmonary hypoplasia; and the physical features of flat face, beaked nose, and low-set ears. The ears appear big because they are simple in structure. There may also be heterotopic brain malformations.

61. **What are the causes of the oligohydramnios sequence?**
    1. Obstructive uropathy
       - PUVs
       - Prune-belly syndrome (PBS)

2. Renal anomalies
   - Bilateral renal agenesis
   - Bilateral renal cystic dysplasia
   - Renal tubular dysgenesis
   - Autosomal recessive polycystic kidneys
   - Autosomal dominant polycystic kidneys
3. Chronic leakage of amniotic fluid

62. **What are the inheritance patterns for conditions causing the oligohydramnios sequence?**
    - **PUVs:** Sporadic
    - **PBS:** Sporadic
    - **Bilateral renal agenesis:** Sporadic, recessive, or dominant
    - **Bilateral renal cystic dysplasia:** Sporadic, recessive, or dominant
    - **Renal tubular dysgenesis:** Sporadic or recessive
    - **Autosomal recessive polycystic kidneys:** Recessive (chromosome 6p21)
    - **Autosomal dominant polycystic kidneys:** Dominant (chromosome 16p)

63. **What are the causes of small kidneys in neonates?**
    Inherited or congenital
    - Renal hypoplasia
    - Renal dysplasia
    - Oligomeganephronic hypoplasia
    Acquired
    - Renal venous thrombosis (kidneys are initially large)
    - Renovascular accidents

64. **How are small kidneys diagnosed? How do they present clinically?**
    In utero
    - Oligohydramnios
    - Fetal ultrasound
    At birth
    - As part of a syndrome
    - Oligohydramnios sequence
    - Polydipsia, polyuria
    Infancy
    - Failure to thrive
    - Urinary tract infection

HYPERKALEMIA IN PREMATURE INFANTS

65. **What is the definition of *hyperkalemia*?**
    Hyperkalemia is a high serum potassium concentration in the blood of ≥ 6.7 mEq/L.

66. **What are the two ways that hyperkalemia develops in premature infants?**
    Hyperkalemia develops in a premature infant either from a positive potassium balance arising from increased intake or reduced excretion of potassium, or from a shift of potassium from the intracellular fluid (ICF) space to the ECF space.

67. **What is the incidence of hyperkalemia in premature infants?**
   In infants weighing ≤1000 gm, the incidence ranges from 15% to 50%. However, some studies
   may have overstated the problem because a hemolytic specimen can artificially elevate the value
   of serum potassium reported by the laboratory.

68. **What is nonoliguric hyperkalemia?**
   Nonoliguric hyperkalemia is a rise in the serum potassium concentration (≥6.7 mEq/L) in the
   absence of a falling or low urine output. In contrast with older children, infants with nonoliguric
   hyperkalemia do not demonstrate a lower rate of urine production than age- and weight-matched
   control subjects.

69. **What is the pathophysiology of nonoliguric hyperkalemia?**
   In a premature infant, hyperkalemia can develop from a state of positive potassium balance or
   an internal shift of potassium. Although premature infants have some difficulty in excreting a
   potassium load, nonoliguric hyperkalemia develops in the first 72–96 hours of life when
   potassium intake is minimal. Therefore, excess administration of potassium is not an important variable. Most infants who develop nonoliguric hyperkalemia are in a state of *negative
   potassium balance*. In affected infants, the ratio of intracellular to extracellular potassium is
   significantly lower than in control subjects. In addition, infants with nonoliguric hyperkalemia
   are in a state of volume contraction, and their levels of Na^+,K^+-ATPase are lower. Therefore,
   nonoliguric hyperkalemia is likely due to a shift of potassium from the intracellular fluid space
   to the ECF space.

70. **What are the consequences of hyperkalemia in a premature infant?**
   Most of the time, there are minimal untoward effects, but an occasional infant may develop
   tachyarrhythmias. With very elevated potassium levels, bradyarrhythmias can occur that
   are extremely problematic to reverse. These are usually seen with potassium levels above
   9 mEq/L.

71. **What are the available treatments for nonoliguric hyperkalemia?**
   - Continuous infusion of insulin
   - Treatment with sodium bicarbonate
   - Na^+,K^+ exchange resins
   - Calcium infusions
   Note: None of these strategies have been studied rigorously or proved to be efficacious.

72. **What is the role of insulin and glucose in reducing serum potassium levels?**
   The reported mechanisms of action are complicated and not well understood.
   - Although insulin transports glucose into the cell, it is not the primary mechanism for shifting
     potassium.
   - Insulin induces the enzyme Na^+,K^+-ATPase, which is independent of glucose.
   - Glucose is needed to prevent hypoglycemia and not to transport potassium.
   - The efficacy of glucose and insulin in affected infants has not been proved.

73. **What is the role of hydration in infants with nonoliguric hyperkalemia?**
   Hyperkalemic infants have urinary indices that indicate a state of prerenal volume contraction.
   When serum potassium values rise above 6 mEq/L and serum creatinine and blood urea nitrogen levels increase in a proportionate fashion, fluid intake should be increased by 25–30%. By
   improving the intravascular volume status, a greater potassium load is delivered at the glomerular level, resulting in higher potassium excretion.

KEY POINTS: HYPERKALEMIA

1. About 15–50% of extremely-low-birth-weight neonates will manifest hyperkalemia (potassium > 6.7 mEq/L) at some point during their hospital course.

2. Hyperkalemia commonly results from overadministration of potassium and must be carefully monitored.

3. Both tachyarrhythmias and bradyarrhythmias may develop with hyperkalemia, depending on the level of potassium in the blood.

4. Hyperkalemia may be a life-threatening emergency. Treatment includes diuretics, sodium bicarbonate, calcium, insulin, and glucose.

RENAL TUBULAR ACIDOSIS

74. **What is the normal serum bicarbonate level for gestational age?**
During the first year of life, the plasma concentration of bicarbonate is approximately 22 ± 1.9 mEq/L, compared with 26 ± 1.0 mEq/L in adults. The bicarbonate concentration is lower in term infants (20 ± 2.8 mEq/L) and even lower in preterm infants (17 ± 1.2 mEq/L), with two standard deviations including values as low as 14.5 mEq/L. Children generally have a bicarbonate level of 23 ± 1.0 mEq/L.

75. **How well do premature infants reabsorb bicarbonate?**
Preterm infants have a depressed renal threshold for bicarbonate. A close negative correlation has been found between bicarbonate threshold and urinary sodium excretion, suggesting that the limited renal capacity to reabsorb sodium may account for the low bicarbonate threshold in premature infants. However, the reabsorption of bicarbonate in the proximal tubule is generally complete in preterm infants, with maximal reabsorptive rates comparable to adult tubules (2.5–2.6 mEq/dL glomerular filtrate). Thus, in early life, the intrinsic capacity of the proximal tubule to reabsorb bicarbonate appears adequate to handle the filtered load of bicarbonate. Bicarbonate reabsorption will improve if the extracellular volume is allowed to contract.

76. **Do infants excrete more or less titratable acid and ammonia per kilogram of body weight compared with older children?**
The titratable acid excretion rate in term infants younger than 1 month old is about one half and the ammonium excretion rate about two thirds that of older children and adults. Preterm infants have even lower rates. Net acid excretion rates (titratable acid plus ammonium) are lower than in infants older than 1 month. After 1 month of age, the net acid excretion rate in term infants is similar to that in older children and adults when expressed per 1.73 m^2. Preterm infants also increase their rates of titratable acid and ammonium excretion with maturation, but these rates still remain lower than in term infants, even up to the age of 4 months.

77. **What are the signs and symptoms of renal tubular acidosis (RTA)?**
RTA usually presents with nonspecific symptoms such as failure to thrive, lethargy, vomiting, and tachypnea. The hallmark of this syndrome is the presence of hyperchloremic metabolic acidosis. The most common cause of hyperchloremic metabolic acidosis is not related to the kidney but is caused by diarrhea with loss of base in the stool. This is also a form of RTA-rectal tubular acidosis.

78. **What are the different types of RTA?**
    - **Type 1:** Impairment of distal acidification
    - **Type 2:** Impairment of bicarbonate reclamation
    - **Type 3:** Combination of types 1 and 2 (now rarely diagnosed as a separate entity)
    - **Type 4:** Secondary to a lack of or insensitivity to aldosterone
    All four types are associated with a hyperchloremic, normal anion gap acidosis.

79. **How does one make the diagnosis of the different types of RTA?**
    - Because *proximal RTA* (classic type II) results from a defect in reabsorption of filtered bicarbonate by the proximal renal tubule, the diagnosis is made by showing reduced bicarbonate reabsorption when the serum bicarbonate level is normal.
    - *Distal RTA* (classic type I) is characterized by the inability to acidify the urine adequately. Thus, the diagnosis is made by demonstrating an inability to lower the urine pH below 5.5 in the setting of metabolic acidemia.
    - *Type IV RTA* results from a deficiency of aldosterone or tubular unresponsiveness to its effects. As a result of the aldosterone deficiency or insensitivity to its effects, hyperkalemia ensues because of decreased excretion and impairs ammonium generation. Titratable acid excretion is less impaired, and patients with type IV RTA can acidify the urine to a pH of 5.5 in acidotic situations. Thus, if metabolic acidosis is present and the serum potassium level is high (>5 mEq/L) with a urinary pH <5.5, one should consider the possibility of type IV RTA. Plasma renin and aldosterone should be measured after salt restriction or furosemide administration to determine whether there is a deficiency or resistance to aldosterone.

80. **What is late metabolic acidosis?**
    The term *late metabolic acidosis* is used to describe premature infants who have poor weight gain and hyperchloremic metabolic acidosis that appeared in the second to third weeks of life. The acidosis is the result of formula that contains excessive metabolic acid precursors that overload the immature kidney's ability to excrete them. With the current formulas for premature infants, late metabolic acidosis has largely disappeared.

81. **What type of RTA is seen in Fanconi syndrome?**
    Fanconi syndrome is a global disorder of proximal tubular function, including bicarbonate reabsorption. Type II RTA is the kind of RTA seen in Fanconi syndrome.

82. **What type of RTA is seen in congenital adrenal hyperplasia?**
    Type IV RTA.

83. **What type of RTA is associated with pseudohypoaldosteronism?**
    Pseudohypoaldosteronism is an inherited unresponsiveness to aldosterone due to a receptor defect. Type I pseudohypoaldosteronism is an autosomal recessive trait that presents in infancy with volume contraction, hyponatremia, hyperkalemia, metabolic acidosis, and severe salt wasting. Patients with this trait have type IV RTA.

84. **Describe the usual causes of type IV RTA in neonates.**
    - Obstructive uropathy
    - Adrenal insufficiency
    - 21-hydroxylase deficiency (congenital adrenal hyperplasia [CAH])
    - Type I pseudohypoaldosteronism

85. **How low can a premature infant reduce the urine pH?**
    During the first 3 weeks of life, a premature infant can reduce the urine pH only to 6.0 ± 0.1. After 1 month, the urine pH can be reduced to 5.2 ± 0.4.

OBSTRUCTIVE UROPATHY

86. **What is the differential diagnosis of antenatal hydronephrosis?**
    - Anomalous ureteropelvic junction/ureteropelvic junction obstruction
    - Ectopic ureter
    - PUVs
    - Multicystic kidney
    - PBS
    - Retrocaval ureter
    - Urethral atresia
    - Primary obstructive megaureter
    - Hydrocolpos
    - Nonrefluxing, nonobstructed megaureter
    - Vesicoureteral reflux
    - Midureteral stricture
    - Ectopic ureterocele
    - Pelvic tumor
    - Cloacal abnormality
    - Idiopathic

    Elder JS: Antenatal hydronephrosis: Fetal and neonatal management. Pediatr Clin North Am 44:1301, 1997.

87. **What does the postnatal evaluation of a neonate with an abnormal prenatal ultrasound include?**
    A renal and bladder ultrasound should be performed to evaluate renal length, degree of caliectasis, parenchymal thickness, presence or absence of ureteral dilation, and bladder wall thickening, and to determine whether a dilated posterior urethra or a ureterocele is present. If hydronephrosis is present, a voiding cystourethrogram and a renal scan (DTPA or MAG-3) are recommended to exclude vesicoureteral reflux and obstruction, respectively. The latter two studies may be postponed for 4–6 weeks so long as there is no significant bilateral disease or pathology affecting a solitary kidney. Prophylactic antibiotic therapy with amoxicillin, 50 mg daily, is recommended until studies are complete.

88. **What if the initial renal ultrasound yields normal results?**
    Relative oliguria in the first 48 hours of life can cause transient normalization of the renal ultrasound at the time of discharge. Because studies have shown significant pathology even with normal neonatal ultrasound, antibiotic prophylaxis and repeat ultrasound are recommended.

89. **What is ureteropelvic junction obstruction? How is it diagnosed and managed?**
    Ureteropelvic junction obstruction is the most common cause of hydronephrosis in children. Diagnosis requires the presence of hydronephrosis (ultrasound with dilated renal pelvis in the absence of a dilated ureter) and determination of significance by the use of diuretic renography. Many cases are managed expectantly. Pyeloplasty, excision of the stenotic segment, is usually necessary in cases in which neonates have an abdominal mass, bilateral hydronephrosis, or a solitary kidney.

90. **What is a ureterocele? How does it cause obstruction?**
    A ureterocele is a cystic dilatation of the distal end of the ureter. It is obstructive because it may extend through the bladder neck (ectopic) but may remain entirely within the bladder (intravesical). Ureteroceles affect girls more than boys and are usually associated with the upper pole of a completely duplicated collecting system, although in some cases the ureter may drain a single collecting system. Ultrasound shows hydronephrosis in the upper pole, dilated ureter, and the ureterocele in the bladder.

KEY POINTS: OBSTRUCTIVE UROPATHY

1. Some fetuses appear to have obstructive uropathy on ultrasound that often resolves before birth.

2. Male patients with obstructive uropathy should be considered to have PUVs until proven otherwise.

3. Prompt treatment of PUVs does not always ensure normal renal function subsequently.

POSTERIOR URETHRAL VALVES

91. **What is a PUV?**
PUVs are classified as type 1 or type 3, based on the cause of obstruction. A type 1 PUV is the most common (95%) and represents an obstructing membrane extending from the verumontanum at the base of the prostatic urethra to the more distal anterior portion of the membranous urethra. This membrane contains only a small opening through which urine can pass; as the urine flows, the membrane billows out in a windsock fashion as a one-way flap valve causing obstruction. The degree of obstruction varies, depending on the size of the opening of the membrane. A type 3 valve is less common (5%) and is caused by a thin transverse membrane across the urethra, which develops from incomplete dissolution of the urogenital diaphragm, causing urinary obstruction.

92. **Describe the most common presentation of a PUV.**
Currently, antenatal ultrasound demonstrating bilateral hydroureteronephrosis, a dilated, thick-walled bladder with poor emptying, and occasionally oligohydramnios are the most common presentations. If not detected antenatally, a PUV presents variably, based on the degree of urinary obstruction. Palpable abdominal masses, including a distended bladder, ureter, or renal pelvis, suggest urinary tract obstruction and PUV. Respiratory distress or pulmonary hypoplasia, renal insufficiency or failure, or urosepsis may all be presenting signs of PUVs in newborns. If missed in the neonatal period, urinary obstruction from valves can present later in life as diurnal enuresis due to bladder dysfunction.

93. **Name some consequences of PUVs.**
    - Glomerular and renal tubular dysfunction causing renal insufficiency, poor urinary concentrating ability, and polyuria
    - Urinary tract dilatation, including hydroureteronephrosis and bladder dilatation, and secondary to obstruction, polyuria, bladder dysfunction, and vesicoureteral reflux
    - Vesicoureteral reflux, which is found in one third to one half of boys with valves
    - Bladder dysfunction, including a wide spectrum ranging from bladder atony (poor contractility), to bladder instability (hyperactive bladder with frequent bladder contractions), to poor bladder compliance due to thickening of the bladder wall, to inability to store normal urine volumes
    - Valve bladder syndrome, which is a constellation of findings including renal tubular dysfunction, polyuria, ureteral obstruction, bladder dysfunction, and incontinence

94. **Does intervention after fetal diagnosis ultimately improve renal function?**
There is no evidence that intervention ultimately improves renal function. Fetal intervention, including vesicoamniotic shunt placement, is performed when progressive oligohydramnios is noted on serial fetal ultrasounds to improve amniotic fluid levels. Oligohydramnios is detrimental to pulmonary development and may cause pulmonary hypoplasia. Correcting oligohydramnios is thought to allow better expansion of the chest wall and lung development,

lessening the chance of pulmonary hypoplasia, but it has not been conclusively shown to affect overall renal function.

95. **Which conditions can be confused with PUVs on fetal ultrasound?**
    - PBS
    - Severe bilateral vesicoureteral reflux with distended bladder

96. **Which conditions are associated with improved prognosis?**
    Conditions that allow decompression of the urinary tract (i.e., "pop-off" mechanism) have a better prognosis. Such conditions include bladder diverticular formation; bladder ascites; and valves, unilateral reflux, and dysplasia (VURD) syndrome. Urinary ascites is caused by transudation of urine across a renal calyceal fornix into the peritoneal cavity and relief of obstruction. VURD syndrome is noted when one kidney refluxes with subsequent renal dysplasia on that side, offering protection for the contralateral kidney.

97. **What fetal findings are associated with good postnatal renal function?**
    - Normal/moderately decreased level of amniotic fluid
    - Normal/slightly increased renal parenchymal echogenicity by fetal sonography
    - Fetal urinary chemistries:
      - Sodium, <100 mEq/L
      - Chloride, <90 mEq/L
      - Osmolarity, <210 mOsm
      - Urinary output, >2 mL/h

HEMATURIA

98. **Is hematuria ever a normal finding in the newborn infant?**
    No! Hematuria is never physiologic, but it can be a common finding in sick premature infants.

99. **How is hematuria typically defined?**
    There are ≥5 red blood cells per high power field.

100. **What are the causes of hematuria in the newborn infant?**
     - Perinatal asphyxia
     - Renovascular accident (renal vein or renal artery thrombosis)
     - Neoplasia
     - Obstructive uropathy
     - Coagulopathies
     - Urinary tract infection
     - Trauma (most often suprapubic aspiration)
     - Congenital malformation, including polycystic disease

101. **How should infants with hematuria be evaluated?**
     - Exclude other causes of red urine, such as urates, porphyrins, bile pigments, myoglobin, and hemoglobin.
     - Obtain a microscopic evaluation on a fresh specimen (when examination is delayed, red blood cells can hemolyze).
     - Decide whether the blood comes from upper or lower tracts (the presence of dysmorphic red cells or casts indicates parenchymal renal disease).
     - Exclude extraurinary sources of blood, such as vaginal, rectal, or perineal sources.
     - Obtain a urine culture if infection is suspected.
     - Perform a renal ultrasound study if hematuria is persistent.

- Exclude a coagulopathy.
- Determine blood urea nitrogen and creatinine levels.

CONGENITAL NEPHROTIC SYNDROME

102. **What is the definition of** *congenital nephrotic syndrome*?
The term *congenital nephrotic syndrome* is used to describe a patient who develops the nephrotic syndrome during the first 3 months of life. Nephrotic syndrome is a constellation of abnormalities that includes (1) nephrotic-range proteinuria, defined as a urinary protein excretion >100 mg/m^2 body surface area/24 h, calculated from a timed urine collection, or a ratio of urine protein concentration (mg/dL)/urine creatinine concentration (mg/dL) >2.0–2.5, calculated from a single spot urine; (2) nephrotic range hypoalbuminemia with serum albumin concentrations <2.5 gm/dL; (3) hyperlipemia, determined from the results of measurements of serum cholesterol and/or triglyceride concentrations; and (4) peripheral edema that may be present in many patients.

103. **Newborns may have proteinuria that occurs without complete nephrotic syndrome. How does one interpret isolated proteinuria?**
Abnormal proteinuria is defined as urine protein excretion >100 mg/m^2 body surface area/24 h, calculated from a timed urine collection, or a ratio of urine protein (mg/dL)/urine creatinine (mg/dL) >0.2, calculated from a spot urine specimen. Normally, preterm infants are more likely to have proteinuria than are term infants. Abnormal proteinuria can occur in newborns as a result of various pathologic processes, including chronic volume depletion, congestive heart failure, and interstitial nephritis due to antibiotic administration. However, nephrotic-range proteinuria, as defined above, suggests significant damage to glomerular epithelial cells caused by some pathologic process. Therefore, discovery of nephrotic-range proteinuria, even in the absence of the full nephrotic syndrome, should prompt an aggressive evaluation.

104. **Describe the disease that can cause congenital nephrotic syndrome in the first 3 months of life.**
By contrast with older children with nephrotic syndrome whose underlying renal pathology is most often minimal change disease, newborns and infants who develop nephrotic syndrome are likely to suffer from a genetically determined disease. The most common cause is congenital nephrotic syndrome of the Finnish type, an autosomal recessive disease that is most common among Finns, although cases have been reported from all over the world. A less common cause of congenital nephrotic syndrome is diffuse mesangial sclerosis (DMS). DMS seems to have a genetic basis, but the exact mode of inheritance is unknown. Patients with DMS tend to develop nephrotic syndrome at an older age than do patients with the Finnish type.

Other renal lesions that can cause neonatal nephrotic syndrome may be associated with malformations that are not inherited in a known mendelian fashion. An example is Denys-Drash syndrome, a combination of ambiguous or female external genitalia with gonadal dysgenesis, a 46,XY genotype, and a predilection for the development of nephroblastoma.

Congenital infections may also cause nephrotic syndrome in a neonate. Congenital syphilis is the most common infectious association, but hepatitis B, HIV, and cytomegalovirus infections have also caused congenital nephrotic syndrome. Many patients with congenital nephrotic syndrome due to a congenital infection demonstrate depressed serum concentrations of one or more components of the complement system.

105. **What prenatal or perinatal abnormalities should alert the perinatologist to the possibility that a newborn may have or may develop congenital nephrotic syndrome?**
Most patients with congenital nephrotic syndrome of the Finnish type (CNF gene map locus 19q13.1) had a large placenta (mean placental/fetal weight, 0.4) and were born preterm and

small for gestational age. Prenatal evaluation of the mother of a patient with congenital nephrosis, Finnish variant (CNF) will have demonstrated elevated concentrations of alpha-fetoprotein in both the amniotic fluid and the mother's blood. These abnormalities are not observed in mother-infant pairs afflicted with other forms of congenital nephrotic syndrome. Infants with nephrotic syndrome due to congenital syphilis exhibit the stigmata of congenital lues.

106. **Which evaluation is appropriate for a newborn with the nephrotic syndrome?**

The evaluation should be, as usual, driven by the differential diagnosis. Although the most likely underlying diagnosis is congenital primary glomerular disease, causes of secondary nephrotic syndrome should be pursued. A careful physical examination and renal/pelvic imaging (ultrasonogram) will identify any abnormalities of the external genitalia, the internal reproductive organs, or the kidneys, such as nephroblastomatosis or Wilms' tumor, that may suggest Denys-Drash syndrome or other malformation syndromes associated with congenital nephrotic syndrome. A family history of consanguinity, fetal or neonatal demise, or renal failure may be useful in suggesting a genetic cause for the nephrotic syndrome. Blood should be drawn to measure the levels of serum complement and complement components and to uncover evidence of prenatal infection with syphilis, hepatitis B or C, HIV, cytomegalovirus, *Toxoplasma gondii*, or malaria. If the imaging and serologic evaluations are unrevealing, a renal biopsy should be performed to make a diagnosis and, thereby, to guide future management.

107. **What is the prognosis for children who develop nephrotic syndrome in the newborn period?**

As a group, patients who develop nephrotic syndrome in the newborn period have a grim prognosis. The majority will die before reaching the age of 3 years. The complications of congenital nephrotic syndrome that are responsible for the morbidity and mortality include bacterial infections and developmental delay (which are especially common among patients with congenital nephrotic syndrome), growth failure, thrombotic events, acute or chronic renal failure, complications of renal transplantation, and Wilms' tumor among patients with Denys-Drash syndrome.

NEPHROCALCINOSIS

108. **How is the diagnosis of nephrocalcinosis usually made in an infant?**

Nephrocalcinosis is usually suggested by the findings on a renal ultrasound of a hyperechoic renal medulla, commonly in a very-low-birth-weight infant. Nephrocalcinosis results from microscopic calcification in the medullary portion of the kidney but often is accompanied by hyperechoic foci in the calyces, which represent renal calculi as well. Nephrocalcinosis can present with hematuria or urinary tract infection, but it is usually an incidental finding.

109. **A 6-week-old premature infant of 28 weeks' gestation with bronchopulmonary dysplasia is found to have nephrocalcinosis. The infant has been treated for several weeks with Lasix. Is long-term furosemide therapy the only known cause of nephrocalcinosis in infancy?**

The association of long-term Lasix therapy and nephrocalcinosis has been well recognized since the original description by Hufnagle et al. in 1982. There are, however, other diagnostic considerations for infants with nephrocalcinosis, which are outlined in Table 8-5.

110. **Hypercalciuria is an important diagnostic consideration in an infant with nephrocalcinosis. What is the normal range for calcium excretion in infants?**

The value for hypercalciuria, if defined as calcium excretion of greater than the 95th percentile for an age-matched cohort, is different in infants compared with older children. In infants

TABLE 8-5.	DIAGNOSTIC CONSIDERATIONS FOR INFANTS WITH NEPHROCALCINOSIS	
Normocalcemic Hypercalciuria	**Hypercalcemic Hypercalciuria**	**Normocalciuric Nephrocalcinosis**
Furosemide therapy	Hyperparathyroidism	Primary hyperoxaluria
Bartter syndrome	Hypophosphatasia	Enteric hyperoxaluria
Distal renal tubular acidosis	Williams syndrome	Renal candidiasis
Hyperprostaglandin E	Idiopathic infantile hypercalcemia	Long-term acetazolamide therapy
Subcutaneous fat necrosis	Dystrophic calcifications	

Adapted from Karlowicz MG, Adelman RD: Renal calcification in the first year of life. Pediatr Clin North Am 42:1397–1413, 1995.

younger than 7 months old, the 95th percentile for urinary calcium/creatinine (mg/mg) was reported by Sargent et al. to be 0.86, and in children 7–18 months old, the value was 0.60. In another study, very-low-birth-weight infants with nephrocalcinosis had a mean urinary calcium/creatinine of 0.49 compared with 0.11 in control subjects. The relatively low calcium excretion in the controls of this study conflicted with the much higher levels in the first study and are in the range described for older children. This discrepancy has resulted in confusion in the evaluation of infants with nephrocalcinosis.

111. **What is the suggested therapy for an infant with nephrocalcinosis?**
Treatment of the primary cause can be important in cases not caused by long-term furosemide therapy. In infants being given furosemide, substitution of a thiazide diuretic for furosemide can decrease the calcium excretion and result in shrinkage of calculi and improvement of the medullary nephrocalcinosis. The long-term prognosis has been correlated to the course of the urinary calcium excretion.

112. **What is the long-term prognosis in infants with nephrocalcinosis?**
Long-term studies of premature infants with nephrocalcinosis have suggested that 30–50% of the children continue to have evidence of renal calcification up to 5 years after diagnosis. There is some evidence of a slightly decreased GFR and tubular function, but some of these findings may be the result of a premature birth and not specific for the history of nephrocalcinosis.

HYPERTENSION

113. **Discuss the environmental and technical factors that can affect blood pressure measurements in the newborn.**
Various factors alter the relationship between blood pressure as recorded on the neonatal intensive care unit (NICU) flow sheet and the patient's true average baseline blood pressure. For example, blood pressure readings are affected by the patient's position (pressures measured when the patient is supine are slightly higher than those obtained when the patient is prone), by recent medical manipulations, or by recent feeding. Cuff inflation, by itself, can stimulate the startle response that can cause a transient increase in blood pressure. In addition, body geography has an impact on blood pressure measurements: pressures measured in the legs are normally somewhat higher than those measured in the arms.

114. **Which newborns have hypertension?**

This question is often difficult to answer. There are published data about the normal ranges of systolic and diastolic blood pressures for term newborns and premature infants at various gestational ages. These data, however, were derived from blood pressure measurements that were obtained randomly, without respect to the patient's state of alertness or agitation.

A single random recording of elevated blood pressure may not have clinical significance because it may not exemplify the patient's average blood pressure. A more representative blood pressure measurement is recorded when the infant has not been fed or manipulated for 90 minutes before the evaluation; further refinement is achieved when several blood pressure measurements are made over a period of 5–10 minutes.

The diagnosis of hypertension should be made only if the systolic and diastolic blood pressures are above the 95th percentile on at least three separate blood pressure measurements recorded at 2-minute intervals during a time when the infant is quiet and otherwise undisturbed.

115. **What is the most common cause of hypertension among patients in the NICU?**

Historically, the most common cause of hypertension among patients in the NICU was renal artery thrombosis due to thrombotic emboli that are released from an umbilical artery catheter (UAC). The thrombotic lesions usually occur in the peripheral circulation of one kidney, although there may be bilateral lesions. In the most serious situation, segmental thrombosis may propagate backward and occlude one or both main renal arteries.

More recently, extremely-low-birth-weight infants with bronchopulmonary dysplasia appear to develop hypertension in the absence of clear evidence of renal artery occlusion at a rate higher than that seen with renal thrombosis. The etiology in many of these cases cannot be determined, and it may appear even after NICU discharge. Extremely-low-birth-weight infants who have been hospitalized for a prolonged period should therefore have routine blood pressure measurements made during their well-baby visits throughout the first year of life. This is often neglected by pediatricians because of the difficulty in obtaining an accurate determination in these tiny babies.

116. **What is the blood pressure profile of a patient whose hypertension is due to a complication related to a UAC?**

Most patients who develop hypertension as a result of complications from a UAC are normotensive until the UAC is pulled. When the UAC is removed, hypertension often develops abruptly. The onset of hypertension in this situation coincides with the embolization of renal vessels by clots that are sheared from the tip of the catheter during its withdrawal.

117. **What is the treatment of choice for newborns with hypertension related to a complication from the UAC?**

UAC-related hypertension is generated by high circulating concentrations of angiotensin II. Angiotensin II production can be blocked by use of drugs that inhibit angiotensin-converting enzyme (ACE) inhibitors. Captopril, given at 0.5 mg/kg/day divided into three or four daily doses, is often able to normalize blood pressure. The daily dose may be increased to 2–4 mg/kg, if needed. Other ACE inhibitors such as enalapril or lisinopril may be used with equally beneficial effects, but dosing of these drugs for very small patients may be problematic for pharmacists. In such instances, hydralazine in a dose of 0.15–0.6 mg/kg/dose may be helpful.

118. **What role do endocrine hormones play in neonatal hypertension?**

Most cases of hypertension in newborns are due to excessive circulating concentrations of hormones that cause hypertension as a result of their ability to increase peripheral vascular resistance and/or by virtue of their ability to cause salt and water retention.

Renin produced by the kidney in response to either UAC-related renal artery thrombosis or to congenital renal artery stenosis generates angiotensin I. Angiotensin I is converted to angiotensin II by action of ACE that is present in the kidney, lung, placenta, brain, and other organs. Angiotensin II has multiple effects when it circulates in the blood, including increased peripheral vascular resistance, augmented production and release of aldosterone by the adrenal glands, and stimulation of thirst and salt craving. All of these angiotensin II actions cause an increase in blood pressure.

Rare endocrine disorders such as virilizing adrenal hyperplasia due to 11β-hydroxylase deficiency and primary hyperaldosteronism may cause neonatal hypertension due to overproduction of mineralocorticoid (desoxycorticosterone in the case of 11β-hydroxylase deficiency; aldosterone in patients with hyperaldosteronism). The overproduction of mineralocorticoid in these diseases causes hypertension via inappropriate renal salt and water retention. There may also be a mineralocorticoid-mediated hypokalemic metabolic alkalosis.

Prenatal or postnatal exposure to exogenous steroids (e.g., betamethasone, prednisone, or methylprednisolone) can, likewise, cause hypertension in newborns.

119. **What abnormality of the physical examination of a hypertensive infant suggests that coarctation of the aorta may be the cause of the elevated blood pressure?**
Despite the conventional wisdom that coarctation of the aorta is associated with a cardiac murmur and absent femoral pulses, many newborns with aortic coarctation do not fit the mold. In hypertensive infants, it is crucial to measure blood pressure in both upper and lower extremities. Coarctation of the aorta should be suspected if the systolic pressure in the leg is more than 10 mmHg lower than the systolic pressure in the arms.

KEY POINTS: HYPERTENSION

1. Neonatal hypertension during or after NICU hospitalization is not rare and should be monitored in all patients.

2. Hypertension related to umbilical catheterization usually occurs during treatment or immediately after removal of the catheter.

3. Hypertension unrelated to catheters typically will appear later during NICU hospitalization in an extremely-low-birth-weight infant with chronic lung disease.

4. Coarctation of the aorta needs to be considered in any neonate with hypertension.

RENAL VEIN THROMBOSIS

120. **Renal vein thrombosis (RVT) occurs rarely among newborn infants. Most cases are idiopathic. What are some maternal and infant factors that increase the risk of RVT?**
Maternal factors known to increase the risk of RVT in the newborn include diabetes mellitus, elevated levels of immunoglobulin G anticardiolipin antibody, and activated protein C resistance. In addition, one should be cautious with infants born to mothers who have required anticoagulation during pregnancy for thrombotic disorders.

Infants with hemoglobin SS or inherited thrombophilic disorders, such as a deficiency of protein S, protein C, or antithrombin III, have an increased risk of RVT. Newborns who are otherwise healthy may develop RVT if they have experienced perinatal asphyxia, an episode of sepsis, or hyperosmolarity and dehydration due to, for example, administration of intravenous radiocontrast or fluid losses as a result of vomiting or diarrhea.

121. **What signs and symptoms suggest the occurrence of RVT in a newborn?**

A clinician should suspect the diagnosis of RVT if a newborn develops hematuria (often gross hematuria) in association with a swollen kidney, palpable as a flank mass, and abrupt or progressive elevation of the plasma creatinine concentration. One should be especially cautious if these abnormalities are accompanied by thrombocytopenia. RVT may not, however, always induce dramatic clinical or laboratory changes. For example, a newborn with RVT may produce urine that is clear yellow; microscopic hematuria with or without proteinuria may be the only urinary abnormality. Even when the RVT does not cause major changes in the urinalysis, however, there is usually a measurable deterioration of renal function, thrombocytopenia, and perhaps a transient elevation of blood pressure.

122. **Which imaging studies are helpful, and which may be harmful, when one is trying to diagnose RVT?**

Renal ultrasonography is a useful tool. It is noninvasive and usually identifies areas of the kidney that are affected by RVT. The renal parenchyma that experiences obstruction to venous drainage appears swollen and hyperechoic.

Renal scans using intravenous injections of technetium DTPA or technetium dimercaptosuccinic acid demonstrate perfusion defects in the areas that are drained by the thrombosed renal vessels. These scans, however, do not provide anatomic detail, nor are they able to differentiate between arterial and venous renovascular disease. Furthermore, the utility of renal scans is limited by the fact that they generally require the sick infant to be transported from the neonatal unit to the nuclear medicine department.

Because RVT may be caused by serum hyperosmolarity, intravenous administration of hypertonic radiocontrast agents may be ill-advised. Therefore, the clinician should avoid ordering studies such as intravenous pyelography or computed tomography that may require administration of intravenous contrast agents.

123. **Which fluid and electrolyte abnormalities may occur in an infant with RVT?**

Infants with RVT commonly experience a period of renal insufficiency that results in the following fluid and electrolyte abnormalities:
- Oliguria, fluid retention, and hyponatremia
- Metabolic acidosis
- Hyperphosphatemia
- Hypocalcemia

124. **Is there a role for thrombectomy or nephrectomy of kidneys with RVT?**

Neither thrombectomy nor nephrectomy has a role. Thrombectomy is unlikely to provide benefit because most cases of RVT begin in the peripheral renal venous circulation; therefore, removal of any clot that may be present in the main renal vein is not likely to restore venous drainage to the bulk of the affected renal parenchyma. Some advocate attempting thrombectomy when bilateral RVT also involves the inferior vena cava; however, there is little evidence to support the notion that the procedure, even in the direst circumstances, improves either long-term patient survival or ultimate renal function.

Because many, if not most, kidneys with RVT ultimately recover some function as a result of recanalization of thrombosed vessels, nephrectomy of the affected kidney in the acute or subacute phase of RVT should be discouraged. Evidence is unsubstantiated that nephrectomy improves patient survival, and it certainly leads to a decrease in functional nephron mass.

125. **Is thrombolytic (e.g., urokinase, tissue plasminogen activator) or anticoagulant therapy useful in neonates with RVT?**

The usefulness of thrombolytic or anticoagulant therapy must be qualified by such terms as *maybe* or *sometimes*.

Infusion of thrombocytic agents, either locally or systemically, has been used with some success in patients with RVT or with renal arterial thrombosis. The risk of hemorrhagic complications, however, is significant. Because thrombolysis and venous recanalization occur as part of the normal resolution of RVT, it is not clear that pharmacologic thrombolytic therapy carries a favorable risk-benefit ratio.

Anticoagulant intervention aimed at prevention of extension of RVT into previously uninvolved venous structures may be appropriate for some patients, particularly those who have congenital thrombophilic disorders. The prothrombotic factors that lead to RVT formation and propagation in most newborns can be eliminated without anticoagulant therapy (e.g., hyperosmolarity, dehydration). However, anticoagulants may protect infants with intrinsic abnormalities of the coagulation cascade from experiencing secondary thrombotic events.

PRUNE-BELLY SYNDROME

126. What is PBS?

Prune-belly syndrome (PBS) consists of (1) absent or decreased abdominal musculature, causing the abdomen of the recumbent newborn to appear wrinkled or prune-like; (2) undescended testes; and (3) abnormalities of the kidneys and urinary tract (Fig. 8-3).

127. What are the most common urinary tract anomalies that occur in patients with PBS?

From bottom to top, the most common urinary tract anomalies are the following:
1. The bladder neck is patulous.
2. The bladder is capacious. The bladder wall may be thickened, but the internal contour of the bladder is smooth, without trabeculations or diverticuli. Often the bladder communicates with a patent urachus.
3. Ureteral abnormalities commonly consist of irregular dilatations and narrowings, usually most dramatic in the lower ureteral segments.
4. The kidneys are often small, with or without dilation of the collecting system.

Of importance, the anatomic abnormalities of the urinary tract in patients with PBS may be due to primary, intrinsic, and diffuse defects of embryologic development of the structures

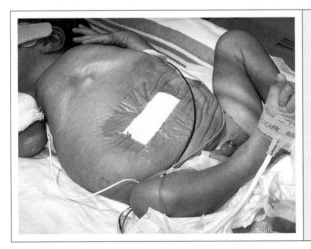

Figure 8-3. Prune-belly syndrome.

involved, which are different from the discrete lesions of obstruction or reflux that may occur in the urinary tract of otherwise normal newborns, although they may appear similar to those that occur in PBS. For example, the large, thick-walled bladder of patients with PBS may occur in the absence of bladder outlet obstruction, although the bladder may bear a resemblance to that of a patient with PUVs. Likewise, although ureteral dilatation in otherwise normal infants is commonly associated with vesicoureteral reflux or obstruction, a similar ureteral lesion in a patient with PBS may occur in the absence of reflux or obstruction.

128. **What important anomalies outside the genitourinary system occur more commonly among patients with PBS than among otherwise healthy neonates? What are their causes?**
Patients with PBS often have problems that are related to pulmonary hypoplasia; hip dislocation or subluxation; talipes equinovarus; congenital cardiac disease, especially atrial septal defect, ventricular septal defect, and tetralogy of Fallot; and gastrointestinal anomalies.

   The urologic/renal dysfunction in patients with PBS is almost certainly responsible for some of the nonurologic complications. For example, oligohydramnios, a common complication of PBS pregnancies, accounts for the pulmonary hypoplasia, the hip dislocation or subluxation, and the talipes equinovarus that may be seen in these newborns. It is uncertain how the components of PBS cause the excess prevalence of other anomalies that occur in the heart and in the gastrointestinal tract.

129. **Which diagnostic studies assist the neonatologist in evaluating a child with PBS?**
A newborn with PBS requires an exhaustive evaluation of the urinary tract anatomy. The aim of the evaluation is to identify the extent of anatomic abnormalities and, more importantly, to diagnose lesions that may require urgent intervention. Therefore, the initial work-up should include (1) abdominal and pelvic ultrasonography to provide a basic road map of the genitourinary anomalies and (2) voiding cystourethrography to diagnose vesicoureteral reflux and reflux into a patent urachus. Either diagnosis, vesicoureteral reflux or patent urachus, mandates initiation of antibiotic prophylaxis. If the infant is stable enough to be transported, other imaging studies significantly enhance understanding of the genitourinary pathology. Computerized axial tomograms of the abdomen, performed before and after intravenous administration of radio-contrast material, will usually reveal more anatomic detail than ultrasound and, in addition, they provide a qualitative assessment of comparative renal function (i.e., right versus left kidney). Renal scan using DTPA localizes any points of obstruction between the kidneys and the bladder and provides a quantitative estimate of the comparative function of the two kidneys.

   Because an infant with PBS may also harbor gastrointestinal and cardiac anomalies, the wise neonatologist will order an upper gastrointestinal tract series with small bowel follow-through, a barium enema, an electrocardiogram, and an echocardiogram.

130. **What is the role for surgical intervention in patients with PBS?**
Every newborn with PBS should be evaluated by a pediatric urologist. However, intervention during the newborn period should be limited to the least invasive procedures available and should be used only when necessary to relieve high-grade obstruction in the urinary tract. More extensive genitourinary reconstructive procedures should be postponed to a later date and, in fact, may not be necessary at all. There is considerable controversy about whether surgical intervention is appropriate in boys with PBS when their genitourinary anomalies are not associated with obstruction or vesicoureteral reflux.

   At some point, the surgeon must deal with the intra-abdominal cryptorchidism. Orchidectomy, as a means to prevent testicular neoplasia, is an option because the reproductive potential of boys with PBS is probably low. An alternate approach is to relocate the abdominal testes into the scrotum by one of a variety of complex surgeries. In any case, these surgical interventions can wait until the infant is several months old.

Surgical plication of the lax abdominal musculature is important for the psychological well-being of patients with PBS, but this cosmetic reconstruction should probably not be performed in a newborn.

131. **What are other names for PBS?**
PBS is also known as *Eagle-Barrett syndrome* and as *triad syndrome*. Eagle and Barrett should not be awarded historic primacy because their 1950 report of nine cases of PBS reiterated a description of the syndrome that had been published by R.W. Parker some 55 years earlier. The term *triad syndrome* may be appropriate, although it is neither specific nor descriptive.

132. **Parents almost always smile when they see that their infant has dimples. Some dimples, however, can constantly remind parents that their child has PBS. Where are these dimples?**
Many patients with PBS have dimples on the lateral aspect of the knees and/or elbows.

CYSTIC KIDNEY DISEASE

133. **What is the definition of *multicystic renal disease*?**
A multicystic kidney is the result of abnormal metanephric differentiation. There is no continuity between glomeruli and calyces, and the kidney does not function. The contralateral kidney may be normal, absent, hydronephrotic, ectopic, or dysplastic.

134. **What is the definition of *renal cystic dysplasia*?**
Renal cystic dysplasia involves unilateral or bilateral, usually cystic kidneys with disorganized architecture. It often contains ectopic tissues (e.g., cartilage, muscle) and results in reduced renal function.

135. **What is the definition of *polycystic renal disease*?**
With polycystic renal disease, there are many cysts in both kidneys, no dysplasia, and continuity between glomeruli and calyces. The kidneys are often large.

136. **Describe the management of autosomal recessive polycystic kidney disease in a neonate.**
- Offer parents the option of withdrawal of life support.
- Treat the hyponatremia with furosemide.
- Treat the hypertension with an ACE inhibitor.
- Ventilate; drain pneumothoraces.
- Perform uninephrectomy, if there is massive nephromegaly, for adequate enteral feeding.
- Perform bilateral nephrectomy, if massive nephromegaly is present, for better ventilation.
- Order peritoneal dialysis in cases of chronic renal failure.

137. **What is the prognosis of autosomal recessive polycystic kidney disease?**
1. Life-table survival rates calculated from birth:
   - 86% alive at 3 months
   - 79% alive at 1 year
   - 51% alive at 10 years
   - 46% alive at 15 years
2. Patients who survive to age 1 year: 82% alive at 10 years

138. **What is the probability of requiring antihypertensive treatment?**
The probability of requiring antihypertensive treatment is 39% at 1 year and 60% at 15 years of age.

139. **Name some additional complications that can occur in infants with autosomal recessive polycystic disease.**
   - Bleeding from gastroesophageal varices
   - Hypersplenism with combinations of anemia, leukopenia, and thrombocytopenia
   - Urinary tract infections in 30%
   - Growth retardation in 25%
   - Rare cases of cholangiocarcinoma

140. **Can autosomal dominant polycystic kidney disease present in the neonate?**
   Patients with polycystic kidney disease and patients with a maternal history of tuberous sclerosis may have polycystic kidneys in the neonatal period.

141. **What are the indications for liver and renal biopsies in neonates with polycystic kidneys?**
   There are no indications for biopsies in these patients. Careful evaluation with ultrasonography is sufficient for diagnostic and treatment purposes.

142. **In which conditions may there be an association between abnormal kidneys and congenital hepatic fibrosis?**
   Congenital hepatic fibrosis and polycystic kidneys
   - Autosomal recessive polycystic kidneys
   - Autosomal dominant polycystic kidneys
   Congenital hepatic fibrosis and hereditary tubulointerstitial nephritis
   - Juvenile nephronophthisis
   - Bardet-Biedl syndrome
   - Jeune's syndrome (asphyxiating thoracic chondrodystrophy)
   Congenital hepatic fibrosis and hereditary renal dysplasia
   - Meckel's syndrome
   - Chondrodysplasia syndromes
   - Renal-hepatic-pancreatic cystic dysplasia (Ivemark's syndrome)
   - Zellweger syndrome

EXTROPHY

143. **What are the correct terms for the developmental defect shown in Fig. 8-4?**
   The correct terms for the developmental defect shown in Fig. 8-4 are *bladder exstrophy* and *epispadias*.

144. **When does this developmental defect occur?**
   Bladder closure takes place between the sixth and eighth weeks of fetal life.

145. **When should the exstrophy-epispadias complex be repaired?**
   Bladder exstrophy should be closed in the first 48 hours of life to ensure the best possible technical results for achieving long-term continence.

146. **Should one be concerned with upper urinary tract anomalies in children with bladder exstrophy?**
   No. The upper urinary tract is almost always normal in these children. Evaluation of these children should include assessment of the hips, however, because some of them will have hip dysplasia.

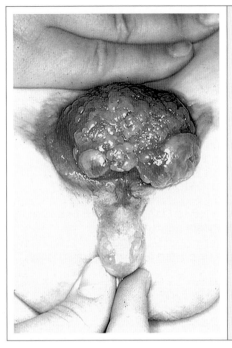

Figure 8-4. Exstrophy of the bladder and epispadius.

147. **What is the risk of recurrence in subsequent pregnancies?**
The risk is no greater than that for the general population, which is 1:50,000 live births.

148. **True or false: the exstrophy-epispadias complex is decreasing in incidence.**
True. The reasons are not entirely clear; however, it appears that the widespread use of prenatal ultrasonography and elective termination have had a significant impact on the incidence of bladder exstrophy worldwide.

HYPOSPADIAS

149. **What is the developmental defect shown in Fig. 8-5?**
The developmental defect shown in Fig. 8-5 is called *hypospadias.*

150. **Does the child shown in Fig. 8-5 need immediate surgical attention?**
No. Surgical correction is best done somewhere between 6 and 12 months of life, assuming there are no additional medical issues.

151. **When during development did this lesion occur?**
Penile development takes place between 12 and 15 weeks of gestation.

152. **Hypospadias in association with bilateral nonpalpable gonads demands what kind of evaluation?**
Chromosomal evaluation is mandatory in infants with hypospadias and nonpalpable gonads. One must rule out virilizing congenital adrenal hyperplasia to prevent errors in gender assignment and to avoid a risk of a salt-losing crisis in the infant.

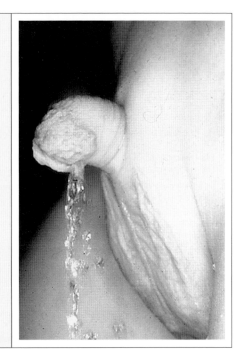

Figure 8-5. Hypospadius.

153. How common are other genitourinary abnormalities in infants with distal hypospadias?
Rare. There is no greater incidence of other genital urinary anomalies in infants with distal hypospadias than in other infants.

154. What is happening to the incidence of hypospadias?
The incidence of hypospadias is increasing nationwide. The reason is not entirely clear, but it may have to do with increasing maternal age and increasing incidence of in vitro fertilization.

BIBLIOGRAPHY

1. Bauer K, Boverman G, Roithmaier A, et al: Body composition, nutrition, and fluid balance during the first two weeks of life in preterm neonates weighing less than 1500 grams. J Pediar 118:615–620, 1991.

2. Bauer K, Götz M, Roithmaier A, et al: Postnatal weight loss in ventilated premature infants below 1500 g: Significance of renal and extrarenal fluid loss. Monatsschrift Kinderheilkunde 139:452–456, 1991.

3. Bauer K, Versmold H: Postnatal weight loss in preterm neonates < 1599 g is due to isotonic dehydration of the extracellular volume. Acta Paediatr Scand Suppl 360:37–42, 1989.

4. Bell EF, Acarregui MJ: Restricted versus liberal fluid intake for preventing morbidity and mortality in preterm infants (Cochrane Review). In The Cochrane Library, Issue 4. Chichester, UK, John Riley & Sons, CD003665, 2001.

5. Bell EF, Warburton D, Stonestreet BS, Oh W: Effect of fluid administration on the development of symptomatic patent ductus arteriosus and congestive heart failure in premature infants. N Engl J Med 302:598–604, 1980.

6. Bell EF, Warburton D, Stonestreet BS, Oh W: High-volume intake predisposes premature infants to necrotizing enterocolitis [letter]. Lancet 2:90, 1979.

7. Cendron M, Elder JS, Duckett JW: Perinatal urology. In Gilenwater JY, Grayhack JT, Howards SS, Duckett JW (eds): Adult and Pediatric Urology, 3rd ed. St. Louis, Mosby, 1996, pp 2075–2169.

8. Clark DA: Time of first void and first stool in 500 newborns. Pediatrics 60:457–459, 1977.

9. Dell RB: Normal acid-base regulation. In Winters RW (ed): The Body Fluids in Pediatrics, 1st ed. Boston, Little, Brown, 1973.

10. Duncan BW, Adzick NS, Longaker MT, et al: In utero arterial embolism from renal vein thrombosis with successful postnatal thrombolytic therapy. J Pediatr Surg 26:741–743, 1991.

11. Edelmann CM Jr, Rodriguez-Soriano J, Boichis H, et al: Renal bicarbonate reabsorption and hydrogen ion excretion in normal infants. J Clin Invest 46:1309–1317, 1967.

12. Elder JS: Antenatal hydronephrosis: Fetal and neonatal management. Pediatr Clin North Am 44:1299–1321, 1997.

13. Ellis EN, Arnold WC: Use of urinary indexes in renal failure in the newborn. Am J Dis Child 136:615–617, 1982.

14. Fick GM, Gabow PA: Hereditary and acquired cystic disease of the kidney. Kidney Int 46:961–964, 1994.

15. Fukuda Y, Kojima T, Ono A, et al: Factors causing hyperkalemia in premature infants. Am J Perinatol 6:76–79, 1989.

16. Gasser B, Mauss Y, Ghnassia JP, et al: A quantitative study of normal nephrogenesis in the human fetus: Its implications in the natural history of kidney changes due to low obstructive uropathies. Fetal Diagn Ther 8:8:371–384, 1993.

17. Gaudio KM, Siegel NJ: Pathogenesis and treatment of acute renal failure. Pediatr Clin North Am 34:771–787, 1987.

18. Glick PL, Harrison MR, Golbus MS, et al: Management of the fetus with congenital hydronephrosis II: Prognostic criteria and selection for treatment. J Pediatr Surg 20:376–387, 1985.

19. Goble MM: Hypertension in infancy. Pediatr Clin North Am 40:105–114, 1993.

20. Gonzalez ET: Posterior urethral valves and other urethral anomalies. In Campbell MF, Walsh PC, Retik AB (eds): Campbell's Urology, 4th ed. Philadelphia, W.B. Saunders, 1998, pp 2069–2091.

21. Gruskay J, Costarino AT, Polin RA, et al: Nonoliguric hyperkalemia in the premature infant weighing less than 1000 grams. J Pediatr 113:381–386, 1988.

22. Hammarlund K, Nilsson GE, Öberg PÅ, Sedin G: Transepidermal water loss in newborn infants. Part I: Relation to ambient humidity and site of measurement and estimation of total transepidermal water loss. Acta Paediatr Scand 66:553, 1977.

23. Hammarlund K, Sedin G, Strömberg B: Transepidermal water loss in newborn infants. Part VIII: Relationship to gestational age and post-natal age in appropriate and small for gestation infants. Acta Paediatr Scand 72:721–728, 1983.

24. Hartnoll G, Bétrémieux P, Modi N: Randomized controlled trial of postnatal sodium supplementation on body composition in 25 to 30 week gestation age infants. Arch Dis Child 82:F24–F28, 2000.

25. Hawdon JM, Ward Platt MP, Aynsley-Green A: Prevention and management of neonatal hypoglycemia. Arch Dis Child 70:F54–F65, 1994.

26. Heimler R, Doumas BT, Jendrzejcak BM, et al: Relationship between nutrition, weight change, and fluid compartments in preterm infants during the first week of life. J Pediatr 122:110–114, 1993.

27. Holbeck CC: Understanding the different values in electrolyte measurements. In Skurp A (ed): http://www.bloodgas.com. Copenhagen, Technology, Radiometer A/S, 2002.

28. Hood VL, Tannen RL: Protection of acid-base balance by pH regulation of acid production. N Engl J Med 339:819–826, 1998.

29. Hoover DL, Duckett JW: Posterior urethral valves, unilateral reflux and renal dysplasia: A syndrome. J Urol 128:994–997, 1982.

30. Hufnagle KG, Khan SN, Penn D, et al: Renal calcifications: A complication of long-term furosemide therapy in preterm infants. Pediatrics 70:360–363, 1982.

31. Ing FF, Starc TJ, Griffits SP, Gersony WM: Early diagnosis of coarctation of the aorta in children: A continuing dilemma. Pediatrics 98:378–382, 1996.

32. Jee LD, Rickwood AM, Turnock RR: Posterior urethral valves: Does prenatal diagnosis influence prognosis? Br J Urol 72:830–833, 1993.

33. Kaplan BS, Fay J, Shah V, et al: TM autosomal recessive polycystic kidney disease. Pediatr Nephrol 3:43–49, 1989.

34. Karlowicz MG, Adelman RD: Renal calcification in the first year of life. Pediatr Clin North Am 42:1397–1413, 1995.

35. Kjartansson S, Arsan S, Hammarlund K, et al: Water loss from the skin of term and preterm infants nursed under a radiant heater. Pediatr Res 37:233–238, 1995.

36. Libenson MH, Kaye EM, Rosman NP, Gilmore HE: Acetazolamide and furosemide for posthemorrhagic hydrocephalus of the newborn. Pediatr Neurol 20:185–191, 1999.

37. Lorenz JM: Fluid and electrolyte management during the first week of life. In Fletcher J, Polin RA (eds): Workbook in Practical Neonatology, 3rd ed. Philadelphia, W.B. Saunders, 2000.

38. Lorenz JM: Fluid and electrolyte therapy in the newborn infant. In Burg FD, Polin RA, Ingelfinger JR, Gershon A (eds): Current Pediatric Therapy 17. Philadelphia, W.B. Saunders, 2002.

39. Lorenz JM, Kleinman LI, Ahmed G, Markarian K: Phases of fluid and electrolyte homeostasis in the extremely low birth weight infant. Pediatrics 96:484–489, 1995.

40. Lorenz JM, Kleinman LI, Disney TA: Renal response of newborn dogs to potassium loading. Am J Physiol 251:F513–F519, 1986.

41. Lorenz JM, Kleinman LI, Kotagal UR, Reller MD: Water balance in very low birth weight infants: Relationship to water and sodium intake and effect on outcome. J Pediatr 101:423–432, 1982.

42. Machin GA: Diseases causing fetal and neonatal ascites. Pediatr Pathol 4:195–211, 1985.

43. Malone TA: Glucose and insulin versus cation-exchange resin for the treatment of hyperkalemia in very low birth weight infants. J Pediatr 118:121–123, 1991.

44. Moore RD: Effects of insulin upon ion transport. Biochim Biophys Acta 737:1–49, 1983.

45. Nawankwo MU, Torenz JM, Gardiner JC: A standard protocol for blood pressure measurement in the newborn. Pediatrics 99:E10, 1997.

46. Ogborn MR: Polycystic kidney disease—a truly pediatric problem. Pediatr Nephrol 8:762–767, 1994.

47. Peters CA: Obstruction of the fetal urinary tract. J Am Soc Nephrol 8:653–663, 1997.

48. Riesenfeld T, Hammarlund K, Sedin G: Respiratory water loss in relation to gestational age in infants on their first day of life. Acta Paediatr 84:1056–1059, 1995.

49. Rodriguez-Soriano J: Bartter and related syndromes: The puzzle is almost solved. Pediatr Nephrol 12:315–327, 1998.

50. Rosendaal FR: Thrombosis in the young: Epidemiology and risk factors. A focus on venous thrombosis. Thromb Haemost 78:1–6, 1997.

51. Roy S, Dillon MJ, Trompeter RS, Barratt TM: Autosomal recessive polycystic kidney disease: Long-term outcome of neonatal survivors. Pediatr Nephrol 11:302–306, 1997.

52. Sargent JD, Stukel TA, Kresel J, Klein RZ: Normal values for random urinary calcium to creatinine ratios in infancy. J Pediatr 123:393–397, 1993.

53. Schwartz GJ, Haycock GB, Edelmann CM Jr, Spitzer A: Late metabolic acidosis: A reassessment of the definition. J Pediatr 95:102–107, 1979.

54. Shaffer SG, Bradt SK, Hall RT: Postnatal changes in total body water and extracellular volume in preterm infants with respiratory distress syndrome. J Pediatr 109:509–514, 1986.

55. Shaffer SG, Bradt SK, Meade VM, Hall RT: Extracellular fluid volume changes in very low birth weight infants during the first 2 postnatal months. J Pediatr 111:124–128, 1987.

56. Shaffer SG, Kilbride HW, Hayen LK, et al: Hyperkalemia in very low birth weight infants. J Pediatr 121:275–279, 1992.

57. Shaffer SG, Meade VM: Sodium balance and extracellular volume regulation in very low birth weight infants. J Pediatr 115:285–290, 1989.

58. Shaffer SG, Weismann DN: Fluid requirements in the preterm infant. Clin Perinatol 19:233–250, 1992.

59. Simon DB, Lifton RP: The molecular basis of inherited hypokalemic alkalosis: Bartter's and Gitelman's syndrome. Am J Physiol 271:F961–F966, 1996.

60. Singhi S, Sood V, Bhakoo ON, Ganguly NK: Effects of intrauterine growth retardation on postnatal changes in body composition of preterm infants. Indian J Med Res 102:275–280, 1995.

61. Singhi S, Sood VI, Bhakoo NK, Kaur A: Composition of postnatal weight loss & subsequent weight gain in preterm infants. Indian J Med Res 101:157–162, 1995.

62. Stefano JL, Norman ME: Insulin therapy for nonoliguric hyperkalemia in the extremely low birth weight infant: Is it effective? [abstract]. Pediatr Res 31:66A, 1992.

63. Stefano JL, Norman ME: Nitrogen balance in extremely low birth weight infants with nonoliguric hyperkalemia. J Pediatr 123:632–635, 1993.

64. Stefano JL, Norman ME, Morales MC, et al: Decreased erythrocyte Na$^+$,K$^+$-ATPase activity associated with cellular potassium loss in extremely low birth weight infants with nonoliguric hyperkalemia. J Pediatr 122:276–284, 1993.

65. Stonestreet BS, Bell EF, Warburton D, Oh W: Renal response in low-birth-weight neonates: results of prolonged intake of two different amounts of fluid and sodium. Am J Dis Child 137:215–219, 1983.

66. Svenningsen NW: Renal acid-base titration studies in infants with and without metabolic acidosis. Pediatr Res 8:659–672, 1974.

67. Tan KL: Blood pressure in very low birth weight infants in the first 70 days of life. J Pediatr 112:266–270, 1988.

68. Van der Wagen A, Okken A, Zweens J, Zijlstra WG: Composition of postnatal weight loss and subsequent weight gain in small for dates newborn infants. Acta Paediatr Scand 74:57–61, 1985.

CHAPTER 9

GASTROENTEROLOGY AND NUTRITION

Roy Proujansky, MD, and Peter C. Wilmot, DO

DEVELOPMENT OF THE GASTROINTESTINAL SYSTEM

1. How does the primitive gut develop in the fetus?

Folding occurs along the embryo in a cephalocaudal progression that results in the incorporation of some of the endodermal-lined yolk sac into the embryo, which in turn results in the creation of the primitive gut. The cephalic portion will become the foregut, and the caudal parts will become the hindgut (Fig. 9-1).

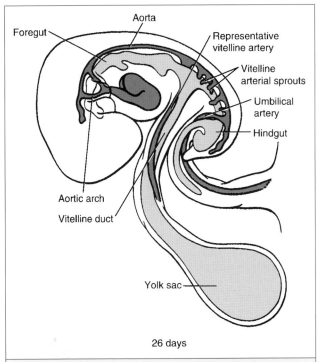

Aorta

Foregut

Representative vitelline artery

Vitelline arterial sprouts

Umbilical artery

Hindgut

Aortic arch

Vitelline duct

Yolk sac

26 days

Figure 9-1. The foregut, midgut, and hindgut of the primitive gut tube are formed by the combined action of differential growth and lateral and cephalocaudal folding. The foregut and hindgut are blind-ending tubes that terminate at the buccopharyngeal and cloacal membranes, respectively. The midgut is at first completely open to the cavity of the yolk sac. (From Larsen WJ, Sherman LS, Potter SS, Scott WJ [eds]: Human Embryology, 3rd ed. New York, Churchill Livingstone, 2001, p 237.)

2. **When does the lung bud separate the esophagus?**
   At about 4 weeks of gestation, the lung buds appear on the ventral surface of the foregut. This out-pocketing from the esophagus will eventually separate completely, forming separate walls known as the *esophagotracheal septum*. This separation is critical, and any remnant in connection leads to esophageal atresia and/or a tracheoesophageal fistula. The most common type of developmental abnormality as a result of this splitting is proximal esophageal atresia and a distal esophagotracheal fistula.

3. **When does the liver develop?**
   The liver forms at about the third week of gestation as an outgrowth, known as the *hepatic diverticulum* or *liver bud,* of the endodermal epithelium of the foregut. This connection grows and narrows to form the bile duct to connect the developing liver to the foregut. A small ventral outgrowth forms that will develop into the gallbladder and connecting cystic duct. The intrauterine failure to develop a complete biliary tree can lead to extrahepatic biliary atresia of embryonic or fetal form, which occurs in 10–35% of all cases.

   Harber BA, Russo P: Biliary atresia. Gastroenterol Clin North Am 32:891–911, 2003.

4. **How does the pancreas develop?**
   The pancreas develops in two separate locations as a bud from the endodermal-lined foregut. The dorsal pancreas develops from a bud on the dorsal surface opposite the developing biliary tree. The dorsal pancreatic bud is located within the dorsal mesentery and grows with a central dorsal pancreatic duct draining to the foregut through the minor papilla. The ventral pancreatic bud develops close to the developing bile duct. When the duodenum rotates to become C-shaped, the bud is rotated onto the dorsal surface along the dorsal pancreas in a position immediately below and behind it. The two developing pancreas parts grow together, and the dorsal pancreatic duct fuses with the ventral pancreas to form the main pancreatic duct (of Wirsung) draining through the major papilla into the duodenum (Fig. 9-2).

5. **What is the clinical significance of the embryologic development of the pancreas?**
   If the connection from the dorsal pancreas continues to drain directly into the duodenum via this secondary drainage system (the accessory pancreatic duct of Santorini), the condition is known as *pancreas divisum*. This connection drains through the minor papilla at a separate location. Any variation in this process can lead to completely separated drainage to a duplicate drainage of the pancreas. The clinical significance of this condition is the higher risk of pancreatitis in patients with pancreatic duct anomalies.

6. **What is the significance of the rotation of the midgut?**
   During the sixth week of gestation, the small intestines and the colon herniate into the umbilical cord due to the rapid growth of the liver. The intestine then rotates about a central axis formed by the superior mesenteric artery. This counterclockwise rotation is completed, and the intestine migrates back into the abdominal cavity to be fixed in position. This rotation results in the colon being located anterior to the small intestines with the cecum being located in the right lower quadrant. An interruption during this physiologic herniation and rotation will result in abnormalities. When the gut fails to return to the abdominal cavity, an omphalocele is formed. This abnormality occurs in approximately 2.5 in 10,000 births. There is a high rate of associated developmental defects, such as cardiac abnormalities, spinal defects, and chromosomal abnormalities. When the midgut fails to rotate completely, the inappropriately positioned small bowel attachment points can lead to twisting on the superior mesenteric artery and can lead to vascular insufficiency and volvulus. The gold standard for diagnosis remains the upper gastrointestinal tract series that shows the duodenal C-loop crossing to the left of midline at a level equal to or greater than the pylorus.

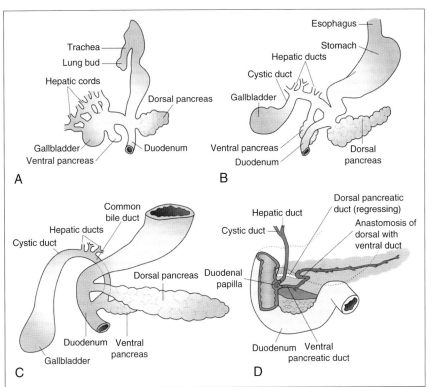

Figure 9-2. Development of the pancreatic primordial from the ventral aspect. **A,** In the fifth week. **B,** In the sixth week. **C,** In the seventh week. **D,** In the late fetus, showing fusion of the dorsal and ventral pancreatic ducts and regression of the distal portion of the dorsal duct. (From Carlson BM: Human Embryology and Developmental Biology, 2nd ed. St. Louis, Mosby, 1999, p 338.)

7. **How does the hindgut develop?**
   The hindgut forms the most distal part of the primitive gut. It develops into the distal third of the transverse colon and the upper part of the rectal canal. Initially, the urogenital system and the hindgut join together in the cloaca. The two systems separate from each other, and the rectal canal fuses with the surface to form an open pathway that will form the anus and rectum. Any abnormalities with this development can result in a continued connection, urorectal fistula, between the urologic and gastrointestinal tracts. When the anorectal canal fails to fuse with the surface, a rectoanal atresia occurs with resulting imperforate anus. Imperforate anus occurs in 1 in 50,000 live births and has a high incidence of other associated birth defects.

8. **What is the enteric nervous system (ENS)?**
   The ENS is the nervous system that regulates intestinal smooth muscle to control gastrointestinal motility. The ENS is composed of a complex network of ganglia that function independently from the central nervous system. The system works independently, but it can be influenced by vagal and pelvic nerves of the parasympathetic nervous system and spinal nerves. It functions to regulate the interstitial cells of Cajal, which function as the pacemaker cells for coordinated smooth muscle contractions.

KEY POINTS: GASTROINTESTINAL DEVELOPMENT

1. The most common form of transesophageal fistula is proximal esophageal atresia with a distal tracheoesophageal fistula.

2. Although most cases of biliary atresia are due to a destructive, perinatal inflammatory process, a subset appears to be due to a prenatal developmental abnormality of the extrahepatic biliary tree.

3. Rotational abnormalities of pancreas development can be observed either as an annular pancreas presenting with obstruction or as ductal abnormalities presenting with pancreatitis later in childhood.

4. Delayed passage of meconium should raise consideration of both anatomic abnormalities (e.g., variants of imperforate anus) and motility disorders (e.g., Hirschsprung's disease).

MECONIUM

9. What is meconium?
Meconium is the material and secretions created by and/or swallowed by the fetus in the gastrointestinal tract while in utero. It contains ingested amniotic fluid, lanugo, intestinal cells, bile salts and pigments, and pancreatic enzymes.

10. When is meconium normally passed in a term infant?
Normally, the initial passage of meconium occurs within the first 12 hours after birth. Meconium passage will occur in 99% of term infants and 95% of premature infants within 48 hours of birth.

11. What is the significance of the lack of passage of meconium at the normal time?
When meconium is not passed by 48 hours of life, the possibility of an anatomic or neuromuscular abnormality must be considered.

FETAL GROWTH AND ASSESSMENT

12. Why is it important to routinely monitor fetal growth during pregnancy?
Intrauterine growth is one of the most important signs of fetal well-being and one of the most reliable indicators of the pathologic conditions that affect the mother and the fetus during pregnancy. In addition, alterations in fetal growth have great implications in the acute and long-term management of the fetus and the newborn infant.

13. What do the terms low birth weight (LBW), very low birth weight (VLBW), and extremely low birth weight (ELBW) indicate?
- **LBW:** <2500 gm
- **VLBW:** <1500 gm
- **ELBW:** <1000 gm

This classification is clinically relevant because neonatal morbidity and mortality are strongly correlated with the infant's gestational age and birth weight.

14. What are the most common causes of intrauterine growth restriction (IUGR)?
Intrinsic (fetal causes)
- Constitutional
- Genetic
- Toxic

- Infectious
- Teratogenetic
- Behavioral
- In-uterine constraint

Extrinsic (maternal/placental) causes

- Maternal age < 16 years or > 35 years
- Maternal illness
- Placental dysfunction
- Multiple gestation
- Demographic

15. **What causes neonates to be large for gestational age?**

Infants with birth weight above the 90th percentile of the intrauterine growth chart are classified as *large for gestational age*. Maternal diabetes is the most common cause of fetal growth acceleration due to the induction of fetal hyperinsulinism during gestation. Other causes include fetal hydrops (edema), Beckwith-Wiedemann syndrome, transposition of the great vessels, and maternal obesity.

16. **Is it clinically useful to classify small-for-gestational-age infants as symmetric or asymmetric?**

Infants who are symmetrically growth retarded have proportionally reduced size in weight, length, and head circumference. This type of growth retardation starts early in pregnancy, and it is often secondary to congenital infection, chromosomal abnormalities, and dysmorphic syndromes. Most IUGR babies, however, are asymmetrically growth retarded with the most severe growth reduction in weight, less severe length reduction, and relative head sparing. Asymmetric IUGR is caused by extrinsic factors that occur late in gestation such as pregnancy-induced hypertension. Infants with asymmetric IUGR have a better long-term growth and developmental outcome than symmetric IUGR infants.

MEDICAL PROBLEMS OF THE GROWTH-RESTRICTED INFANT

17. **What are the long-term risks of IUGR?**

- **Development:** Because this group is heterogeneous, the outcome is dependent on perinatal events, the etiology of growth retardation, and the postnatal socioeconomic environment. In general, the asymmetric growth-retarded baby does not show significant differences in intelligence or neurologic sequelae but does demonstrate differences in school performance related to abnormalities in behavior and learning.
- **Health effects:** An increased risk of hypertension is found in adolescents and young adults. Growth-retarded infants with a low ponderal index are at increased risk from syndrome X (non–insulin-dependent diabetes mellitus, hypertension, and hyperlipidemia) and death from cardiovascular disease by the age of 65 years (Barker hypothesis).
- **Growth:** Fetuses that experienced growth failure after 26 weeks' gestation (asymmetric growth retardation) exhibit a period of catch-up growth during the first 6 months of life. However, their ultimate stature is frequently less than an appropriate-for-gestational-age (AGA) baby.

CALORIC REQUIREMENTS

18. **What is the significance of energy balance?**

Energy, being neither created nor destroyed, conforms to classic balance relationships. Energy balance is a state of equilibrium when energy intake equals expenditure plus losses. If energy intake exceeds expenditure plus losses, the infant is in positive balance, and excess calories are stored. If energy intake is less than expenditure plus losses, the infant is in negative balance, and calories are mobilized from body stores. Maintenance or basal energy requirements are the energy needs required to cover basal metabolic rate or resting energy expenditure; total energy expenditure in infants is the sum of the energy required for basal metabolic rate, activity, thermoregulation, diet-induced thermogenesis, and growth. The energy balance equation may be stated as follows:

$$\text{Gross energy intake} = \text{energy excreted} + \text{energy expended} + \text{energy stored or}$$
$$\text{Metabolizable energy} = \text{energy expended} + \text{energy stored}$$

19. **What are the caloric requirements for LBW infants?**
LBW infants require at least 120 cal/kg/day, partitioned to approximately 75 cal/kg/day for resting expenditure and the remainder for specific dynamic action (10 cal/kg/day), replacement of inevitable stool losses (10 cal/kg/day), and growth (25 cal/kg/day) (Table 9-1).

20. **What is the respiratory quotient (RQ), and what is its significance?**
The RQ is the ratio of the volume of CO_2 produced to the volume of O_2 consumed per unit of time (VCO_2/VO_2). This ratio varies with the type of nutrient oxidized. In addition, the energy produced varies with the type of substrate burned. Thus, various substrates will differ in RQs, and varying proportions of different nutrients will result in different energy production per liter of O_2 consumption or CO_2 production. The RQs and caloric equivalents of O_2 and CO_2 for carbohydrate, fat, and protein are shown in Table 9-2.

21. **What is the energy cost of growth?**
The energy cost of growth includes the energy used for synthesis of new tissues (e.g., absorption, metabolism, and assimilation of fat and protein) and the energy stored in these new tissues. The energy cost of growth varies with the type of tissue added during growth. The precise caloric requirements for growth are unknown. A wide range of values for energy cost of growth

TABLE 9-1. CALORIC REQUIREMENTS OF LOW-BIRTH-WEIGHT INFANTS

	Requirements (in cal/kg/day)
Resting[*]	50–75
Specific dynamic action	5–8% of total intake
Stool losses	10% of total intake
Growth	25–45
Total[†]	85–142

[*]Estimate includes caloric expenditure for maintenance of basal metabolism plus activity and response to cold stress.
[†]Includes sum of resting and growth requirements for specific dynamic action and replacement of stool losses plus an increment of 15–18%.

TABLE 9-2. RQS AND CALORIC EQUIVALENTS

	RQ	Energy Produced/L of O_2 (kcal)	Energy Produced/L of CO_2 (kcal)
Carbohydrate	1.00	5.0	5.0
Fat	0.71	4.7	6.6
Protein	0.80	4.5	5.6

in neonates has been determined (1.2–6 kcal/gm of weight gain). Separate evaluations of energy expenditure requirement for fat and protein deposition in premature newborns estimate that 1 gm of protein deposition requires 7.8 kcal, and 1 gm of fat requires 1.6 kcal.

CARBOHYDRATE REQUIREMENTS

22. **How can carbohydrate requirements be estimated in newborn infants?**
    Strict carbohydrate requirements are difficult to estimate because glucose, a preferred metabolic fuel for many organs (including the brain), is synthesized endogenously from other compounds. Several methods have been used to assess carbohydrate requirements in neonates:
    - Breast milk intake of lactose (assuming breast milk provides optimal intakes of all nutrients)
    - Constant infusion of labeled glucose to determine the rates of glucose production and oxidation (as a reflection of overall carbohydrate metabolism)
    - Altering the amount of the carbohydrate intake in the diet and determining its effect on energy metabolism and nitrogen retention

23. **The rate of endogenous glucose production in neonates has been estimated to range from 4 to 6 mg/kg/min. Do these values represent the ideal carbohydrate intake in neonates?**
    No. The rates of endogenous glucose production should be regarded only as the *minimal* carbohydrate requirement because of the methods and conditions in which these measurements were performed. These studies were done in neonates under basal or resting metabolic conditions and during fasting periods. In addition, they did not take into account the energy cost of physical activity, growth, and thermal effect of feeding. Higher values ranging from 5.8 to 6.8 mg/kg/min have been used as guidelines for the initiation of glucose infusion in neonates receiving parenteral nutrition.

24. **What problems can be associated with excessive carbohydrate intake?**
    Excessive intake of carbohydrate in infant feedings may lead to delayed gastric emptying, emesis, diarrhea, and abdominal distention due to excessive gas formation. The excessive administration of intravenous glucose, at rates exceeding 13.8 mg/kg/min, may be associated with metabolic complications such as hyperglycemia, glycosuria, and osmotic diuresis. In addition, the excessive glucose metabolized is stored mainly as fat.

25. **Why do infant formulas contain comparable amounts of lactose and glucose polymers?**
    - Premature infants have a limited ability to digest lactose because intestinal lactase does not reach maximal activity until near term.
    - Glucose polymers are well digested and absorbed by premature infants.
    - The use of glucose polymers allows the osmolarity of the formula to remain low, even at high caloric density of 24 kcal/30 mL (<300 mOsm/L).

26. **What is the metabolic fate of the lactose malabsorbed by the small intestine?**
    The malabsorbed lactose is fermented in the colon, forming various gases such as carbon dioxide, methane, and hydrogen and short-chain fatty acids such as acetate, propionate, and butyrate. These short-chain fatty acids are absorbed in the colon, reducing energy losses in the stools and maintaining the nutrition and function of the colon. Despite these putative benefits of lactose fermentation, there are metabolic concerns that result from the reduced digestion and absorption of lactose in the small intestine such as:
    - Decreased insulin secretion and a reduced effect on protein synthesis
    - Lower adenosine triphosphate formation when lactose is fermented to acetate instead of following the glucose metabolic pathways
    - Possible increased risk of necrotizing enterocolitis

PROTEIN REQUIREMENTS

27. **What are the essential amino acids?**
    The amino acids that cannot be synthesized in the body are regarded as essential amino acids:
    - Leucine
    - Threonine
    - Phenylalanine
    - Isoleucine
    - Methionine
    - Tryptophan
    - Valine
    - Lysine
    - Histidine

28. **Which of the amino acids are considered conditionally essential for the preterm infant?**
    Cysteine, tyrosine, and taurine are essential because of immaturity of the enzymes (decreased activity) involved in their synthesis.

29. **What is the whey-to-casein ratio of cow's milk and human milk protein?**
    The whey-to-casein ratio of cow's milk protein is 18:82 and that of human milk protein is 60:40.

30. **How does the whey-to-casein ratio change during lactation?**
    The ratio of whey to casein is about 90:10 at the beginning of lactation and rapidly decreases to 60:40 (or even 50:50) in mature milk.

31. **What is the predominant whey protein in human milk and cow's milk?**
    The predominant whey protein in cow's milk is β-lactoglobulin, and the predominant whey protein in human milk is α-lactalbumin.

32. **What are the non-nutritive roles of protein in human milk?**
    - Whey proteins are known to be involved in the immune response (immunoglobulins), lactose synthesis (α-lactalbumin), and other host defenses (lactoferrin).
    - Casein phosphopeptides are believed to enhance the absorption of minerals.
    - Casein fragments are thought to increase intestinal motility.
    - Glycoproteins may promote the growth of certain beneficial bacteria.

33. **Name the methods used for determining protein requirements.**
    - Factorial method (based on reference data of infant body composition)
    - Balance method (protein intake = protein retention + inevitable protein losses)
    - Indices of protein nutritional status (e.g., plasma albumin and transthyretin concentrations; protein intake required to maintain these indices within an acceptable range)
    - Stable isotope tracer techniques (insight into how metabolism changes with clinical state or nutritional status and thus an assessment of protein requirement)

34. **What is a lactobezoar?**
    Lactobezoars are intragastric masses composed of partially digested milk curd (i.e., casein, fat, and calcium). Rarely seen now, lactobezoars were reported in LBW infants (<2000 gm) fed casein-predominant formulas.

35. **What is the protein requirement of term and preterm infants?**
    The recommended protein intake for term infants is 2–2.5 gm/kg/day and for preterm infants is 3–4 gm/kg/day.

36. **What factors may affect protein use in the neonate?**
    - Energy intake
    - Quality of protein intake
    - Intake of other nutrients
    - Infections and stress

37. **What is the protein content of currently available formulas?**
    1. **Term formulas**
       - Milk-based formulas (e.g., Similac Advance, Enfamil LIPIL, Good Start Supreme): 2.1–2.8 gm/100 kcal
       - Soy-based formulas (e.g., Similac Isomil Advance, Enfamil Prosobee LIPIL, Good Start Supreme Soy): 2.3–2.5 gm/100 kcal
    2. **Preterm formulas** (e.g., Similac Special Care, Enfamil Premature LIPIL): 2.5–2.9 gm/100 cal
    3. **Follow-up formulas for LBW weight infants** (e.g., Similac NeoSure Advance, EnfaCare LIPIL): 2.6–2.8 gm/100 kcal

38. **What is the rate of protein loss in premature infants who receive only 10% dextrose and water in the immediate newborn period?**
    ELBW infants (<1000 gm) who receive only glucose lose 1.2 gm/kg/day. More mature infants lose protein at a slower rate (0.9 gm/kg/day at 28 weeks and 0.7 gm/kg/day at 31 weeks). Any protein deficits that are accrued must be replaced.

39. **How can the protein losses be minimized?**
    Early provision of protein (1.0–1.5 gm/kg/day) along with minimal calories (30 cal/kg/day) can stem the protein losses in ELBW infants.

40. **How do protein requirements differ when protein is delivered parenterally versus enterally?**
    Protein requirements are higher parenterally because preterm infants retain only 50% of amino acids administered intravenously but 70–75% of formula or human milk protein.

41. **What is the ideal calorie-to-protein ratio to ensure complete assimilation of protein?**
    - **Enteral feedings:** ~30 cal/gm of protein
    - **Parenteral feedings:** 20–30 cal/gm of protein (based on limited data)

LIPID REQUIREMENTS

42. **What are the beneficial effects of lipid emulsions in a premature infant?**
    - Provision of calories (in a calorically dense form)
    - Prevention of essential fatty acid deficiency

43. **In human milk, what is the percentage of calories provided by fat?**
    Between 40% and 55%.

44. **What is the source of fat in breast milk?**
    Most of the fat in breast milk is formed from circulating lipids derived from the mother's diet. A small amount of fat is synthesized by the breast itself, with that percentage increasing in women receiving a low-fat, high-carbohydrate diet.

45. **What structural features of fatty acids improve enteral absorption?**
    - Shorter-chain-length to medium-chain triglycerides are absorbed more efficiently than long-chain triglycerides.
    - Fatty acids with double bonds are absorbed more efficiently.

46. **What are the energy contents of long-and medium-chain triglycerides?**
    - Long-chain triglycerides: 9 cal/gm
    - Medium-chain triglycerides: ~7.5 cal/gm

47. **What is the energy cost of synthesizing fat from carbohydrate?**
    Synthesis of fat from glucose requires about 25% of the glucose energy invested in synthesis. In comparison, synthesis of fat from fat requires only 1–4% of the energy invested.

48. **What fatty acids are essential for fetuses and premature infants?**
    All humans have a requirement for linoleic and linolenic acid. These are 18-carbon, omega-6 and omega-3 fatty acids, respectively. Linoleic and linolenic acid serve as precursors for long-chain polyunsaturated fatty acids (LCPUFAs) such as arachidonic (a 20-carbon omega-6 fatty acid), eicosapentaenoic (a 20-carbon omega-3 fatty acid), and docosahexaenoic acid (a 22-carbon omega-3 fatty acid). LCPUFAs are essential components of membranes and are particularly important in membrane-rich tissues such as the brain. In addition, eicosapentaenoic and arachidonic acids are precursors for prostaglandins, leukotrienes, and other lipid mediators. The fetus receives essential fatty acids (including LCPUFAs) transplacentally, and breast-fed babies receive them in breast milk. Vegetable oil–based formulas do not contain LCPUFAs, and the ability of preterm infants to synthesize LCPUFAs from linoleic and linolenic acid may be limited.

49. **What are the current recommendations for LCPUFA supplementation?**
    In Europe, the recommendation is that formulas designed for preterm infants contain LCPUFAs in addition to linoleic and linolenic acid. Because of a concern about the effect of LCPUFA supplementation on postnatal growth, a similar recommendation has not been made in the United States.

50. **What are the side effects of LCPUFA depletion?**
    - **Omega-6 LCPUFA:** Reduced growth
    - **Omega-3 LCPUFA:** Alterations in electroretinogram responses, reduced visual acuity, and possible cognitive abnormalities

51. **What is the advantage of supplying calories as lipid rather than carbohydrate in infants with chronic lung disease?**
    The RQ of lipids is lower than that of carbohydrate. Therefore, the use of lipid infusions should theoretically decrease CO_2 production in infants with bronchopulmonary dysplasia.

52. **What is the advantage of using a 20% lipid emulsion versus a 10% lipid emulsion in newborn infants?**
    Twenty-percent lipid emulsions are cleared from the circulation more rapidly than 10% emulsions. Ten-percent lipid emulsions contain proportionately more emulsifier (egg yolk phospholipid). In 10% emulsions, the phospholipid-to-triglyceride ratio is 0.12, and in 20% emulsions the ratio is 0.06. The excess phospholipid forms bilayer vesicles that extract free cholesterol from peripheral cell membranes to form lipoprotein X. Lipoprotein X is cleared very slowly from the circulation (half-life, 2 days).

53. **What is the maximum acceptable triglyceride level in infants receiving lipid emulsions, and how often should they be checked?**
    The maximum level is 150 mg/dL. Routine monitoring of serum triglycerides is necessary because they are being advanced.

TOTAL PARENTERAL NUTRITION: MONITORING AND COMPLICATIONS

54. **What is the usual distribution of nutrients in total parenteral nutrition (TPN) solutions used for neonates?**
TPN is written with a calorie distribution of 8–10% from amino acids, 30–40% from lipid emulsions, and 50–60% from dextrose.

55. **What are the metabolic advantages of using different regimens containing high carbohydrate (67%) and low fat (5%) or low carbohydrate (34%) and high fat (58%)?**
There are none. The administration of TPN solutions containing a moderate carbohydrate (60%) to fat (32%) ratio has been shown to result in a higher nitrogen retention rate than that of the unbalanced regimens.

Nose O, Tipton JR, Ament ME, Yabuuchi H: Effect of energy source on changes in energy expenditure, respiratory quotient and nitrogen balance during total parenteral nutrition in children. Pediatr Res 21:538–541, 1987.

56. **Hyperglycemia is a common complication observed in ELBW infants receiving parenteral nutrition. Should insulin infusions be provided routinely to these infants?**
In most infants, hyperglycemia is a transient problem and resolves when the rate of glucose or lipid administration is reduced. Insulin infusions have been used for infants weighing <1000 gm who develop hyperglycemia (serum glucose level in excess of 150 mg/dL) and glycosuria during the course of parenteral nutrition, *providing low glucose infusion rates* (<12 mg/kg/min). In these infants, insulin infusions at rates of 0.04–0.1 U/kg/h have been shown to improve glucose tolerance and to promote weight gain, compared with control infants.

Collin JW, Hoppe M: A controlled trial of insulin infusion and parenteral nutrition in extremely low birth weight infants with glucose intolerance. J Pediatr 118:921–927, 1991.

57. **The clearance of intravenous fat emulsions in neonates is improved by all of the following measures except: *A,* increasing the period of infusion from 8 to 24 hours; *B,* adding a low dose of heparin to the tpn solutions (1 u/ml); *C,* exposing the fat emulsions to ambient light or to phototherapy lights; *D,* using 20% instead of 10% lipid emulsions.**
C. Exposure of lipid emulsions to ambient or to phototherapy lights increases the formation of triglyceride hydroperoxide radicals but does not enhance lipid clearance. Lipid clearance in neonates is improved by prolonging the infusion period, by adding heparin to TPN solutions (which releases lipoprotein lipase from capillary endothelial cells), and by using 20% lipid emulsions, which contain a lower phospholipid content than 10% lipid emulsions.

58. **Why do premature infants who receive prolonged courses of parenteral nutrition develop osteopenia resulting in pathologic bone fractures?**
The development of osteopenia during the course of TPN in premature infants is believed to result from the inability to provide the calcium and phosphorus required for proper bone mineralization. The solubility of calcium and phosphorus in TPN solutions can be improved by providing a high amino acid intake and by the supplementation of cysteine hydrochloride. These measures allow for a greater but still inadequate intake of calcium and phosphorus. The administration of calciuric diuretics such as furosemide, the use of postnatal steroids, and the development of cholestatic liver disease further aggravate calcium homeostasis in these patients. The intravenous administration of vitamin D does not prevent the occurrence of TPN-induced osteopenia.

59. **Which of the trace elements in TPN solutions can be potentially toxic for patients with cholestatic liver disease?**
Copper and manganese. Both of these trace elements are metabolized in the liver and primarily excreted in bile. Therefore, the chronic administration of trace elements in patients with cholestasis can potentially result in toxic states. Manganese and copper supplements should be withheld from TPN solutions when hepatic cholestasis is present. Monitoring of serum levels of copper and manganese is indicated in patients with cholestasis who require a prolonged course of TPN.

60. **What is the most common complication of TPN administered by peripheral vein catheters?**
The accidental infiltration of TPN solution into the subcutaneous fat tissue resulting in skin necrosis. This complication can be minimized by lowering the osmolality of TPN solution through the administration of dextrose concentrations not exceeding 10% and by the concomitant administration of lipid emulsions.

61. **What is the most common cause of bacterial infection in neonates receiving TPN by central vein catheter?**
Staphylococcus epidermidis remains the most common cause of bacterial sepsis during the course of TPN. Other organisms include *Staphylococcus aureus, Escherichia coli, Pseudomonas* species, *Klebsiella* species, and *Candida albicans*. TPN-related infections are more common in the smallest and sickest infants receiving prolonged courses of TPN via a central catheter. The rate of these infections can be reduced by aseptic preparation of TPN solutions and by avoiding the use of the TPN catheter for blood transfusions, administration of medications, and blood sampling. Most importantly, TPN should be discontinued (and central lines removed) when "full" enteral volume feedings have been achieved (~100 mL/kg/day).

ENTERAL NUTRITION

62. **What is the carbohydrate source in human milk and in term and preterm formulas?**
Lactose is the major source of carbohydrate in human milk and in formulas for term infants. The preterm formulas contain a mixture of lactose and glucose polymers to compensate for the developmental lag in the intestinal mucosal lactase activity. Glycosidase enzymes involved in the digestion of glucose polymers are active in preterm infants.

63. **Why is the fat absorption of preterm infants lower than that of term infants?**
The lower fat absorption reported in preterm infants is attributed to their relative deficiency of pancreatic lipase and bile salts.

64. **Why is the fat of human milk well absorbed by preterm infants?**
The human milk triglyceride molecule has palmitic acid in the β position and is more easily absorbed compared with triglyceride molecules of cow's milk, vegetable fats, and animal fats that have palmitic acid in the α position. The presence of human milk lipase also improves fat absorption.

65. **When should soy protein–based formulas be used for feeding infants?**
Soy formulas are recommended for the following:
- Infants with congenital lactase deficiency and galactosemia (soy formulas are lactose free)
- Infants with allergy to cow's milk protein
- Infants of parents requesting a vegetarian-based diet

66. **What essential amino acid is added to soy-based infant formulas?**
Because soy protein has low concentrations of methionine, this amino acid is added to all soy-based formulas.

67. **When can preterm infants be nippled successfully?**
The success of feeding a preterm infant by nipple is dependent on the ability of the infant to coordinate sucking and swallowing, which develops at about 33–34 weeks of gestational age.

68. **Why may transpyloric feedings result in fat malabsorption?**
Transpyloric feedings may result in fat malabsorption as a result of bypassing the lipolytic effect of gastric lipase.

69. **Why are early minimal enteral feedings recommended for preterm infants receiving parenteral nutrition?**
Gastrointestinal hormones, gastrin, enteroglucagon, and pancreatic polypeptide may have a trophic effect on the gut. Postnatal surges of these hormones occur in preterm infants receiving minimal enteral feedings. Minimal enteral feeding has also been reported to produce more mature small intestinal motor activity patterns in preterm infants. Thus, early minimal enteral feedings given along with parenteral nutrition may improve subsequent enteral feeding tolerance and may shorten the time to achieve full enteral intake.

70. **What are the reported advantages of feeding human milk to preterm infants over the commercially available infant formulas?**
   - A lower incidence of necrotizing enterocolitis in preterm infants fed human milk
   - Faster gastric emptying in preterm infants fed human milk compared with those fed bovine milk–derived formulas
   - Improved long-term cognitive development, which has been correlated with human milk feedings in preterm infants

71. **Does human milk meet the nutritional requirements of preterm infants (birth weight < 1500 gm)?**
Growth rates of preterm infants fed banked human milk or their own mother's milk are lower than that of infants fed preterm formulas. In addition, the calcium and phosphorus content of human milk is insufficient to support adequate skeletal mineralization. Supplementation of human milk with available human milk fortifiers that provide protein, calcium, phosphorus, sodium, zinc, and vitamins helps overcome the nutritional inadequacies. Newly designed preparations of pooled human breast milk (Prolacta) do contain adequate calories and minerals for growth.

BREAST-FEEDING

72. **What are the determinants of milk volume (milk production)?**
Initially, hormonal factors (prolactin and oxytocin) affect the synthesis and secretion of milk. Once milk "comes in," tight junctions close, and lactation shifts from endocrine control to autocrine control, or control driven by milk removal. The frequency of breast-feeding then becomes the most important factor affecting the continuation of adequate milk production. The term infant should receive at least 8–12 feedings per day in the first week and more than 6 per day thereafter. So that the volume of residual milk is minimized, mothers should alternate the breast they start on the next feeding. Maternal diet and fluid intake rarely affect milk volume. In severe malnutrition, there *may* be diminished milk production.

73. **How can milk production be increased?**
There are no magic potions or medications that increase milk production. If mothers are producing a low milk volume, the administration of metoclopramide will occasionally increase serum prolactin and increase milk production. Unfortunately, there are side effects of this medication, including sedation and extrapyramidal neurologic signs. Oxytocin will not increase milk production, but it may help milk ejection (once milk already has been synthesized). Herbal remedies have been advocated, but no data are available that determine their efficacy or risk. Fatigue and

stress also affect milk production adversely. A small percentage of women (2–5%) have lactation insufficiency and cannot produce adequate quantities of milk.

74. **What are the contraindications for breast-feeding?**
    - **Galactosemia**
    - **Substance abuse/use:** Cocaine, narcotics, and stimulants.
    - **Miliary tuberculosis:** Avoid breast-feeding until adequate therapy has been received for about 2 weeks.
    - **Human immunodeficiency virus (HIV):** This contraindication has far-reaching global concerns. In the United States, women who test positive for HIV should not breast-feed. The risk-benefit ratios must be determined for particular populations. Efforts are underway to determine the risk-benefit ratio and cost-benefit ratio for the use of antiretroviral therapy along with breast-feeding or the use of infant formula in high-risk populations.
    - **Medications:** Only a few medications are incompatible with breast-feeding:
      - □ Bromocriptine (suppresses lactation)
      - □ Amiodarone
      - □ Ergotamine
      - □ Thiouracils
      - □ Chemotherapeutic agents
      - □ Metronidazole
      - □ Radiopharmaceuticals
      - □ Klonapin
      - □ Phenindione
      - □ Salts containing bromide and gold
      - □ Amantadine

75. **Does energy expenditure differ between breast-fed and formula-fed infants?**
    In studies of AGA gavage-fed infants, there was significantly lower energy expenditure in the infants fed human milk compared with those fed formula.

    Lubetzky R, Vaisman N, Mimouni F, Dollberg S: Energy expenditure in human milk–versus formula-fed preterm infants. J Pediatr 143:750–753, 2003.

76. **A mother has breast-fed her 5-week-old infant exclusively. She now calls with a concern that she has recently noticed a burning pain in her nipple during breast-feeding. You examine the mother and note some erythema of her areola. You diagnose a fissure and advise her to use dry heat and a few drops of milk on her areola after breast-feeding. She calls back in a few days saying that the pain is increasing. What other diagnosis should you consider?**
    This is not an uncommon presentation for a *Candida* infection of the nipple. You should have the mother bring her infant to your office and examine the infant for evidence of perioral thrush. If present, the baby should be treated with an oral medication and the mother with an antifungal.

77. **A mother calls you and explains that she is worried because her 4-day-old baby is not receiving enough breast milk. How do you assess whether a newborn is receiving sufficient amounts of breast milk during the first week after birth?**
    Understand why the mother is concerned. Some of the following factors should influence your decision either to see the mother and baby or to reassure the mother over the phone: frequency of feeding (8–12 times in 24 hours, no interval longer than 4 hours), urine output (light yellow–stained diapers), and stool output (no more meconium stools after day 3). Some practitioners use the following rough guide for urine and stool output in the first week: minimum of one urine output in the first 24 hours, two to three in the next 24 hours, about four to six on day 3, and six to eight on day 5; stools should be one per day on days 1 and 2, two per day on day 3, and four or more afterward. The mother should sense that her milk has "come in" between the second and fourth days postpar-

tum. The baby should have established feeding activities, such as lip smacking and rooting. You should hear swallows, and the baby should be satisfied after a feeding. Feeding activities, however, vary widely. Some adequately hydrated infants are sleepy and need coaching with feedings. If a mother experiences leaking from one breast while the child is nursing at the other, her milk supply is usually quite adequate. Weighing an infant before and after feeding can provide an accurate assessment of milk intake. The technique requires an electronic scale and strict attention to details such as not unwrapping the infant or changing diapers before the reweighing is done.

78. **You see a 5-day-old male infant in the office for a routine check after early hospital discharge. The mother reports no particular problems; he is much easier to manage than she thought a newborn would be. She is breast-feeding every 3 hours but lets him sleep at night (last night he slept for 6 hours). About once a day she notes that he has dark yellow urine in his diaper. He had a dark green, tarry stool yesterday. The mother thinks her milk has "come in," but she acknowledges no signs of engorgement. You examine the infant and note jaundice to the level of the umbilicus and dry skin, but moist mucous membranes. He is responsive and alert. You examine the mother and note that her breasts are moderately engorged. The infant's body weight is 11 ounces below his birth weight of 7 pounds, 8 ounces. You check his serum bilirubin concentration, which is 11 mg/dL. There is no blood group incompatibility. How would you manage this case, and what would you advise the mother?**
You should observe a breast-feeding to ensure that the baby has a good latch-on to the breast and is able to suck and swallow. You advise the mother to breast-feed every 2 hours and to supplement the baby with formula. As the baby takes more milk from the breast, he will take less formula and will wean himself. You do not advise water supplements. The baby needs calories. His bilirubin level should decline. If the mother had not been making milk, you might suggest that she mechanically express her milk after every feeding to increase stimulation. You must schedule a return visit in 24–48 hours to assess the infant.

79. **What is the most variable nutrient in human milk?**
Fat is the most variable content of all nutrients in human milk. The fat content rises slightly during lactation, increases from the beginning (foremilk) to the end (hindmilk) of the feeding, varies among women (probably a direct effect of body fat stores), and varies over the course of the day. If the mother does not completely empty her breast after feeding, the baby will not receive all the calories (fat). Mothers using mechanical methods to express their milk may not completely empty the breast.

80. **Breast-feeding a premature infant can be a challenge. How do you advance from tube-feeding to breast-feeding in a premature infant?**
Note the sucking and swallowing ability of the infant. Parental skills, infant feeding cues, and timing of feedings should also be considered. Begin one breast-feeding in place of a tube feeding or in addition to the tube feeding. If the latch-on is good and clinical signs of sucking, swallowing, and some drooling of milk are noted, then continue the process each day. It is not accurate to withdraw milk from an indwelling feeding tube to assess milk intake from breast-feeding, since gastric emptying from the stomach after a human milk feeding is rapid. Furthermore, clinical signs of feeding activity and maternal assessment of breast emptying are inexact measures of milk intake and may not reflect small amounts consumed. Weighing the infant before and after breast-feeding is the most accurate way to assess milk intake.

Meier P, Lysakowski TY, Engstrom JL: The accuracy of test weighing for preterm infants. J Pediatr Gastroenterol Nutr 10:62–65, 1990.

81. **Do mothers benefit from breast-feeding?**
Postpartum weight loss and uterine involution may be more rapid with breast-feeding. The postpartum amenorrhea during lactation is an acknowledged method of child spacing,

especially for 4–6 months. This technique is most reliable if breast-feeding is practiced around the clock. Several reports now suggest that women who breast-fed their infants had a decreased incidence of premenopausal breast cancer and ovarian cancer. Women who breast-fed their infants also may have a decreased incidence of osteoporosis.

Labbok MH: Health sequelae of breastfeeding for the mother. Clin Perinatol 26:491–503, 1999.

VITAMINS AND TRACE NUTRIENTS

82. **A 2-month-old preterm infant (with an estimated gestational age of 26 weeks) develops osteopenia of prematurity and fractures of both humeri. The infant is receiving 400 units of vitamin D/day. Should the dose of vitamin D be increased?**
No! Contrary to earlier theory, osteopenia of prematurity results primarily from inadequate intake of mineral substrate (calcium and phosphorus) and not vitamin D. High doses of vitamin D do not appear to aid in the prevention or treatment of osteopenia of prematurity. Infants born prematurely are at risk for developing osteopenia because of limited accretion of bone mass in utero (fetal accretion rates for calcium and phosphorous range from 92 to 119 mg/kg/day and 59 to 74 mg/kg/day, respectively). Preterm infants often receive limited intravenous and enteral calcium until full enteral feedings are established. Diuretics and steroids, as well as physical inactivity, have a negative effect on bone mineralization. To mimic fetal accretion, an enteral intake of 120–230 mg/kg/day of calcium and 60–140 mg/kg/day of phosphorus is recommended for preterm infants. This amount is provided by 150 cc/kg/day of premature infant formula or fortified breast milk.

83. **A 6-week-old infant is recovering from necrotizing enterocolitis that necessitated resection of two thirds of the jejunum and placement of an ileostomy. When enteral feedings are restarted, the drainage from the ileostomy becomes excessive. The infant is growing poorly (despite an adequate caloric intake) and develops vesiculobullous and eczematous lesions around the eyes, mouth, and genitals. What mineral deficiency should be considered?**
Infants with abnormal gastrointestinal losses (persistent diarrhea, excessive ileostomy drainage) may be at risk for zinc deficiency because fecal loss is the major excretory route. Signs of zinc deficiency include poor wound healing, poor linear growth, decreased appetite, hair loss, depressed immune function, and skin lesions.

84. **What are the causes of zinc deficiency in LBW infants?**
   - Poor zinc stores
   - Increased requirement for growth
   - Prolonged intravenous nutrition containing inadequate zinc
   - Abnormally low zinc content of mother's milk
   - Supplements of iron or copper compete with zinc for absorption

   Adapted from Atkinson SA, Zlotkin S: Recognizing deficiencies and excesses of zinc, copper, and other trace elements. In Tsang RC, Zlotkin SH, Nichols BL, Hansen JW (eds): Nutrition During Infancy, 2nd ed. Cincinnati, Digital Educational Publishing, 1997.

85. **The requirements for what nutrient are increased under phototherapy?**
Riboflavin is a photosensitive vitamin, and requirements may be increased in infants being treated with phototherapy.

86. **Is fluoride an essential nutrient for a newborn infant?**
Although fluoride has been considered "beneficial for humans," it is unproven whether it is essential. Fluoride supplementation is not recommended from birth because of questions concerning whether the benefit of fluoride warrants the risk of dental fluorosis. Commercial infant formulas do not contain fluoride.

KEY POINTS: GROWTH AND NUTRITION

1. The parents of IUGR infants should be aware that significant catch-up growth will occur in the first year of life but that ultimate stature may be less than that of an AGA infant.

2. Lactose malabsorption is extremely uncommon in infants unless they have had a significant insult to the intestinal mucosa (e.g., infection, short gut) or have the very rare disorder of congenital lactase deficiency.

3. The infant with an ostomy should be carefully monitored for excessive sodium losses and zinc deficiency, both of which can impair growth.

4. A critical nutritional goal for the infant with short gut syndrome is to advance enteral feeds as rapidly as tolerated to enable intestinal adaptation and discontinuation of TPN.

87. **What is the scientific rationale for administering vitamin A to prevent bronchopulmonary dysplasia (BPD)?**
    - Lung differentiation is affected by vitamin A.
    - Vitamin A deficiency causes replacement of mucus-secreting epithelium by stratified squamous keratinizing epithelium in the trachea and bronchi.
    - Bronchopulmonary dysplasia has been associated with vitamin A deficiency in VLBW preterm infants.
    - Premature birth deprives the newborn infant of the supply of retinol (vitamin A).
    - The histopathology of bronchopulmonary dysplasia includes findings commonly seen with vitamin A deficiency (e.g., loss of ciliated cells and keratinizing metaplasia).

88. **What are the concentrations of water-soluble vitamins in mature human milk, and how do they compare with the recommended dietary allowances for healthy term infants?**
    See Table 9-3.

TABLE 9-3. WATER-SOLUBLE VITAMINS IN MATURE HUMAN MILK		
	Human Milk	**AAP, CON* (units/100 kcal)**
Thiamin (μg)	31 (21–36)	40
Riboflavin (μg)	56 (42–85)	60
Niacin (mg)	0.29 (0.27–0.34)	0.25 (0.8)
Vitamin B_6 (μg)	20 (15–30)	35
Pantothenic acid (mg)	0.6 (0.3–1.0)	0.3
Biotin (μg)	0.7 (0.6–1.1)	1.5
Folate (μg)	7 (6–12)	4
Vitamin B_{12} (μg)	0.10 (0.07–0.16)	0.15
Vitamin C (mg)	8 (5–13)	8

*Committee on Nutrition of the American Academy of Pediatrics
Adapted from Schanler RJ: Who needs water soluble vitamins? In Tsang RC, Zlotkin SH, Nichols BL, Hansen JW (eds): Nutrition During Infancy, 2nd ed. Cincinnati, Digital Educational Publishing, 1997.

IRON REQUIREMENTS

89. **How long can iron stores meet the needs of term, LBW, and preterm infants before supplementation is necessary?**
The quantity of iron stored is proportional to the birth weight of the infant. On average, the iron stores in a term infant can meet the infant's iron requirement until 4–6 months of age and that of LBW and preterm infants until 2–3 months of age. Transfused infants, however, likely have greater iron stores.

90. **What are the daily dietary iron requirements for term, LBW, and preterm infants?**
The estimated daily requirement is 1 mg/kg/day for term infants and 2–4 mg/kg/day for LBW and preterm infants.

91. **Do breast-fed infants require iron supplementation?**
Although the bioavailability of iron in breast milk is high (because of the presence of lactoferrin, which enhances iron absorption), the content is relatively low. Additional sources of iron are recommended for breast-fed infants after 4–6 months of age.

92. **What is the iron content of hemoglobin?**
Each gram of hemoglobin contains 3.4 mg of iron.

93. **Where is iron absorbed, and what factors can influence iron absorption?**
Dietary iron is absorbed in the duodenum and the proximal jejunum. Absorption is influenced by iron need and also by the dietary source. The majority of the dietary iron (in plant foods and fortified food products) is non-heme iron. Ascorbic acid enhances the absorption of non-heme iron, and calcium, phytates, manganese, and polyphenols decrease it.

94. **Do premature infants need more or less iron than term infants?**
Overall, premature infants need more iron than term infants during their first postnatal year. The reason for this increased need stems from two factors. First, iron is accreted primarily during the last trimester. The fetus maintains a fairly steady level (75 mg of elemental iron per kilogram of body weight) during this period. At 24 weeks' gestation, the fetus has 37.5 mg of total body iron, whereas at term the newborn has 225 mg. Therefore, premature birth results in significantly reduced total body iron. Second, premature infants exhibit a more rapid rate of growth per kilogram of body weight than the term infant. Iron intake must increase to support the increase in hemoglobin mass. Thus, whereas the term newborn needs approximately 1 mg/kg of iron per day, the preterm infant needs between 2 and 4 mg/kg/day. The more premature the infant, the greater the need.

95. **What groups of term neonates are at increased risk of low iron stores at birth?**
Growth-retarded infants and infants of diabetic mothers are at risk for reduced iron stores. Fifty percent of IUGR infants and 65% of infants of diabetics have cord serum ferritin concentrations below the fifth percentile (60 μg/L). In growth-restricted infants, the etiology is probably related to impaired placental transport of nutrients. The pathophysiology of low iron stores in infants of diabetic mothers is more complex. Chronic maternal hyperglycemia results in chronic fetal hyperglycemia and hyperinsulinemia, both of which increase the oxygen consumption of the fetus by approximately 30%. Chronic fetal hypoxia leads to increased erythropoietin secretion and secondary polycythemia, which in turn requires increased iron delivery. Each extra gram of hemoglobin synthesized by the fetus requires an additional 3.49 mg of elemental iron delivered by the placenta. The human placenta is apparently not capable of up-regulating placental transport to that extent, leaving the fetus dependent on its accreted iron stores to support the expanding fetal blood volume. The result is that iron is redistributed away from storage and nonstorage

tissues and into the red cell mass. It does not appear that either group needs additional dietary iron postnatally, suggesting that the neonatal intestine avidly absorbs iron.

Chockalingam UM, Murphy E, Ophoven JC, et al: Cord transferrin and ferritin values in newborn infants at risk for prenatal uteroplacental insufficiency and chronic hypoxia. J Pediatr 111:283–286, 1987.

Stonestreet BS, Goldstein M, Oh W, Widness JA: Effect of prolonged hyperinsulinemia on erythropoiesis in fetal sheep. Am J Physiol 257:R1199–R1204, 1989.

Widness JA, Susa JB, Garcia JF, et al: Increased erythropoiesis and elevated erythropoietin in infants born to diabetic mothers and in hyperinsulinemic rhesus fetuses. J Clin Invest 67:637–642, 1981.

96. **What is the effect of recombinant human erythropoietin (rhEPO) on the iron needs of the premature infant?**
Erythropoietin increases the need for iron by up to threefold to 6 mg/kg/day. In the national collaborative trial of rhEPO for preterm infants, 6 mg/kg/day maintained steady ferritin concentrations over the duration of the study. Studies of erythropoietin given to sheep of varying degrees of iron sufficiency demonstrated that the degree of hemoglobin response is directly related to the iron sufficiency of the animal.

Shannon KM, Keith JF 3rd, Mentzer WC, et al: Recombinant human erythropoietin stimulates erythropoiesis and reduces erythrocyte transfusions in very low birth weight preterm infants. Pediatrics 85:1–8, 1995.

97. **True or false: premature infants are iron overloaded at hospital discharge.**
This is a trick question. In fact, preterm infants could be iron deficient, iron neutral, or iron overloaded. Preterm AGA infants start with approximately 75 mg of iron per kilogram of body weight. This amount of iron is considered sufficient for the neonatal period, and iron supplementation probably should not begin until the preterm infant is at least 2 weeks of age. Preterm infants are born with very immature antioxidant systems, and there is concern that large doses of iron could overwhelm the system and lead to disease that is related to oxidant stress (e.g., retinopathy of prematurity, bronchopulmonary dysplasia). On the other hand, the rapid growth rate of preterm infants results in a rapid expansion of the blood volume, and iron is required to support this growth. Those who are born at low gestational ages, who have a benign neonatal course, and who are fed a low-iron diet (e.g., breast milk without iron supplementation) are at high risk of using all the available stores soon after discharge. These infants need to have their iron and hemoglobin status checked earlier than the usual 9 months of age recommended for term infants. In contrast, a sick preterm infant who requires multiple transfusions to maintain cardiovascular stability may be at high risk for iron overload. Preterm infants can have ferritin concentrations of 500 µg/dL at discharge, suggesting significant iron loading of the liver.

98. **Is placental iron transport dependent on maternal iron status, fetal iron status, or both?**
Both. Early studies clearly establish a relationship between maternal iron stores as indexed by her ferritin concentration and the infant's cord serum ferritin concentration. This relationship appears to be particularly strong when the mother is suffering from profound iron deficiency. However, lesser degrees of iron deficiency do not seem to influence fetal iron status. In fact, the fetus manages to maintain iron sufficiency in the face of maternal iron deficiency. Conversely, certain fetuses can become iron deficient in spite of maternal iron sufficiency. This occurs when placental iron transport is disturbed by utero-placental vascular insufficiency (resulting in IUGR) and when fetal iron demand exceeds placental iron transport ability. The latter is seen in pregnancies complicated by diabetes mellitus and chronic fetal hypoxia with augmented secondary fetal erythropoiesis.

99. **How can the fetus increase placental transport of iron?**
In pregnancies complicated by fetal iron deficiency as indexed by a low cord serum ferritin concentration or decreased placental iron content, the expression of iron transport proteins such

as the transferrin receptor is increased on the apical (maternal-facing) membrane of the syncy-tiotrophoblast. Studies have shown that this up-regulation is most likely in response to the iron status of the syncytiotrophoblast. This up-regulation is achieved by intracellular iron regulatory proteins that bind transferrin receptor mRNA, stabilizing it to produce more copies of the receptor and leading to greater iron transport. Thus, the fetus appears to regulate its own iron accretion! A similar system has been described for the transport of certain amino acids by the placenta.

Bergamaschi G, Bergamaschi P, Carlevati S, Cazzola M: Transferrin receptor expression in the human placenta. Haematologica 754:220–223, 1990.

Georgieff MK, Berry SA, Wobken JA, Leibold EA: Increased placental iron regulatory protein-1 expression in diabetic pregnancies complicated by fetal iron deficiency. Placenta 20:87–93, 1999.

Petry CD, Wobken JD, McKay H, et al: Placental transferrin receptor in diabetic pregnancies with increased fetal iron demand. Am J Physiol 267:E507–E514, 1994.

GASTROESOPHAGEAL REFLUX

100. How common is gastroesophageal reflux (GER)?
Gastroesophageal reflux is seen in up to 50% of infants with recurrent emesis.

101. What is the course of GER in a healthy infant?
During infancy, GER is very common. Recurrent vomiting is the most common manifestation of reflux in this age group and is usually effortless. It is clinically evident in 50% of infants in the first 3 months of life. Only 5–10% of children have reflux at the age of 1 year of life. There is gradual resolution of vomiting by the age of 1–2 years of life. If regurgitation has not resolved by 24 months of age, further evaluation is recommended.

102. What does the term *happy spitter* signify?
These infants have uncomplicated GER. They have no concerning signs or symptoms and have effortless, painless vomiting. Weight gain is normal and the children develop normally. Reassurance/education and anticipatory guidance are generally the only needed interventions.

103. What are the red flags of GER disease (GERD) in infants?
- Bilious vomiting
- Hematemesis
These findings should suggest an alternative diagnosis to GERD.

104. What is the differential diagnosis for GERD in infants and children?
A key point is differentiating GERD from the causes of recurrent or persistent vomiting:
Gastrointestinal obstruction
- Pyloric stenosis
- Malrotation with intermittent volvulus (Fig. 9-3)
- Intermittent intussusception
- Intestinal duplication
- Hirschsprung's disease
- Antro/duodenal web
- Incarcerated hernia
Gastrointestinal disorders
- Gastroparesis
- Gastroenteritis
- Eosinophilic esophagitis/gastroenteritis
- Food allergy or intolerance
- Achalasia
- Peptic ulcer disease

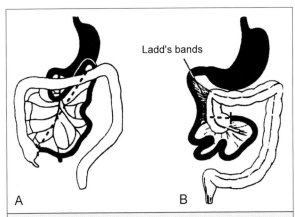

Figure 9-3. **A,** The cecum descends into the right lower quadrant. Note the normal broadness of the small bowel mesentery *(dashed line)*. **B,** In malrotation, the duodenal loop lacks 90 degrees of its normal 270-degree rotation, and the cecocolic loop lacks 180 degrees of its normal rotation.

Neurologic problems: Increased intracranial pressure
Infectious disorders
- Sepsis
- Meningitis
- Urinary tract infection
- Hepatitis
- Pneumonia
Metabolic/endocrine disorders
- Galactosemia
- Urea cycle defects
- Hereditary fructose intolerance
- Amino and organic acidemias
- Congenital adrenal hyperplasia
- Maple syrup urine disease
Renal disorders
- Obstructive uropathy
- Renal insufficiency
Toxic causes
Cardiac disorder: Congestive heart failure

105. **What diagnostic tests are available to evaluate GER?**
See Table 9-4.

106. **What are nonmedical treatment options for GER?**
- Smaller volume feeds given more frequently
- Thickened formula
- Avoidance of seated or supine positions after feeding
- Elevation of the head of the crib
- Elimination of second-hand smoke (which causes relaxation of the lower esophageal sphincter)
- Trial of cow's milk protein–free formula

Infants with GER can be placed in an upright position for at least 30 minutes after meals and elevating the head of the crib to 30–45 degrees. Placing the child seated in a car seat in the home should be avoided. Thickening of the formula with rice cereal and/or commercial thickening agents may

TABLE 9-4.   DIAGNOSTIC TESTS FOR THE EVALUATION OF GER

Test	Advantages	Disadvantages
Upper gastrointestinal tract	Evaluates for structural or anatomic abnormalities.	Has a limited period of observation (<1 hour) so that true significance of reflux may not be captured. Is neither sensitive nor specific enough for diagnosis of GER often.
Gastroesophageal scintigraphy	Evaluates for gastric emptying, reflux, and aspiration. Looks over a longer period (1–2 hours) so that frequency and degree of aspiration can be better quantified. Can look for evidence of aspiration by showing traces in lungs.	Only examines period of time after feeding bolus given. May also underestimate if inappropriate feed volume or composition used. Lacks a standardized technique and age-specific normative data.
pH probe	Evaluates for pH changes. Can look over extended period (12–24 hours) to better obtain true quantity of reflux. Can be done in conjunction with other clinical and physical monitoring to try to correlate with episodes. No restrictions on activity during the test.	If feeding frequency too often and/or inadequate termination of acid suppression prior to test, may not record acid from stomach. Will test for acid reflux episodes only. Is a more invasive testing method.
Impedance probe	Evaluates for pH changes and impedance. Will test for acid and nonacid reflux episodes. Can look over extended period (12–24 hours) to better obtain true quantity of reflux. Can be done in conjunction with other clinical and physical monitoring to try to correlate with episodes. No restrictions on activity during the test.	Is a more invasive testing method.
Esophagogas-troduodenoscopy	Evaluates visual and histologic mucosal abnormalities of the esophagus, stomach, and duodenum.	Is a more invasive testing method.

help to decrease the amount of regurgitation and lessen irritability. It is recommended to start with 1 teaspoon per ounce of formula, and this may be increased to 1 tablespoon per ounce as needed. Lastly, modification of the feeding schedule to offer smaller feeds at a more frequent interval can help to decrease the gastric distension and regurgitation of less frequent larger feeds.

107. **What are the medical treatments of GER?**

Pharmacologic

- Antacids
- Prokinetic agents (e.g., metoclopramide, bethanechol, erythromycin)
- H_2-receptor antagonists (e.g., ranitidine, cimetidine, famotidine, nizatidine)
- Proton-pump inhibitors (e.g., omeprazole, lansoprazole, esomeprazole, pantoprazole, rabeprazole)
- Surface agents (sucralfate gel)

Surgical

- Transpyloric feeding tubes
- Fundoplication
- Pyloroplasty

EOSINOPHILIC GASTROINTESTINAL DISORDERS

108. **What are eosinophilic enteropathies?**

Eosinophilic enteropathies are eosinophilic inflammatory conditions that can be present throughout the entire gastrointestinal tract. The inflammatory process is characterized by the selective infiltration of large numbers of eosinophils into the bowel mucosa and/or smooth muscle. The initial trigger for this process is unknown.

109. **What is the differential diagnosis for eosinophils in the gastrointestinal lining in newborns?**

The differential diagnosis includes idiopathic eosinophilic gastroenteritis, formula protein intolerance, GERD, and normal variation.

110. **How does this process present in neonates?**

This disease process can present as failure to thrive, diarrhea, malabsorption, regurgitation and irritability (identical to GER), and colitis. In neonates, the protein found in cow's milk or soy protein may be the offending antigen for the inflammatory process. When this occurs, the process is called *dietary protein–induced colitis, milk protein colitis, enteritis,* and so forth. A common presentation is an infant who has a history of irritability, diarrhea including mucus and blood, poor weight gain or failure to thrive, and some degree of anemia. It is the most common cause of bloody stools in the first year of life. The second common presentation in neonates is that of reflux that does not respond to therapeutic management. In this clinical picture, the neonate has symptoms of GER and irritability that do not improve as expected despite appropriate medical and nonmedical therapeutic interventions.

111. **What is the prognosis of eosinophilic colitis in the neonate?**

Eosinophilic colitis in infants has a very good prognosis. The vast majority of patients are able to tolerate milk protein by the age of 1–3 years. There have been some studies that associate eosinophilic colitis with the later development of inflammatory bowel disease, but this association has been questioned.

112. **What treatment options are available?**

Multiple medications have been tried and used depending on the location of the involved portion of the gastrointestinal tract. These medications mostly work by attempting to modify the immune response. These medications include systemic steroids, protein pump inhibitors, histamine receptor-2 blockers, topical steroids, antacids, cromolyn, leukotriene antagonists, sucralfate, and prokinetics if secondary dysmotility is noted. Elimination from the diet of the offending milk or soy protein allergen is accomplished in neonates by changing to a protein-hydrolyzed or amino acid formula or, on occasion, by eliminating milk from the maternal diet for breast-fed infants.

KEY POINTS: INFLAMMATORY GASTROINTESTINAL DISORDERS

1. Features of gastroesophageal reflux and allergic esophagitis may be clinically similar; the latter should be considered when standard antireflux therapy is ineffective.

2. Allergic colitis is a relatively common cause of rectal bleeding and bloody stools in the otherwise healthy-appearing infant.

3. The presence of *Clostridium difficile* toxin in stools is a common finding in healthy infants.

4. Hirschsprung's disease can be associated with an inflammatory enterocolitis that can be quite severe.

MALABSORPTION

113. **What is an easy method of differentiating between osmotic and secretory diarrhea?**
Patients with secretory diarrhea continue to have diarrhea even after they are not fed enterally. The laboratory method of differentiating between osmotic and secretory diarrhea is the measurement of the osmotic gap in the stool, which is achieved by measuring the stool osmolarity and sodium and potassium concentrations in a random sample of stool. Normal fecal osmolality is 290 mOsm/kg H_2O, and the normal osmotic gap is <40 mEq/L.

$$\text{Osmotic gap} = \text{Fecal osmolality} - 2 \times ([\text{Na}] + [\text{K}])$$

Osmotic gap and Na and K concentrations are expressed as mEq/L and fecal osmolality as mOsm/kg H_2O.

114. **What are the most common causes of lactose malabsorption?**
Almost any process damaging the mucosa of the small intestine can result in malabsorption of lactose due to secondary lactase deficiency. The most common cause of secondary lactase deficiency is mucosal damage due to infection (e.g., postviral damage). Lactase enzyme has the lowest activity of any brush border disaccharidases and is localized at the tip of the villus, thus making it vulnerable to brush border injury at the time of infection. It is the first enzyme to be affected and the last one to recover after mucosal damage.

115. **What are the stool characteristics of carbohydrate malabsorption? Why does diarrhea occur?**
Stools in carbohydrate malabsorption are acidic, with a pH of less than 5.5 (due to fermentation), and are positive for reducing substances (sugar). Reducing substances will be negative in the stool in the face of carbohydrate malabsorption, if the sugar is not a reducing sugar (e.g., sucrose). In that situation, the stool sample will need to be hydrolyzed with 0.1 N HCl and boiled briefly to break up the sucrose before being tested.
The malabsorbed carbohydrate induces an osmotic fluid shift in the small intestine, resulting in an increase in fluid delivery to the colon. There, the carbohydrate is fermented by colonic bacterial flora to organic acids such as lactic acid, yielding an increase in the osmolality beyond the colon's salvage capacity. Colonic bacteria ferment carbohydrate in a process known as colonic scavenging. The main by-products of fermentation are short-chain fatty acids, which can be used as a source of energy by the epithelial cells of the colon.

116. **Is a 72-hour fecal fat collection useful for detecting fat malabsorption in the neonate?**
The 72-hour fecal fat collection is only useful if patients are receiving a diet containing long-chain fat as the only source of fat in the diet. The standard method used for quantitation of fat

does not detect medium-chain triglycerides. A 72-hour dietary record must be obtained simultaneously so that the coefficient of fat absorption can be obtained.

117. **What is the coefficient of fat absorption in infants younger than 6 months of age?**
The coefficient is 85%.

118. **How common is primary lactase deficiency in neonates?**
Contrary to common belief, primary or congenital lactase deficiency is a very rare disease with only a few dozen cases reported in the literature. The disease is manifested by severe diarrhea while the infant is receiving a lactose-containing formula or breast-feeding, and it starts within the first few hours or days of life.

119. **What is microvillus inclusion disease?**
This very rare congenital disease is often quoted as a cause of severe neonatal diarrhea. The major manifestation is severe secretory diarrhea unresponsive to the withdrawal of oral diet. Diagnosis is based on a small bowel biopsy where shortened enterocyte microvilli with microvillus inclusions are seen on electron microscopy. The etiology is unknown, and prognosis is poor.
Other uncommon causes of congenital diarrhea include autoimmune enteropathy, enterocolitis associated with Hirschsprung's disease, primary lactase deficiency, congenital chloride diarrhea, congenital sodium diarrhea, primary bile acid malabsorption, and enterokinase deficiency.

120. **What is the cause of diarrhea in a neonate fed exclusively Pedialyte?**
If other causes of diarrhea (e.g., infections) are excluded, congenital glucose/galactose malabsorption is a possibility since the carbohydrate in Pedialyte is dextrose (a form of glucose monohydrate). Glucose/galactose malabsorption is an autosomal recessive disease caused by a missense mutation in the SGLT1 gene resulting in a complete loss of Na^+-dependent glucose transporter, which mediates glucose absorption in the brush border of the intestine. The treatment is elimination of glucose and galactose from the diet.

121. **Is there a test to assess the absorptive integrity of the small intestine?**
The D-xylose absorption test is a useful tool frequently used for the evaluation of small intestine integrity and to screen for carbohydrate malabsorption. d-Xylose is a 5-carbon sugar handled similarly to natural 6-carbon sugars via high-efficiency proximal small bowel uptake. It is not metabolized and is rapidly excreted in the urine. Thus, it is ideally suited to test the most basic of carbohydrate pathways. The test is performed in a fasting patient who is given 14.5 gm/m^2 of d-xylose orally as a 10-gm% solution. One hour later, a serum level of the d-xylose is measured. Small intestinal biopsies can be used to confirm anatomic disruption of the mucosal surface or reduced disaccharidase levels to complement the functional absorptive results obtained from a d-xylose test.

122. **A 21-year-old pregnant woman was diagnosed with polyhydramnios. A prenatal ultrasound study demonstrated distended loops of small intestine. The baby was delivered at 33 weeks' gestation by cesarean section, and at the time of delivery the amniotic fluid was noted to contain yellow-green stool. On day 2 of life, the infant developed a hypochloremic metabolic alkalosis and loose stools. A stool sample contained high concentrations of chloride. What is the most likely diagnosis in this case?**
The following features of this case suggest a diagnosis of congenital chloride diarrhea:
- High concentrations of fecal chloride (exceeding the sum of sodium and potassium)
- Polyhydramnios
- Distended loops of bowel on a prenatal ultrasound
- Prematurity

This is an autosomal recessive disease caused by a defect in the chloride-bicarbonate exchange transport system in the ileum and colon resulting in a lifelong secretory diarrhea. The diagnosis is made by the high concentration of fecal chloride. Treatment consists of fluid and electrolyte replacement—initially intravenously, and then orally. If the condition is diagnosed and treated early, the prognosis is excellent.

123. **What are the anatomic causes of gastric outlet obstruction in neonates and infants?**
   - Hypertrophic pyloric stenosis
   - Antral and pyloric membranes
   - Eosinophilic gastroenteritis
   - Aberrant pancreatic tissue
   - Duplication of antrum or duodenum
   - Pyloric channel ulcer
   - Pyloric atresia

124. **What type of surgery is typically performed in complicated cases of meconium ileus?**
   In 1957, Bishop and Koop described the technique of resection of the dilated ileal segment and proximal end-to-distal side ileal anastomosis with distal ostomy, also known as the *Bishop-Koop ileostomy*. This procedure minimizes contamination, allows for anastomosis between appropriately sized bowel segments, provides access to the distal bowel for decompression and irrigation, and allows for bedside closure of the stoma once the obstruction has resolved. Various irrigating solutions have been used, including normal saline, Gastrografin, hydrogen peroxide, and 2–4% solutions of *N*-acetylcysteine. Figures 9-4 and 9-5 illustrate the typical findings of meconium ileus with obstruction and the technique of the Bishop-Koop ileostomy.

125. **What is the operative approach if the patient has meconium ileus with suspected intestinal perforation?**
   If the infant has had a perforation with peritonitis, one must determine the degree of peritonitis. If perforation occurs just before delivery, meconium ascites without calcification is present, whereas if it occurs several weeks or months before delivery, calcification and dense adhesions develop. Occasionally a fibrous wall forms around the meconium, leading to a pseudocyst, often referred to as *giant cystic meconium peritonitis*. Operative repair of the obstruction can be difficult because of the adhesions, which are usually quite vascular. The goal is relief of the obstruction and, if possible, restoration of bowel continuity or creation of a Bishop-Koop ileostomy

KEY POINTS: INHERITED DISORDERS OF ABSORPTION AND MOTILITY

1. An infant who continues to stool significantly in the absence of oral intake should be evaluated for an inherited or acquired secretory process.

2. Congenital disorders of carbohydrate malabsorption that cause significant diarrhea in the infant are extremely rare.

3. The diagnosis of cystic fibrosis should be considered in any infant with meconium ileus.

4. An abnormal stooling pattern in an infant with Down syndrome should raise the possibility of Hirschsprung's disease.

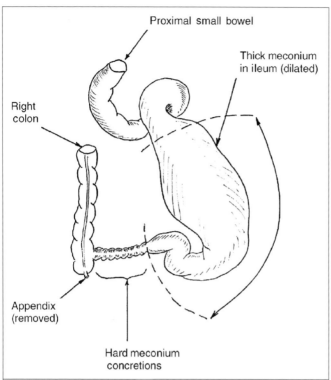

Proximal small bowel

Thick meconium in ileum (dilated)

Right colon

Appendix (removed)

Hard meconium concretions

Figure 9-4. Typical appearance, at the time of operative exploration, of a neonate with meconium ileus that failed nonoperative management. Note the dilated ileum proximal to the point of obstruction. Thick and viscous meconium is found in the dilated segment, and hard meconium pellets are found in the segment of ileum that is causing the complete mechanical obstruction. The massively dilated bowel must be resected.

(temporary). Ostomy closure is usually safe 6–8 weeks later. TPN may be necessary if inadequate bowel length is available for feeding.

126. **In newborns, what are the three most common gastrointestinal manifestations of cystic fibrosis?**
   - *Meconium ileus* is the earliest clinical manifestation of cystic fibrosis. Between 10% and 20% of patients with cystic fibrosis develop intestinal obstruction in utero during the last trimester of development. Abdominal distention is marked with no passage of meconium. The obstruction is secondary to the mass of extremely thick, tenacious meconium, which adheres to the wall of the distal small bowel and impacts the lumen.
   - The most common complication is *volvulus* of meconium-laden loops, frequently associated with ischemia, necrosis, perforation, and peritonitis. Twisted devitalized loops may become adherent, lose their continuity with the intestinal lumen, and form a gelatinous pseudocyst.
   - Spillage of meconium into the peritoneal cavity following antenatal intestinal perforation results in the development of *meconium peritonitis*. Meconium peritonitis may be seen before birth on ultrasound and presents as calcifications of the abdomen during the newborn period.

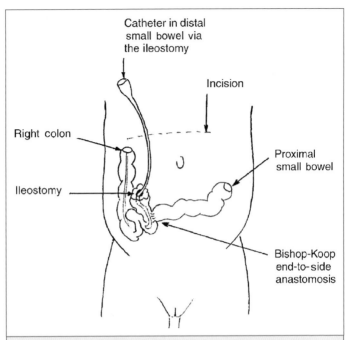

Figure 9-5. Creation of the Bishop-Koop ileostomy after segmental ileal resection for management of meconium ileus. A catheter can be placed in the ileostomy for postoperative irrigation of the distal ileum and colon that still contain thick and partially obstructing meconium.

SHORT GUT SYNDROME

127. **What is short gut syndrome?**

The newborn intestine is approximately 200–300 cm in length. Traditionally, the definition of short gut was less then 75 cm of total small bowel, thus an approximate loss of about half of the small bowel. Short gut syndrome is the constellation of symptoms, signs, and metabolic and nutritional alterations associated with a physiologically significant loss of gut. The overall prognosis would depend on what specific sections were lost and the overall remaining bowel function, including the following:

- Amount of remaining small intestine
- Whether it is proximal (jejunal) or distal (ileal)
- Whether the ileocecal valve is resected
- Whether the colon is resected
- Degree of intestinal adaptation
- Presence of residual bowel disease

128. **What are the mechanisms responsible for diarrhea in short gut syndrome?**

- **Decreased absorptive surface area**
- **Rapid transit time**
- **Bacterial overgrowth**
- **Hypersecretion and impaired regulation of gut motility**
- **Decreased absorption of bile salts:** The unabsorbed bile salts are deconjugated by anaerobic bacteria causing inhibition and even net secretion of water and electrolytes

- **Steatorrhea:** Secondary to decreased availability of bile salts
- **Loss of the ileocecal valve:** This permits reflux of colonic bacteria contributing to bacterial overgrowth
- **Colonic resection:** The colon is where most fluid reabsorption occurs

129. **What problems may be associated with enteral feeding in patients with short gut syndrome?**

Enteral feeds should be initiated early and aggressively advanced as tolerated to promote intestinal adaptation and help to diminish the complications associated with TPN. Formula is given via a feeding tube at a continuous rate initially to maximize absorption during advancement. There are no conclusive data that one type of formula or breast milk is ideal, and many different regimens have been used successfully. The major limiting factor in the formulas is the amount of carbohydrate. Unabsorbed sugars increase the osmotic load in the colon and cause an osmotic diarrhea that can lead to significant water loss and acidosis. The excessive malabsorption is accompanied by an increase in stool volume (stool outputs greater then 40–50 mL/kg/day), positive reducing substances, and a stool pH <5.5.

130. **What are the long-term complications of short gut syndrome?**
    - TPN-related liver disease
    - Nutrient deficiencies
    - Small bowel bacterial overgrowth
    - Catheter-related sepsis
    - Motility disturbances
    - Gastric acid hypersecretion
    - d-Lactic acidosis
    - Renal stones and gallstones

IMPERFORATE ANUS

131. **How is imperforate anus diagnosed?**

Imperforate anus is often diagnosed in the nursery as the nursing staff attempts to obtain a rectal temperature from the neonate or during the newborn examination. Rectal atresia might be missed during the examination because the anal opening can appear normal. However, failure to pass meconium and increasing abdominal distension should warrant further evaluation.

132. **How frequent is imperforate anus associated with other abnormalities?**

Associated spinal and genitourinary anomalies are rather common, occurring in 20–50% of imperforate anus cases. Imperforate anus may be seen as part of the vertebral defects, imperforate anus, tracheoesophageal fistula, and radial and renal dysplasia (VATER) or vertebral abnormalities, anal atresia, cardiac abnormalities, tracheoesophageal fistula and/or esophageal atresia, renal agenesis and dysplasia, and limb defects (VACTERL) association. The evaluation of an infant with imperforate anus includes looking for other associated anomalies.

133. **What tests determine initial management of an infant with imperforate anus?**

The initial testing needs to include a complete physical examination and a urine analysis. If the baby has a flat bottom without a well-developed gluteal fold or has meconium in the urine, a colostomy is indicated. Conversely, in the setting of a bucket handle deformity or meconium staining in the perineal midline, a minimal anorectoplasty is indicated without colostomy. In girls, only demonstration of a perineal fistula will avoid a colostomy. These decisions are all made after 16–24 hours to permit increased luminal pressures to force meconium through a fistula so that it is noted on examination. In all cases, an abdominal ultrasound should be obtained to rule out other anomalies.

- **Colostomy not required:** Perineal (cutaneous) fistula.
- **Colostomy required:** Rectourethral fistula (bulbar or prostatic), rectovesical fistula, imperforate anus without fistula, rectal atresia

HIRSCHSPRUNG'S DISEASE

134. When and by whom was Hirschsprung's disease first classically described?
The classical description of Hirschsprung's disease is attributed to Harold Hirschsprung, a pathologist, who described this condition in two children in 1888. This abnormality occurs in 1 in 5,000 live births. Males are four times more likely to be affected then females.

135. Why does Hirschsprung's disease occur?
The parasympathetic fibers that innervate the colonic bowel wall (to form the myenteric [Auerbach's] and the submucosal [Meissner's] nervous plexi) are derived from neural crest cells in the neural folds. During embryologic life, the cells migrate along the bowel in a cranial to caudal migration providing innervation. If during this migration the progression stops, then Hirschsprung's disease results. The result is a lack of parasympathetic innervation that allows the intestine to relax via release of nitric oxide from the postganglionic nerve fibers. Approximately 80% of the time the progression stops in the rectum, and only 20% involve the total bowel and/or small bowel.

136. How is Hirschsprung's disease diagnosed?
The diagnosis of Hirschsprung's disease can be made with a barium enema, rectal suction, or surgical full-thickness biopsy or by anorectal manometry. The initial test of choice is the unprepared barium enema. The test looks for the classic finding of a transition zone where the distal noninnervated section of bowel is smaller then the more proximal dilated bowel. The transition zone will occur in a location dependent on when the neurons stopped normal progression. The diagnosis by pathologic examination uses rectal biopsies to look for evidence of nerve cells directly. The biopsy will show absence of ganglion cells or presence of nerve cell hypertrophy or increased acetylcholinesterase with special staining. Anorectal manometry can be used to demonstrate the absence of the normal rectoanal inhibitory reflex that is present in the internal anal sphincter when innervated by the parasympathetic plexi.

137. Is there a genetic component to the disease?
Approximately 10% of children have a family history, especially with longer-segment Hirschsprung's disease. A higher incidence occurs in children with Down syndrome and other genetic abnormalities. Recent studies indicate the presence of mutations in the RET proto-oncogene in 17–38% of children with short-segment disease and in 70–80% of those with long-segment disease. Additional genes linked to the RET activation pathway and other mechanisms have now been identified.

138. What are the complications after surgical repair of Hirschsprung's disease?
- Obstruction
  - Mechanical obstruction
  - Incomplete resection of aganglionic bowel segments
  - Motility disorder
  - Functional megacolon
  - Internal sphincter achalasia
- Enterocolitis
- Incontinence

GASTROINTESTINAL HEMORRHAGE

139. **How does one determine whether swallowed maternal blood is the cause for gastrointestinal bleeding in the neonate?**
This determination is made using the Apt-Downey test. For this test, 1 part stool is mixed with 5 parts water and centrifuged for 2 minutes to separate out fecal material. The supernatant is removed, and 1 mL of 0.25 N (1%) sodium hydroxide is mixed with the 5 mL of supernatant. After 2 minutes there is a color change; if the hemoglobin is fetal the color stays pink, and if it is adult it turns yellow-brown.

140. **What are the sources of neonatal gastrointestinal bleeding?**
See Table 9-5.

TABLE 9-5. SOURCES OF NEONATAL GASTROINTESTINAL BLEEDING	
Hematemesis, Melena	**Hematochezia**
Swallowed maternal blood	Swallowed maternal blood
Stress ulcers, gastritis	Dietary protein intolerance
Duplication cyst	Infectious colitis
Vascular malformation	Necrotizing enterocolitis
Coagulopathy: vitamin K deficiency, DIC	Hirschsprung's disease with enterocolitis
Hemophilia	Duplication cyst
Maternal idiopathic thrombocytopenic purpura	Vascular malformations
	Coagulopathy: vitamin K deficiency, DIC
Maternal NSAID use	Hemophilia
	Maternal idiopathic thrombocytopenic purpura
	Maternal NSAID use

DIC = Disseminated intravascular coagulopathy, NSAID = nonsteroidal anti-inflammatory drug.

141. **What are some of the risk factors and clinical features that help distinguish necrotizing enterocolitis (NEC) from other causes of gastrointestinal bleeding in the neonate?**
NEC tends to be more common in premature infants and often occurs in those who have experienced some type of perinatal stress such as hypoxia, need for mechanical ventilation, and sepsis. The addition of gross or occult blood in stools, feeding intolerance, abdominal distension, bilious emesis, and lethargy should all lead to the consideration of NEC in the differential diagnosis.

142. **What is the first step in the management of an acutely ill infant with significant gastrointestinal bleeding?**
The key initial step is to obtain stable intravenous access to manage patient resuscitation. Particularly with hematemesis, the rapidity and severity of gastrointestinal bleeding can be significant, and the need for urgent intravenous access should not be underestimated. Once the ABCs of resuscitation have taken place, it is appropriate to focus on diagnosis and etiology.

NECROTIZING ENTEROCOLITIS

143. What is necrotizing enterocolitis (NEC)?

NEC is a disease of unknown origin that primarily affects premature infants (20% are term infants) after the onset of enteral alimentation during convalescence from the common cardiopulmonary disorders associated with prematurity. Manifestations cover a broad spectrum from mild abdominal distension with hematochezia to a fulminant septic shock–like picture with transmural necrosis of the entire gastrointestinal tract (NEC totalis).

144. Which infants are at risk for developing NEC?

NEC typically occurs in infants with a corrected gestational age of 30–32 weeks and at a time when most premature infants are progressing on enteral feedings. Onset of NEC is unusual on the first day of life and highly uncommon among infants who have not received enteral feeds. NEC may occur sporadically, but often patients are clustered in place and time. Although an infectious etiology is often sought, no consistent agent has been isolated from reported epidemics.

Many associated risk factors have been suggested that are not necessarily associated with the pathogenesis of NEC. Thus, when investigated in carefully controlled studies, risk factors such as perinatal asphyxia, respiratory distress syndrome, umbilical catheters, patent ductus arteriosus, hypotension, and anemia have not been demonstrated to be more common among patients who developed NEC than among unaffected age-matched control subjects. The most dominant risk factor for NEC is the degree of immaturity.

145. How are breast milk–fed infants thought to be protected from NEC?

Breast milk may reduce the risk of NEC. Breast milk offers many nutritive advantages in addition to protective immunologic substances. Milk macrophages and phagocytes, immunoglobulins A and G, and immunocompetent T and B lymphocytes may offer a protective advantage to the mucosa. These components potentiate the effect of complement components (C3 and C4), lysozyme, lactoferrin, and secretory immunoglobulin A. Breast milk contains hormones (e.g., thyroid, thyroid-stimulating hormone, prolactin, steroid), enzymes (e.g., amylase, lipase), and growth factors (endothelial growth factor). Breast milk also favors the growth of *Lactobacillus bifidus* and promotes a healthy gut flora.

146. What feeding risk factors have been associated with the development of NEC?

The absence of NEC in utero suggests an absolute requirement for gut colonization in its pathogenesis. Host luminal pH, proteases, oxygen tension, temperature, and osmolarity of enteral feedings have been implicated in the pathogenesis of NEC. The volume of milk fed to infants may also predispose them to NEC. Excessively rapid increments of milk feeding may overcome the infant's intestinal absorptive capability (especially in the presence of altered motility), resulting in malabsorption.

Large-volume milk feedings that are increased too rapidly during the feeding schedule may place undue stress on a previously injured or immature intestine. Two studies have shown that volume increments in excess of 20–25 mL/kg/day have been associated with NEC, whereas another two studies have shown the safety of 30–35 mL/kg/day increments. Therefore, volume increments should not be more than 20–35 mL/kg/day and should be based on normal clinical examination, physiologic stability, and absence of feeding intolerance.

147. What is the gas in pneumatosis intestinalis?

Malabsorbed carbohydrates contribute to enhanced intestinal bacterial gas production, resulting in abdominal distension. This gas dissects into the submucosa and subserosa, producing pneumatosis intestinalis; it is 30–40% hydrogen gas. High intraluminal pressure from gaseous distension may reduce mucosal blood flow, producing secondary intestinal ischemia.

148. **What infective agents are associated with NEC?**

In many cases of NEC, no infective agent is identifiable. Bacteria identified by positive blood cultures are seen in only 20–30% of patients with NEC. *S. epidermidis* is the most common organism, followed by gram-negative bacilli such as *E. coli* and *Klebsiella* species. Epidemics have been associated with a single pathogen such as *E. coli, Klebsiella* species, *Salmonella* species, *S. epidermidis, Clostridium butyricum, Coronavirus* species, *Rotavirus* species, and enteroviruses. NEC has also been associated with fungal sepsis. NEC may also result from an enterotoxin-mediated illness, such as toxins produced by *Clostridium* species or *S. epidermidis.* It is important to emphasize that, unlike in adults, *Clostridium difficile* and associated toxins are found in the intestinal tracts of many neonates who are entirely asymptomatic. The asymptomatic carrier state in some infants may be due to differences in intestinal immaturity, local differences in the intestinal milieu, absence of toxin-related receptors, or other protective factors.

149. **What are the criteria for considering the diagnosis of NEC?**

NEC is a common cause of systemic inflammatory response syndrome in neonates. Based on systemic signs, intestinal signs, and radiologic signs, staging of NEC is performed as shown in Table 9-6.

TABLE 9-6. STAGING OF NEC			
Stage	**Systemic Signs**	**Intestinal Signs**	**Radiographic Signs**
IA (suspect NEC)	Temperature instability, apnea, bradycardia, lethargy	Increased gastric residuals, mild abdominal distension, emesis, guaiac-positive stools	Normal or mild intestinal dilatation, mild ileus
IB (suspect NEC)	Same as IA	Bright red blood per rectum	Same as IA
IIA (definite NEC)	Same as IA	Same as IA and IB plus diminished or absent bowel sounds ± abdominal tenderness	Intestinal dilation, ileus, pneumatosis intestinalis
IIB (definite NEC)	Same as IIA plus mild acidosis and mild thrombocytopenia	Same as IIA plus definite abdominal tenderness, ± abdominal cellulites, or right lower quadrant mass, absent bowel sounds	Same as IIA ± portal vein gas ± ascites
IIIA (advanced NEC)	Same as IIB, plus hypotension, bradycardia, severe apnea, combined respiratory and metabolic acidosis, DIC, neutropenia, anuria	Same as IIB plus signs of generalized peritonitis, marked tenderness, distension, abdominal wall erythema	Same as IIB, definite ascites
IIIB (advanced NEC, severely ill, bowel perforated)	Same as IIIA, sudden perforation	Same as IIIA, sudden increased distension	Same as IIB plus pneumoperitoneum

DIC = Disseminated intravascular coagulopathy.

150. **A 1000-gm infant, born at 28 weeks' gestation, had an initial course characterized by respiratory distress syndrome and suspected sepsis. He was initially treated with surfactant and mechanical ventilation. The antibiotics were stopped after 3 days because the blood culture results were negative. On day 5, he was placed on nasal continuous positive airway pressure until day 18. He began enteral gavage feeds on day 5, at 20-cc/kg/day increments, and finally achieved "full feeds" (150 cc/kg/day) by day 20. He then developed an increased frequency of apnea and bradycardia associated with temperature instability. The gavage feeds were held because of increasing gastric residuals, presence of blood in stools, and abdominal distension. What should be done next?**

This infant falls into stage IB because of the temperature instability, apnea and bradycardia, increased gastric residuals, presence of blood in stools, and abdominal distension. An abdominal x-ray is recommended to view bowel gas pattern. We expect to see dilated bowel loops. Management includes the following: (1) consultation with a pediatric surgeon, (2) withdrawing all enteral feeds, (3) gastric decompression by placing an orogastric tube to suction, and (4) beginning antibiotics after appropriate cultures. Meanwhile, TPN is necessary. It is important to carefully follow up with this infant to monitor for progression to NEC and to exclude other diagnostic possibilities that may mimic NEC at this age.

151. **One day after beginning appropriate management, the same infant (*see* question 150) develops persistent abdominal distension, right lower quadrant tenderness, and diminished bowel sounds. The abdominal radiographs are shown in Figs. 9-6 and 9-7. How do you interpret these signs? What should be done next?**

At this stage, the infant is showing definite signs of NEC (stage II). This is evidenced by failure to recover from earlier stage and worsening intestinal signs such as diminished bowel sounds, distension of the abdomen, guarding, and abdominal tenderness. These clinical findings may herald the beginning of dilated viscus, submucosal or subserosal dissection of air, and peritonitis. Such an infant should be regarded as having NEC and is moderately ill. The radiograph in Fig. 9-6 shows grossly dilated bowel loops and submucosal and subserosal pneumatosis intestinalis. Management at this stage includes careful monitoring for worsening of clinical status (e.g., metabolic acidosis and thrombocytopenia) and continuing antibiotics for a minimum of

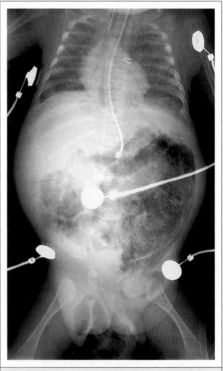

Figure 9-6. Abdominal radiograph 1 day after treatment for NEC stage IB. (Courtesy of Dr. Jack Sty, Department of Pediatric Radiology, Children's Hospital of Wisconsin, Medical College of Wisconsin, Milwaukee, WI.)

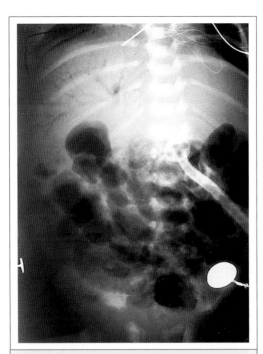

Figure 9-7. Abdominal radiograph of same infant 8 hours later. (Courtesy of Dr. Jack Sty, Department of Pediatric Radiology, Children's Hospital of Wisconsin, Medical College of Wisconsin, Milwaukee, WI.)

7–10 days. However, the second radiograph in Fig. 9-7 confirms the worsening status, manifested by portal vein gas (within the liver). NEC in this infant is progressing. At this stage, it is imperative to anticipate the possibility of intestinal perforation. Management at this stage includes correction of hypovolemia and metabolic acidosis using colloids and sodium bicarbonate, respectively. If NEC does not progress further, 2 weeks of appropriate antibiotics would suffice.

152. **Twenty-four hours later, the infant's condition deteriorates suddenly. He develops generalized abdominal tenderness and periumbilical erythema. An arterial blood gas determination shows a pH of 7.10, PCO_2 of 80 mmHg, PO_2 of 32 mmHg, HCO_3- of 12 mEq/L, and a base deficit of 16. The blood count is remarkable for a platelet count of 22,000/uL. The abdominal radiography is shown in Fig. 9-8. How do you interpret these signs? What should be the approach to the management of this infant?**
The infant at this stage has advanced NEC and is severely ill. This condition is characterized by worsening hypotension, a combined respiratory and metabolic acidosis, thrombocytopenia, and anuria. Thrombocytopenia usually represents a consumptive thrombocytopenia with or without intestinal perforation. The sudden deterioration is ominous for a bowel perforation, and progressive abdominal distension with erythema signifies worsening peritonitis and pneumoperitoneum. The lateral decubitus abdominal radiograph is remarkable for worsening pneumatosis and free air (*see* Fig. 9-8).

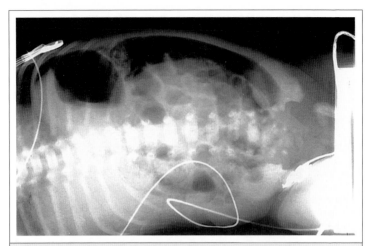

Figure 9-8. Abdominal radiograph of advanced NEC. (Courtesy of Dr. Jack Sty, Department of Pediatric Radiology, Children's Hospital of Wisconsin, Medical College of Wisconsin, Milwaukee, WI.)

This infant needs vigorous fluid resuscitation with colloids (i.e., fresh frozen plasma, albumin) and cellular products (i.e., packed red cells, platelets). Inotropic support using dopamine and epinephrine drips may be needed. Surgical exploration is indicated in this setting to facilitate abdominal decompression and salvage the viable bowel. If it is difficult to ventilate the infant at this stage, an abdominal paracentesis may be helpful.

153. **When is surgery indicated in an infant with NEC? What are the complications of performing surgery on an infant with advanced NEC with bowel perforation?**
Absolute indications for surgery include pneumoperitoneum and intestinal gangrene (as evidenced by positive results of abdominal paracentesis). Relative indications include progressive clinical deterioration (metabolic acidosis, ventilatory failure, oliguria, thrombocytopenia), fixed abdominal mass, abdominal wall erythema, portal vein gas, and persistently dilated bowel loop.

The postoperative complications occurring immediately after surgery are usually related to the stoma (retraction, prolapse, or peristomal hernia) or wound (infection, dehiscence, enterocutaneous fistula). Rarely, intra-abdominal abscesses, recurrence of NEC, and bowel obstruction can develop. Chronic complications result from the dysfunctional ostomies, strictures, or short gut syndrome.

154. **A 30-week-gestation male infant had been diagnosed with stage IIA NEC and was appropriately managed medically for 10 days. He subsequently tolerated feeds poorly. The stooling pattern was reported as normal (small green stools). Different formulas and prokinetics were tried without any positive result. An abdominal x-ray revealed what was reported as a "gassy abdomen." Treatment with antibiotics was begun again, and feedings were held for 3 days. A sepsis work-up bore negative results at 3 days. Feedings were then resumed with an elemental formula. The same feeding-intolerance pattern prevailed. What are the diagnostic considerations in this infant?**
Recovery after NEC occurs by second intention. Areas of patchy necrosis often heal by fibrosis and stricture formation. The repair process also involves the peritoneum, resulting in adhesions. An upper gastrointestinal contrast radiograph may show a prolonged transit time and gross

dilation of jejunum consistent with more distal stricture formation. A lower gastrointestinal contrast x-ray may be necessary to identify strictures in the large bowel. At laparotomy, he was found to have multiple strictures, which were resected and ultimately resulted in a short bowel syndrome.

155. **A 3500-gm term female infant born after an uncomplicated pregnancy was discharged home from the newborn nursery after a normal transition. She was fed exclusively with breast milk. On her seventh day of life, she presented acutely with bilious emesis. The clinical examination was remarkable for a pulse rate of 180 beats/min, respiratory rate of 70/min, mean blood pressure of 30 mmHg, abdominal distension, and marked tenderness with diminished bowel sounds. She passed a dark bloody stool. Laboratory study results were notable for an arterial blood gas of pH 7.15, PCO$_2$ level of 30 mmHg, PO$_2$ level of 120 mmHg, and HCO$_3^-$ level of 10 mEq/L. The complete blood count was remarkable for a hematocrit level of 24 and platelet count of 400,000/uL. What is the approach to management in this infant? How would you establish a diagnosis in this infant?**

The infant's exam is compatible with acute abdomen, and she has signs of hypovolemia and shock. She needs fluid resuscitation and correction of metabolic acidosis. Because sepsis is a common entity in the neonatal period, antibiotics are indicated after obtaining blood cultures. A nasogastric tube should be placed and the stomach decompressed. An abdominal x-ray reveals gassy distended bowel loops with fluid levels. An upper gastrointestinal contrast radiograph is shown in Fig. 9-9. The contrast fails to flow distally, suggesting intestinal obstruction, and in this case it looks like a pig-tail. A diagnosis of volvulus is highly likely in this infant, and surgical exploration should be considered.

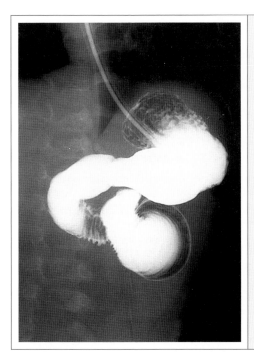

Figure 9-9. Upper gastrointestinal contrast radiograph. (Courtesy of Dr. Jack Sty, Department of Pediatric Radiology, Children's Hospital of Wisconsin, Medical College of Wisconsin, Milwaukee, WI.)

156. **How do you differentiate NEC from volvulus? In what conditions is pneumatosis intestinalis seen?**

    Table 9-7 summarizes the features that differentiate NEC from volvulus. Apart from NEC, pneumatosis intestinalis is also seen in midgut volvulus, acute or chronic diarrhea, postoperative gastrointestinal surgery, Hirschsprung's disease, short bowel syndrome, mesenteric thrombosis, postcardiac catheterization, structural disease of the hindgut (colonic atresias and stricture, imperforate anus), and intestinal malignancies.

TABLE 9-7. NEC DIFFERENTIATED FROM VOLVULUS		
Characteristics	**NEC**	**Volvulus**
Preterm	90%	30%
Onset by 2 weeks	90%	60%
Male:female ratio	1:1	2:1
Associated anomalies	Rare	25–40%
Bilious emesis	Unusual	75%
Grossly bloody stools	Common	Less common
Pneumatosis intestinalis	90%	2%
Marked proximal obstruction	Rare	Common
Thrombocytopenia without DIC	Common	Rare

Modified from Kliegman R: Necrotizing enterocolitis: differential diagnosis and management. In Polin RA, Yoder MC, Burg FD (eds): Workbook in Practical Neonatology, 2nd ed. Philadelphia, W.B. Saunders, 1993, pp 449–470, with permission.

NEONATAL HEPATITIS

157. **What are the components of neonatal biliary disease?**

    Any disease process in the neonate with altered bile acid transport or biliary structure is a biliary disease. The clues to its presence include cholestasis (elevated serum bile acids), conjugated hyperbilirubinemia, and altered serum levels of enzymes from biliary inflammation or obstruction (e.g., gamma glutamyl transferase [GTT] and alkaline phosphatase).

158. **What is cholestatic jaundice?**

    Conjugated bilirubin >2.0 mg/dL or exceeding 15% of the total bilirubin is referred to as *direct hyperbilirubinemia* and is a clinical indicator of cholestatic jaundice. Cholestatic jaundice is always physiologically abnormal and warrants a medical evaluation. Note that biliary disease can present with or without cholestatic jaundice.

159. **What are the causes of direct hyperbilirubinemia?**

    The mechanisms include:
    - Impaired bilirubin metabolism secondary to parenchymal disease of the liver
    - Inherited disorders of bilirubin excretion
    - Mechanical obstruction to biliary flow, both intrahepatic and extrahepatic
    - Excessive bilirubin loads such as may occur in massive hemolysis

160. **When should an infant's fractionated bilirubin be obtained?**

    Evaluation of jaundice persisting beyond the normal physiologic period (2 weeks) in newborns must always include a fractionation of bilirubin.

161. **How should the evaluation of cholestatic jaundice in infants be approached?**
Neonatal cholestasis can be a manifestation of (1) extrahepatic biliary disease, (2) intrahepatic biliary disease, or (3) hepatocellular disease. All can present with similar symptoms. Therefore, differentiation based on history and physical examination alone is usually not helpful.

The physician should embark on a diagnostic evaluation that will promptly identify clinical conditions amenable to therapy (Table 9-8) and where delay in treatment could be tragic (e.g., sepsis; urinary tract infection; hypothyroidism; biliary atresia; and congenital metabolic disorders treated with special diets such as galactosemia, hereditary fructose intolerance, and tyrosinemia).

TABLE 9-8. TREATABLE CAUSES OF NEONATAL CHOLESTASIS

Infectious	Surgical	Metabolic	Other
Urinary tract infection	Biliary atresia	Galactosemia	Hypothyroidism
Sepsis	Choledochal cyst	Hereditary fructose intolerance	Neonatal iron storage disease
	Cholelithiasis	Tyrosinemia	TPN
	Biliary strictures		Bile acid synthetic disorders
	Duct perforation		Histiocytosis X
	Congenital duct anomalies		
	Mass (neoplasia)		
	Intestinal obstruction		

162. **What tests should be obtained during the initial evaluation of neonatal cholestasis?**
See Table 9-9.

TABLE 9-9. TESTS FOR THE INITIAL EVALUATION OF NEONATAL CHOLESTASIS

Test	Indication
Blood	
Fractionation of bilirubin	Detect cholestatic jaundice
CBC	To rule out sepsis
Blood cultures (as clinically indicated)	To rule out sepsis
Hepatic function panel	Abnormal in hepatobiliary disease
TSH/T_4	To rule out hypothyroidism
Coagulation studies	Liver synthetic function
Urine	
Urinalysis and culture	(+) reducing sugar: galactosemia
	(±) protein: galactosemia, hereditary fructose intolerance, tyrosinemia
	(+) culture: UTI, sepsis
Abdominal ultrasound	(+) choledochal cyst, stones, masses, and stricture
Diisopropyl immodiacetic acid (DISIDA)	Nonexcreting in biliary atresia, delayed uptake and (+) excreting in neonatal hepatitis

163. **When should the infant be referred to a gastroenterologist?**

As soon as cholestatic jaundice is diagnosed and sepsis ruled out, a gastroenterologist should be consulted. The tests mentioned in the previous question can be scheduled, but no time should be spent waiting for results. In most cases, the final diagnosis requires that a liver biopsy be performed. The hepatologist will conduct a broad laboratory evaluation to make a diagnosis so that therapy can be initiated. In addition to medical therapy, preventive therapy can be provided through genetic counseling. Time is of the essence to identify treatable causes of cholestasis and because early intervention in biliary atresia affects prognosis.

164. **What is spontaneous bile duct perforation?**

Spontaneous perforation of the bile ducts is a rare occurrence but has been documented in infants between 4 and 12 weeks of age. The cause is currently unknown. It most often occurs at the point of joining of the cystic duct to the common bile duct. Infants can present with lethargy, nonbilious vomiting, acholic stools, mild jaundice, dark urine, abdominal distension, and a mildly elevated conjugated hyperbilirubinemia. Definitive diagnosis can be made with a hepatoiminodiacetic acid (HIDA) scan or abdominal paracentesis.

165. **How do the bile salt transporter defects present?**

This group of conditions is collectively known as *progressive familial intrahepatic cholestasis.* They typically present as neonatal cholestasis but individually have distinct clinical, laboratory, and histologic features that differentiate them (Table 9-10).

BILE DUCT AND BILIARY ATRESIA

166. **A 6-week-old healthy, term breast-fed infant was noted to be jaundiced at the routine well-care visit. She was growing well. Examination of the abdomen revealed a palpable liver (1 cm below right costal margin) and spleen (2 cm below left costal margin). Her history revealed that she had pigmented stools. Total and direct bilirubin levels were 6.9 and 4.3 mg/dL, respectively. Other findings include: alanine aminotransferase (ALT), 138 u/L; aspartate aminotransferase (AST), 120 u/L; alkaline phosphatase (ALK), 205 u/L; gamma-glutamyl transferase (GGT), 420 u/L; albumin, 3.0 gm/dL; and prothrombin time (PT) 13.9 sec. Ca, PO_4, and Mg were normal; complete blood count, urinalysis, and culture had normal results. What do the lab results suggest, and which further tests need to be performed?**

Apart from ruling out sepsis and urinary tract infection, the above tests are nondiagnostic. The liver enzymes and PT are useful for following the course of hepatic function. Other tests should be performed:

- **Ultrasound:** This is a quick noninvasive test for detecting causes of extrahepatic cholestasis (e.g., choledochal cysts, biliary stones, tumors). Finding a gallbladder on ultrasound does not rule out biliary atresia.
- **Radionuclide scans (DISIDA):** Good hepatic uptake of radionuclide with absence of excretion into the gut lumen is suggestive of an obstructive process such as biliary atresia. Delayed excretion may also occur in hepatitis.

167. **The ultrasound revealed hepatosplenomegaly, and no gallbladder was seen. The DISIDA scan showed normal uptake but no excretion at 24 hours. A liver biopsy specimen was obtained, which showed intrahepatic cholestasis with proliferation of the bile ducts. Is the evaluation now complete for making a definitive diagnosis?**

The evaluation is very suggestive of biliary atresia; however, this can be confirmed only by performing an intraoperative cholangiogram. Other causes of neonatal cholestasis such as Alagille

TABLE 9-10.   BILE SALT TRANSPORTER DEFECTS

	Symptoms	Gene Mutation	Distinguishing Hallmark	Liver Biopsy	Prognosis
PFIC type I (Byler's disease)	Elevated AST/ALT Severe pruritus Jaundice Growth failure Cholelithiasis Fat-soluble vitamin deficiencies Recurrent epistaxis	FIC1 gene	Severe cholestasis Low-to-normal GGT levels Normal cholesterol levels	Liver histology shows cholestasis and progression of cirrhosis but no ductal proliferation Canalicular bile appears coarse and granular on EM	Variable progression
PFIC type II	Similar to PFIC I except more rapidly progressive cholestasis and liver disease	BSEP gene	Severe cholestasis Low to normal GGT levels Normal cholesterol levels	Liver histology shows cholestasis and progression of cirrhosis but no ductal proliferation Giant cells Canalicular bile appears filamentous or amorphous on EM	Rapidly progressive
PFIC type III	Similar to PFIC I but more variable in presentation and clinica course than other two types	MDR2 gene	High GGT levels Markedly reduced bile phospholipids	Portal fibrosis and bile duct proliferation	Variable progression

PFIC = Progressive familial intrahepatic cholestasis, EM = electron microsopy.

syndrome may clinically mimic biliary atresia and may only be differentiated by intraoperative cholangiogram.

168. **What are the causes of extrahepatic neonatal cholestasis?**
    In general, these lesions lead to the extrahepatic obstruction of bile flow from the liver to the duodenum. These processes lead to bile buildup in the duct, causing inflammation and damage to the liver. The result is elevations of GGT and alkaline phosphatase consistent with biliary duct damage and varying degrees of elevation of liver enzymes and direct hyperbilirubinemia. Examples of extrahepatic bile duct disorders include the following:

- Biliary atresia
- Choledochal cyst and choledochocele
- Biliary hyperplasia
- Bile duct perforation
- Neonatal sclerosing cholangitis

169. **What are the causes of pediatric elevations of GGT?**
See Table 9-11.

TABLE 9-11. CAUSES OF PEDIATRIC ELEVATIONS OF GGT	
Disease	**Variation of GGT**
Extrahepatic biliary atresia	Increased to 10 times upper limit
Alagille syndrome	Increased 3–20 times upper limit
Sclerosing cholangitis	Increased 50–100 times upper limit
PFIC types I and II	Normal to decreased
PFIC type III	Increased
Bile acid disorders	Normal

170. **Is it critical to make an early diagnosis of biliary atresia?**
The effectiveness of surgical therapy (Kasai operation) for biliary atresia is dependent on age at surgery. Best outcomes are achieved when intervention is before 8–10 weeks. Biliary atresia is the leading indication for liver transplantation in children.

171. **A 10-week-old former 34-week premature, breast-fed boy was referred for evaluation of jaundice and elevated liver enzymes. His test results indicated a conjugated bilirubin, 3.8 mg/dL; ALK 650 u/L; AST, 120 u/L; ALT, 138 u/L; and GGT, 1200 u/L. During the newborn period, he had mild respiratory distress syndrome, was treated for sepsis, and received TPN for 7 days. He was discharged home on breast-milk feeds at the age of 3 weeks. How should the evaluation proceed?**
The laboratory results show a disproportionately elevated serum GGT and ALK, suggesting biliary disease. However, because the clinical manifestations of neonatal cholestasis are independent of etiology, the initial basic evaluation should be as described in Table 9-9.

172. **A careful physical exam revealed the patient in question 171 had a prominent forehead, small chin, and a systolic heart murmur consistent with peripheral pulmonary stenosis. The ultrasound had normal results. The DISIDA scan showed excretion at 24 hours. Is this sufficient for making the diagnosis of Alagille syndrome?**
A liver biopsy is necessary to confirm the diagnosis. Alagille syndrome is also referred to as *syndromic bile duct paucity*. It needs to be differentiated from biliary atresia. During infancy, histology may show bile duct proliferation. However, in later childhood and adulthood, the liver histology commonly shows bile duct paucity. The genetic defect has been identified as Jagged 1 (JAG1) located on chromosome 20p12. Inheritance occurs in an autosomal dominant pattern. Alagille syndrome is the most common form of familial intrahepatic cholestasis and consists of five characteristics:

- **Chronic cholestasis:** Associated with hypercholesterolemia and paucity of intralobular bile ducts
- **Congenital heart disease:** Peripheral pulmonic stenosis is the most common

- **Bone defects:** Including vertebrae
- **Eye findings:** Posterior embryotoxon
- **Typical facies:** Frontal bossing, deep-set eyes, bulbous tip of nose, and pointed chin

173. **What clinical conditions are associated with cholelithiasis?**
   - Hemolytic disease
   - TPN
   - Diuretic use
   - Short bowel syndrome
   - Small bowel bacterial overgrowth
   - Sepsis

174. **What are common mistakes in the evaluation of an infant with neonatal cholestasis?**
   - Attributing all jaundice beyond the physiologic period in healthy infants to breast milk
   - Not fractionating bilirubin
   - Not performing the basic evaluation in an expedited fashion
   - Relying on the clinical history and physical exam to make a diagnosis
   - Delayed referral to a specialist

175. **What is extrahepatic biliary atresia?**
   Extrahepatic biliary atresia is the term given to idiopathic progressive obliteration or discontinuity of the extrahepatic biliary tree in infancy. The process is a progressive destruction of the biliary tree. Two forms are recognized based on when the obliteration occurs.
   The *embryonic/fetal* type of biliary atresia occurs in 10–35% of cases:
   - Direct hyperbilirubinemia seen at birth and no true jaundice-free period after physiologic jaundice
   - More often associated with congenital malformations
   - Bile duct remnants are often not seen at time of surgery
   The *perinatal* type of biliary atresia occurs in 65–90% of cases:
   - Direct hyperbilirubinemia occurs at 4–8 weeks of age
   - Jaundice-free period after physiologic jaundice
   - Bile duct remnants are often seen at the time of surgery

   Hinds R, Davenport M, Mieli-Vergani G, Hadzic N: Antenatal presentation of biliary atresia. J Pediatr 144:43–46, 2004.

KEY POINTS: LIVER DISEASE

1. Direct hyperbilirubinemia is *always* abnormal.

2. The key to the evaluation of an infant with cholestatic jaundice is early assessment of treatable causes.

3. Significant hypoglycemia or coagulopathy in an infant with cholestatic jaundice may be an important sign of significant hepatocellular disease.

4. Do not forget silent urinary tract infection as an important, treatable cause of cholestatic jaundice in the infant.

176. **What are the demographics of extrahepatic biliary atresia?**
   Biliary atresia occurs in 1 in 10,000–15,000 live births, with females affected 1.4 times more frequently than males. Approximately 10–20% of infants with biliary atresia will have associated

anomalies (syndromic biliary atresia), including splenic abnormalities (polysplenia or asplenia), malrotation, and situs inversus.

177. **What are the typical presenting clinical features of an infant with extrahepatic biliary atresia?**
The usual presentation is that of an otherwise healthy infant who develops jaundice between 4 and 8 weeks of age. If an infant appears ill (e.g., vomiting, acidosis, failure to thrive), metabolic (nonobstructive) causes of jaundice should be considered promptly.

178. **What are the typical radiographic findings in extrahepatic biliary atresia?**
   - **Ultrasound:** Hepatic parenchyma may be normal, and the gallbladder and common bile duct are generally not visualized. It is important to note that the gallbladder may not be visualized in healthy infants because of contraction; nonvisualization of the gallbladder should not be considered diagnostic of biliary atresia. The main purpose of ultrasound in this setting is to rule out an obstructing choledochal cyst.
   - **DISIDA scan:** There should be uptake of the radiotracer by the hepatic parenchyma, although uptake may be delayed (due to associated hepatocyte injury). In biliary atresia, absolutely no contrast will reach the bowel even after 12–24 hours; contrast will ultimately appear in the kidneys and urinary bladder as it is cleared through the urinary tract.

179. **What are the typical histopathologic findings in extrahepatic biliary atresia?**
Liver biopsy is the final step in preoperative diagnosis of biliary atresia. The biopsy will demonstrate proliferation of bile ducts and bile plugs in response to extrahepatic obstruction. The main purpose of the biopsy is to differentiate between obstructive and nonobstructive causes of cholestasis. A variable amount of fibrosis will also be present, depending on the age of the infant and the rapidity of progression of the disease process.

180. **How do the radiologic and histopathologic findings in biliary atresia compare with those of neonatal hepatitis?**
See Table 9-12.

TABLE 9-12.	BILIARY ATRESIA VERSUS NEONATAL HEPATITIS		
Study	**Biliary Atresia**	**Neonatal Hepatitis**	**Other Disorders of Interest**
Ultrasound	Nonvisualization of the gallbladder, common bile duct	Normal gallbladder and common bile duct, occasional nonvisualization of gallbladder and common bile duct	Choledochal cyst
DISIDA scan	Good or delayed uptake of tracer with no excretion of tracer into the bowel	Delayed uptake of tracer, excretion into the bowel occurs	Will detect a bile leak in the rare setting of spontaneous rupture of the biliary tree
Liver biopsy	Proliferation of the bile ducts, bile plugs in the ducts, fibrosis of the portal tracts or cirrhosis, formation of hepatic acini (rosettes), and variable inflammation	Inflammation of the hepatic parenchyma, giant cell transformation of the hepatocytes common in infants, cholestasis	Wide variety of specific abnormalities suggestive of other specific diseases

181. **What is the natural history of untreated biliary atresia?**
Untreated biliary atresia is uniformly fatal within 2 years, with a median survival of 8 months. Untreated biliary atresia leads to biliary cirrhosis, portal hypertension, esophageal varices, failure to thrive, and liver failure, and death can occur due to any of a number of complications.

182. **What is appropriate surgical and medical therapy for biliary atresia, and how does therapy affect survival?**
   - **Surgical:** If the liver biopsy is suggestive of biliary atresia, the infant undergoes exploratory laparotomy and an intraoperative cholangiogram. If biliary atresia is confirmed, an attempt to restore biliary drainage by the Kasai procedure (i.e., hepatic portoenterostomy) is made. A loop of bowel is anastomosed directly to the hepatic capsule at the porta hepatis after resection of the fibrous biliary remnants. Bowel continuity is restored by formation of a Roux-en-Y intestinal anastomosis. The success of the procedure depends on the age of the infant at operation and the experience of the surgeon. Long-term survival rates may exceed 60% for infants younger than 2 months of age at the time of portoenterostomy, compared with only 25% for those older than 2 months of age. The first sign of a successful portoenterostomy is the passage of green (bile stained), rather than acholic, stools. A retrospective study of 81 patients in the United States noted a success rate of approximately 38% with the Kasai procedure alone.
   - **Medical:** Any child with biliary atresia, regardless of the status of portoenterostomy, should be treated for chronic liver disease and its potential complications. Infants should receive fat-soluble vitamin supplementation. Many infants require supplemental tube feedings, particularly if the portoenterostomy is unsuccessful. Good nutritional status will optimize the infant's survival if liver transplantation becomes necessary.

   Wildhaber BE, Coran AG, Drongowski RA, et al: The Kasai portoenterostomy for biliary atresia: a review of a 27-year experience with 81 patients. J Pediatr Surg 38:1480–1485, 2003.

183. **What are the potential complications of the Kasai portoenterostomy?**
Specific complications include failure to achieve drainage, ascending cholangitis where drainage is achieved, and biliary cysts at the portoenterostomy site.

184. **What are the therapeutic options that exist for children who do not undergo portoenterostomy or in whom drainage is not achieved?**
Liver transplantation is the only definitive therapy and has an approximately 80% expected 5-year survival rate.

185. **Other than biliary atresia, what are the causes of obstructive jaundice in infancy?**
Choledochal cysts and spontaneous perforation of the extrahepatic biliary tree are two causes of obstructive jaundice in infancy. Cholelithiasis is not a major cause of biliary obstruction in infancy, although gallstones may be seen as incidental findings on ultrasound of premature infants and occasionally even on prenatal ultrasound.

186. **What are the demographics and presentation of choledochal cysts?**
Choledochal cysts are rarer than biliary atresia, with estimates of incidence ranging from 1 in 13,000 to 1 in 2,000,000 live births. Girls are affected four times more frequently than boys. The classic triad of abdominal pain, mass, and jaundice occurs in fewer than 20% of cases. Choledochal cysts may present as jaundice, mass, vomiting, fever, and even pancreatitis. Fewer than half of choledochal cysts present in infancy.

187. **What are the types of choledochal cysts?**
   - **Type I:** Diffuse enlargement of the common bile duct (the majority fall in this category)
   - **Type II:** Diverticular cyst
   - **Type III:** Choledochocele

- **Type IV:** Multiple cysts of the intrahepatic and extrahepatic biliary tree
- **Type V:** Caroli's disease

ABDOMINAL MASSES

188. **What is the origin of most neonatal abdominal masses?**
Over half of all abdominal masses in the neonate arise from the urinary tract.

189. **List the two most common causes of abdominal masses of urologic origin in the neonate.**
- Hydronephrosis secondary to ureteropelvic junction obstruction
- Multicystic kidney disease

190. **A pregnant women has an antenatal ultrasound scan that reveals an intra-abdominal mass in the fetus. Are any special arrangements necessary for the timing and mode of delivery?**
No.

191. **How do the location and other physical examination characteristics of the common abdominal masses in newborn infants provide clues for their identification?**
Physical examination may significantly narrow the diagnostic possibilities, even if it does not provide an absolute answer (Table 9-13). Of note:
- Large masses may fill the entire abdomen, making it impossible to determine the site of origin on examination.

TABLE 9-13. COMMON ABDOMINAL MASSES IN NEONATES

Mass Location	Examples	Characteristics
Lateral mass	Multiple kidney or hydronephrosis	Smooth, moderate mobility, transilluminates
	Renal tumor	Smooth, minimally mobile, does not transilluminate
	Neuroblastoma	Irregular contour, minimally mobile, frequently crosses midline
Midabdominal	Mesenteric cyst	Smooth, mobile, transilluminates
	Gastrointestinal duplication cyst	Smooth, mobile, does not transilluminate; may be associated with obstruction
	Ovarian cyst	Smooth, mobile, transilluminates
Upper abdominal mass	Hepatic tumors	Hard, immobile, does not transilluminate
	Choledochal cyst	Smooth, immobile, does not transilluminate; may be associated with jaundice
Lower abdominal mass	Hydrometrocolpos	Smooth, immobile, does not transilluminate; may be associated with imperforate hymen
Lower abdominal mass	Bladder	Smooth fixed; associated with lower urinary obstruction
	Urachal cyst	Smooth, fixed to abdominal wall, extends to umbilicus
	Sacrococcygeal teratoma	Hard, fixed, does not transilluminate; often associated with external sacral component

- Hard, nodular masses are usually malignant tumors.
- A highly mobile mass is usually a mesenteric cyst, a duplication, or an ovarian cyst.

BIBLIOGRAPHY

1. Bishop HC, Koop CE: Mangement of meconium ileus: Resection, Rous-en-Y anastamosis, and ileostomy irrigation with pancreatic enzymes. Ann Surg 145:410–414, 1957.
2. Kleinman RE (ed): Pediatric Nutrition Handbook, 5th ed. Elk Grove, IL, American Academy of Pediatrics, 2004.
3. Spitzer AR (ed): Intensive Care of the Fetus and Neonate, 2nd ed. Philadelphia, Elsevier, 2005.
4. Walker WA, Goulet O, Kleinman RE, et al (eds): Pediatric Gastrointestinal Disease: Pathophysiology, Diagnosis, Management, 4th ed. Hamilton, Ontario, BC Decker, 2004.

CHAPTER 10

GENETICS

Wendy K. Chung, MD, PhD

1. **What are the most common major congenital anomalies in the United States?**
   Anencephaly and spina bifida, occurring with a prevalence of about 0.5–2.0/1000 live births.

2. **Should an asymptomatic infant with a single umbilical artery have a screening ultrasound scan done for renal anomalies?**
   This point has been argued for years. A single umbilical artery is a rare phenomenon. In one study of nearly 35,000 infants, examination of the placenta showed that only 112 (0.32%) had a single umbilical artery. All 112 underwent renal ultrasonography, and 17% had abnormalities (45% of which persisted). A more recent study demonstrated that left umbilical arteries tend to be absent more often than right umbilical arteries when only a single artery is present. In addition, there was a high incidence of associated congenital malformations in nearly 25% of the infants diagnosed prenatally with a single umbilical artery. Because of the rarity of the condition and the increased association of abnormalities, patients with single umbilical arteries probably should receive a screening renal ultrasound.

   Burke WG, Clarke TA, Mathews TG, et al: Isolated single umbilical artery: The case for routine renal screening. Arch Dis Child 68:600–601, 1993.

   Geipel A, Germer U, Welp T, et al: Prenatal diagnosis of single umbilical artery: Determination of absent side, associated anomalies, Doppler findings, and perinatal outcome. Ultrasound Obstet Gynecol 15:114–117, 2000.

3. **Excluding chromosomal analysis, what laboratory test results suggest that a woman is carrying a fetus with trisomy 21 syndrome?**
   There is some variation in the accuracy of diagnosis, depending on the tests used and the timing of the screening. In the mid-trimester of gestation, the combination of low levels of maternal serum alpha-fetoprotein (AFP) and unconjugated estriol and elevated levels of human chorionic gonadotropin (hCG; the so-called "triple screen") can identify 69% of fetuses with Down syndrome with a false-positive rate of 5–10%. The addition of nuchal translucency screening improves diagnosis to about 80–85%. Some preliminary evidence from proteomic screening for Down-specific biomarkers, however, suggests that this approach may eliminate the triple or quadruple screen in the near future, improving the accuracy of diagnosis to near 100% with an extremely low false-positive rate. Abnormal screening test results can prompt definitive studies of chromosomal analysis.

4. **Which other conditions may be detected by a raised amniotic fluid AFP level?**
   - Multiple gestation
   - Intrauterine fetal death
   - Omphalocele and gastroschisis
   - Bowel and esophageal atresias
   - Turner's syndrome (cystic hygroma)
   - Meckel's syndrome
   - Congenital nephrosis (Finnish type)
   - Sacrococcygeal teratoma
   - Bladder exstrophy
   - Focal dermal hypoplasia/aplasia cutis congenita

5. **A woman who had a positive triple screen in the second trimester and normal fetal ultrasound results, but declined amniocentesis, delivers a healthy-appearing infant. What further studies are indicated based on the triple screen?**
    None. A positive triple screen is a screening test, *not* a diagnostic test. If the infant looks healthy without features of Down syndrome or other anomalies, no further testing is necessary. Chromosome tests do not need to be done on a normal-appearing infant just because the triple test result was abnormal.

6. **First-trimester screening for aneuploidy is becoming available. What is being measured, and how reliable is this new method?**
    Pregnancy-associated plasma protein (PAPP-A), free hCG, and ultrasound nuchal translucency are being used. PAPP-A is the single best serum marker in early pregnancy found to date. Its levels decrease by more than one half on average in a Down syndrome pregnancy. Low PAPP-A may also be associated with trisomy 18. hCG levels are approximately doubled in Down syndrome.

    Measurement of nuchal translucency thickness between 10 and 13 weeks' gestation has been shown to identify about 75% of fetuses with Down syndrome. Higher detection rates are obtained by combining free hCG, PAPP-A, and nuchal thickness—up to 85% detection of Down syndrome with a 5% false-positive rate.

7. **How would you evaluate a newborn with Down syndrome to ensure you are discharging a healthy infant? What serious abnormalities could one expect to find?**
    - Order a chromosome study on peripheral blood (G-banding) to rule out translocation or mosaicism.
    - Perform a cardiac evaluation (40% of infants with Down syndrome have congenital heart disease, with the most common defect being an atrioventricular canal).
    - Ensure there is no bowel obstruction. Duodenal atresia, duodenal web, and Hirschsprung's disease are more common in Down syndrome. Anal stenosis may mimic Hirschsprung's disease.
    - Assess hearing.
    - Check eyes for cataracts, nystagmus, and strabismus.
    - Monitor feeding and sucking.
    - Perform a thyroid screen (state screen).
    - Refer for genetic counseling and early intervention.

KEY POINTS: COMMON CAUSES OF BIRTH DEFECTS

1. Chromosomal disorders (aneuploidy, deletions, duplications)

2. Maternal diabetes

3. Insufficient maternal micronutrients (folic acid and neural tube defects)

4. Teratogenic exposures

5. Maternal infection

6. Inborn errors of metabolism

7. Monogenic disorders

8. Multifactorial (cleft lip and cleft palate)

9. Developmental deformation

10. Developmental disruption

8. **A macrosomic infant is born with an omphalocele and large tongue. What would you anticipate monitoring closely in this baby, and why?**
This baby may have Beckwith-Wiedemann syndrome and may be at risk for hypoglycemia. Other signs of Beckwith-Wiedemann syndrome include grooves on the ear lobes, hemihypertrophy, and visceromegaly. These children are at risk for Wilms' tumor and hepatoblastoma and should be monitored with an abdominal ultrasound and AFP every 4 months for the first 6 years of life.

9. **What is the difference between an omphalocele and gastroschisis?**
Omphalocele
   - This midline anterior abdominal well defect is covered by a transparent sac consisting of amnion and peritoneum with Wharton's jelly between them.
   - Intra-abdominal viscera is herniated through the umbilical ring. The size varies with contents.
   - The umbilical cord inserts into the sac.
   - Other malformations are present in 67% of cases.
   - This defect can be associated with chromosome abnormalities, especially trisomy 13.
   Gastroschisis
   - The umbilical cord is attached to the abdominal wall to the left of the defect. There is a normal umbilical cord insertion.
   - Herniated organs usually consist of thickened loops of small intestine with no membranous covering. The intestine floats freely in the amniotic fluid in utero.
   - Fifteen percent of cases of gastroschisis are associated with other major malformations.
   - It is not commonly found in fetuses with chromosome abnormalities.

10. **What are the most common syndromes associated with congenital diaphragmatic hernia?**
Congenital diaphragmatic hernia is an associated inherited condition in the following syndromes:
   - Fryns syndrome
   - Donnai syndrome
   - Cornelia de Lange's syndrome
   - Beckwith-Wiedemann syndrome
   - Simpson-Golabi-Behmel syndrome
   - Denys-Drash syndrome
   - Pallister-Killian syndrome (mosaic tetrasomy 12p)
   - Perlman syndrome
   - Aneuploidy/chromosomal disorders

11. **An infant is born with the following features: puffiness of the dorsum of the hands and feet, excessive skin at the nape of the neck with a low posterior hairline, a broad chest and widely spaced nipples, cardiac and aortic defect, cubitus valgus, and renal anomaly. What is your differential diagnosis?**
   - Turner's syndrome
   - Noonan's syndrome

12. **How would you work up the baby in question 11?**
   - Chromosome study on peripheral blood (G-banding)
   - Hearing evaluation
   - Genetic testing for Noonan's syndrome (PTPN11 gene) if chromosomes are normal
   - Cardiac evaluation
   - Renal ultrasound
   - Referral for genetic counseling and early intervention

KEY POINTS: PRINCIPLES OF BIRTH DEFECTS

1. Single minor anomalies such as an isolated simian crease are common and not necessarily associated with an underlying genetic problem. However, as the number of minor anomalies increases, the likelihood of an underlying genetic diagnosis also increases.

2. Susceptibility for some birth defects such as cleft lip and palate are multifactorial and due to a combination of genetic and environmental factors.

3. The findings of intrauterine growth restriction and/or birth defects should warrant investigation into genetic, infectious, and teratogenic etiologies.

4. The most common birth defect is a neural tube defect.

---

13. **How is *fetal growth restriction* defined?**

    Fetal growth restriction is the failure of a fetus to achieve its growth potential. In practice, measures of size relative to the population mean for gestational age and sex are used. Fetal growth retardation is variably defined as an infant who is either below the 10th percentile or less than two standard deviations (SDs) below the population mean for that gestational age and sex.

14. **Intrauterine growth restriction (IUGR) has many causes. What approach would you use to evaluate a newborn with IUGR?**

    - Establish whether the growth restriction is proportionate or disproportionate.
    - Perform a detailed physical examination for anomalies or dysmorphic features.
    - If dysmorphic or multiple anomalies are present, chromosome studies are indicated.
    - Take a detailed pregnancy history to look for teratogenic exposures, smoking, infection history, or maternal illness (e.g., hypertension and preeclampsia).
    - Viral studies and antibody titers should be ordered as indicated.
    - Uncontrolled maternal phenylketonuria can be associated with IUGR and microcephaly.
    - An infant with disproportionate IUGR should be worked up for skeletal dysplasia or metabolic bone disease.
    - Proportionate IUGR may be associated with many dysmorphic syndromes that may be recognized by a geneticist.
    - Placental examination for size and infarction and placental genetic studies should be performed for confined placental mosaicism (CPM) and uniparental disomy (UPD).

15. **What is CPM?**

    The abnormal cell line in this condition is "confined" either to the cytotrophoblast or chorionic stroma cells of the placenta and is not present in the fetus itself. This situation may be discovered when an abnormal karyotype results from chorionic villous sampling (CVS) reflecting the placenta, but the fetus appears to be healthy and amniocentesis is normal. The diagnosis of CPM postnatally is usually made retrospectively by follow-up studies on the infant or fetus, placenta, and membranes. CPM may be associated with growth impairment in chromosomally normal fetuses. It may increase the risk of a spontaneous abortion. Overall, there appears to be a low risk of adverse pregnancy outcome with CPM.

16. **What is UPD?**

    UPD occurs when both members of a chromosome pair are derived solely from one parent in a diploid offspring. Many cases of UPD are the result of resolved trisomies in which the individual was initially trisomic but lost one of the extra chromosomes and ended up with two chromosomes from the same parent. The disomy may be two copies of the same chromosome (i.e., isodisomy) or one copy of each of the given parent's chromosomes (i.e., heterodisomy).

17. **What conditions are associated with UPD?**
    - Maternal UPD 15 is associated with Prader-Willi syndrome, whereas paternal UPD 15 is associated with Angelman's syndrome.
    - Paternal UPD 11 is associated with Beckwith-Wiedemann syndrome.
    - Maternal UPD 7 has been seen in some cases of Russell-Silver syndrome.
    - Paternal UPD 6 causes growth retardation (sometimes severe) and transient neonatal diabetes.
    - Maternal UPD 16 is associated with growth retardation and variable congenital anomalies but a generally good prognosis.

18. **What conditions are commonly diagnosed by fluorescent in situ hybridization (FISH)?**
    - DiGeorge syndrome
    - Williams syndrome
    - Prader-Willi syndrome
    - Angelman's syndrome
    - Wilms' tumor, aniridia, genitourinary (GU) anomalies, and retarded growth and development (i.e., WAGR syndrome)
    - Kallmann's syndrome
    - Smith-Magenis syndrome
    - Miller-Dieker syndrome

19. **Is FISH a more sensitive way to detect microdeletions, or is it simply a faster way?**
    Whereas deletions are sometimes detectable on a karyotype, submicroscopic deletions cannot be visualized even on high-resolution chromosome banding. These deletions can be detected by FISH. In this technique, a DNA probe specific for the chromosomal region of interest is hybridized to the chromosomes. A fluorescent signal is attached to the probe so that the number of copies of the DNA corresponding to the probe can be determined for each cell. Normally, two copies of each region, one on each chromosome, should be present. If a deletion has occurred, only one of the copies will be seen. This technique has aided in the diagnosis of microdeletion syndromes that were formerly difficult to detect because of their small size.

20. **When is FISH most useful in clinical practice?**
    An example of the use of FISH is for rapid prenatal diagnosis of trisomies on amniotic fluid or chorionic villi, using interphase cells from cultured specimens and probes for the most common chromosomal abnormalities (13, 18, 21, X, and Y). Although interphase FISH for prenatal diagnosis has low false-positive and false-negative rates, it is considered investigational and is used only in conjunction with standard cytogenetic analysis. FISH is also useful in diagnosing the genetic syndromes noted in question 18.

21. **What is subtelomeric FISH analysis? To whom should this test be offered?**
    This is a series of FISH probe panels that cover the region near the ends of all the chromosomes (i.e., subtelomeres) to detect genomic imbalances due to deletions or duplications. This region of the chromosomes is genetically dense and difficult to resolve by conventional cytogenetics; therefore, deletions of this region are more readily detected by FISH. Patients with dysmorphic features, multiple congenital anomalies, and/or mental retardation who have a normal karyotype should have this test.

KEY POINTS: CHROMOSOMAL DEFECTS

1. The risk of aneuploidy increases with advanced maternal age; however, the majority of aneuploid births are to mothers who are not of advanced maternal age. The majority of trisomies are a result of maternal meiotic errors; however, almost half of Klinefelter cases are due to errors in paternal meiosis.

2. Screening for Down syndrome with a combination of noninvasive ultrasound markers of nuchal translucency and maternal serum markers allows for >95% sensitivity in detecting Down syndrome.

3. Microdeletions are too small to be resolved by a karyotype and require fluorescence in situ hybridization. The majority are de novo and not inherited. They are associated with a variety of clinical syndromes such as DiGeorge syndrome, Williams syndrome, Angelman's syndrome, Miller-Dieker syndrome, Smith-Magenis syndrome, and Kallmann's syndrome.

4. Balanced translocations have the total correct amount of DNA. If the balanced translocation is inherited, the phenotype in the child is predicted to be that of the balanced translocation carrier parent. If the translocation is de novo, there is an approximately 15% chance it will be associated with a phenotypic consequence such as a birth defect, cognitive impairment, or medical problem.

5. UPD means that for one set of chromosomes, both chromosomes were inherited from the same parent. If genes on that chromosome are imprinted, this can produce specific clinical symptoms such as Prader-Willi syndrome. UPD cannot be detected by a standard karyotype but can be detected with other molecular genetic techniques.

---

22. **The geneticist cannot be reached, and you have to evaluate an intrauterine fetal demise. What do you do?**
    - Obtain the pregnancy history and a family history.
    - Take photographs and obtain an x-ray (i.e., babygram) of the fetus.
    - Do a detailed clinical exam of the fetus.
    - Perform a skin biopsy for fibroblasts, to allow chromosome studies, genetic studies, and possible metabolic studies.
    - Examine the placenta, and culture the placenta or fetal membranes if available.
    - If possible, obtain blood samples from the cord or perform a cardiac puncture for immunoglobulin M and cultures if you suspect a congenital infection.
    - Obtain autopsy permission (freeze liver, heart, and muscle from autopsy for additional metabolic studies, if indicated).

23. **What is anophthalmia?**
    Anophthalmia is the medical term used to describe the absence of the globe and ocular tissue from the orbit. *Anophthalmia* and *microphthalmia* are often used interchangeably because, in most cases, the magnetic resonance imaging (MRI) or computed tomography (CT) scan shows some remnants of either the globe or surrounding tissue. Anophthalmia may be unilateral or bilateral and is often associated with other anomalies. There are many causes of anophthalmia including single gene mutations, syndromes, chromosome abnormalities, and teratogenic exposures. Anophthalmia is rare, with an incidence of about 1 in 10,000.

24. **How would you evaluate a newborn with anophthalmia?**
    - Ophthalmology evaluation and referral to an oculoplastic surgeon and ocularist
    - CT scan or MRI of brain and globe to determine whether any ocular tissue is present and whether the optic nerve is present; brain anomalies may help point to a specific diagnosis

- Genetic evaluation
- Renal ultrasound
- Chromosome study, G-banding
- Referral to early intervention and nearest school for the blind
- Parent support group information can be obtained from the Alliance of Genetic Support Groups, 800-336-GENE

25. **What are the main advantages of CVS over amniocentesis?**

CVS is the aspiration of chorionic villi via a transcervical catheter or transabdominal needle using ultrasound guidance. The main advantage of CVS is that it can be done between 10 and 12 weeks of gestation compared with the usual 16-week timing for amniocentesis. This permits the termination of pregnancy at a significantly earlier date in the event of major chromosomal or genetic anomalies. CVS does not permit analysis of the amniotic fluid AFP levels, so screening for neural tube defects must be performed with maternal serum AFP and ultrasound.

26. **What are the major characteristics of the three major chromosomal malformations: trisomy 21, trisomy 18, and trisomy 13?**

See Table 10-1.

TABLE 10-1. COMMON AUTOSOMAL TRISOMIES			
Feature	Trisomy 21	Trisomy 18	Trisomy 13
Eponym	Down syndrome	Edward's syndrome	Patau's syndrome
Tone	Hypotonia	Hypertonia	Hypotonia or hypertonia
Live-born incidence	1/800	1/8000	1/15,000
Cranium/brain	Mild microencephaly, flat occiput, three fontanels	Microcephaly, prominent occiput	Microcephaly, sloping forehead, occipital scalp defects, holoprosencephaly
Eyes	Upslanting, epicanthal folds, speckled iris (Brushfield spots)	Small palpebral fissures, corneal opacity	Microphthalmia, hypotelorism, iris coloboma, retinal dysplasia
Ears	Small, low-set, over-folded upper helix	Low-set, malformed	Low-set, malformed
Facial features	Protruding tongue; large cheeks; low, flat nasal bridge	Small mouth, micrognathia	Cleft lip and palate
Skeletal	Clinodactyly fifth digit, gap between toes 1 and 2, excess nuchal skin, short stature	Clenched hand, absent fifth finger distal crease, hypoplastic nails, short stature, thin ribs	Postaxial polydactyly, hypoconvex fingernails, clenched hands
Cardiac defect	40%	60%	80%
Survival	Long-term	90% die in first year	80% die in first year
Other	Abnormal palate, single palmar crease (i.e., simian crease)	Rocker bottom feet, dermatoglyphic arch pattern	Polycystic kidneys

27. **What is the chance that a newborn with a simian crease has Down syndrome?**
A single transverse palmar crease is present in 4% of normal newborns. Bilateral palmar creases are found in 1%. These features occur twice as commonly in males than in females. However, 50–55% of newborn infants with Down syndrome have a single transverse crease. Since Down syndrome occurs in 1/800 live births, the chance that a newborn with a simian crease has Down syndrome is only 1 in 60.

28. **What is the expected intelligence and personality of a child with Down syndrome?**
The IQ range is generally 35–65, with a mean reported IQ of 54. Occasionally, the IQ may be higher. Intelligence deteriorates in adulthood, with clinical and pathologic findings consistent with advanced Alzheimer disease. Autopsy results from the brains of deceased adults with Down syndrome reveal both neurofibrillary tangles and senile plaques, as found in Alzheimer disease. By age 40, the mean IQ is 24. Children with Down syndrome are generally affectionate and docile. They tend toward mimicry and are noted usually to enjoy music, having a good sense of rhythm. However, 13% have serious emotional problems, and their coordination is usually poor.

29. **Why is the maternal age of 35 years at delivery chosen as the cutoff for recommending amniocentesis for chromosome analysis?**
There is a well-known association between advanced maternal age and trisomies (including XXY; XXX; and trisomies 13, 18, and 21). Most cases of Down syndrome involve nondisjunction at meiosis I in the mother. This may be related to the lengthy stage of meiotic arrest between oocyte development in the fetus and ovulation, which may occur as much as 40 years later (Table 10-2).

TABLE 10-2. ASSOCIATION BETWEEN MATERNAL AGE AND RISK OF TRISOMY 21 SYNDROME

Maternal Age (years)	Approximate Risk
30	1/1000
35	1/365
40	1/100
45	1/50

30. **What percentage of babies with Down syndrome are born to women over the age of 35?**
Only 20% of babies are born to mothers with advanced maternal age. Although their individual risk is higher, women in this age bracket account for only 5% of all pregnancies in the United States.

Haddow JE, Palomaki GE, Knight GJ, et al: Prenatal screening for Down syndrome with use of maternal serum markers. N Engl J Med 327:588–593, 1992.

31. **What percentage of cases of Down syndrome are due to translocations?**
Of all cases of Down syndrome, 3.3% are due to unbalanced Robertsonian translocations in which a third copy of chromosome 21 is present, attached to an acrocentric chromosome. The chance of translocation Down syndrome is two to three times greater in children of younger mothers (6–8% of mothers younger than 30). One of three infants with translocation Down syndrome will have a parent with a Robertsonian translocation. Two thirds of the time, translocation Down syndrome occurs as a de novo event in the infant.

32. **What is the overall recurrence risk of Down syndrome?**
In chromosomally normal women under the age of 40, the recurrence risk for Down syndrome is 1% (assuming the father's chromosomes are also normal). Above age 40, the risk of having a child with Down syndrome increases, primarily as a function of maternal age. If the mother carries a translocation, the recurrence risk is 10–15%. If the father carries a translocation, the recurrence risk is 2–5%. One theory for this observed discrepancy between maternal and paternal rates of translocation Down syndrome is hindered motility of chromosomally abnormal sperm.

33. **With what genetic abnormality is advanced paternal age associated?**
De novo point mutations.

KEY POINTS: MONOGENIC CONDITIONS

1. Genetic susceptibility to some neurologic conditions that are dominantly inherited is due to expansion of triplet repeats. The likelihood of repeat expansions depends on the sex of the transmitting parent and is specific to each disease. For instance, triplet repeats in the gene for myotonic dystrophy are more likely to expand when transmitted maternally, whereas the triplet repeats in the gene for Huntington's disease are more likely to expand when transmitted paternally.

2. The majority of monogenic conditions affecting children are autosomal recessively inherited.

3. Genes encoding mitochondrial proteins can be found either in the mitochondrial genome and be maternally inherited or found within the nuclear genome and autosomal recessively inherited.

4. Genetic mosaicism may be detectable by differences in skin pigmentation that appear as swirls.

5. Genetic testing is currently clinically available for more than 2500 disorders.

34. **Which is technically correct: *Down's syndrome* or *Down syndrome*?**
In 1866, John Langdon Down, physician at the Earlswood Asylum in Surrey, England, described the phenotype of a syndrome that now bears his name. However, it was not until 1959 that it was determined that this disorder is caused by an extra chromosome 21. The correct designation is *Down syndrome.*

35. **What genetically inherited disease has the highest known mutation rate per gamete per generation?**
Neurofibromatosis. The estimated mutation rate for this disorder is 1×10^{-4} per haploid genome. The clinical features are café-au-lait spots and axillary freckling in childhood, followed by development of neurofibromas in later years. There is approximately a 10% risk of malignancy with this condition, and learning disabilities are common.

36. **Which disorders with ethnic and racial predilections most commonly warrant maternal screening for carrier status?**
See Table 10-3.

37. **Why are mitochondrially encoded disorders transmitted from generation to generation by the mother and not the father?**
Mitochondrial DNA abnormalities (e.g., many cases of ragged red fiber myopathies) are passed on from the mother because mitochondria are present in the cytoplasm of the egg and not the

sperm. Transmission to males or females is equally likely; however, expression is variable because mosaicism with normal and abnormal mitochondria in varying proportions is very common.

Johns DR: Mitochondrial DNA and disease. N Engl J Med 333:638–644, 1995.

TABLE 10-3. SCREENING FOR GENETIC DISORDERS

Disorder	Ethnic or Racial Group	Screening Marker
Tay-Sachs disease	Ashkenazi Jewish, French-Canadian	Decreased serum hexosaminidase A concentration, direct mutation analysis of nexosominidase A
Sickle cell anemia	Black, African, Mediterranean, Arab, Indian, Pakistani	Presence of sickling of cells in hemolysate, followed by confirmatory hemoglobin electrophoresis
α- and β-thalassemia	Mediterranean, southern and southeastern Asian, Chinese	MCV <80 mm^3, followed by hemoglobin concentrations
Cystic fibrosis	All ethnicities; more common among caucasians	Direct mutation analysis of CFTR

CFTR = cystic fibrosis transmembrane conductance regulator, MCV = mean corpuscular volume.

38. **Are all mitochondrial diseases encoded by DNA in the mitochondria?**
No. The protein found in the mitochondria and therefore mitochondrial diseases can be encoded within the nucleus or the mitochondria. Those encoded within the nuclear genome are most commonly autosomal recessively inherited.

39. **Which syndromes are associated with advanced paternal age?**
Advanced paternal age is associated with new dominant mutations. The assumption is that the increased mutation rate is due to accumulation of new mutations from many cell divisions. The more cell divisions, the more likely that an error (mutation) will occur. The mutation rate in fathers >50 years is five times higher than the mutation rate in fathers <20 years of age. New, common autosomal dominant mutations that have been recently mapped and identified are achondroplasia (Shiang et al., 1994), craniosynostosis (Wilkie et al., 1995), neurofibromatosis, and Marfan syndrome (Dietz et al., 1991).

Dietz HC, Cutting GR, Pyeritz RE, et al: Marfan syndrome caused by a recurrent de novo missense mutation in the fibrillin gene. Nature 352:337–339, 1991.

Shiang R, Thompson LM, Zhu YZ, et al: Mutations in the transmembrane domain of FGFR3 cause the most common genetic form of dwarfism, achondroplasia. Cell 78:335–342, 1994.

Wilkie AO, Slaney SF, Oldridge M, et al: Apert syndrome results from localized mutations of FGFR2 and is allelic with Crouzon syndrome. Nature Gen 9:165–172, 1995.

40. **What is the most common genetic disease that is lethal within the first year of life?**
Spinal muscular atrophy, an autosomal recessively inherited disease of the anterior motor neuron associated with decreased reflexes and progressive neuromuscular degeneration.

41. **What is the H$_3$O of Prader-Willi syndrome?**
Hyperphagia, **h**ypotonia, **h**ypogonadism, and **o**besity. Up to 75% of patients have a paternal microdeletion on the long arm of chromosome 15. The gene(s) responsible for Prader-Willi

syndrome are subject to parental imprinting. Imprinting is the process by which expression of a gene depends on whether it has been inherited from the mother or the father (Deal, 1995). The gene(s) associated with Prader-Willi syndrome are maternally imprinted, meaning that loss of the paternal copy will result in the phenotype of Prader-Willi (Knoll et al., 1989; Robinson et al., 1991). A closely related area of the long arm of chromosome 15 is maternally imprinted, and loss of the maternal copy leads to Angelman's syndrome (Chan et al., 1993). Angelman's syndrome is characterized by severe developmental delay, abnormal ataxic gait, seizures, inappropriate laughter, and jerking movements, especially of the arms.

Chan CTJ, Clayton-Smith J, Cheng XJ, et al: Molecular mechanisms in Angelman syndrome: A survey of 93 patients. Am J Med Genet 30:895–902, 1993.

Deal CL: Parental genomic imprinting. Curr Opin Pediatr 7:445–458, 1995.

Knoll JHM, Nicholls RD, Magenis RE, et al: Angelman and Prader-Willi syndromes have a chromosome 15 deletion but differ in parental origin of the deletion. Am J Med Genet 32:285–290, 1989.

Robinson WP, Bottani A, Xie YG, et al: Molecular, cytogenetic, and clinical investigations of Prader-Willi syndrome patients. Am J Hum Genet 49:1219–1234, 1991.

42. Name the two most common forms of dwarfism recognizable at birth.

Twenty-one different skeletal dysplasia syndromes were classified at the International Nomenclature of Constitutional Diseases of Bone meeting as *recognizable at birth*. The most common is thanatophoric dwarfism, a lethal chondrodysplasia characterized by flattened, U-shaped vertebral bodies, telephone receiver–shaped femurs, macrocephaly, and redundant skin folds causing a pug-like appearance. Thanatophoric means *death-loving* (an apt description). The incidence is 1 in 6400 births.

Achondroplasia is the most common viable skeletal dysplasia, occurring 1 in 26,000 live births. Its features are small stature (mean adult height, 4 feet 2 inches), macrocephaly, depressed nasal bridge, lordosis, and a trident hand. Some patients develop hydrocephalus due to a small foramen magnum. Radiographic findings include narrowing of the interpedicular distance as one proceeds caudally. Both achondroplasia and thanatophoric dysplasia are due to mutations in fibroblast growth factor receptor 3. In achondroplasia, the mutation is in the transmembrane domain, whereas the mutation in thanatophoric dysplasia is either in the intracellular domain (type 2) or in the extracellular domain (type 1).

Tavormina PL, Shiang R, Thompson LM, et al: Thanatophoric dysplasia (types 1 and 2) caused by mutations in fibroblast growth factor receptor 3. Nature Gen 9:321–328, 1995.

43. What chromosomal abnormality is found in cri du chat syndrome?

Cri du chat syndrome is due to a deletion of material from the short arm of chromosome 5 (i.e., 5p-) that causes many problems including growth retardation, microcephaly, and severe mental retardation. Patients have a characteristic cat-like cry in infancy from which the syndrome derives its name. In 85% of cases, the deletion is a de novo event. In 15%, it is due to malsegregation from a balanced parental translocation.

44. What are the syndromes and malformations associated with congenital limb hemihypertrophy?

- Russell-Silver syndrome
- Conradi-Hünermann syndrome
- CHILD syndrome (**c**ongenital **h**emidysplasia with **i**cthyosiform **e**rythroderma and **l**imb **d**efects)
- Klippel-Trénaunay-Weber syndrome
- Beckwith-Wiedemann syndrome
- Neurofibromatosis

One of every 32 patients with isolated hemihypertrophy is at risk for developing Wilms' tumor or hepatoblastoma. For this reason, renal and abdominal ultrasound and AFP should be followed every 4 months until 6 years of age as screening for patients with hemihypertrophy.

45. Which genetic disorders are associated with hypoplastic left heart syndrome?
Most newborns with hypoplastic left heart syndrome have this defect as an isolated abnormality, but several syndromes with which this congenital heart malformation is a component have been identified: Down syndrome, Turner's syndrome, Smith-Lemli-Opitz syndrome, trisomy 13, trisomy 18, and Ivemark's syndrome. Before extensive reconstructive surgery is attempted, it may be prudent to obtain a chromosomal analysis in cases where other malformations are noted. There is no question, however, that one of the major ethical dilemmas that confronts all neonatologists is the extent to which one embarks on surgical repair of a variety of defects when one has chromosomal aberrations, especially those with known limited life expectancy.

KEY POINTS: GENETIC CARE IN PREGNANCY

1. Standard genetic care in pregnancy should include evaluation of the family history, screening for hemoglobinopathies, offering carrier testing for cystic fibrosis, and evaluating for aneuploidy including noninvasive testing such as nuchal translucency and serum screening, and/or invasive testing such as chorionic villus sampling or amniocentesis. Certain populations or individuals should be offered specific genetic testing for monogenic disorders based on their personal or family history or their ethnicity.

2. When taking a family history, one should gather information about the number and relationships of family members with birth defects, growth problems, mental retardation, serious medical problems (especially those at a young age), auditory or visual impairment, ethnicity, and consanguinity.

3. Prenatal genetic testing can be performed by chorionic villus sampling or amniocentesis. There is a chance that a genetic abnormality could be identified by chorionic villus sampling that is confined to the placenta (CPM) that will have little bearing on the fetus if the placenta develops normally.

4. Carrier screening for cystic fibrosis is currently offered to all couples contemplating pregnancy or currently pregnant, regardless of ethnicity.

5. The sensitivity of carrier screening for diseases like cystic fibrosis depends critically on the ethnicity of the patient.

46. In the evaluation of a stillborn infant, how does the general appearance of the fetus suggest a likely etiology?
A fresh embryo or fetus implies a rapid expulsion after intrauterine or intrapartum death. These fetuses are usually without major anomalies and have normal karyotypes. Common causes of death are placental abruption, cord accidents, and infection. A macerated fetus indicates prolonged retention and is more likely to be associated with structural malformations or chromosomal anomalies.

47. In which fetal and infant deaths are autopsies strongly advised?
- Infants with external or suspected internal structural abnormalities
- Infants with no obvious cause of death
- Macerated fetuses
- Infants with IUGR
- Infants with nonimmune hydrops
- Families with a previous unexplained loss

In addition to an autopsy, other studies that should be considered include chromosomal analysis, skeletal radiographs, placental and cord histologic studies, titers for congenital infection, and, if hydropic, evaluation for a hemoglobinopathy (e.g., α-thalassemia), or possible metabolic storage disease.

Curry CJR: Pregnancy loss, stillbirth, and neonatal death. Pediatr Clin North Am 39:157–192, 1992.

48. **How should women with recurrent pregnancy loss be evaluated?**
Couples with recurrent pregnancy loss, defined as three or more losses, should be considered for the following evaluations:
- Cytogenic analysis of both parents to rule out mosaicism or a balanced translocation
- Hysterosalpingography to rule out malformations of the uterine cavity (e.g., congenital, diethylstilbestrol-induced, myomas, and intrauterine synechiae)
- Infectious work-up for *Mycoplasma* species, *Chlamydia* species, and other pathogens
- Immunologic evaluation for antiphospholipid antibody, anticardiolipin antibody, and antinuclear antibody (e.g., systemic lupus erythematosus)
- Hormonal-endometrial biopsy or progesterone level analysis to rule out a luteal phase defect
- Thyroid function tests
- Thrombophilia
- Evaluation of any suspected systemic illnesses

It is particularly important to initiate these studies before pursuit of any in vitro fertilization approach because the pregnancy may be adversely affected again with a number of these problems.

49. **How are structural dysmorphisms categorized?**
- **Malformation:** A problem of poor formation (likely genetically based) in which the abnormality is present at the onset of development (e.g., hypoplastic thumbs of Fanconi's anemia).
- **Disruption:** An extrinsic destructive process interferes with previously normal development (e.g., amniotic banding causing limb abnormalities).
- **Deformation:** An extrinsic mechanical force causes abnormalities, which are usually asymmetric (e.g., breech position causing tibial bowing and positional club feet).
- **Dysplasia:** An abnormal cellular organization or function that generally affects only a single tissue type (e.g., cartilage abnormalities that result in achondroplasia).

50. **What is the difference between a major and a minor malformation?**
Major malformations are unusual morphologic features that cause significant cosmetic, medical, or developmental consequences for the patient. Minor anomalies are features that do not have associated medical problems. Approximately 14% of newborns will have a minor malformation, whereas only about 2–3% will have a major malformation.

51. **Describe the most common associations.**
- **CHARGE: C**oloboma of the eye, **h**eart defects, **a**tresia of the choanae, **r**etardation (mental and growth), **g**enital anomalies (in males), **e**ar anomalies. Some cases of CHARGE association are due to mutations in the gene chromodomain helicase DNA-binding protein 7.
- **VATER: V**ertebral, **a**nal, **t**racheo**e**sophageal, **r**enal or **r**adial anomalies.
- **VACTERL:** VATER anomalies plus **c**ardiac and **l**imb anomalies.

52. **What malformations and conditions are associated with oligohydramnios?**
In early pregnancy (<4 months), the majority of amniotic fluid is produced by transudation through the placental membranes and fetal skin. Later in pregnancy, the bulk of amniotic fluid arises from fetal urination and fetal lung fluid production. At term, the fetus swallows approximately 500 mL of amniotic fluid per day and urinates an equivalent amount. Fetal urine production increases rapidly from 3.5 mL/h at 25 weeks to 25 mL/h at term. Any malformation that leads to impaired urine production will cause oligohydramnios, including renal dysplasia,

renal agenesis, and bladder outlet obstruction. When uteroplacental insufficiency occurs, the fetus is often faced with poor nutritive and volume support. The fetus becomes intravascularly depleted, leading to increased fluid conservation and decreased urine output, causing oligohydramnios. Oligohydramnios is often associated with IUGR.

53. **What are the causes of polyhydramnios?**
The etiology of polyhydramnios may be broken down into maternal causes (30%), fetal causes (30%), and idiopathic causes (40%). Maternal disorders, such as diabetes, erythroblastosis fetalis, and preeclampsia, are often associated with excess amniotic fluid. Fetal disorders that commonly predispose to polyhydramnios are central nervous system (CNS) anomalies (e.g., anencephaly, hydrocephaly, neurologic disorders), gastrointestinal disorders (e.g., tracheo-esophageal fistula, duodenal atresia), fetal circulatory disorders, and multiple gestation. The etiology for polyhydramnios in fetuses with CNS and upper gastrointestinal tract anomalies is presumed to be impaired fetal swallowing ability.

54. **What causes Potter's syndrome?**
Potter's syndrome has come to be synonymous with fetal malformations caused by extreme oligohydramnios. A lack of amniotic fluid leads to fetal compression; a squashed, flat face; club-bing of the feet; pulmonary hypoplasia; and, commonly, breech presentation. Normal fetal lung development is dependent on in utero "breathing" and production of fetal lung fluid. In the absence of amniotic fluid, pulmonary hypoplasia occurs and is the cause of death for most fetuses with Potter's syndrome. The underlying mechanism in Potter's syndrome was initially reported to be renal agenesis or renal dysplasia. However, bladder outlet obstruction and pro-longed premature rupture of the membranes may also cause this sequence. Some prefer that Potter's syndrome be defined solely as renal agenesis.

Often, these children present in the neonatal period with severe respiratory distress begin-ning shortly after birth. Pneumothorax is common because high ventilatory pressures are often used in an attempt to initiate gas exchange. Survival rarely lasts longer than a few hours in the most severe cases.

55. **If an infant is born with Potter's syndrome, why should the parents undergo a renal ultrasound?**
Renal agenesis is thought to be a sporadic or multifactorial condition, although autosomal dominant inheritance with variable expression (i.e., unilateral renal agenesis in a parent) has also been postulated. For this reason, obtaining a renal ultrasound on parents of a child with renal agenesis is advised. If the parents have normal renal evaluations, the empirically determined recurrence risk is approximately 3%. If one of the parents has unilateral renal agenesis, the recurrence risk may be as high as 50% because of a presumed autosomal dominant gene.

56. **How do clinodactyly, syndactyly, and camptodactyly differ?**
   - **Clinodactyly:** Curvature of a toe or finger (usually the fifth) due to hypoplasia of the middle phalanx, which is the last fetal bone to develop in the hands and feet. Normal curvature can consist of up to 8 degrees of in-turning. Curvature beyond this is considered a minor anomaly.
   - **Syndactyly:** An incomplete separation of fingers (usually third and fourth) or toes (usually second or third).
   - **Camptodactyly:** Abnormal persistent flexion of fingers or toes.

57. **Are preauricular ear tags a significant finding?**
Preauricular pits and tags are minor anomalies that occur in about 0.3–1.0% of persons, with a wide variance in frequency among racial groups. They are twice as common in females as in males and can be inherited as an autosomal dominant trait. They are believed to represent

remnants of early embryonic bronchial cleft or arch structures. As isolated findings, they do not warrant additional evaluations.

58. **What is the proper way to test for low-set ears?**
    This designation is made when the upper portion of the ear (i.e., helix) meets the head at a level below a horizontal line drawn from the lateral aspect of the palpebral fissure. The best way to measure is to align a straight edge between the two inner canthi and determine whether the ears lie completely below this plane. In normal persons, approximately 10% of the ear is above this plane.

    Feingold M, Bossert VM: Normal values for selected physical parameters: An aid to syndrome delineation. In Bergsma D (ed): The National Foundation-March of Dimes Birth Defects Series 10:9. White Plains, NY, March of Dimes Birth Defects Foundation, 1974, pp 1–16.

59. **Why do the sclerae of patients with osteogenesis imperfecta appear blue?**
    Osteogenesis imperfecta is a disease of bone, in which the affected neonate with osteogenesis imperfecta type II or III often manifests severe fractures prenatally, at birth, or shortly after birth. Although the disease has several levels of severity, in its most problematic forms growth is significantly impaired and life expectancy is very short. The primary component of sclera in humans is collagen. Given that abnormal collagen formation is the underlying defect in many of these disorders, it is not surprising that in osteogenesis imperfecta types I, II, and III and many other connective tissue diseases, the sclerae are abnormally thin and transparent. The bluish color of the sclera in patients with connective tissue (especially collagen) diseases is thought to be due to visualization of the bluish-colored uvea (the eye layer behind the retina) as seen through a more transparent sclera.

60. **What is the inheritance pattern of cleft lip and palate?**
    Most cases of cleft lip and palate are inherited in a polygenic or multifactorial pattern. The male-to-female ratio is 3:2, and the incidence in the general population is approximately 1 in 1000. The recurrence risk after one affected child is 3–4%; after two affected children, it rises to 8–9%.

61. **How can hypertelorism be rapidly assessed?**
    If an imaginary third eye would fit between the eyes, hypertelorism is possible. Precise measurement involves measuring the distance between the center of each eye's pupil. This is a difficult measurement in newborns and uncooperative patients because of eye movement. In practice, the best way to determine hypotelorism or hypertelorism is to measure the inner and outer canthal distances, then plot these measurements on standardized tables of norms.

62. **Which syndromes are associated with colobomas of the iris?**
    Colobomas of the iris are due to abnormal ocular development and embryogenesis. They are frequently associated with chromosomal syndromes, most commonly trisomy 13, 4p-, 13q-, and triploidy. In addition, they may be commonly found in the CHARGE association, Goltz syndrome, and Rieger's syndrome. Whenever iris colobomas are noted, chromosome analysis is recommended.

63. **How large is the posterior fontanel in a healthy term infant?**
    In 97% of term infants, the posterior fontanel is normally fingertip-sized or smaller. Large posterior fontanels can be seen in infants with congenital hypothyroidism, skeletal dysplasias, or increased intracranial pressure.

64. **On which side does a newborn "crown" usually sit?**
    In the fetus, hair follicles on the skin surface grow downward during weeks 10–16. During this time, the brain and scalp expand outward in a dome-like fashion, pulling the follicles in different directions, and at 18 weeks when the hair erupts, patterns are set. The "crown," or

parietal hair whorl, is the focal point of this outgrowth. At birth, it is usually a few centi-
meters anterior to the posterior fontanel. Fifty-five percent of single parietal scalp whorls
are left of midline (presumably secondary to the larger size of the left brain), 30% are right-
sided, and 15% are midline. Five percent of normal persons have bilateral hair whorls.
Abnormal positioning of the hair whorl (particularly a posterior location) can be seen in
microcephaly.

KEY POINTS: RISK OF RECURRENCE

1. The risk of having an affected child with an autosomal recessive condition if both parents are
   carriers is 25%.

2. The risk of having an affected child with an autosomal recessive condition after having three
   previously affected children (if both parents are carriers) is still 25%. Each pregnancy is an
   independent event.

3. The risk of having a child with Duchenne's muscular dystrophy if the mother is a carrier is
   25%. None of the girls will be affected for this X-linked disorder, but 50% of the boys will be
   affected.

4. A karyotype should be determined for every baby with Down syndrome to determine whether
   the condition was caused by an inherited translocation of chromosome 21, since this would
   significantly increase the risk of recurrence for the parents.

65. **How does mosaicism develop?**
    Mosaicism is the possession of multiple genetically different cell lines in a single person. Most
    chromosomal mosaicism involves the sex chromosomes and occurs because of defects in mito-
    sis in an early embryo. Normally, chromosomes duplicate and separate equally in mitotic divi-
    sion. Mosaicism can occur when the chromosomes fail to separate (mitotic nondisjunction) or
    fail to migrate (anaphase lag). In general, the greater the proportion of abnormal cell lines, the
    more abnormal the phenotype. The earlier in embryonic development an abnormal cell is
    established, the higher the percentage of abnormal cells in that person.

66. **What causes chimerism in infants?**
    The term *chimera* is derived from the Greek mythologic monster that, according to Homer, had
    the head of a lion, body of a goat, and tail of a dragon. In cytogenetic parlance, chimerism is the
    presence of two or more cell lines in a person that are derived from two separate zygotes. The
    most common cause of chimerism is the mixing of blood from unlike-sexed twins, resulting in a
    karyotype of 46,XX/46,XY. Chimerism can also result from the admixture of cells from a nonvi-
    able twin into a surviving fetus or, most rarely, from incorporation of two zygotes into a single
    embryo.

67. **What is the risk of having a child with a recessive disorder when the parents are
    first or second cousins?**
    First cousins may share more than one deleterious recessive gene. They have ⅛ of their genes
    in common, and their progeny are homozygous at 1/16 of their gene loci. Second cousins have
    only 1/32 of their genes in common. The risk that consanguineous parents will produce a child
    with a severe or lethal abnormality is 6% for first-cousin marriages and 1% for second-cousin
    marriages.

68. **How does a reciprocal translocation differ from a Robertsonian translocation?**
A chromosome translocation is a transfer of chromosomal material between two (or more) nonhomologous chromosomes. The exchange is usually reciprocal (the two segments trading places). The genetic content of the person is therefore complete but rearranged. A Robertsonian translocation represents a special variety of chromosome translocation in which the long arms of two acrocentric chromosomes (13, 14, 15, 21, or 22) fuse at their centromeres. The breaks may occur within, above, or below the centromeres. The short arms are usually lost, but this does not produce an abnormality because the genetic material on the short arms of acrocentric chromosomes occurs in multiple copies throughout the genome. A phenotypically normal person with a Robertsonian translocation has only 45 chromosomes inasmuch as the long arms of two acrocentric chromosomes are fused into one.

69. **How can an autosomal recessive disease occur when only one parent is a carrier?**
UPD is an inheritance pattern in which a child receives two identical chromosomes from one parent and none from the other. The most likely explanation is an abnormality in meiosis whereby one gamete receives an extra copy of a homologous chromosome due to an error in separation. This gamete with two copies from one parent then unites with the gamete of the other parent. If the second gamete lacks that particular chromosome (i.e., nullisomic gamete), a normal karyotype results. If the second gamete contains that particular chromosome, a trisomic zygote results. During embryonic development, this trisomy may be lost, resulting in a normal karyotype. UPD has been reported in some patients with Prader-Willi, Angelman's, and Beckwith-Wiedemann syndromes as well as cystic fibrosis.

70. **46,XY, t(4:8)(p21; q22)—what does it all mean?**
    - **46:** Normal number of chromosomes.
    - **XY:** Genetic male.
    - **t(4:8):** The first set of parentheses refers to the chromosomes. The symbol in front indicates the change: *t* stands for reciprocal translocation, *del* for deletion, *dup* for duplication, and *inv* for inversion.
    - **(p21; q22):** The second set of parentheses refers to the bands on the chromosomes. The short arm symbol is *p;* the long arm symbol is *q.*
    In this case, a genetic male with a normal number of chromosomes has a reciprocal translocation between the short arm of chromosome 4 at band 21 and the long arm of chromosome 8 at band 22.

71. **What are the features of the four most common sex chromosome abnormalities?**
See Table 10-4.

72. **Is it possible to get identical twins of different sexes?**
Yes. If anaphase lag (loss) of a Y chromosome occurs at the time of cell separation into twin embryos, a female fetus with karyotype 45,X (Turner's syndrome) and a normal male fetus (46,XY) result.

73. **What are the possible placental appearances for monozygotic twins? For dizygotic twins?**
Monozygotic twins can be monochorionic monoamniotic, monochorionic diamniotic, or dichorionic diamniotic. Dizygotic twins will be dichorionic diamniotic.

74. **Of the four most common types of sex chromosomal abnormalities, which is identifiable at birth?**
Only infants with Turner's syndrome have physical features easily identifiable at birth.

TABLE 10-4.	CHARACTERISTICS OF SEX CHROMOSOME DISORDERS			
	47,XXY	47,XYY	47,XXX	45,X
	(Klinefelter's Syndrome)			(Turner's Syndrome)
Frequency of live births	1/2000	1/2000	1/2000	1/800
Maternal age association	Yes	No	Yes	No
Phenotype	Tall, eunuchoid habitus, underdeveloped secondary sex characteristics, gynecomastia	Tall, severe acne, indistinguishable from healthy males	Tall, indistinguishable from healthy females	Short stature, web neck, shield chest, pedal edema at birth, coarctation of aorta
IQ and behavior	80–100; behavioral problems	90–100; aggressive behavior	90–110; behavioral problems	Mildly deficient to normal IQ, spatial-perceptual problems
Reproductive function	Extremely rare	Common	Common	Extremely rare
Gonad	Hypoplastic testes, Leydig cell hyperplasia, Sertoli cell hypoplasia, seminiferous tubule dysgenesis, few spermato-genic precursors	Normal size testes, normal testicular histology	Normal size ovaries, normal ovarian histology	Streak ovaries with deficient follicles

75. **Describe the similarities and differences between Turner's syndrome and Noonan's syndrome.**
   - Similarities include short stature, web neck, cardiac defects, low posterior hairline, broad chest, wide-spaced nipples, edema of the dorsum of the hands and feet, and cubitus valgus.
   - Differences are summarized in Table 10-5.

76. **What is the most common inherited form of mental retardation?**
   Fragile X syndrome.

77. **What is the nature of the mutation in fragile X syndrome?**
   When the lymphocytes of an affected male are grown in a folate-deficient medium and the chromosomes examined, a substantial number of X chromosomes demonstrate a break near the distal end of the long arm. This site, the fragile X mental retardation-1 gene (FMR-1), was identified and sequenced in 1991. At the center of the gene is a repeating trinucleotide sequence (CGG) that, in normal persons, repeats 6–45 times. However, in carriers, the sequence expands to 50–200 times (called a *premutation*), and in fully affected persons, it expands to 200–600 copies. These longer sequences cause malfunctioning of the gene. The repeat expansion is most

sensitively and accurately determined by Southern blot analysis. Males as well as females can be affected, although it is an X-linked disorder.

TABLE 10-5. DIFFERENCES BETWEEN TURNER'S SYNDROME AND NOONAN'S SYNDROME

Turner's Syndrome	Noonan's Syndrome
Females only	Both males and females
Chromosomal disorder (45,X)	Normal chromosomes (autosomal dominant); 50% due to mutations in PTPN11
Near-normal IQ	Mental deficiency
Coarctation the most common cardiac defect	Pulmonary stenosis the most common cardiac defect
Amenorrhea and sterility	Normal menstrual cycle in females

78. **What diseases have been successfully treated by in utero hematopoietic stem cell transplantation or in utero gene therapy?**
Although there have been at least 26 human cases of in utero hematopoietic stem cell transplantation to date, the only clear successes have been in patients with severe combined immunodeficiency syndrome. Effective reconstitution of the immunodeficiency was achieved by using 34-enriched bone marrow transplantation to the fetus.

79. **What are the most common genetic causes of aniridia?**
Isolated aniridia is most commonly caused by mutations in PAX6 and is prognostically associated with a multitude of ophthalmologic abnormalities that significantly impair vision but do not result in involvement of other organ systems. A contiguous gene deletion of 11p13 can produce syndromic aniridia associated with WAGR syndrome (Wilms' tumor, aniridia, GU anomalies, and retarded growth and development). When initially diagnosing a neonate with aniridia, it may not be obvious at birth whether this will be isolated or syndromic, and genetic testing for these two disorders is useful to determine the prognosis and the potential for associated problems.

80. **What findings on ultrasound scan may suggest the diagnosis of aneuploidy?**
Short femurs, IUGR, congenital heart disease, pyelectasis, echogenic cardiac focus, echogenic bowel, choroid plexus cyst, and cystic hygroma.

81. **What disorder should be considered in a neonate with a maternal history of acute fatty liver of pregnancy or hypertension, elevated liver enzymes, and low platelet (HELLP) syndrome?**
Long-chain hydroxyacyl-CoA dehydrogenase (LCHAD), a fatty acid oxidation disorder.

82. **What types of congenital heart disease are classically associated with DiGeorge syndrome?**
Conotruncal defects such as tetralogy of Fallot, interrupted aortic arch, truncus arteriosus, and ventricular septal defects.

83. **What other features are associated with DiGeorge syndrome?**
Cleft lip, cleft palate, hypothyroidism, hypocalcemia due to hypoparathyroidism, immunodeficiency with thymus hypoplasia and altered T cell function, failure to thrive, and developmental delay.

84. **What inborn errors of metabolism are associated with birth defects?**
Smith-Lemli-Opitz syndrome (congenital heart disease and GU anomalies), peroxisomal disorders (congenital heart disease, epiphyseal stippling, renal cysts, CNS malformations), congenital disorders of glycosylation (CNS malformations, renal cysts, GU anomalies), and fatty acid oxidation disorders (renal cysts, hypertrophic cardiomyopathy, CNS malformations including cerebellar hypoplasia).

85. **What disorders are associated with triplet repeat expansions?**
Fragile X syndrome, myotonic dystrophy, Huntington's disease, spinocerebellar ataxia, and spinal bulbar muscular atrophy (Kennedy's disease).

86. **What genetic disorders should you suspect in the severely hypotonic neonate?**
Prader-Willi syndrome, congenital myopathy or muscular dystrophy, myotonic dystrophy, and inborn error of metabolism.

87. **If you suspect a baby has congenital myotonic dystrophy, which parent would you examine for symptoms, and what would you look for?**
You would examine the mother for evidence of a myopathic face, difficulty with speech or swallowing, myotonia and inability to release her grip, or cataracts. The AGC/CTG repeat size is unstable and much more likely to expand when transmitted through a female than through a male. As the repeat increases in size, the severity increases, and age of onset decreases.

88. **If there is a maternal history of long QT syndrome, what should be done for the neonate?**
If the long QT syndrome is genetically based, it is most likely to be autosomal dominantly inherited, putting the baby at 50% risk of long QT syndrome. The baby should be screened by electrocardiography, and the QTc interval should be calculated. If prolonged greater than 440 msec, the baby should be started on β blockers. Additionally, genetic testing is now available for long QT syndrome, a genetically heterogeneous disorder caused by mutations in at least six currently known genes. Once a familial mutation is identified, the baby can be tested to determine whether he or she has inherited the mutation. Electrocardiographic screening is not perfectly sensitive, especially in children. Therefore, when possible, genetic screening of the at-risk child should always be performed to increase the sensitivity and specificity of screening. Additionally, medical management and risk of sudden cardiac death is dependent on which of the genes is affected and is definable only with genetic testing.

BIBLIOGRAPHY

1. Burke WG, Clarke TA, Mathews TG, et al: Isolated single umbilical artery: The case for routine renal screening. Arch Dis Child 68:600–601, 1993.

2. Chan CTJ, Clayton-Smith J, Cheng XJ, et al: Molecular mechanisms in Angelman syndrome: A survey of 93 patients. Am J Med Genet 30:895–902, 1993.

3. Curry CJR: Pregnancy loss, stillbirth, and neonatal death. Pediatr Clin North Am 39:157–192, 1992.

4. Deal CL: Parental genomic imprinting. Curr Opin Pediatr 7:445–458, 1995.

5. DeBiasio P, Siccardi M, Volpe G, et al: First-trimester screening for Down syndrome using nuchal translucency measurement with free p-hCG and PAAP-A between 10 and 13 weeks of pregnancy: The combined test. Prenat Diagn 19:360–363, 1999.

6. Dietz HC, Cutting GR, Pyeritz RE, et al: Marfan syndrome caused by a recurrent de novo missense mutation in the fibrillin gene. Nature 352:337–339, 1991.

7. Enns G, Cox V, Goldstein, et al: Congenital diaphragmatic defects and associated syndromes, malformations, and chromosome anomalies: A retrospective study of 60 patients and literature review. Am J Med Genet 79:215–225, 1998.

8. Flake A, Roncarolo MG, Puck J, et al: Treatment of X-linked severe combined immunodeficiency by in utero transplantation of paternal bone marrow. N Engl J Med 335:1806, 1996.

9. Flake AW, Zanjani ED: In utero hematopoietic stem cell transplantation: Ontogenic opportunities and biologic barriers. Blood 94:2179–2191, 1999.

10. Geipel A, Germer U, Welp T, et al: Prenatal diagnosis of single umbilical artery: Determination of absent side, associated anomalies, Doppler findings, and perinatal outcome. Ultrasound Obstet Gynecol 15:114–117, 2000.

11. Haddow JE, Palomaki GE, Knight GJ, et al: Prenatal screening for Down syndrome with use of maternal serum markers. N Engl J Med 327:588–593, 1992.

12. Hurst L, McVean G: Growth effects of uniparental disomies and the conflict theory of genomic imprinting. TIG 13:436–442, 1997.

13. James D: Diagnosis and management of fetal growth retardation. Arch Dis Child 65:390–394, 1990.

14. Johns DR: Mitochondrial DNA and disease. N Engl J Med 333:638–644, 1995.

15. Knoll JHM, Nicholls RD, Magenis RE, et al: Angelman and Prader-Willi syndromes have a chromosome 15 deletion but differ in parental origin of the deletion. Am J Med Genet 32:285–290, 1989.

16. Kohn DB, Parkman R: Gene therapy for the newborn. FASEB J 11:635–639, 1997.

17. Lam YH, Tang MH: Second-trimester maternal serum inhibin: A screening for fetal Down syndrome in Asian women. Prenat Diagn 19:463–467, 1999.

18. McCullough L, Chervenek F: Ethics in Obstetrics and Gynecology. New York, Oxford University Press, 1994.

19. Milunsky A (ed): Genetic Disorders and the Fetus: Diagnosis, Prevention, and Treatment, 3rd ed. Baltimore, MD, Johns Hopkins University Press, 1998.

20. Rimion DL, Connor JM, Pyeritz RE (eds): Emery and Rimion's Principles and Practice of Medical Genetics, 3rd ed. New York, Churchill Livingstone, 1997.

21. Robinson WP, Bottani A, Xie YG, et al: Molecular, cytogenetic, and clinical investigations of Prader-Willi syndrome patients. Am J Hum Genet 49:1219–1234, 1991.

22. Romano G, Pacilio C, Giordano A: Gene transfer technology in therapy: Current applications and future goals. Stem Cells 17:191–202, 1999.

23. Shiang R, Thompson LM, Zhu YZ, et al: Mutations in the transmembrane domain of FGFR3 cause the most common genetic form of dwarfism, achondroplasia. Cell 78:335–342, 1994.

24. Stevenson RE, Hall J, Goodman R (eds): Human Malformations and Related Anomalies. Oxford Monographs on Medical Genetics, No. 27. New York, Oxford University Press, 1993.

25. Wald NJ, Watt HC, Hacksaw AK: Integrated screening for Down syndrome based on tests performed during the first and second trimesters. N Engl J Med 341:461–467, 1999.

26. Wilkie AO, Slaney SF, Oldridge M, et al: Apert syndrome results from localized mutations of FGFR2 and is allelic with Crouzon syndrome. Nature Gen 9:165–172, 1995.

27. Yang EY, Cass DL, Sylvester KG, et al: Fetal gene therapy: Efficacy, toxicity, and immunologic effects of early gestation recombinant adenovirus. J Pediatr Surg 34:235–241, 1999.

28. Zanjani ED, Anderson WF: Prospect for in utero human gene therapy. Science 285:2084–2088, 1999.

CHAPTER 11

HEMATOLOGY

Sujit Sheth, MD

DEVELOPMENTAL HEMATOPOIESIS

1. **What is the evolution of the hematopoietic process during intrauterine development?**
   Hematopoiesis in the developing embryo begins at approximately 2 weeks postconception. It begins in the yolk sac, but as the gut develops, hematopoiesis is gradually taken over by the liver and spleen. This continues until the late second trimester, when the bone marrow develops and begins producing cells. By the mid third trimester, most hematopoietic activity is in the bone marrow, but stem cell rests may still be found in the liver and spleen.

KEY POINTS: HEMATOPOIETIC DEVELOPMENT

1. Production: yolk sac → liver and spleen → bone marrow.

2. Hemoglobin: embryonic → fetal → adult.

3. The oxygen dissociation curve of Hb F is shifted to the left to enhance oxygen uptake in utero.

4. Maturation of cell lines goes from larger cells to smaller cells.

---

2. **How do the different cell lines differentiate?**
   All cell lineages derive from the pluripotent stem cells. These are uncommitted and self-renewing. Under the influence of various cytokines, the pluripotent stem cells initially differentiate into colony-forming units (CFUs) that are capable of multiplication and maturation. There are three types: CFU-GM (granulocytes and monocytes), CFU-mega (megakaryocytes and platelets), and CFU-e (erythrocytes). The latter change to burst-forming units–erythrocytes, then mature through the erythroblast; early, intermediate, and late normoblast; and finally reticulocyte stage, into mature red blood cells (RBCs). CFU-GM cells similarly differentiate to produce myeloid precursors (e.g., promyeloblasts, myelocytes, metamyelocytes, and bands), which mature into neutrophils, eosinophils, basophils; and platelet precursors (megakaryocytes), which mature to form platelets (Fig. 11-1).

3. **What is the structure and function of hemoglobin?**
   Hemoglobin is a tetramer of globin chains, usually of two distinct types, bound to a heme moiety. For example, adult hemoglobin consists of two α chains and two β chains. The function of hemoglobin is to transport oxygen and carbon dioxide to and from the tissues, respectively. This is primarily a function of the heme portion of the molecule.

4. **How do the hemoglobins evolve during intrauterine development?**
   Embryonic hemoglobins are present in the first 8 weeks of intrauterine development. These consist of Hb Gower 1 ($\zeta_2\varepsilon_2$), Hb Gower 2 ($\alpha_2\varepsilon_2$), and Hb Portland ($\zeta_2\gamma_2$). These are replaced by fetal hemoglobin (Hb F–$\alpha_2\gamma_2$). By 30–32 weeks of intrauterine life, adult hemoglobin (Hb

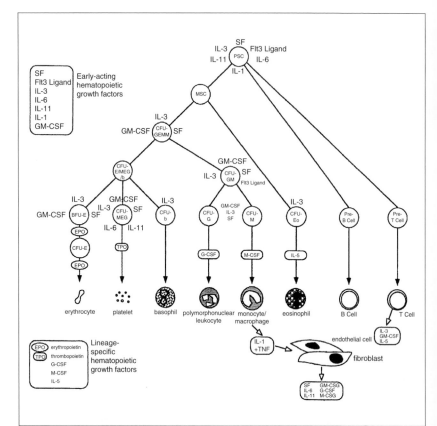

Figure 11-1. Major cytokine sources and actions. Cells of the bone marrow microenvironment, such as macrophages (mP), endothelial cells (ec), and reticular fibroblastoid cells (fb), produce macrophage colony-stimulating factor (M-CSF), granulocyte macrophage colony-stimulating factor (GM-CSF), interleukin (IL) 6, and probably Steel factor (SF: cellular sources not yet precisely determined) after induction with endotoxin (ma) or IL-1/TNF (ec, fb). T cells produce IL-3, GM-CSF, and IL-5 in response to antigenic and IL-1 stimulation. These cytokines have overlapping actions during hematopoietic differentiation, as indicated, and for all lineages optimal development requires a combination of early- and late-acting factors. PSC = pluripotent stem cells, MSC = myeloid stem cells, TNF = tumor necrosis factor. (From Seiff CA, Nathan DG, Clark SC: The anatomy and physiology of hematopoiesis. In Nathan DG, Orkin SH [eds]: Nathan & Oski's Hematology of Infancy and Childhood, 5th ed. Philadelphia, W.B. Saunders, 1997.)

A–$\alpha_2\beta_2$) begins to be produced, and at birth a term infant has approximately 20–30% Hb A and the remainder is mostly Hb F (Fig. 11-2).

5. **How does fetal hemoglobin differ from adult hemoglobin?**
Fetal hemoglobin differs from adult hemoglobin primarily in its binding affinity for oxygen. The PO_2 at which 50% of hemoglobin is saturated is termed the P_{50}. The curve for fetal hemoglobin is said to be shifted to the left of the adult curve (a lower P_{50}), representing the greater affinity of fetal hemoglobin for oxygen at any given PO_2. This higher affinity for oxygen binding facilitates extraction from the maternal adult hemoglobin but also results in decreased oxygen release to

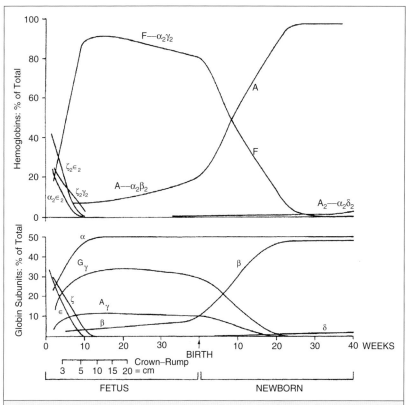

Figure 11-2. Changes in hemoglobin tetramers *(top)* and in globin subunits *(bottom)* during human development from embryo to early infancy. (From Bunn HF, Forget BG: Hemoglobin: Molecular, Genetic, and Clinical Aspects. Philadelphia, W.B. Saunders, 1986.)

the tissues. The latter is not a disadvantage since fetal tissues use oxygen primarily for growth; metabolic functions are mostly handled by the mother.

Factors that shift the hemoglobin oxygen curve to the right (and thereby increase oxygen delivery to tissues) include increased temperature, increased $PaCO_2$, increased red cell 2, 3-diphosphoglycerate content, and increased hydrogen ion concentration (decreased pH).

6. **How do the red cells change during development?**
   As with all cell lines, RBCs become smaller as they mature. The "primitive" megaloblast-like cells in the yolk sac are very large (~180 fl). By birth, however, the red cell size (mean corpuscular volume [MCV]) decreases to 110–120 fl. The hemoglobin content also changes from being predominantly fetal to a mixture of fetal and adult. The RBC life span in the fetal and neonatal period is 90 days, compared with 120 days in older children and adults. In addition, fetal RBCs express the i antigen (adult red cells express the I antigen).

7. **What are the normal values for hemoglobin level, MCV, and reticulocyte count in preterm and term neonates on the first day of life?**
   See Table 11-1.

TABLE 11–1. RED CELL VALUES ON FIRST POSTNATAL DAY

	Gestational Age (weeks)							
	24–25	26–27	28–29	30–31	32–33	34–35	36–37	Term
Hemoglobin (gm/dL)	9.4 ± 1.5	19.0 ± 2.5	19.3 ± 1.8	19.1 ± 2.2	18.5 ± 2.0	19.6 ± 2.1	19.2 ± 1.7	19.3 ± 2.2
MCV (fl)	135 ± 0.2	132 ± 14.4	131 ± 13.5	127 ± 12.7	123 ± 15.7	122 ± 10.0	121 ± 12.5	119 ± 9.4
Reticulocyte (%)	6.0 ± 0.5	9.6 ± 3.2	7.5 ± 2.5	5.8 ± 2.0	5.0 ± 1.9	3.9 ± 1.6	4.2 ± 1.8	3.2 ± 1.4

Data derived from Zaizov R, Matoth Y: Red cell values on the first postnatal day during the last 16 weeks of gestation. Am J Hematol 1:275–278, 1976.

KEY POINTS: ANEMIA

1. Physiologic anemia reaches its nadir at about 6 weeks in premature infants and 8 weeks in term infants.

2. The primary causes of hemolytic anemia are immune defects (ABO, Rh), membrane defects (spherocytosis), and enzyme deficiencies (G6PD).

3. The most common causes of anemia in the neonatal intensive care unit are bleeding and iatrogenic causes.

4. The basic work-up for anemia should include CBC, type and Coombs' tests, reticulocyte count, review of a blood smear, and serum bilirubin measurement.

5. Treatment for anemia includes transfusion, administration of EPO, and minimizing blood drawing.

PHYSIOLOGIC ANEMIA

8. **How does the site of blood sampling affect hemoglobin and hematocrit?**
Capillary samples obtained by heel stick shortly after birth have hemoglobin levels that are on average 3.6 gm/dL higher than corresponding venous samples. The ratio of the capillary hematocrit to the venous hematocrit is 1.21 at 26–30 weeks' gestation and decreases to 1.12 in term infants and 1.02 at 5 days of age in healthy infants. It is particularly important to remember that the differences between capillary and venous hemoglobins are most pronounced in sick, premature infants in whom anemia is most likely to be a clinical problem. Thus, unexpected changes in the hemoglobin level in such infants should prompt consideration of the site of sampling.

9. **What is physiologic anemia?**
The phrase *physiologic anemia of infancy* is actually a misnomer that describes the normal, nonpathologic drop in hemoglobin and hematocrit experienced by term and preterm infants. Expansion of the lungs after birth improves oxygen availability and tissue oxygen delivery, resulting in near cessation of red cell production in both term and preterm infants. Serum erythropoietin (EPO) concentrations decrease to 0–10 mU/mL. Reticulocyte (retic) counts drop from 6% to 10% at birth to <1% by day 3–5. As a result, the hemoglobin gradually decreases to a nadir of approximately 10–11 gm/dL by 8–10 weeks of age in the term infant and 9–10 gm/dL by 4–8 weeks in the preterm infant. At this point, there is stimulation of erythropoiesis from an increase in EPO production, and the hemoglobin rises to infant levels as below.

10. **How do RBC indices change during the first months of life?**
Changes in RBC indices are shown in Table 11-2. The hemoglobin, hematocrit, MCV, and mean corpuscular hemoglobin decrease gradually in the first 1–3 months of life, whereas the mean corpuscular hemoglobin concentration remains relatively unchanged.

ANEMIA IN THE FETUS AND NEWBORN

11. **You are asked to evaluate a 10-week-old healthy infant who was born at term and found on a totally unnecessary but nonetheless complete blood count (CBC) to have a hemoglobin level of 9.8 gm/dL. Is further work-up of this "anemia" necessary?**
The mean hemoglobin level at 10 weeks for a term infant is 11.2 gm/dL, and two standard deviations extend the lower limit of the normal range to 9.4 gm/dL. A number of children with slightly

TABLE 11-2. POSTNATAL CHANGES IN RED BLOOD CELL (RBC) INDICES IN TERM INFANTS

RBC Indices	Birth (cord blood)	Days		Weeks			Months					
		1	3	1	2	4	2	3	4	6	9	12
Hgb (gm/dL)	16.5 (13.0)	18.5 (14.5)	18.6 (16.5)	17.5 (13.5)	16.6 (13.4)	13.9 (10.7)	11.2 (9.4)	11.5 (9.5)	12.2 (10.3)	12.6 (11.1)	12.7 (11.4)	12.7 (11.3)
Hct (%)	51 (42)	56 (45)	55	54 (42)	53 (41)	44 (33)	35 (28)	35 (29)	38 (32)	36 (31)	36 (32)	37 (33)
RBC (×10^{12}/L)	4.7 (3.9)	5.3 (4.0)	5.6	5.1 (3.9)	4.9 (3.9)	4.3 (3.3)	3.7 (3.1)	3.8 (3.1)	4.3 (3.5)	4.7 (3.9)	4.7 (4.0)	4.7 (4.1)
MCV (fl)	108 (98)	108 (95)	110 (104)	107 (88)	105 (88)	101 (91)	95 (84)	91 (74)	87 (76)	76 (68)	78 (70)	78 (71)
MCH (pg)	34 (31)	34 (31)	36.7	34 (28)	33.6 (30.0)	32.5 (29)	30.4 (27)	30 (25)	28.6 (25)	26.8 (24)	27.3 (25)	26.8 (24)
MCHC (gm/dL)	33 (30)	33 (29)	33.1	33 (28)	31.4 (28.1)	31.8 (28.1)	31.8 (28.3)	33 (30)	32.7 (28.8)	35 (32.7)	34.9 (32.4)	34.3 (32.1)

Values represent mean (values in parentheses are −2 standard deviations). Hgb = Hemoglobin, Hct = hematocrit MCH = mean corpuscular hemoglobin, MCHC = mean corpuscular hemoglobin concentration. (Data from Saarinen UM, Siimes MA: Developmental changes in red blood cell counts and indices of infants after exclusion of iron deficiency by laboratory criteria and continuous iron supplementation. J Pediatr 78:412–416, 1978; and Rudolph A [ed]: Pediatrics, 16th ed. New York, Appleton-Century-Crofts, 1977. Reproduced from Ohls RK: Developmental erythropoiesis. In Polin RA, Fox WW [eds]: Fetal and Neonatal Physiology. Philadelphia, W.B. Saunders, 1998, p 1767.)

lower Hb levels at this age may have had low-grade ABO incompatibility at birth, which has led to a low-grade chronic hemolysis. In the absence of specific symptoms or signs of an underlying disorder, a work-up of a hemoglobin level of 9.8 gm/dL is likely to be unrewarding.

12. **In terms of etiology, how is anemia classified in the newborn infant?**
As in children and adults, causes of neonatal anemia can be classified into three broad categories: decreased production, increased destruction, and blood loss.

13. **What are the causes of decreased RBC production in a neonate?**
The most common causes of decreased RBC production include infections (congenital or postnatally acquired) and drug-induced suppression of the erythroid marrow. Rarer causes include some inborn errors of metabolism, Diamond-Blackfan anemia, congenital leukemia, Down syndrome, osteopetrosis, and transient erythroblastopenia of the newborn. Iron deficiency is rare in newborns, unless the mother is very severely iron deficient. Etiologies of increased RBC destruction include immune-mediated hemolysis (e.g., Rh, ABO, or minor blood group incompatibility, maternal autoimmune disease), membrane defects (e.g., spherocytosis, elliptocytosis, pyropoikilocytosis), enzyme defects (e.g., glucose-6-phosphate dehydrogenase [G6PD] or protein kinase deficiency), hemoglobinopathies (e.g., thalassemias), and acquired disorders (e.g., bacterial sepsis, congenital infections, disseminated intravascular coagulation [DIC], microangiopathic anemia). Infants with the thalassemia syndromes may be anemic at birth because of ineffective erythropoiesis; characteristically, this anemia is microcytic. Blood loss is so common that it deserves its own questions.

14. **Blood loss is the most common cause of anemia in an ill newborn. Where can you find the lost blood?**
In the laboratory, where it has been sent for multiple tests. Unfortunately, micromethods are not routinely available for all tests at most medical centers. In very sick infants, it is very useful to maintain a log of all blood drawn. Withdrawing 1 mL of blood from a 1000-gm infant is equivalent to taking 70 mL of blood from an adult!

15. **What are the causes of blood loss in an infant other than phlebotomy?**
Occult antenatal hemorrhage, obstetric accidents, placenta or umbilical cord malformations, and internal hemorrhage are the major categories of blood loss once excessive phlebotomy has been eliminated. Causes of antenatal hemorrhage include fetomaternal bleeding (e.g., abdominal trauma, traumatic amniocentesis, placental tumors) and twin-to-twin transfusions. Obstetric causes of blood loss include abruptio placentae, placenta previa, incision of the placenta during cesarean section, rupture of the umbilical cord or an anomalous vessel, and hematoma of the cord or placenta. Blood loss in the neonatal period may be due to intracranial hemorrhage; giant cephalohematoma; subgaleal hematoma; retroperitoneal, renal, or adrenal hemorrhage; a ruptured liver or spleen; or gastrointestinal bleeding.

16. **What are the most useful initial laboratory studies in evaluating the anemic newborn?**
Review of the peripheral smear is the most useful single study. The MCV, reticulocyte count, and other indices may give you valuable information as well. The size and shape of the RBCs often provide valuable information. Microcytosis will point to iron deficiency or thalassemia; excessive polychromasia or increased nucleated red cells suggest a destructive process or compensated blood loss; spherocytes suggest spherocytosis or ABO incompatibility; blister cells suggest G6PD deficiency; and schistocytes or fragments suggest a microangiopathic anemia as is seen in DIC or renal failure. The presence of blasts suggests leukemia. However, the interpretation of the peripheral blood smear of the newborn is complex and best done by someone with an experienced pair of eyes. Normal findings at this age, including target cells; spherocytes; variation in

RBC size and shape; and occasional young, blast-looking lymphocytes, may resemble disease-related findings. Additional laboratory tests, such as a direct antiglobulin test (DAT or direct Coombs' test) and the Kleihauer-Betke preparation are helpful in more conclusively identifying specific causes of anemia such as alloimmunization and fetomaternal bleeding.

17. **Can you diagnose anemia in utero? If so, how can you treat it?**
    Percutaneous umbilical blood sampling (PUBS) allows the evaluation of fetal blood as early as 18 weeks' gestation. In addition, studies have shown that noninvasive Doppler evaluation of elevated flow velocities in the fetus' cranial circulation may indirectly indicate anemia. Anemia in the fetus may be treated with intrauterine transfusion. Blood is administered through the umbilical vein or into the peritoneal cavity. Fetal anemias that are sometimes managed with transfusions in utero include severe immune hemolysis (Rh incompatibility), homozygous α-thalassemia, severe fetomaternal bleeding or twin-to-twin transfusion, and parvovirus B19 infection-associated red cell aplasia. Stem cell transplantation in utero is currently being evaluated for certain inherited hematologic diseases such as thalassemia and sickle cell anemia.

IMMUNE HEMOLYTIC ANEMIAS

18. **Who was the first person to describe hemolytic disease of the newborn?**
    Luoyse Bourgeois, a French midwife, described a set of twins with hemolytic disease of the newborn in 1609. The first twin was born hydropic and died shortly after birth, and the second twin died of kernicterus.

19. **Who first suggested the term *Erythroblastosis fetalis*?**
    Diamond and coworkers coined the term *erythroblastosis fetalis* in 1932 to describe infants with a hemolytic anemia, extramedullary hematopoiesis, hepatosplenomegaly, and an outpouring of immature erythroblasts. In addition, they showed that hydrops fetalis, icterus gravis, and kernicterus were different manifestations of the same disease.

20. **What is erythroblastosis fetalis?**
    In this condition, antibody-mediated hemolysis in a fetus leads to severe anemia ultimately resulting in hydrops fetalis. Hydrops is due to a combination of extramedullary hematopoiesis leading to liver dysfunction and hypoalbuminemia, decreased plasma osmotic pressure, poor tissue oxygen delivery, capillary leak, and heart failure from severe anemia. In the classic scenario, an RhD-negative woman (15% of Caucasians, 5% of African-Americans, and <1% of Asians) carrying an RhD-positive fetus is sensitized (usually from a previous pregnancy, but rarely during a first pregnancy) and produces anti-RhD antibodies, which cross the placenta and cause immune hemolysis in the fetus. Other Rh and minor blood group antigens occasionally cause isoimmunization and significant fetal hemolysis. Before 1968, the incidence of erythroblastosis fetalis, or hemolytic disease of the newborn, was 6 per 1000 births, with a mortality as high as 25%.

21. **What is the Rh blood system?**
    In the Rh blood group system, three pairs of antigens are present on the surface of the RBC (Cc, Ee, and Dd). The presence of "D" signifies Rh positivity, and "d" signifies the absence of this antigen. The antigens are inherited from each parent as a set of three. Cde and cDE are the most common genotypes. There are 43 other combinations of antigens in the Rh system, which are alleles of Cc, Ee, and D. The D^u antigen is an allele of D. The D^u antigen is weakly antigenic and is depressed by the presence of C on the opposite chromosome. Only rarely will the D^u antigen lead to isoimmunization.

22. **What is RhoGAM and how effective is it at preventing Rh disease?**
    The introduction of RhoGAM (high-titer anti-D immune globulin) to prevent RhD isoimmuniza-tion in pregnancy dramatically decreased the incidence of erythroblastosis fetalis. RhoGAM is given as an intramuscular injection to RhD-negative women (unless the father is known to be RhD-negative as well) at 28 weeks' gestation, immediately after birth, and in situations in which there is a high risk of fetomaternal bleeding (including spontaneous or induced abortion, mis-carriage, ectopic pregnancy, chorionic villous sampling, amniocentesis, percutaneous umbilical blood sampling, abdominal trauma, and placental abruption). The anti-D antibody binds to fetal RhD-positive RBCs in the maternal circulation and decreases the load of foreign antigen presented to the maternal immune system. Since RhoGAM was introduced, the incidence of immune hemolytic disease of the newborn has declined to 6 per 10,000 births, and with advances in perinatal and neonatal care, the mortality has declined to less than 5%.

23. **Since RhoGAM is so effective, why do women still get sensitized?**
    Women may get sensitized if the situation is not recognized, and they do not receive the anti-D titer, or receive an inadequate dose. For example, women who have early first-trimester fetal losses may not even realize that they were pregnant and thus do not receive the anti-D titer. Blood transfusions during childhood may also sensitize a mother when she reaches the child-bearing years.

24. **When an Rh-sensitized fetus is identified, what should be done?**
    A blood type and antibody screen are routinely performed on every woman in the first trimester of pregnancy. If the anti-D titer is greater than 1:8 or if the fetus shows signs of hydrops or poly-hydramnios on ultrasound, amniocentesis or PUBS is performed. PUBS allows fetal RhD typing (in cases in which the father is heterozygous [Dd]) and measurement of fetal hematocrit, reticu-locyte count, and Coombs' test. In cases in which the fetus is RhD positive, amniotic fluid optical density (OD) analysis can be used to predict the severity of hemolysis. Bilirubin released into the amniotic fluid causes an increase in the OD at a wavelength of 450 nm. Using curves first devel-oped in 1961 by Liley, the change in amniotic fluid OD_{450} over time may be plotted and used in conjunction with other tests such as ultrasonography to determine when intervention is required to prevent or treat hydrops fetalis. Intrauterine fetal blood transfusions are performed in cases of severe hemolytic anemia.

25. **What is now the most common cause of immune hemolytic anemia in newborns?**
    Since RhoGAM became widely available, ABO incompatibility has become the most common cause of immune-mediated hemolysis in newborns. An ABO set-up occurs when a woman who is blood type O delivers a baby who is blood type A, B, or AB. A type A or B mother may also produce antigens against the opposite blood type. ABO set-up occurs in about 15% of all pregnancies. Persons with blood type O can produce a significant amount of immunoglobulin (Ig) G against A and B antigens. Unlike IgM, this IgG does cross the placenta.

26. **Which is worse, O-A or O-B incompatibility?**
    "B is Bad, but A is Awful." The A antigen is more antigenic than B, and anti-A antibodies tend to cause more severe hemolysis.

27. **If 15% of all pregnancies have an ABO set-up, why do only 3% have ABO hemolytic disease?**
    The reasons for this phenomenon are many: maternal anti-A and anti-B antibodies may be IgG, IgM, or IgA, and the titer of IgG is variable; RBCs of newborns have less than one third the number of A and B antigenic sites compared with adult RBCs, and their sparse distribution contributes to low antibody binding. In contrast to Rh antigens, A and B antigens are found on many tissues besides RBCs (maternal antibody may be taken up in the placenta or in other

tissues in the baby after birth); anti-A and anti-B antibodies do not bind complement on neonatal cells and thus cause less severe hemolysis in neonates than in adults.

28. **How would you manage a newborn whose mother is blood type O?**
A general recommendation is to send cord blood for typing and DAT (Coombs') testing on all babies of blood type O mothers. The DAT on cord blood is positive (often only weakly so) in about 30% of ABO-incompatible pregnancies. Blood drawn directly from the baby is less likely to be DAT positive, especially after the first day of life.

A serum bilirubin or transcutaneous bilirubin should be obtained from:
- All babies who appear jaundiced in the first 24 hours of life.
- Those who are DAT positive.
- Those who are ABO incompatible and are being discharged early (before day 3 of life).
- Those in whom clinical assessment of jaundice may be difficult.

   Note: Even in the presence of a positive DAT result, only about 10% of newborns will require treatment for hyperbilirubinemia. On the other hand, a significant number of newborns with an ABO set-up who have a negative DAT result will also require phototherapy. If the DAT result is negative but hemolysis is suspected, a more sensitive assay may be done, which involves eluting RBC-bound antibodies and testing against a panel of cells of known RBC antigens.

29. **What clinical and laboratory features distinguish hemolytic disease due to Rh and ABO incompatibility?**
See Table 11-3.

30. **What follow-up care is required for neonates with immune hemolytic disease?**
Babies with significant hyperbilirubinemia should have a hearing screen performed before nursery discharge. In addition, a significant anemia may develop between 4 and 10 weeks of age (particularly in cases of Rh isoimmunization). Late anemia is generally well tolerated, and

TABLE 11-3.   CLINICAL AND LABORATORY FEATURES OF RH AND ABO HEMOLYSIS IN THE NEWBORN

	Rh	ABO
Incidence	0.06% of pregnancies	3% of pregnancies
First pregnancy affected	Rare (<5%)	Frequent (50%)
Subsequent pregnancies	Increasing severity	Not predictable
In utero hemolysis, hydrops	Common	Rare
Hepatomegaly	Moderate to severe	Mild or absent
Anemia at birth	Yes	No
Jaundice at birth	Possible	No
Jaundice by 24 hours	Yes	Yes
Direct Coombs' test	Strongly positive	Weakly positive
Reticulocytosis	Moderate to severe	Mild
Microspherocytosis	No	Yes
Need for exchange transfusion	50–70%	<10%
Late anemia	Frequent	Uncommon

transfusion is rarely indicated unless signs of cardiorespiratory compromise are present. Early iron supplementation should be considered, except in babies who received intrauterine transfusions (who should have adequate iron stores).

31. **What is the course of a newborn who received intrauterine RBC transfusions?**
Babies born to mothers with high antibody titers who received intrauterine transfusions must be very closely monitored. At birth, virtually all of the circulating RBCs are transfused. All new RBCs that the infant makes will be bound with antibody and hemolyzed. Thus, once the transfused cells age and are removed from the circulation, these infants may become profoundly anemic. They often require several transfusions until the passively transferred antibody disappears over time, and the new RBCs that the infant is making are able to survive.

32. **What other antigens besides RhD and the ABO group may cause hemolytic disease of the newborn?**
The majority of cases of minor blood group incompatibility are due to the antigens Kell, E, and c (which are about 1% as potent as the D antigen), and a small percentage of cases are caused by M or Duffy (<0.1% as potent as D). Hemolytic disease caused by the Kell antigen can be particularly severe ("Kell kills"). Management is the same as that for RhD disease.

NONIMMUNE HEMOLYTIC ANEMIAS

33. **How do fetal RBC membranes differ from those in older children and adults?**
Fetal red cells carry the i antigen on the surface, whereas adult RBCs carry the I antigen. Fetal RBC membranes are more permeable to monovalent cations and contain less Na+, K+-adenosine triphosphatase (ATPase), as well as less phospholipid and cholesterol. This makes them more prone to shear stresses and more susceptible to fragmentation. It may also account for the lower life span of RBCs in the neonate compared with adults.

34. **What is hereditary spherocytosis (HS)?**
HS is a congenital hemolytic anemia due to abnormalities in the membrane proteins (spectrin or ankyrin). The abnormal proteins allow the RBC to swell to a spherical shape (compared with the normal biconcave shape), making traversing the capillary beds more difficult for these less plastic cells. This results in hemolysis in the spleen (extravascular) and anemia. It is inherited in an autosomal dominant manner, but the parents may both be normal as the penetrance of the gene defect is variable. It may cause anemia to a widely variable degree. In the newborn period, HS usually presents as prolonged hyperbilirubinemia.

35. **How is HS diagnosed?**
HS is diagnosed based on the family history, the presence of spherocytes on the peripheral smear, a mild normocytic anemia, an increased mean corpuscular hemoglobin concentration, and an elevated osmotic fragility.
Note: About 25% of patients with HS will have a normal osmotic fragility test when freshly isolated cells are tested. However, incubation of the RBCs for 24 hours will bring out the abnormalities.

36. **Which condition in neonates is often difficult to differentiate from HS?**
ABO incompatibility. Both conditions may have anemia, hyperbilirubinemia, microspherocytes, and an altered osmotic fragility test result.

37. **How does a deficiency of G6PD affect RBCs?**
    G6PD is necessary to maintain the generation of reduced nicotinamide adenine dinucleotide phosphate (NADPH), which keeps glutathione in a reduced state. Glutathione is important for the maintenance of sulfhydryl groups and the prevention of oxidative damage. Mature RBCs are unable to synthesize G6PD. In G6PD deficiency, the half-life of RBCs is reduced to approximately 10–15 days.

38. **Does G6PD deficiency cause jaundice in newborn infants?**
    Neonatal jaundice is more common in infants with G6PD deficiency but is not invariably observed. The increased incidence of hyperbilirubinemia does not correlate with the risk of anemia. Therefore, differences in hepatic metabolism (and not hemolysis) may account for the risk of hyperbilirubinemia.

39. **How is G6PD deficiency diagnosed?**
    G6PD deficiency is inherited as an X-linked trait. A family history may help pinpoint the diagnosis. In the newborn period, there is a persistence of reticulocytosis, indicating ongoing hemolysis. This may contribute to hyperbilirubinemia. Definitive diagnosis is made based on a RBC G6PD enzyme assay. If this test is done after a hemolytic episode when the reticulocyte count is high, a false-normal level may be obtained (since younger cells have higher levels of the enzyme).

40. **What are the characteristic features of pyruvate kinase deficiency?**
    Infants with pyruvate kinase deficiency have anemia at birth, invariably develop prolonged hyperbilirubinemia, and will typically have a very high nucleated RBC count. The latter is pathognomonic since mature RBCs have almost no enzyme and cannot survive, and it is the normal RBCs that perform most RBC functions. Similar to G6PD deficiency, the erythroid marrow is markedly hypertrophied.

ABNORMALITIES OF HEMOGLOBIN PRODUCTION

41. **Which abnormalities of hemoglobin production are clinically apparent at birth?**
    Hemoglobin is comprised of two pairs of globin chains. Alpha-globin is made during most of fetal life as well as during infancy and adulthood. Therefore, all forms of α-thalassemia, including α-thalassemia trait (one or two α gene deletions), hemoglobin H disease (three α gene deletions), and homozygous α-thalassemia with hydrops fetalis (all four α genes deleted) may be apparent in the newborn period.
    Disorders of the β-globin gene cluster produces abnormalities in the β, γ, δ, and ϵ chains. Of these, the relevant chains are β and γ. Disorders of γ globin production (γ-thalassemia) may cause a microcytic anemia in the fetus and newborn that subsequently resolves, whereas disorders of β globin production (β-thalassemia) or β-globin structure (sickle cell disease) may be silent at birth but will reveal themselves at an older age. However, β-globin abnormalities, usually clinically silent at birth, may be unmasked by circumstances resulting in excessive destruction or loss of fetal RBCs, such as blood group incompatibility or intrauterine blood loss, by accelerating the production of RBCs with adult hemoglobin.

42. **What is the earliest time that these abnormalities can be diagnosed?**
    Many of these abnormalities can be diagnosed prenatally. Fetal DNA obtained by amniocentesis or chorionic villus sampling can be used. Of course, this is only done if there is a family history or the parents are found to be at risk for having such a child based on their blood counts. Postnatal diagnosis can also easily be made on newborn screening or electrophoresis. The presence of Hb S and the absence of Hb A at birth is diagnostic of sickle cell disease or sickle-β zero thalassemia. The presence of only Hb F at term is indicative of homozygous α-thalassemia, and the presence of Hb H suggests Hb H disease or homozygous α-thalassemia.

43. **Is screening for sickle cell anemia in high-risk populations cost-effective?**
Yes. Several studies have confirmed that neonatal diagnosis and follow-up can reduce mortality.

44. **Why isn't sickle cell disease symptomatic in newborn infants?**
Newborn infants have predominantly Hb F, which does not sickle. When the level of Hb F drops and the predominant hemoglobin is Hb S, the RBCs will begin to sickle, and the infant will begin to have symptoms. This generally begins at 2–3 months of age.

45. **What are the effects of hemoglobin A and F on polymerization of Hb S?**
Both Hb A and Hb F (Hb F more than Hb A) delay polymerization of sickle hemoglobin, allowing more time for the conditions that precipitated the sickling to reverse and for the hemoglobin to become soluble again.

46. **What complications must be anticipated when a woman with sickle cell disease becomes pregnant?**
The mother may experience an increase in severity and frequency of painful crises, increase in severity and frequency of chest syndrome, exaggeration of physiologic anemia of pregnancy, toxemia, or even death (<1%). In addition, there is a higher risk of spontaneous abortion, prematurity, and intrauterine growth restriction in the fetus.

47. **What are the manifestations of the α-thalassemia syndromes?**
   - **Silent carrier:** One of four α-globin genes is inactivated. The MCV may be somewhat lower in these infants, and some Hb Barts (γ chain tetramer) may be present in the cord blood sample.
   - **α-Thalassemia trait:** Two of four α-globin genes are inactivated. Levels of Hb Barts are increased (4–6%) during the neonatal period. Affected infants develop a persistent mild microcytic anemia.
   - **Hemoglobin H disease:** Three of four α-globin genes are inactivated. These infants have a moderate microcytic anemia and Hb H (β chain tetramer-β_4) on electrophoresis. They are at risk for developing gallbladder disease and symptoms from the anemia.
   - **Hydrops fetalis:** All four α-globin genes are inactivated. Prenatal ultrasound may show hydropic changes, and intrauterine transfusions may be necessary to allow normal development. If they are not transfused, these infants are stillborn or die shortly after birth, and their blood contains only Hb Bart's (γ_4), Hb H (β_4), and small amounts of hemoglobin Portland ($\zeta_2\gamma_2$).

48. **Why is it important to make the diagnosis of α-thalassemia trait?**
The diagnosis of α-thalassemia trait is generally one of exclusion. It is easier to make this diagnosis at birth because of the presence of Bart's hemoglobin (γ_4) and microcytosis. In older children, it is necessary to exclude iron deficiency and β–thalassemia trait to make this diagnosis. Analysis of the α genes is now available, but only at a few centers. If the diagnosis is not made, these children may be inappropriately treated for long periods of time.

49. **What is hemoglobin Constant Spring?**
Some silent carriers of α-thalassemia produce small quantities of an unusual hemoglobin called *Constant Spring*. This hemoglobin was named after a small Jamaican town in which the first family known to carry the gene resided.

50. **What is methemoglobin (MetHb), and how does the body deal with it?**
MetHb is formed when the ferrous ion of the heme moiety is oxidized to the ferric form, destroying the oxygen-carrying capacity of heme. MetHb's presence also causes a shift in the oxygen dissociation curve to the left, reducing the transfer of oxygen to the tissues. In normal RBCs, a small amount of MetHb is constantly being formed, but the level remains low (<1% of total Hb) because of the presence of two enzyme systems, the NADH-dependent

cytochrome b_5 MetHb reductase system and NADH diaphorase. Cytochrome b_5 reductase uses NADH to reduce cytochrome b_5, which in turn reduces MetHb to Hb. A small amount of MetHb is reduced to hemoglobin by NADPH diaphorase. The latter mechanism is enhanced by methylene blue, the standard treatment for methemoglobinemia. Cellular antioxidants such as vitamin C and glutathione may reduce MetHb to Hb nonenzymatically.

51. **What agents result in the production of MetHb?**
MetHb production can be increased by *endogenous* oxidants, mainly nitric oxide (NO). Endogenous NO is produced during an inflammatory response (e.g., with sepsis or diarrheal diseases). Exposure to *exogenous* oxidants (e.g., drugs, food preservatives [sodium nitrite], and nitrites and nitrates in the water) has also been implicated. Typically, well water in farming communities is contaminated by nitrites and nitrates leached from minerals or from nitrogen-enriched fertilizers. Bacteria present in the water may degrade nitrates to nitrites. Drugs reported to cause methemoglobinemia include local anesthetics such as prilocaine (EMLA) and benzo-caine, as well as dapsone, primaquine, amyl nitrite, isobutyl nitrite, NO, and nitroglycerin.

52. **Why is methemoglobinemia more common in infants?**
During the period up to 6 months of age, there is a relative deficiency of NADPH diaphorase. This deficiency not only predisposes persons to methemoglobinemia but also leads to a lack of response to methylene blue. Fetal hemoglobin is more sensitive to oxidation than adult hemoglobin.

CONGENITAL ANEMIAS

53. **What are the inherited syndromes in which hematologic manifestation is a major component?**
Table 11-4 briefly describes some of these genetic syndromes.

54. **What is Diamond-Blackfan anemia (DBA)?**
DBA, also called *congenital hypoplastic anemia* or *constitutional red cell aplasia,* is a hetero-geneous disorder primarily involving the erythroid progenitor cells. This results in a progressive macrocytic anemia that begins in infancy. The genetic abnormality appears to be a mutation in the gene that encodes the ribosomal protein S19 (located on chromosome 19q), which may play an important role in erythropoiesis and embryogenesis.

55. **What are the clinical and laboratory manifestations of DBA? How is it treated?**
Affected children present most often in infancy with severe anemia. About one third of them have one or more congenital defects such as craniofacial dysmorphism, skeletal anomalies, congenital heart and urogenital defects, and mental retardation. There is usually growth retardation as well. Laboratory tests show a severe macrocytic anemia with reticulopenia, a normal white cell count, and normal or increased platelet count. There is a decrease or absence of erythroid precursors in the marrow. A majority of patients respond to corticosteroids, most in the long term, but those who do not or who stop responding need transfusions or stem cell transplantation. These persons have a predisposition to leukemia and solid tumors such as osteogenic sarcoma and breast and hepatocellular carcinoma.

56. **What is Fanconi's anemia? What are its clinical and laboratory features?**
Fanconi's anemia is a syndrome in which persons have a defect in DNA repair. They may have a variety of systemic abnormalities including skeletal anomalies and abnormalities in the eyes, ears, genitourinary system, face, and skin. They almost always present with aplastic anemia, usually within the first decade of life. Affected children demonstrate macrocytic anemia, with i antigen expression on the RBCs and elevated levels of Hb F.

TABLE 11-4. INHERITED SYNDROMES IN WHICH HEMATOLOGIC MANIFESTATIONS ARE A MAJOR COMPONENT

Syndrome	Genetics	Manifestations
Diamond-Blackfan anemia	AR, AD, or sporadic	Skeletal anomalies, hypoplastic anemia responsive to steroids
Fanconi's anemia (FA)	AR, FANC gene abnormalities, DNA repair defect	Skeletal anomalies, pancytopenia, predisposition to malignancies
Pearson's syndrome	XL, AR, mitochondrial abnormalities	Exocrine pancreas, liver and kidneys affected, pancytopenia
Osteopetrosis	AR	Developmental delay, ocular abnormalities, neuro-degeneration, pancytopenia
Congenital dyserythropoietic anemia (CDA)	AR	Macrocytic anemia
Thrombocytopenia with absent radii (TAR)	AR	Abnormal radial elements, variable thrombocytopenia
Kostmann's syndrome neutropenia with infections	AR	Severe congenital
Shwachman-Diamond syndrome	AR	Small for gestational age, malabsorption, failure to thrive, neutropenia, aplastic or leukemic transformation

AD = Autosomal dominant, AR = autosomal recessive, XL = X-linked.

The diagnosis is made based on the family history, skeletal anomalies, and a lack of normal DNA repair when chromosomes are stressed with agents such as DEB or mitomycin C. The treatment is supportive, and stem cell transplantation has been performed successfully for aplasia. These persons also have a predisposition to malignancies.

ANEMIA OF PREMATURITY

57. **What is anemia of prematurity?**
Infants born before completing 32 weeks of gestation are prone to developing anemia. This is a normochromic, normocytic anemia that resolves by the postnatal age of 3–6 months.

58. **What is the pathophysiology of anemia of prematurity?**
The pathogenesis of the anemia is not completely clear. Possible contributors include shortened RBC life span, hemodilution from a rapid gain in weight postnatally, and inadequate RBC production. Preterm infants are not able to respond normally to the drop in hemoglobin by producing EPO. The erythroid marrow is extremely sensitive to EPO and in its absence remains quiescent. The switching of the site of EPO production in the premature infant (from the liver to the kidney) may also be an issue.

59. **What is the clinical picture of anemia of prematurity?**
This condition is seen typically in infants born at 32 weeks of gestation or less. It generally begins between the first and third month of life. Three phases have been described: an early phase in which the hemoglobin actually drops, a maintenance phase in which the low hemoglobin is maintained for 1–3 weeks, and a phase of true anemia, with a continued drop in hemoglobin wherein tissue oxygenation is not maintained.

60. **How is this condition treated?**
Anemia of prematurity is not responsive to nutritional support with iron, folate, or vitamin E. Transfusions may be necessary if the infant is ill or has cardiovascular manifestations of anemia. EPO has been used with mixed results in this condition. A recent meta-analysis concluded that, if used appropriately, it does reduce the need for transfusion in these infants. It must always be administered with iron supplements.

TRANSFUSION THERAPY

61. **How often are samples required in the blood bank for an infant who needs multiple transfusions?**
Infants younger than 4 months old are unable to produce RBC alloantibodies on exposure to allogeneic RBCs. As a result, if a neonate's initial sample for type and crossmatching of RBC demonstrates no evidence of a maternally derived alloantibody, further pretransfusion testing is not required until the child is older than 4 months of age. In contrast, older children and adults may produce new alloantibodies despite adequate crossmatching, and so fresh samples must be sent to the blood bank every 3 days.

KEY POINTS: TRANSFUSIONS IN NEONATES

1. Transfusion components for neonates include RBCs, fresh frozen plasma, platelets, cryoprecipitate, and factor concentrates.

2. Neonates must get irradiated, leukocyte-depleted, CMV-negative products.

3. A single donor should be used as much as possible—split the donated units.

62. **Should infants receive type O RhD-negative RBCs exclusively during the neonatal period?**
Infants can be safely transfused with ABO/Rh type-specific blood. O RhD-negative blood is the so-called universal donor blood type and can be safely transfused without establishing an infant's ABO/Rh type. The practice of transfusing only type O RhD-negative RBCs to infants is unnecessary and will only deplete the availability of this resource for emergency transfusion of infants, older children, and adults.

63. **The storage of RBCs is associated with progressive leakage of K+ out of the erythrocyte into the extracellular fluid. Under what circumstances is transfusion of stored RBCs associated with hyperkalemia that might be dangerous to the infant transfusion recipient?**
The storage of RBCs is associated with progressive leakage of K+ and hemoglobin out of the erythrocyte into the extracellular fluid. The transfusion of RBCs that have been stored for >1 week has resulted in hyperkalemia and death due to arrhythmia after neonatal exchange transfusion or when large volumes of RBCs have been transfused. In these clinical situations,

RBCs intended for transfusion should have been stored for <1 week or, alternatively, can be washed to remove extracellular potassium.

64. **What is the best way to avoid transfusions in the first week of life in an otherwise healthy preterm very-low-birth-weight infant?**
KBIB (keep the blood inside the baby). Minimize phlebotomy losses.

65. **How should neonates be transfused RBCS?**
Newborns should receive ABO/Rh-specific packed RBCs. All blood products should be pre-leukofiltered, cytomegalovirus (CMV) negative, and irradiated. RBCs should be transfused in aliquots of 5–15 mL/kg body weight, unless the transfusion is perioperative or an exchange transfusion. Infants who are likely to need multiple such aliquots should receive these from a designated unit that is set aside for them. This will minimize exposure to multiple donors. The duration of transfusion should be approximately 1–3 hours.

66. **What types of transfusion-associated complications may be caused by donor white blood cells (WBCs), and how can they be prevented?**
Adverse reactions caused by passenger or contaminating WBCs include:
- Sensitization to human leukocyte antigen (HLA)
- Febrile transfusion reactions
- CMV transmission
- Transfusion-associated graft-versus-host disease (TA-GVHD)

Although HLA sensitization and febrile transfusion reactions are unusual in infants, transfusion-transmitted CMV and TA-GVHD are associated with serious, sometimes life-threatening outcomes. Although many physical methods for removing passenger WBCs exist, the most practical methods for leukoreduction use filters that remove WBCs by adhesion. Filtration is classified according to log reduction of WBCs in the component. Reducing the number of WBCs by 1–2 logs is usually effective in preventing febrile transfusion reactions, whereas HLA alloimmunization and prevention of transfusion-associated CMV requires a 3–4-log reduction per unit.

67. **Which neonates are at a risk for transfusion-transmitted CMV disease, and how can it be prevented?**
Infants born to seronegative mothers with birth weights of <1200 gm are at highest risk for transfusion-transmitted CMV infection. Transmission can result in asymptomatic viruria, pneumonia, or sepsis. The risk of acquiring CMV from a transfusion correlates with the number of CMV-positive donors to which an infant is exposed. Between 40% and 90% of healthy blood donors have the antibody to CMV.

Transfusion of cellular components from a donor negative for CMV antibody until recently was the best strategy for preventing CMV in those at risk. Because CMV resides in leukocytes, the risk of transmitting CMV through cellular blood products can be minimized through leukoreduction filtration (to a residual WBC of $<1 \times 10^6$ WBC/mL). Leukoreduction results in a component with risk of transmitting CMV comparable to blood from donors who are CMV negative; that is, both leukoreduced and CMV AB-negative components are considered CMV safe.

68. **What is TA-GVHD, and how can it be prevented?**
TA-GVHD is caused by the transfusion of viable lymphocytes contained in cellular blood products to recipients unable to recognize the lymphocytes as foreign. Patients at risk for TA-GVHD fall into two categories: (1) those who are immunodeficient and (2) those who are otherwise healthy but receive cellular products from close biologic relatives. In either case, when the passenger lymphocytes engraft, they are capable of proliferation and may attack the host, causing diarrhea, liver damage, and bone marrow failure. Because TA-GVHD has a high mortality and morbidity, prevention is key. TA-GVHD is not completely prevented by leukoreduction of blood products but rather by gamma irradiation (dose = 2500 rads per component). This becomes particularly important during exchange transfusions.

69. **What is fresh frozen plasma (FFP), and what are the indications for its use in the newborn?**

FFP is the noncellular portion of blood that is separated from the donated unit of fresh blood soon after it is collected and then frozen. It is a rich source of all of the coagulation factors, both procoagulant and anticoagulant. It is used to replenish all the coagulation factors in situations when these are lost (e.g., massive hemorrhage or exchange transfusion), when they are not being produced (e.g., hepatic failure), or when they are being consumed (e.g., DIC). It may also be used to replenish specific factors that may be deficient, such as fibrinogen factor; factors X, XI, and XIII; and von Willebrand's factor. (Deficiency of factors VIII and IX is treated with specific factor concentrates, but FFP may be used if these conditions are suspected but have not been confirmed.) The dose of FFP is 10–20 mL/kg. The half-life varies depending on the factor deficiency for which it is being given, varying from 4 (factor VII) to 60 hours (fibrinogen).

70. **What is cryoprecipitate, and when should it be used?**

Cryoprecipitate is the portion of FFP that remains solid at 4°C when FFP is being thawed. It is a rich source of fibrinogen, factor VIII, von Willebrand's factor, and factor XIII. In the newborn period, it is primarily used to replenish fibrinogen. One unit of cryoprecipitate is 15–20 mL and contains about half as much fibrinogen as a whole unit of FFP, which is about 150–180 mL.

71. **What is the difference between a random-donor unit of platelets and a single-donor unit? Aren't both types of platelets derived from one donor?**

Both platelet products are taken from one volunteer donor. Random-donor platelets are those separated from 1 unit of whole blood. One unit of random-donor platelets contains at least 5.5 $\times 10^{10}$ platelets and is approximately 40 mL in volume. One dose of platelets for a thrombocytopenic infant can usually be supplied from a random-donor unit. Single-donor platelets (also called *platelets* or *apheresis*) are derived from one donor and are harvested using a hemapheresis technique, which allows for the collection of larger units containing at least 3×10^{11} platelets. Single-donor platelets are appropriate for the transfusion requirements of a thrombocytopenic adult.

72. **What is the expected rise following a platelet transfusion? What is the average survival of these platelets?**

A single unit of random-donor platelets should raise the platelet count (checked at 1 hour after transfusion) by 70,000–100,000, depending on the weight of the infant. On average these platelets will last 1–2 days, with a gradual drop. However, if there is a consumptive process ongoing, such as DIC or the infant is post surgery, the count may drop more rapidly.

ERYTHROPOIETIN

73. **What is the source of EPO in the fetus?**

Since maternal EPO does not cross the placenta in humans, erythropoiesis in utero is solely controlled by EPO produced by the fetus. EPO is made primarily by the fetal liver, although small amounts are produced by the fetal kidney during mid and late gestation. It is not known what factors regulate the switch of EPO production from the liver to the kidney around the time of birth. This switch may occur during the physiologic anemia of infancy and may contribute to the anemia of prematurity.

74. **How do the pharmacokinetics of EPO differ between preterm newborns and adults?**

Data from pharmacokinetic studies in newborn humans and animals indicate that neonates have 2–4 times the volume of distribution and 3–4 times the clearance of EPO. Thus, higher doses must be administered to infants than would be required for adults.

75. **How is EPO administered to newborns?**
    EPO must be administered intravenously or subcutaneously. Intramuscular administration is not recommended. EPO has sometimes been added to total parenteral nutrition solutions and administered over 24 hours. It must be kept in mind that EPO is a very large molecule that is somewhat fragile. Therefore, the vial must not be shaken before administration. Various doses as well as different schedules have been used, from daily to alternate day to weekly, with mixed results. It is generally recommended that iron supplementation be administered along with EPO therapy.

76. **What laboratory tests should be ordered to determine whether EPO is effective?**
    A reticulocyte or "retic" count is the best measure of active erythropoiesis. To determine whether EPO is effective, a comparison between a baseline retic count and one obtained 7–10 days after the start of EPO therapy will help determine whether erythropoiesis has been stimulated. It usually takes 2–4 weeks to see the rise in hemoglobin, assuming that blood losses (from phlebotomy or otherwise) have been minimized.

77. **What are the main indications for EPO use in newborns?**
    Multiple studies have shown that EPO and iron therapy reduce the transfusion requirements in anemia of prematurity. EPO therapy may also be indicated in the postoperative state, if there is ongoing blood loss, and in renal failure. In all these situations, it must be administered in conjunction with iron supplementation.

POLYCYTHEMIA

78. **What are the common causes of polycythemia in a newborn?**
    Primary polycythemia results from a variety of conditions, including those associated with chronic fetal hypoxia, such as preeclampsia, severe maternal heart disease, and maternal smoking. It is also observed in growth-restricted infants; infants of diabetic mothers; infants born at high altitudes; and infants with thyrotoxicosis, congenital adrenal hyperplasia, chromosomal anomalies (13, 18, or 21) and Beckwith-Wiedemann syndrome. The most common secondary cause is delayed clamping of the umbilical cord. Other secondary causes include dehydration, congenital cyanotic heart disease, twin-to-twin transfusion, maternal-fetal transfusion, and, occasionally, overzealous or inadvertent overtransfusion of RBCs.

79. **What is twin-to-twin transfusion?**
    The classic signs of twin-to-twin transfusion are disparate growth and weight between the infants, and disparate hematocrit values. One twin is polycythemic, and the other is anemic. There exists an inverse, linear correlation between hematocrit and pulmonary blood flow. Therefore, the polycythemic twin often has very low pulmonary blood flow and increased pulmonary vascular resistance, accounting for the need for supplemental oxygen. Reduction of the hematocrit will increase pulmonary blood flow and eliminate the need for oxygen. The anemic twin may have mild congestive heart failure resulting from anemia. A simple transfusion or partial exchange transfusion with packed RBCs is indicated to increase the hematocrit.

80. **What clinical manifestations should be anticipated in a polycythemic infant?**
    Clinically, these infants look ruddy and plethoric. Infants with polycythemia may exhibit decreased urine output (from decreased renal plasma flow), hyperbilirubinemia and thrombocytopenia (from sludging), and cardiomegaly and respiratory distress from circulatory overload. Nonspecific symptoms may include a weak suck, lethargy, respiratory distress, jitteriness (from hypocalcemia), irritability, hypotonia, vomiting, and hepatosplenomegaly. There is an increased incidence of hypoglycemia in infants with polycythemia.

81. **What is the pathophysiology of cerebral damage in these infants?**
Polycythemia reduces cerebral blood flow. However, the reduction in cerebral blood flow is not secondary to hyperviscosity but is a physiologic response to the increase in arterial oxygen content resulting in normal cerebral oxygen delivery and metabolism. The decreased cerebral blood flow does not cause cerebral hypoxia. Therefore, it should not be surprising that studies have failed to show any benefit in long-term neurologic function by reducing the hematocrit. Lastly, several epidemiologic studies have suggested that it is the other events that occur in association with polycythemia (e.g., asphyxia) that cause the brain injury. Rather, polycythemia is a marker for fetal or perinatal distress and hypoxia.

82. **A heel stick hematocrit was sent that was 76%. You are concerned about polycythemia and hyperviscosity. What should you do?**
Obtain a central hematocrit.

83. **How does one manage the care of these infants?**
The goal of therapy is to reduce the hematocrit by performing a partial exchange transfusion. Any infant with a hematocrit level above 70% should be treated. This will correct the hyperviscosity; however, other manifestations may take a few hours to days to resolve. Symptomatic infants with central hematocrit between 65% and 70% are also considered for a partial exchange transfusion. In the interim, it is important to monitor the metabolic abnormalities and correct them.

84. **Should screening for polycythemia be done in every newborn infant?**
In a healthy term newborn with a normal examination, there are no data to support the efficacy of obtaining a screening hematocrit. No etiologic link between polycythemia and neurologic injury has ever been established, and in population studies of asymptomatic polycythemic infants, all had normal long-term neurologic function.

NEUTROPHIL ABNORMALITIES

85. **How do neutrophils develop and circulate in the healthy fetus/neonate?**
Neutrophils are produced by clonal maturation of progenitors in the bone marrow. The morphologically recognizable neutrophil precursors (myeloblasts, promyelocytes, and myelocytes) are capable of cell division and are collectively termed the *neutrophil proliferative pool*. The maturing neutrophils in the marrow that have lost mitotic capacity (metamyelocytes, band neutrophils, and segmented neutrophils) constitute a ready reserve, termed the *neutrophil storage pool*. Once neutrophils are released from the marrow into the blood, they become apportioned to one of two interchangeable pools, the *circulating* or the *marginated* pool. Together, these two blood pools of neutrophils are termed the *total blood neutrophil pool*.

86. **What constitutes neutropenia in a neonate?**
In the healthy newborn, the total WBC count is commonly higher than in an older child, with a predominance of mononuclear cells (lymphocytes and monocytes). However, the absolute number of neutrophils is generally above 1500/mm^3. Neutropenia is defined as an absolute neutrophil count less than 1500/mm^3.

87. **What are the causes of neutropenia in neonates?**
Neutropenia in the neonatal period may be classified based on the etiology into the following groups:

- **Diminished production of neutrophils in the marrow:** Infants of hypertensive mothers, Rh hemolytic disease, severe congenital neutropenia (Kostmann's syndrome), Shwachman syndrome, reticular dysgenesis, drug or toxin induced
- **Accelerated neutrophil usage or destruction:** Infection, isoimmunization/alloimmune neutropenia, autoimmune neutropenia and chronic benign neutropenia, hypersplenism
- **Excessive neutrophil margination:** Polycythemia, endotoxemia

88. **What is the pathophysiology of neonatal alloimmune neutropenia?**
Neonatal alloimmune neutropenia arises when a mother has IgG antibodies that cross the placenta and react with neutrophil antigens that are foreign to her but are expressed on fetal (and paternal) neutrophils. Immune destruction of fetal neutrophils in the fetal bone marrow and blood can lead to severe fetal and neonatal neutropenia. In compensation for the neutrophil destruction, neutrophil production within the marrow increases, with a shift of the "myeloid erythroid ratio" further to the myeloid side.

89. **What are the common hematologic findings among neonates delivered to women with pregnancy-induced hypertension?**
Hyporegenerative neutropenia, hyporegenerative thrombocytopenia, reticulocytosis, elevated nucleated RBCs, and polycythemia.

90. **What are the indications for the use of cytokines such as granulocyte colony-stimulating factor?**
Regular use of granulocyte colony-stimulating factor is only indicated in the treatment of severe congenital neutropenia that results from Kostmann's or Shwachman syndromes or reticular dysgenesis. Intermittent use may be indicated in autoimmune neutropenia when there is the possibility that the infant may have an infection.

91. **What are some of the hematologic abnormalities that may be seen in a baby with trisomy 21 syndrome?**
Infants with Down syndrome may have a myriad of hematologic abnormalities. They may be polycythemic (with or without congenital heart disease), they may be thrombocytopenic, and they may also have an elevated number of circulating blasts. The latter is called *transient myeloproliferative disorder*. The disorder is usually transient, resolving in most infants by 3 months of age. However, the incidence of leukemia in the first decade of life is increased 10-fold in children with Down syndrome.

THROMBOCYTOPENIA

92. **What is the normal platelet count for a term newborn infant?**
More than 150,000/μL, the same as for an older child or adult.

93. **How does the platelet count tend to vary during the neonatal period?**
Thrombocytopoiesis is not completely effective in the neonatal period. Although healthy newborns usually have platelet counts similar to adults (150,000–450,000/μL), many premature and very-low-birth-weight babies (up to 20%) have platelet counts between 100,000 and 150,000/μL, without apparent cause. Moreover, in cases of infections, the platelet count of infants tends to drop precipitously. Elevated platelet counts (up to 700,000/μL) are often seen between 2 weeks and 6 months of age. In infants, as in older children, thrombocytosis is not associated with increased tendency to thrombosis, and thus it is not of clinical significance. "Neonatal platelets" appear to be functionally normal.

KEY POINTS: PREMATURE AND VERY-LOW-BIRTH-WEIGHT INFANTS

1. Premature and very-low-birth-weight babies may have lower platelet counts than older children or adults.

2. The etiology of thrombocytopenia is decreased production or increased destruction, but it is often multifactorial.

3. Neonatal alloimmune thrombocytopenia can occur in the first pregnancy.

4. Consumptive processes resolve when the underlying problem is corrected.

94. **What are the common causes of thrombocytopenia in newborn infants?**
    Etiologies for thrombocytopenia may be divided into the following categories of causes:
    - Immune-mediated destruction (passively transferred antibody—maternal ITP or lupus, alloimmunization, or actively produced antibody-autoimmune)
    - Infection (consumptive—sepsis/DIC, or decreased production from marrow suppression)
    - Drugs/toxins (marrow suppression)
    - Mechanical destruction (microangiopathic conditions, prosthetic devices, ECHO, dialysis)
    - Genetic (thrombocytopenia with absent radii [TAR]; Fanconi's anemia; congenital amegakaryocytic thrombocytopenia; trisomy 13, 18, or 21 syndrome; Wiskott-Aldrich syndrome; Noonan's syndrome; inborn errors of metabolism such as methylmalonic acidemia, propionic acidemia, isovaleric acidemia)
    - Miscellaneous (thrombosis, necrotizing entercolitis [NEC], perinatal asphyxia, infants of hypertensive others).
    Usually, the etiology is multifactorial, involving a combination of the conditions above.

95. **What physical findings suggest a specific etiology for thrombocytopenia in the neonate?**
    - Blueberry muffin rash (TORCH or viral infection)
    - Absence of radii (TAR syndrome)
    - Palpable flank mass and hematuria (renal vein thrombosis)
    - Hemangioma, often with bruit (Kasabach-Merritt syndrome)
    - Abnormal thumbs (Fanconi's syndrome, but it is unusual for affected infants to be thrombocytopenic at birth)
    - Skin rashes (Wiskott-Aldrich syndrome)
    - Dysmorphic features (trisomy 13, 18, or 21 syndrome)

96. **What is neonatal alloimmune thrombocytopenia (NAIT)?**
    Just as RBCs have surface antigens that make it possible to classify persons into "blood groups," platelets have surface antigens as well. These are now called human platelet antigens (HPAs). There are over 10 different HPAs. NAIT is a platelet incompatibility between mother and fetus analogous to Rh disease. As with Rh disease, the mother makes antibody against "paternal" antigens (most commonly HPA-1a, previously called PLA-1). The antibody crosses the placenta and binds fetal platelets, resulting in their destruction. The antibody can also cause a defect in platelet aggregation.

97. **What is the incidence of NAIT? When should one suspect it?**
    The incidence of NAIT is approximately 1 in 1000–2000 live births. It should be suspected if the thrombocytopenia is unexplained, if the mother has a normal platelet count and is well, if the baby is not sick (other than purpura), if the platelet count is very low ($\leq$50,000/μL), or if there is a

positive family history for thrombocytopenia (firstborn offspring are affected in about half the cases). A disparity in maternal and paternal HPA-1 does not necessarily mean that the mother will produce antibodies. Only 1 in 10–20 women who are HPA-1a negative will make the antibody.

98. **What is the clinical course of NAIT?**
The newborn is generally well but may have some petechiae and may ooze from heel sticks or venipunctures. The platelet count is low at birth and continues to drop over the first few days. It then stabilizes and may rise to normal levels within 1–4 weeks.

99. **How is NAIT managed?**
The key is appropriate diagnosis. Blood from both parents and the infant should be sent for typing and antibody analysis. An ultrasound scan of the head is indicated in all infants with platelet counts less than 50,000/mm^3. If the platelet count is less than 30,000/µL, one should consider giving intravenous immunoglobulin (IVIG) at a dose of 1 gm/kg and methylprednisolone (2 mg/kg/day) until the platelet count rises above 50,000. If the diagnosis has been made prenatally, appropriate platelets or maternal pheresed (and washed) platelets may be prepared in advance for transfusion. Random-donor platelets are not likely to be effective and should be given in larger doses only if there is significant bleeding and typed platelets are not available. Of course, the parents must be counseled regarding future pregnancies, and early testing must be performed.

100. **What are the clinical features of maternal autoimmune thrombocytopenia?**
This diagnosis should be considered when both mother and infant have thrombocytopenia or when there is a history of thrombocytopenia in the mother. It is sometimes difficult to distinguish maternal idiopathic thrombocytopenic purpura (ITP) from gestational thrombocytopenia, but in ITP the count is generally lower and the peripheral smear shows large platelets. In comparison with NAIT, thrombocytopenia is generally milder. The degree of maternal thrombocytopenia is a poor predictor of the degree of neonatal thrombocytopenia. This condition is treated with IVIG and methylprednisolone.

101. **When should platelets be administered to a sick infant with thrombocytopenia?**
In a sick infant without bleeding manifestations, the platelet count should be kept above 25,000/µL. In an infant who is bleeding immediately postoperatively, the platelet count should be kept above 75,000/µL.

DISSEMINATED INTRAVASCULAR COAGULATION

102. **How is DIC defined?**
DIC is as an acquired pathologic process in which there is generalized activation of the coagulation system with widespread fibrin deposition and simultaneous activation of the fibrinolytic system. The entire process occurs within the vascular compartment.

103. **Why are sick newborns particularly susceptible to developing DIC?**
Newborns have an immature reticuloendothelial system and liver that, when compromised, may not be able to clear activated products appropriately. In addition, the tiny size of the blood vessels predisposes the infant to small vessel thrombosis.

104. **What are the major causes of neonatal DIC?**
As defined, DIC is always acquired and always pathologic. The triggers for the activation of the coagulation system include activation of the intrinsic pathway after injury to the vascular endothelium (e.g., sepsis, large hemangiomas, hypotension, hypothermia, hypoxemia, polycythemia, excessive instrumentation or the placement of catheters and tubes), activation of the extrinsic pathway after severe tissue injury (e.g., abruption, preeclampsia, brain injury,

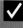

KEY POINTS: DISSEMINATED INTRAVASCULAR COAGULATION

1. DIC in the neonate always results from some underlying pathology.

2. Clotting *and* fibrinolysis are the etiologic keys.

3. Thrombocytopenia and elevated D-dimers are diagnostic for the disease.

4. The problem will not resolve until the underlying disorder is treated.

5. Supportive care includes platelet and FFP transfusions, and heparin if there is a significant thrombus.

surgical procedures, neoplasms, NEC), massive red cell or platelet injury (e.g., intravascular hemolysis, antigen-antibody reactions), and reticuloendothelial system injury.

105. What is the pathophysiology and clinical picture of DIC?
When triggered, the two arms of the coagulation cascade combine to generate increased amounts of thrombin; this gives rise to more fibrin generation, activation of the fibrinolytic system, and plasmin-mediated lysis of this fibrin. In addition, there is activation of platelets by a variety of factors, leading to aggregation and consumption. These processes lead to microvascular thrombosis and a resulting microangiopathic hemolytic anemia. Because of consumption of coagulation factors, there may be a bleeding diathesis as well. The clinical picture may include symptoms related to thrombosis (small or large vessel) or hemorrhage (mucocutaneous or internal) and a mild to moderate intravascular hemolytic process giving rise to anemia (hematuria/hemoglobinuria and hyperbilirubinemia).

106. What is the classic constellation of laboratory abnormalities seen in severe DIC?
Elevated prothrombin time (PT) and partial thromboplastin time (PTT), low platelet count, low fibrinogen, elevated D-dimers, mild to moderate anemia, hyperbilirubinemia, and low levels of all coagulation factors. The peripheral blood smear will show the presence of schistocytes and fewer platelets than normally seen. Schistocytes are thought to be formed when RBCs pass through small blood vessels that are partially occluded or distorted by excess fibrin deposited because of the DIC process.

107. What is the differential diagnosis of DIC?
The differential diagnosis includes hemorrhagic disease of the newborn, a hereditary coagulopathy, hepatic failure, and other causes of isolated thrombocytopenia.

108. What single test can help distinguish DIC from hepatic failure?
Factor VIII level. This factor is thought to be synthesized in vascular endothelial cells, not in the hepatocyte. It is decreased in a state of consumption of coagulation factors, such as DIC, but remains normal in hepatic failure. Note that some factor VIII may be synthesized "in the liver" in endothelial cells rather than in hepatocytes.

109. What are the principles of management of DIC?
- Identify and treat the underlying disease process that is triggering the DIC.
- Closely monitor the laboratory parameters to guide replacement therapy.
- Support with blood products to replace the coagulation factors, platelets, and "natural" anticoagulants that are consumed in DIC. Platelet transfusions, FFP, and cryoprecipitate are typically given. In severe situations where volume is an issue, exchange transfusion with FFP reconstituted fresh red cells may be undertaken. Platelets must be given in addition.

- Maintain optimal oxygenation and perfusion.
- Consider heparin therapy to interrupt the consumptive process. The value of this therapy is controversial in the absence of major vessel thrombosis.
- Provide supplemental vitamin K.

110. What parameters should be monitored, and what are the important values to maintain?
It is important to keep the fibrinogen above 100 mg/dL and the platelet count above 50,000/mm³. If the source of fibrinogen is FFP, all the other coagulation factors will be provided as well. Fibrinogen may also be supplemented with cryoprecipitate, but this should be used only after FFP has been given.

INHERITED DISORDERS OF COAGULATION

111. How does the coagulation system develop in utero and postnatally?
Components of the coagulation system first begin to appear at 10–11 weeks of gestation. All factor levels are low before the fetus is considered viable. When the infant is born, the coagulation system is immature, but it matures rapidly after birth to the adult state. Since almost all the proteins involved in the coagulation system are produced in the liver, immaturity of this organ at birth results in depressed levels of many factors. Furthermore, some of the proteins that are synthesized may have decreased functional activity. The immature system has a different balance between thrombin generation and inhibition of this process. Levels of both the procoagulants (factors II, VII, IX, and X) and anticoagulants (proteins S and C) that are vitamin K-dependent are low. Thus, normal term newborns do not have a bleeding or thrombotic predisposition. At birth, there is a consumption of most factors. Since the metabolic rate is more rapid in newborn infants, the clearance of the coagulation factors is also more rapid. Neonates also have a reduced sensitivity to heparin and require larger doses to achieve anticoagulation.

112. Why is it difficult to assess coagulation in a newborn?
First of all, it is difficult to obtain enough blood and place the specimen quickly enough into the appropriate tube before it clots. In addition, the normal ranges for most coagulation tests are very different in newborns, have a wide range of normal values, and vary by gestational age as well.

KEY POINTS: HEMOPHILIA AND VON WILLEBRAND'S DISEASE

1. Hemophilia A and B are X-linked; hemophilia C is autosomal.

2. A family history may not be present in 25–30% of patients with hemophilia A and B.

3. Von Willebrand's disease affects 0.5–1% of patients and is not clinically significant in the neonatal period unless severe.

4. Factor replacement is available for hemophilia A and B and von Willebrand's disease.

113. What is hemophilia? Are there different types?
Hemophilia is a condition in which the congenital absence of a clotting protein predisposes a person to bleeding. There are three types of hemophilia—A, B, and C—which are caused by differences of factors VIII, IX, and XI, respectively.

114. **What is meant by "severe" hemophilia?**
Hemophilia may also be classified based on the residual factor level at the time of birth. If the level is below 1% of expected, it is severe, 1–5% moderate, and 5–25% mild. Patients with severe hemophilia will have frequent, spontaneous bleeding, such as hemarthrosis. In the mild and moderate phenotypes, bleeding typically occurs only with identifiable trauma.

115. **How is hemophilia inherited? If there is no family history, how is the diagnosis made?**
Hemophilia A or factor VIII deficiency and hemophilia B or factor IX deficiency are inherited in an X-linked recessive manner. These conditions are seen only in males. It is important to remember that in approximately 25–30% of boys with hemophilia, there is no family history (either because the mother is a silent carrier or because it is a new mutation). The rate of spontaneous mutations is significant. Factor XI deficiency is inherited in an autosomal recessive manner and thus affects both sexes. The diagnosis can be made prenatally if there is a family history. If there is no family history, the diagnosis is made by assaying the specific factor levels in newborn male infants with significant bleeding (most often after circumcision).

116. **What are the mechanisms that cause hemophilia A or B in females?**
Hemophilia in females is extremely rare (estimated incidence, 1 in 250 million). There are several described mechanisms:
- She is the homozygous offspring of a hemophiliac male and a carrier female.
- She is a hemophilia carrier with extremely unfavorable "lyonization" such that most of her cells use the X chromosome with the defective gene.
- She has a chromosomal abnormality with only one X chromosome (XO), and that X chromosome has a hemophilia mutation.

In most of these situations, the female embryo or fetus is spontaneously lost and often is not analyzed for the defect. Alternatively, the woman may be genetically normal and may have an acquired inhibitor to factor VIII or IX.

117. **Can a person have a deficiency of both factor VIII and factor IX?**
Since the genes for these factors are adjacent on the X chromosome, a mutation that involved both would be a possibility. However, these mutations are considered to be lethal to the embryo, and no individual has been described with a congenital deficiency of both of these factors.

118. **What fraction of infants born with hemophilia have factor VIII deficiency?**
Eighty to eighty-five percent have hemophilia A, which is a factor VIII deficiency, and 15–20% have hemophilia B, which is a factor IX deficiency. The incidence of hemophilia A is 1 in 5000–6000 live male births, and for hemophilia B the incidence is 1 in 25,000–30,000 live male births.

119. **What percentage of male infants with hemophilia who are circumcised in the neonatal period (before the diagnosis is established) will have unusual or excessive bleeding?**
About 30–50%. The absence of bleeding at routine circumcision does not rule out the diagnosis of severe hemophilia.

120. **How common is intracranial bleeding in infants with hemophilia?**
Quite uncommon. Intracranial hemorrhage occurs in only 1–2% of severe cases, even with vaginal delivery. However, if it does occur, it can have devastating consequences. Hence, if the diagnosis of severe hemophilia is known prenatally, an elective cesarean section may be preferred. The diagnosis is usually anticipated, however, when there has been a prior child or relative born with hemophilia.

121. **What would be the empirical treatment in a newborn with intracranial hemorrhage and an elevated PTT before the factor levels are known?**
Until the specific factor deficiency is elucidated, the best empiric therapy would be to administer FFP. This would contain all of the coagulation factors that could be deficient. Using cryoprecipitate would not provide factor IX or XII. Using specific factor VIII or IX concentrates would not be appropriate without a specific diagnosis.

122. **What coagulation factor deficiencies result in an extremely prolonged PTT but no bleeding diathesis?**
Deficiencies of factor XII, prekallikrein, and high-molecular-weight kininogen. These factors are referred to as *contact factors;* they are critical to initiating the activation of coagulation in the in vitro clotting assays but do not contribute significantly to hemostasis in vivo. Although there is no true factor deficiency, it is important to keep in mind that heparin contamination may result in a prolonged PTT without bleeding.

123. **Should newborn infants be screened for hemophilia if there is a family history? If so, how should this be done?**
If there is a history of hemophilia on the mother's side of the family, it is worth doing a thorough work-up *prenatally.* The mother can be tested to see whether she is a carrier, and if she is, male fetuses should be tested for the same mutation. Postnatally, the specific factor level may be assayed in the baby. Normal ranges for gestational age are available. The activated PTT (aPTT) is not a good screening test. The normal range for aPTT is wider in term newborns than older children and adults, and it becomes even wider after a premature birth. An elevated aPTT does not distinguish between factor VIII and factor IX deficiency. The aPTT may also be within the normal range for a neonate with mild or moderate hemophilia.

124. **What is von Willebrand's disease? Are there different types?**
Von Willebrand's disease is the most common inherited disorder of coagulation, with an estimated prevalence of 0.5–1% in the general population. Von Willebrand's factor is a complex of multimeric proteins synthesized by the vascular endothelium, to bring factor VIII to the site of bleeding and promote platelet aggregation. A deficiency of these factors or an abnormal structure of the proteins results in the disease. There are several different types: type I is a mild quantitative defect, type II is a qualitative defect (several subtypes), and type III is a severe quantitative defect.

125. **How is von Willebrand's disease inherited?**
The most common and mildest forms are autosomal dominant. There are rare recessive variants. The disease is frequently so mild that the family history may be negative, even when one of the parents is actually affected. Only the severe, autosomal recessive forms would be likely to present with bleeding manifestations in the newborn period.

126. **When should one test for von Willebrand's disease if there is a family history? What tests are sent to make the diagnosis?**
Testing a newborn is not recommended because the levels of the von Willebrand's factors may be falsely high in the perinatal period as a result of the effect of maternal hormones. For this reason, infants with type I do not present with bleeding symptoms during this time. Testing is best performed after the age of 6 months and includes assays for factor VIII, von Willebrand's antigen, and the ristocetin cofactor. Further testing of the multimer distribution is warranted if type II is suspected.

127. **How is von Willebrand's disease treated?**
Von Willebrand's factor is contained in FFP, cryoprecipitate, and some human-derived factor VIII complex concentrates such as Humate-P. The recombinant factor VIII concentrates do *not*

contain von Willebrand's factor. If the concentrate is not available, one of the other products may be used.

128. **What coagulation factor deficiency is classically associated with delayed separation of the umbilical cord stump?**

Factor XIII deficiency. Factor XIII stabilizes and cross-links fibrin clots after they are formed. Factor XIII deficiency is a clinical bleeding disorder in which the screening tests, PT, PTT, and platelet count are all normal.

129. **Can factor XIII deficiency cause serious bleeding? How is it treated?**

Factor XIII deficiency may have serious consequences, such as intracranial bleeding. Both FFP and cryoprecipitate have factor XIII and may be used to treat these bleeding episodes. There is no concentrate available.

THROMBOTIC DISORDERS

130. **What are some of the more common inherited disorders of coagulation proteins that may cause a prothrombotic or thrombophilic state?**
   - Antithrombin III deficiency
   - Protein C deficiency
   - Protein S deficiency
   - Activated protein C resistance or factor V Leiden
   - Factor II mutation 20210A

131. **What are the most common causes of thrombosis in the neonate?**

The most common causes of thromboses are not inherited defects. In fact, the presence of lines, grafts, patches, or other instrumentation such as cardiac catheterization or surgery are by far the most common reasons for thrombosis in a newborn. Dehydration may be added to the list, although this is not very common. If any of these predisposing factors are present, a thrombophilia work-up is *not* indicated.

KEY POINTS: THROMBOTIC DISORDERS

1. Etiology is usually related to procedures or foreign bodies and occasionally from inherited thrombophilic states.

2. The recommended anticoagulation involves heparin (UFH or LMWH); neonates need higher doses.

3. Thrombolytic therapy is most effective when used early, but there is a high risk for hemorrhage.

132. **What comprises a basic thrombophilia work-up?**

If a thrombophilia work-up is indicated, blood is sent to assay plasma concentrations of antithrombin III (ATIII), protein C, and protein S, as well as to look for maternally transferred IgG lupus anticoagulant antibodies. Protein S and C and ATIII are all physiologically decreased at birth, with values that rapidly increase in the first days to week of life. Published reference ranges for healthy term and premature infants (30–40 weeks' gestational age for the first 6 months of life) are available with reliable limits that encompass 95% of the population. Factor V

Leiden and prothrombin gene 20210A mutation analyses are also indicated, given their relative frequency in the population. These are both DNA-based tests that are accurate in newborns. The evaluation of parents can be helpful in distinguishing an acquired from a congenital abnormality.

133. How do infants with homozygous protein C or S deficiency present?

The classical clinical presentation of homozygous protein C or S deficiency consists of cerebral or ophthalmic damage that occurred in utero, purpura fulminans within days or hours of birth, and (on rare occasions) large vessel thrombosis. The skin lesions start as small ecchymotic sites that increase in size, develop bullae, and become necrotic. They occur mainly on the extremities but can occur on the buttocks, abdomen, scrotum, and scalp. There is a severe, diffuse DIC with secondary hemorrhagic complications and immeasurable levels of protein C or S.

A second form of homozygous protein C or S deficiency presents with thromboembolic events during early childhood; these infants develop severe skin necrosis when administered warfarin (Coumadin). Protein C or S levels in these patients are detectable and range from ~1% to 20% of normal. If warfarin is used to treat these patients, international normalized ratio values must be maintained at >4, and there is a considerable risk of bleeding. An alternative approach is to use low-molecular-weight heparin (LMWH).

134. How is the care of infants with homozygous protein C or S deficiency managed?

Protein C concentrates are available, but for protein S deficiency, FFP remains the treatment of choice.

135. How does one diagnose thrombosis in newborns?

Although ultrasound is the most commonly used diagnostic test, the sensitivity and specificity of ultrasound is not consistent. In children with thrombi in the upper venous system, ultrasound appears to be sensitive for clots in the jugular and axillary veins, but not in the inferior vena cava, subclavian, and innominate veins, where 80% of the thrombi may be missed. In these situations, computed tomography (CT) scans are more sensitive. The use of the D-dimer assay is a specific and sensitive indicator of a thrombus formation. When used in conjunction, the specificity and sensitivity of the ultrasound/CT and D-dimer assay are very high.

136. What are the indications for thrombolytic therapy?

Thrombolytic therapy is used most commonly to treat arterial thrombi that result from catheters placed in a peripheral artery, aorta, or femoral artery. The decision whether to use thrombolytic therapy is based on certain pieces of clinical information such as age and location of the thrombus and severity of the clinical symptoms. If there is potential loss of limb or critical organ function, thrombolytic therapy should be considered, provided there is no significant bleeding disorder, hemorrhage into the brain, hypertension, or other risk factors. In the presence of these complications, thrombolytic therapy might still be used if the baby's life is at risk.

137. Which is the thrombolytic agent of choice, and when should heparin be started?

Tissue plasminogen activator is the drug of choice, and protocols are available. Heparin therapy is indicated either immediately after an infusion of a thrombolytic (provided the thrombolytic agent is infused for less than 12 hours) or during thrombolytic therapy (for infusions lasting more than 12 hours). Prolonged infusions of thrombolytic therapy (12–24 hours) will consume endogenous plasminogen (already physiologically decreased) and render the patient relatively resistant to thrombolytic therapy. Supplementation of plasminogen should be considered in these instances and can be achieved through the administration of FFP and cryoprecipitate.

138. **How should neonates with thrombi associated with central venous lines be treated?**
In all situations, a determination must be made of how essential the line is for the infant. Additional options include anticoagulation and thrombolytic therapy. Local thrombolytic therapy with either urokinase or tissue plasminogen activator is commonly used and is very effective at restoring line patency. Systemic thrombolytic therapy is rarely indicated because the thrombi are usually old, occur gradually over time, and have little likelihood of lysing. However, a new acute clot in the presence of an old clot may present with a relatively sudden superior vena cava syndrome. In this situation, thrombolytic therapy may be helpful in resolving the acute symptoms. Anticoagulation therapy with either unfractionated heparin (UFH) or LMWH can be very effective in preventing further progression of the thrombus.

ANTICOAGULATION

139. **What are the options for immediate anticoagulation in newborns? What are the pros and cons of each?**
The treatment options are UFH and LMWH. The advantages of UFH are that it is immediate, has a short half-life (30 minutes), and can be easily reversed. This is particularly important for infants in whom an emergent surgical procedure might become necessary, such as babies with congenital heart lesions. However, UFH has the disadvantages of being highly bound to a variety of cells in the body, being more unpredictable in its response, and requiring far more frequent monitoring. LMWH has a more predictable effect, with far less nonspecific binding, and thus requires less monitoring. However, it must be given subcutaneously and has a longer half-life of 4–6 hours. It is not the drug of choice if a surgical procedure is emergent.

140. **How is anticoagulation with heparin different in a newborn compared with an older child?**
Newborn infants are more resistant to the effect of heparin and need higher doses to achieve anticoagulation. This is in part due to the lower levels of circulating antithrombin. It is not uncommon for a neonate to require multiple boluses of UFH and drip rates of 25–40 U/kg/h to maintain anticoagulation. Dosing of LMWH is approximately 50% higher in the newborn.

141. **How is anticoagulation with heparin monitored?**
Anticoagulation with UFH is monitored using a standard aPTT. The therapeutic range is 65–115 seconds. Since LMWH does not affect the aPTT, its efficacy is monitored using the Anti-Xa assay. Blood is drawn 4 hours after the dose has been administered, usually after the fourth dose. The therapeutic range is 0.5–1. This assay may also be used to monitor UFH but is a more specialized assay, and the aPTT is adequate in most instances.

142. **How is the effect of heparin reversed?**
Since UFH has a very short half-life, simply stopping the heparin drip will result in fairly rapid normalization of the aPTT. If this is desired emergently, the specific antidote is protamine sulfate. One milligram is administered for every 100 U of UFH administered in the previous 2 hours. There is no complete antidote for LMWH. Protamine sulfate will reverse approximately 60% of the anticoagulant effect if administered within 4 hours of the LMWH dose. It is given in the same dose as the last enoxaparin dose (within the past 4 hours). It is important to remember that protamine is a fish product and may cause allergic reactions. Furthermore, it has anticoagulant properties of its own, and dosing must be checked carefully.

NEOPLASMS

143. **What biologic variables at the time of diagnosis distinguish congenital or infant leukemia from leukemia in an older child?**
   - Extreme leukocytosis
   - Massive hepatosplenomegaly
   - High incidence of central nervous system leukemia at diagnosis
   - Hypogammaglobulinemia
   - High incidence of coexpression of lymphoid and myeloid phenotypic markers
   - Increased frequency of cytogenetic abnormalities
   - Pseudodiploidy
   - Hypodiploidy
   - Translocations: t(4;11), 11q23 breakpoints involve myeloid/lymphoid leukemia (MLL) gene
   - Five-year event-free survival of 25%

144. **On initial examination, a term male infant is found to have an abdominal mass. A sonogram reveals a right suprarenal mass with calcification. What is the probable diagnosis and course of management?**
   The most likely diagnosis is a neuroblastoma. Neuroblastomas account for >50% of the malignancies diagnosed in the neonatal period. However, their management remains controversial. Although small primary tumors without metastases may regress spontaneously without intervention, a biopsy to assess biologic markers is warranted. If no adverse parameters are found, observation (without medication or chemotherapy) is acceptable. However, if unfavorable characteristics are identified, or if respiratory compromise resulting from massive hepatic involvement is present, chemotherapy or radiotherapy should be instituted.

145. **What prognostic variables in infants with neuroblastoma predict an unfavorable prognosis?**
   See Table 11-5.

TABLE 11-5. UNFAVORABLE PROGNOSTIC VARIABLES IN INFANTS WITH NEUROBLASTOMA	
Prognostic Variable	**Result**
Shimada histopathology	Unfavorable
N-myc amplification	>10 copies
Catecholamines	Increased VMA, HVA
Serum ferritin	Elevated
Neuron-specific enolase	>100 ng/mL
Stage	III, IV
Tumor cell ploidy	Hyperdiploidy
Karyotype	Terminal 1p deletions

VMA = Vanillylmandelic acid, HVA = homovanillylmandelic acid.

146. **On initial examination, a term male infant is found to have an abdominal mass. A sonogram reveals a right renal mass. What is the probable diagnosis and course of management?**
The most likely diagnosis is congenital mesoblastic nephroma, a monomorphous spindle-cell neoplasm that is a congener of Wilms' tumor diagnosed early in life. Ninety percent of congenital mesoblastic nephromas occur during the first 6 months of life. A meticulous, complete nephrectomy with clear surgical margins is required. Careful observation without additional therapy is curative.

147. **A newborn infant with Down syndrome is found to have a WBC count of 150,000/mm³. What course of management would you recommend to the family?**
Although children with Down syndrome have a 20-fold increased risk for developing acute leukemia as infants, they have a propensity for a "transient leukemia." It is prudent to observe the patient and treat with supportive care measures. In the majority of patients with transient leukemia, the blood counts normalize in several weeks to months without treatment.

148. **On examination, a newborn male is noted to have bilateral leukocoria, or "cat's eye reflex" of the retina. An ophthalmologic exam confirms a diagnosis of retinoblastoma. What features characterize hereditary retinoblastoma?**
- Bilateral presentation
- Diagnosis established at an early age
- May be present in newborns
- Occurs in 20–30% of newly diagnosed cases of retinoblastoma
- Ocular tumors are multifocal
- Arise from a mutation in a germinal cell
- Presence of chromosome 13q14 deletion
- Loss of two retinoblastoma gene alleles
- Offspring may be affected
- Increased risk of second malignant neoplasms, particularly sarcomas

149. **A female infant presents with constipation and is found to have a sacrococcygeal mass. What is the most likely diagnosis?**
Germ cell tumor. Approximately 70% of sacrococcygeal germ cell tumors occur in females, and 50% are diagnosed in the neonatal period. At diagnosis, 50% are benign, 30% are malignant, and 20% have immature embryonic elements (although not frankly malignant have malignant potential). Clinically sacrococcygeal masses may be classified in order of frequency as follows:
- **Type I:** Predominantly external with a minimal presacral component
- **Type II:** External with a significant intrapelvic component
- **Type III:** External with a predominant pelvic mass extending into the abdomen
- **Type IV:** Entirely presacral without an external component

150. **Describe the clinical presentation and management of an infant with familial erythrophagocytic lymphohistiocytosis.**
Familial erythrophagocytic lymphohistiocytosis is a rare, poorly understood disease that has an autosomal recessive pattern of inheritance. It is characterized by a positive family history, hemophagocytosis, and defective cellular and humoral immunity. Infants present with irritability, fever, wasting, hepatosplenomegaly, hyperlipidemia, and coagulopathy. Treatment consists of an exchange transfusion, chemotherapy, and an experimental allogeneic bone marrow transplant. The disease is fatal if not treated.

151. What are the clinical manifestations of Langerhans cell histiocytosis?
The clinical presentation of infants and children with Langerhans cell histiocytosis is varied. The spectrum of symptoms ranges from mild discomfort secondary to lytic bone lesions, diabetes insipidus, seborrhea, and chronic otitis media to generalized symptoms of fever, failure to thrive, hepatosplenomegaly, pulmonary compromise, and bone marrow failure. The diagnosis is confirmed by the presence of Birbeck granules and CD1 expression in lesional cells.

BIBLIOGRAPHY

1. Andrew M, deVeber G: Pediatric Thromboembolism and Stroke Protocols. Hamilton, Ontario, B.C. Decker, 1999.
2. Carbonell-Estrany X, Figueras-Aloy J: Anaemia of prematurity: Treatment with erythropoietin. Early Hum Dev 65 Suppl:S63–S67, 2001.
3. Christensen RD (ed): Hematologic Problems of the Neonate. Philadelphia, W.B. Saunders, 2000.
4. Colman RW, Hirsh J, Marder V, Salzman EW (eds): Hemostasis and Thrombosis: Basic Principles and Clinical Practice, 3rd ed. Philadelphia, J.B. Lippincott, 1994.
5. Flake AW, Zanjani ED: In utero transplantation for thalassemia. Ann NY Acad Sci 850:300–311, 1998.
6. Liley AW: Liquor amnil analysis in the management of pregnancy complicated by resus sensitization. Am J Obstet Gynecol 82:1359–1370, 1961.
7. Link MP (ed): Pediatric Oncology. Pediatric Clinics of North America, vol. 44. Philadelphia, W.B. Saunders, 1997.
8. Manno CS: What's new in transfusion medicine? Pediatr Clin North Am 43:793–808, 1996.
9. Monagle P, Andrew M, Halton J, et al: Homozygous protein C deficiency: Description of a new mutation and successful treatment with low-molecular-weight heparin. Thromb Haemostas 79:756–761, 1998.
10. Nathan DG, Orkin SH, Ginsburg D, Look AT (eds): Nathan and Oski's Hematology of Infancy and Childhood. 6th ed. Philadelphia, W.B. Saunders, 2003.
11. Pizzo PA, Poplack DG (eds): Principles and Practice of Pediatric Oncology, 4th ed. Philadelphia, Lippincott-Raven, 2001.
12. Spitzer AR (ed): Intensive Care of the Fetus and Newborn. St. Louis, Mosby, 1996.
13. Vamvakas EC, Strauss RG: Meta-analysis of controlled clinical trials studying the efficacy of rHuEPO in reducing blood transfusions in the anemia of prematurity. Transfusion 41:406–415, 2001.
14. Young NS, Alter BP (eds): Aplastic Anemia: Acquired and Inherited. Philadelphia, W.B. Saunders, 1994.

CHAPTER 12

INFECTION AND IMMUNITY

Mary Catherine Harris, MD, David A. Munson, MD

1. **What is the maternal contribution of immunoglobulin (IG) G to the fetus and newborn infant? How quickly does it disappear postnatally?**
    The IgG content of the fetus and the newborn infant is mainly maternal in origin. Levels of all classes of IgG fall rapidly after birth, and the respective concentrations derived from the maternal placental transfer and active production by the young infant are approximately equal by 2 months postnatal age. By 10–12 months of age, catabolism of passively acquired IgG is complete, and all circulating IgG is produced by the infant (Fig. 12-1).

2. **What are the principal types of IgA in a newborn infant?**
    Because IgA does not cross the placenta, all the IgA in neonatal serum and secretions is derived from the baby. The two principal types are IgA_1 and IgA_2. Some of their properties are summarized in Table 12-1. Despite the presence of circulating IgA_1 at birth, the respiratory and gastrointestinal (GI) tracts remain vulnerable to the entry of infectious organisms in the absence of secretory IgA_2.

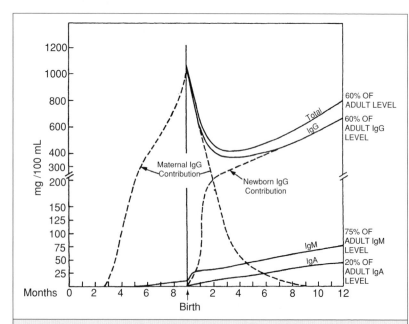

Figure 12-1. Maternal contribution of IgG to fetus and neonate. (From Wilson CB, Lewis DB, Penix LA: The physiologic immunodeficiency of immaturity. In Stiehm R [ed]: Immunologic Disorders in Infants and Children, 4th ed. Philadelphia, W.B. Saunders, 1996, pp 253–295.)

TABLE 12-1. PRINCIPAL TYPES OF IgA IN THE NEONATE

	IgA$_1$	IgA$_2$
IgA subunits	Monomer	Dimer
J-piece and secretory component	Absent	Present
Major site	Serum	Secretions
Presence at birth	Yes	No
Adult levels attained	16 years to adulthood	6–8 years

3. **What are the levels of serum complement at birth relative to the adult?**
Complement components are synthesized as early as 6–14 weeks of gestation. However, levels of virtually all components of both the classic and alternative pathways are reduced at birth in term and preterm newborn infants, with greater deficits noted in the latter. Overall activity and components of the alternative pathway are more consistently decreased than those of the classical pathway. This finding is especially problematic for neonates who are exposed to organisms with polysaccharide capsules such as *Escherichia coli* K1 and group B *Streptococcus* (GBS) and who cannot rely on classical pathway activation due to the lack of specific antibodies. In addition to differences in concentration, functional differences in C3 have also been described, resulting in deficits of opsonization.

4. **What phenomena are responsible for "depletion" or "exhaustion" neutropenia in neonates?**
The precursors of neutrophils, the colony-forming unit–granulocyte macrophage, appear to proliferate at or near the maximal rate in neonates under baseline conditions. Consequently, these cells may not be able to increase their number in response to infection. In addition, the postmitotic storage pool in the bone marrow is small relative to the circulating pool in neonates (approximately 2–3:1) compared with adults (approximately 10–15:1).
   The neutrophil storage pool compartment expands during development. Although the data in humans are not as precise, evidence suggests similar patterns with relatively small pools expanding into large ones with advancing age. Thus, the small neonatal storage pools are rapidly released from the bone marrow in response to infection and cannot be readily replaced by the early neutrophilic precursors that are already in a state of maximal proliferation. As a result, rather than develop neutrophilia as might occur in the adult, the neonate will rapidly develop neutropenia due to exhaustion or depletion of his or her storage pools.

5. **When do thymocytes first appear during fetal life, and what are their stages of development?**
Prothymocytes bearing the CD7 and CD34 surface antigens enter the thymus at approximately 8.5 weeks' gestation. As the separation between the thymic cortex and medulla becomes apparent after 12 weeks, thymocytes localize according to their stage of maturation. Subcapsular thymocytes (type I) are negative for CD3, a molecule whose interaction with T-cell receptors is critical for the function of the latter, as well as negative for CD4 and CD8. Cortical thymocytes (type II) are positive for expression of CD3, CD4, and CD8. During this stage, the process of "positive" and "negative" selection occurs, resulting in selective survival of cells with specificities for a particular repertoire of antigens. Type III thymocytes located in the medulla are CD3 positive and express either CD4 *or* CD8. This latter cell type is the immediate precursor to the peripheral T lymphocyte (Fig. 12-2).

6. **When does cell-mediated immunity mature in the fetus?**
By the twelfth week of gestation, lymphocytes obtained from the human thymus respond to mitogens and foreign histocompatibility antigens. Furthermore, fetal cells stimulated with alloantigens exhibit normal antigen-specific cytotoxicity. In contrast, the phenotypic appearance and proportion of circulating cells are diminished, and the production of some cytokines is reduced in neonates. The most significant defect appears to be a deficiency of memory T cells, which may be responsible for the deficient production of interferon-γ in the neonate.

7. **How do neutrophils in a neonate differ functionally from those in an adult?**
Despite the conflicting data in the literature, there is enough information to demonstrate that neonatal neutrophils are deficient in adherence, deformability, and chemotaxis. These properties would result in a relatively slow influx of neutrophils into sites of microbial invasions, resulting in rapidly progressive infections (Table 12-2).

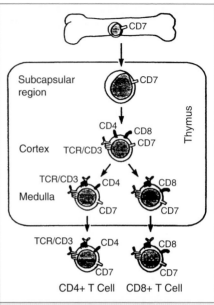

Figure 12-2. Development of thymocytes. (From Lewis DB, Wilson CB: Developmental immunology and role of host defenses in fetal and neonatal susceptibility to infection. In Remington JS, Klein JO [eds]: Infectious Diseases of the Fetus and Newborn Infant, 5th ed. Philadelphia, W.B. Saunders, 2001, pp 25–138.)

8. **Why do newborn infants respond poorly to polysaccharide vaccines or encapsulated bacteria such as GBS?**
The ability of the B lymphocytes to respond to specific antigens develops chronologically and in a manner that depends on whether the response requires T lymphocyte "help." In humans and in mice, the antigens can be divided into three groups based on the nature of the immune response: (1) thymus-dependent (TD) antigens, which include most protein antigens, (2) thymus-independent type 1 (TI-1) antigens, which bind directly to B lymphocytes and do not require T cells at all for antibody production, and (3) thymus-independent type 2 (TI-2) antigens, which are mostly polysaccharides composed of multiple identical subunits and require small numbers of T lymphocytes for antibody production to occur. The response to TI-2 antigens appears last chronologically at approximately 6 months of age, accounting for the poor neonatal response to polysaccharide vaccines and to infection with encapsulated organisms such as GBS. Interestingly, although the *Haemophilus influenzae* type B polyribosol ribitol phosphate (PRP) vaccine is poorly immunogenic in neonates, the coupling of *H. influenzae* polysaccharide to carrier proteins renders it immunogenic by converting it from a TI-2 antigen to a TD antigen, for which responsiveness is already present at birth.

9. **Why are neonates particularly susceptible to infection with viruses such as herpes simplex?**
The defenses against viral infections involve numerous mechanisms, including antibody neutralization of extracellular virus, direct cytolysis of infected cells by natural killer (NK) cells, and antibody-dependent cellular cytotoxicity as well as specific cell-mediated cytotoxicity through T lymphocytes. Neonatal patients have deficits in virtually all of these components.

TABLE 12–2.	NEUTROPHILS IN NEONATES VERSUS ADULTS
Characteristic	**Neonate Function Versus Adult**
Neutrophils in circulation	↑
Neutrophil storage pool	↓
Adherence	↓
Adhesion content and regulation	Abnormal
Deformability	↓
Locomotion	
Random migration	Normal
Chemotaxis	↓
Binding of chemotactic factors	Normal
Signal transduction	Some elements abnormal
Phagocytosis	Normal
Degranulation	Normal
Lactoferrin content	↓
Bactericidal capacity	Normal (↓ during stress) respiratory burst
O_2^-, H_2O_2	Normal or ↑
OH, chemiluminescence	Normal or ↓

Note: Some functions have not been studied thoroughly, and the biochemical basis for most defects is not understood.
Adapted from Speer CP, Johnson RB: Neutrophil function in newborn infants. In Polin RA, Fox WW (eds): Fetal and Neonatal Physiology, 2nd ed. Philadelphia, W.B. Saunders, 1998, pp 1954–1998.

Infants infected at the time of parturition depend on the presence of passively acquired maternal antibody, which will not be present in large quantities in mothers with primary infection, the setting in which the most severe neonatal infection occurs. Insofar as NK cells are concerned, they appear early in gestation and reach normal numbers by mid to late gestation. However, even at term, they are largely immature in phenotype, consisting of 50% CD56-negative cells. These cells are deficient in their ability to kill virus-infected cells and in the ability to produce critical cytokines such as interferon-γ. Furthermore, virus-specific T-cell–mediated immunity is also diminished or delayed in the human neonate with decreased T-cell killing and production of interferon-γ. Consequently, infection with herpes simplex virus (HSV) in the neonate can result in a rapidly progressive, fulminant, and often fatal infection.

10. **In a young infant with prolonged retention of the umbilical cord and recurrent severe infections, what diagnosis should be considered?**
Leukocyte adhesion deficiency type I. This disorder is caused by a mutation in the CD18 gene, whose product is required for the expression of the β_2 integrins on the membranes of leukocytes. This group of surface molecules consists of Mac-1, leukocyte function–associated antigen 1, p 150, 95 (which are heterodimers of CD11a, CD11b, and CD11c, respectively), and CD18 and are essential to the ability of neutrophils to adhere to and migrate within sites of inflammation. As a result, patients with this disorder will demonstrate a virtual absence of neutrophils in inflammatory exudates despite marked elevations of peripheral blood leukocyte counts. Patients with leukocyte adhesion deficiency type I are highly susceptible to life-threatening infections of the skin, mucous membranes, and the GI tract, with the degree of severity

varying with the degree of expression of the β_2 integrins. For example, patients with moderately severe disease who express these molecules at 2.5–6.0% of normal values have been described. Delayed separation of the cord, which normally occurs on the average at 15.0 ± 7.2 days, has been described in some of the most severe patients. Diagnosis can be made through use of specific immunophenotyping reagents to demonstrate the severe reduction in expression of the β_2 integrins.

KEY POINTS: CLINICAL PRESENTATION OF HERPES SIMPLEX VIRUS

1. Skin-eye-mouth (SEM) disease is typically the earliest presentation and has the best prognosis.

2. Systemic infection usually presents in the second or third week of life and can manifest as a severe sepsis syndrome.

3. CNS involvement is typically the latest presentation.

4. There is considerable overlap in the time of onset of these three clinical classifications.

5. Acyclovir should be started in the event of suspicion of any type of HSV infection.

11. **What factors diminish the capacity of neutrophils derived from preterm infants to kill bacterial pathogens?**
Respiratory distress syndrome and sepsis decrease bactericidal activity of neutrophils isolated from preterm infants. A low neutrophil-to-bacterial ratio (1:100) is also associated with decreased bacterial killing. Certain bacterial strains (*E. coli*, *Staphylococcus aureus*, and GBS) are more readily killed by neutrophils isolated from well term neonates and adult subjects than those from preterm infants.

12. **What neutrophil defect causes chronic granulomatous disease?**
Chronic granulomatous disease is due to a variety of molecular defects. The most common one is a mutation in the gene encoding for the subunit of cytochrome b558, which is located on the x chromosome. Cytochrome b558 is part of the NADPH oxidizing complex. Abnormalities in this complex result in inadequate generation of superoxide anion and other reactive oxygen intermediates. Deficiency of these reactive oxygen intermediates results in poor bactericidal activity and recurrent infections. Treatment includes prophylactic antibiotics, aggressive antibiotic treatment of infections, steroids, and interferon-γ. Bone marrow transplantation has been successful.

13. **What is the most common neutrophil defect observed in neonates treated with high doses of glucocorticoids?**
The anti-inflammatory effects of glucocorticoids primarily affect granulocyte trafficking. Neutrophils demonstrate diminished adhesion to vascular endothelium. This may be due in part to diminished endothelial and leukocyte expression of adhesion molecules as a result of decreased macrophage production of proinflammatory mediators (e.g., cytokines, arachidonic acid metabolites, and platelet-activating factor).

14. **Which of the following components of neonatal host defense constitutes the primary barrier to invasive infections?**
A. Neutrophils
B. Macrophages

C. Skin and mucous membranes
D. NK cells
C. Skin and mucous membranes are the primary defense against invading microbes. Neutrophils, macrophages, and NK cells attempt to eradicate those organisms that manage to bypass the primary defense barrier. The high incidence of nosocomial infections in preterm neonates may not be effectively diminished until new strategies that augment skin and mucous membrane defense mechanisms are discovered.

EARLY-ONSET NEONATAL SEPSIS: EPIDEMIOLOGY

15. **How has the use of maternal intrapartum antibiotics altered the incidence of early-onset neonatal sepsis?**
    Since consensus guidelines were developed in 1996 and subsequently revised in 2002, the incidence of early-onset GBS infections has declined by 65% overall with a 75% decline in black infants. During the same time period, however, intrapartum antibiotic administration has been associated with an increased incidence of drug-resistant neonatal sepsis, particularly ampicillin-resistant gram-negative disease in very-low-birth-weight (VLBW) infants (<1500 gm).

16. **Which maternal and neonatal factors increase the infant's risk of early-onset disease?**
    Several obstetric and neonatal factors have been identified that may be associated with an increased risk of neonatal infection. The presence of any of these factors alone is not an indication for a complete sepsis work-up and antibiotic therapy; however, combinations of risk factors are clearly additive and should greatly enhance the suspicion of sepsis (Table 12-3).

TABLE 12-3. RISK FACTORS FOR PERINATALLY ACQUIRED NEONATAL BACTERIAL INFECTION

Maternal	Neonatal
Prolonged rupture of membranes >18–24 hour	Prematurity
Premature rupture of membranes (<37 wk)	Low birth weight (<2500 gm)
Maternal fever ≥100.4°F	Male gender
Maternal chorioamnionitis	5-minute Apgar score <6
Maternal colonization with GBS	
GBS bacteriuria	
Previous infant with invasive GBS disease	
Maternal urinary tract infection at delivery	
Multiple gestation (?)	

Adapted from Eichenwald EC: Perinatally transmitted neonatal bacterial infections. Infect Dis Clin North Am 11:226–239, 1997.

17. **What is the attack rate for neonatal sepsis in the presence of the above risk factors?**
    As a general rule of thumb, presence of a major risk factor (such as premature rupture of fetal membranes or maternal GBS colonization) leads to a sepsis attack rate of about 1% for proven sepsis or 2% for proven or highly suspected sepsis. If a second risk factor is present, the attack rate rises to 4–6% for proven and 10% for proven or highly suspected sepsis. Further risk factors are additive; the presence of three risk factors raises the sepsis risk 25-fold over baseline with no risk factors.

18. **How has the epidemiology of early-onset sepsis changed in a VLBW infant (<1500 gm)?**
     Among VLBW infants, the incidence of early-onset sepsis increases with decreasing gestational age (15 cases/1000 live births versus 2.5 cases/1000 live births in term infants). Compared with data derived before the inception of guidelines for the prevention of GBS disease, there has been a significant reduction in early-onset GBS disease from 5.9 to 1.7 cases per 1000 live births and an increase in *E. coli* sepsis from 3.2 to 6.8 per 1000 live births. Eighty-five percent of the *E. coli* isolates have been resistant to ampicillin. When the years 1991–1993 were compared with 1998–2000, there was also an increase in the incidence of early-onset fungal disease from 0.1 to 0.4 per 1000 live births.

     Stoll BJ, Hansen N, Fanaroff AA, et al: Changes in pathogens causing early-onset sepsis in very-low-birth-weight infants. N Engl J Med 347:240–247, 2002.

19. **What is the mortality associated with sepsis in VLBW infants?**
     Despite improvements in neonatal care and the use of broad-spectrum antimicrobial agents, the mortality for early-onset disease in VLBW neonates is 37%. The mortality is higher with gram-negative than with gram-positive pathogens (41% versus 26%).

20. **What is the distribution of pathogens among term and preterm neonates with early-onset sepsis?**
     Although the increased use of peripartum antibiotics has resulted in an overall decline in early-onset disease, GBS sepsis occurs most commonly in infants >37 weeks' gestational age and with birth weights >2500 gm. In contrast, infants infected with bacteria other than GBS are more likely to be born preterm and with low birth weight.

     Hyde TB, Hilger TM, Reingold A, et al: Trends in incidence and antimicrobial resistance of early-onset sepsis: Population-based surveillance in San Francisco and Atlanta. Pediatrics 110:690–695, 2002.

NOSOCOMIAL SEPSIS

21. **What are nosocomial infections?**
     By definition, these are infections that develop in hospitalized patients that were neither present nor incubating at the time of admission.

22. **What percentage of VLBW infants develop a nosocomial infection?**
     Approximately 25% of VLBW infants will develop one or more episodes of blood culture-proven late-onset sepsis. Rates of infection are inversely related to birth weight and gestational age.

23. **What is the major risk factor for late-onset GBS disease?**
     Prematurity is the major risk factor for late-onset GBS disease. The risk increases for each week of decreasing gestation. Other risk factors include African-American heritage and positive GBS culture in the mother.

     Lin FC, Weisman LE, Troendle J, et al: Prematurity is the major risk factor for late-onset group B streptococcal disease. J Infect Dis 188:267–271, 2003.

24. **What are the most common nosocomial pathogens isolated from VLBW infants?**
     In recent years, coagulase-negative staphylococci (CONS) have emerged as the most frequently isolated pathogens responsible for late-onset sepsis. Other pathogens associated with late-onset sepsis include GBS, *S. aureus*, *E. coli*, *Enterococcus*, *Klebsiella* species, *Enterobacter*, *Pseudomonas aeruginosa*, and fungi (especially *Candida albicans*).

25. **What are the adverse consequences of late-onset infections among VLBW infants?**
    - Patent ductus arteriosus
    - Prolonged length of mechanical ventilation
    - Prolonged need for total parenteral nutrition and need for indwelling catheters
    - Necrotizing enterocolitis
    - Prolonged length of hospitalization
    - Increased cost of care
    - Increased risk of death

26. **What factors distinguish early-onset infections from late-onset infections and late, late-onset infections?**
    See Table 12-4.

TABLE 12-4. CHARACTERISTICS OF EARLY- AND LATER-ONSET INFECTIONS			
Characteristic	Early-Onset	Late-Onset	Late, Late-Onset
Age at onset	Birth to 7 days	7–30 days	>30 days
Maternal obstetric complications	Common	Uncommon	Varies
Prematurity	Frequent	Varies	Usual, especially if birth weight is <1000 gm
Source of organism	Maternal genital tract	Maternal genital tract or environment	Environment/community
Clinical presentation	Multisystem	Multisystem or focal	Multisystem or focal
Mortality rate	10–20%	5–10%	<5%

Adapted from Baker CJ: Group B streptococcal infections. Clin Perinatol 24:59–70, 1997.

27. **What are the major risk factors for late-onset neonatal sepsis?**
    See Table 12-5.

DIAGNOSIS OF NEONATAL SEPSIS

28. **What is the significance of maternal fever (defined as ≥100.4°F)?**
    If the fever is one of a constellation of symptoms for the diagnosis of chorioamnionitis (fever plus two or more other abnormalities including fetal tachycardia, uterine tenderness, foul vaginal discharge, or maternal leukocytosis), there is a significant sepsis risk for the neonate, with reported attack rates ranging from 6% to 20%. However, if the fever is isolated, the sepsis attack rate is low. This issue is further compounded by the use of epidural anesthesia, which is associated with maternal fever without raising the neonatal sepsis rate. If the maternal fever is >101°F, there is a risk of other adverse outcomes for the neonate, including seizures.
    Lieberman E, Lang J, Richardson DK, et al: Intrapartum maternal fever and neonatal outcome. Pediatrics 105:8–13, 2000.

29. **What are the presenting signs and symptoms of neonatal sepsis?**
    The signs and symptoms of neonatal sepsis are protean and nonspecific. Almost any symptom in the neonate may be an indication of sepsis, but there is extensive overlap with

TABLE 12-5. RISK FACTORS FOR LATE-ONSET NEONATAL SEPSIS	
Risk Factor	Comments
Prematurity/low birth weight	Risk of infection is inversely related to gestational age and birth weight.
Intravascular catheters	Intravascular catheters provide a portal of entry for infectious organisms, and risk of infection is directly related to the number of catheter days.
Parenteral nutrition	TPN requires vascular access, which increases risk; intralipids enhance the growth of lipophilic organisms, particularly coagulase-negative staphylococci and *Malassezia furfur.*
Enteral nutrition	Human milk decreases and formula feeding increases risk.
Intubation/ventilation	Endotracheal intubation provides a portal of entry for colonization infection with potential pathogens.
Invasive procedures	Provide portal of entry for organisms by breaking the skin and mucous membrane barriers.
Medications	Dexamethasone and H_2 blocker use increase risk of infection; widespread and prolonged use of broad-spectrum antibiotics may predispose to infections caused by resistant organisms and/or fungi.
Hospitalization	Prolonged length of stay increases risk of exposure to hospital pathogens.
Overcrowding/ understaffing	Increases the likelihood of poor infection control practices (especially poor handwashing), which increase the risk of infection.

TN = Total parenteral nutrition.

other conditions and with normal newborn transitional findings. They include fever, respiratory distress, jaundice, lethargy, irritability, anorexia or vomiting, hypotonia, "not looking well," abdominal distension, hypothermia, hypoglycemia, apnea, seizures, shock, petechiae, and purpura.

30. **With all of these possible signs of sepsis, how does one differentiate sepsis from other conditions, particularly after antibiotics have been started and decisions need to be made regarding duration of treatment?**
Laboratory data are important, including cultures and sepsis screen strategies. It is important to remember that sepsis usually presents with a constellation of signs and symptoms, which usually persist for more than 12 hours even when treated. If signs resolve quickly and one makes a firm diagnosis of a noninfectious condition such as transient tachypnea of the newborn or transitional hypoglycemia, sepsis is unlikely.

31. **How reliable is blood culture in the diagnosis of neonatal sepsis?**
Unfortunately, the sensitivity of the blood culture is not very high in this condition. In patients with well-defined clinical GBS sepsis, only 50% may have positive blood culture results. In studies of neonates who died, the postmortem diagnosis of sepsis was confirmed by premortem blood cultures in only 80% of cases. The current extensive use of maternal antibiotic administration further confounds the reliability of the blood culture.

32. **Should a urine culture be part of the work-up for sepsis in the newborn infant?**
Urine cultures are of low yield in the evaluation of infants with possible early-onset sepsis. However, suprapubic aspiration or bladder catheterization should be performed in all infants in whom late-onset sepsis is suspected.

33. **When should lumbar puncture be performed?**
In retrospective studies, early-onset meningitis was detected in 1–2% of lumbar punctures performed. However, if there are no symptoms of meningitis and the sepsis evaluation is done for nonspecific reasons or for respiratory distress, the incidence of meningitis is either 0% or <1%. On the other hand, Wiswell and colleagues reported that 37% of cases of meningitis would be missed if one relied on symptoms or positive blood culture results and that at least 15% of proven meningitis occurs with a negative blood culture result. Because neonatal meningitis is a low-incidence disease (0.25/1000 live births), an informal meta-analysis of published reports shows that one would need to do at least 1000 lumbar punctures to diagnose one case that would be missed by lack of symptoms or a negative blood culture result.

   One rational approach is to perform a lumbar puncture if there are symptoms of meningitis *or* if sepsis is the leading diagnosis. One would not perform the lumbar puncture if respiratory distress or nonspecific symptoms have led to a sepsis evaluation, but sepsis is a secondary consideration.

   Wiswell TE, Baumgart S, Gannon CM, Spitzer AR: No lumbar puncture in the evaluation for early neonatal sepsis: Will meningitis be missed? Pediatrics 95:803–806, 1995.

34. **Which characteristics of laboratory tests (e.g., sensitivity, specificity, positive predictive accuracy, and negative predictive accuracy) are most important for the diagnosis of neonatal sepsis?**
The ideal laboratory test is one in which sensitivity, specificity, positive predictive accuracy, and negative predictive accuracy are all high. Unfortunately, no tests for sepsis fulfill those criteria. Specificity and positive predictive accuracy are less important because the treatment of neonatal sepsis is relatively benign and unlikely to result in serious medical consequences. Tests with a high negative predictive accuracy are particularly useful because the purpose of laboratory testing is to exclude "disease" in uninfected babies who do not require antibiotics or in whom antibiotics can be discontinued at the earliest possible time.

35. **What is the relevance of C-reactive protein (CRP) in the diagnosis of neonatal sepsis?**
Serum CRP is an acute phase reactant, which becomes elevated in the face of inflammation or infection, with a response time of 6–8 hours. The normal value in the neonate is <1.0 mg/dL. An elevated CRP level 12–24 hours after the onset of possible sepsis has a positive predictive value of only 7–43%, but a negative predictive value of 97–99.5%; thus, CRP is quite useful in ruling out sepsis. A marked elevation of CRP level (>5.0 mg/dL) has a positive predictive value for sepsis of 10%.

   Benitz WE, Han MY, Madan A, Ramachandra P: Serial serum C-reactive protein levels in the diagnosis of neonatal infection. Pediatrics 102:E41, 1998.
   Gerdes JS: Clinicopathologic approach to the diagnosis of neonatal sepsis. Perinatol 18:361–381, 1991.

36. **Can a normal white blood cell (WBC) count, immature-to-total (I:T) neutrophil ratio, neutrophil count, or CRP measurement be used to rule out sepsis on admission?**
Unfortunately not. Neither these nor any other tests can be used to reliably rule out infection in neonates. The usefulness of the tests improves markedly with serial measurements because there have been many cases of sepsis described in which the WBC count or CRP level became abnormal 12–24 hours after the onset of the disease. Furthermore, these

tests can be combined in a sepsis screen in which several parameters are used to improve the diagnostic accuracy.

37. **What clinical factors affect neutrophil counts?**
See Table 12-6.

TABLE 12-6.   CLINICAL FACTORS THAT AFFECT NEUTROPHIL COUNTS

	Total Neutrophils		Total Immature Increase	Increased I:T Ratio	Approximate Duration
Complication	Decrease	Increase			
Maternal hypertension	++++	0	+	+	72 hours
Maternal fever, neonate healthy	0	++	+++	++++	24 hours
≥6 hours intrapartum oxytocin	0	++	++	++++	120 hours
Stressful labor	0	+++	++++	++++	24 hours
Asphyxia (5-minute Apgar score ≤5)	+	++	++	+++	24–60 hours
Meconium aspiration syndrome	0	++++	+++	++	72 hours
Pneumothorax with uncomplicated hyaline membrane disease	0	++++	++++	++++	24 hours
Periventricular hemorrhage, no seizures	+++	+	++	++++	120 hours
Seizures—no hypoglycemia, asphyxia, or central nervous system hemorrhage	0	+++	+++	++++	24 hours
Prolonged (≥4 min) crying	0	++++	++++	++++	1 hour
Asymptomatic blood sugar ≤30 mg/dL	0	++	+++	+++	24 hours
Hemolytic disease	++	++	+++	++	7–28 days
Surgery	0	++++	++++	+++	24 hours
High altitude	0	++++	++++	0	6 hours

+ = 0–25% affected, ++ = 26–50% affected, +++ = 51–75% affected, ++++ = 76–100% affected.
Adapted from Powell K, Marcy M: Laboratory aids in the diagnosis of neonatal sepsis. In Remington JS, Klein JO (eds): Infectious Diseases of the Fetus and Newborn Infant. Philadelphia, W.B. Saunders, 2001, pp 1327–1344.

38. **When evaluating an infant for possible sepsis, when is the best time to obtain a WBC count and differential count?**

Counts obtained immediately after birth are frequently normal because there has not been sufficient time for inflammatory mediators to disturb neutrophil indices. Counts obtained 12–24 hours after birth are more likely to be abnormal in infants with sepsis. In a symptomatic infant (term or preterm), delaying the WBC for 12–24 hours should pose no problem because most symptomatic infants are treated with antibiotics empirically. In these infants, the main issue is whether antibiotics can be discontinued before a full course of treatment is given. In asymptomatic infants, an "early" WBC or differential count should only be obtained if it will influence the decision to begin antibiotics.

39. **What studies are useful in creating a sepsis screen strategy?**

Although diagnostic tests are frequently ordered to identify infants with probable sepsis, their main benefit is to exclude disease in infants with a low probability of infection. A combination of diagnostic tests improves the predictive values over use of a single test. In this strategy, serial sepsis screens that have negative results substantially reduce the likelihood that the infant has sepsis. One suggested sepsis screen is given in Table 12-7. The screen result is considered positive if 2 or more points are present. It is important to recognize that no sepsis screen is perfect, and one should err on the side of caution with neonatal sepsis.

TABLE 12-7. PARAMETERS FOR SEPSIS SCREEN STRATEGY	
Test	Point Value
Absolute neutrophil count <1750/mm^3	1 point
Total WBC <7500 or >40,000/mm^3	1 point
I:T neutrophil ratio ≥0.2	1 point
I:T neutrophil ratio ≥0.4	2 points
CRP+ (≥1.0 mg/dL)	1 point
CRP+ (≥5.0 mg/dL)	2 points

40. **Are cytokine determinations helpful in the diagnosis of neonatal sepsis?**

A number of inflammatory mediators have been investigated as possible diagnostic tests for neonatal sepsis. Interleukin (IL) -6, IL-8, and IL-10 have been found to have a critical role in the inflammatory response during neonatal sepsis; however, none of these mediators has sufficient sensitivity or specificity for the diagnosis of infection in this population. These markers may be most useful in understanding the pathophysiology of infection.

ANTIMICROBIAL THERAPY

41. **Ampicillin is used in conjunction with gentamicin as empiric therapy for early-onset sepsis. Why is ampicillin used?**

Ampicillin is the antimicrobial of choice for treatment of GBS, *Listeria monocytogenes*, and most enterococci. Other β-lactam antibiotics have acceptable activity against GBS, but only ampicillin provides good coverage for *Listeria* organisms and enterococci.

42. **Is cefotaxime an acceptable alternative to gentamicin?**

The third-generation cephalosporins (such as cefotaxime and ceftazidime) have excellent activity against GBS and gram-negative organisms. Some data, however, indicate that resistance of gram-negative organisms developed rapidly when cefotaxime was used for presumptive therapy. In addition, a recent publication has found that there is a higher neonatal mortality rate with the use of cefotaxime compared with gentamicin. Furthermore, the third-generation cephalosporins are not active against *Listeria* and *Enterococcus* species. Therefore, it is prudent to restrict their usage to infants with meningitis due to susceptible gram-negative organisms.

Clark RE, Bloom BT, Spitzer AR, Gerstmann DR: Empiric use of ampicillin and cefotaxime compared to ampicillin and gentamicin is associated with an increased risk of death for neonates at risk for sepsis. Pediatrics 117:67–74, 2006.

43. **What are the theoretical advantages of third-generation cephalosporins?**
   - Toxicity is low.
   - Measurement of serum levels is unnecessary.

   Note: Cefotaxime is the third-generation cephalosporin of choice because it is not excreted in the bile and has been used extensively in neonates.

44. **Why shouldn't ceftriaxone be used in neonates?**
   Ceftriaxone can displace bilirubin from albumin and may increase the risk of kernicterus in a jaundiced infant.

45. **How long should proven bacterial sepsis be treated?**
   There are as many answers to this question as there are neonatologists in the world. The following are commonly accepted guidelines:
   - **Bacterial sepsis with minimal or absent focal infection:** 7–10 days
   - **Gram-negative meningitis:** 21 days
   - **Gram-positive meningitis:** 14 days

   However, in all cases, a negative result from a blood or cerebrospinal fluid (CSF) culture should be documented 48 hours after the institution of antimicrobial therapy.

46. **What is acceptable empiric therapy for late-onset sepsis?**
   Because *Staphylococcus epidermidis* is the most common cause of nosocomial sepsis in neonates, empiric therapy should include vancomycin. This antibiotic is generally paired with an aminoglycoside antibiotic to cover gram-negative organisms.

47. **What are the major adverse reactions to antimicrobials commonly used in neonates?**
   See Table 12-8.

GROUP B STREPTOCOCCAL INFECTIONS

48. **Early-onset GBS disease occurs after maternal GBS colonization. Are there other adverse outcomes of pregnancy associated with maternal GBS colonization?**
   Higher titer colonization is associated with:
   - Early fetal loss
   - Premature rupture of membranes
   - Preterm labor
   - Low birth weight
   - Maternal sepsis
   - Maternal chorioamnionitis

49. **Are special methods needed to isolate GBS?**
   The majority of studies using selective broth media containing antibiotics (e.g., nalidixic acid, gentamicin, colistin) demonstrate at least a twofold greater yield of positive culture results from

TABLE 12–8. ADVERSE EFFECTS OF ANTIBIOTICS

Antibiotic	Adverse Effects
Ampicillin	Rare hypersensitivity reactions[*]
Amphotericin B	Hypokalemia
	Reversible nephrotoxicity due to reduced glomerular filtration rate
Acyclovir	Reversible renal dysfunction caused by the formation of acyclovir crystals in renal tubules[†]
Cefotaxime	Rare, occasional leukopenia
Ceftriaxone	Displaces bilirubin from albumin, resulting in higher bilirubin concentrations
	Gallbladder sludging
Gentamicin	Irreversible ototoxicity and reversible nephrotoxicity
Vancomycin	Rare nephrotoxicity, enhanced by combination with an aminoglycoside
	Red man syndrome (rash and hypotension)[‡]

[*]Hypersensitivity reactions are not commonly seen in the neonatal period.
[†]Adequate hydration helps to prevent this complication.
[‡]Appears rapidly and resolves within minutes to hours. Lengthening infusion time usually eliminates risk for subsequent doses.

genital and rectal sites of adults in comparison to nonselective methods. This is because of the suppression of overgrowth by co-colonizing bacteria. Current guidelines from the Centers for Disease Control and Prevention (CDC) suggest specific procedures for collecting and processing clinical specimens for GBS culture and susceptibility testing. On the other hand, standard laboratory methods for the isolation of GBS from blood and spinal fluid are fully adequate.

50. **Is GBS sexually transmissible?**
Yes. Several studies in the 1970s demonstrated increased efficacy of antepartum treatment to eradicate GBS colonization by concurrent treatment of sexual partners of colonized women, supporting the speculation that these organisms can be sexually transmitted. A definitive study from Japan published in 1999 demonstrated sexual transmission and reinfection during pregnancy in longitudinal studies of couples with a 92% serotype concurrence among infected couples.
   Although it is apparent that GBS is sexually transmissible, epidemiologic data for GBS colonization are significantly different from those of classic sexually transmitted diseases, such as gonorrhea and *Chlamydia trachomatis*. GBS colonization is most common in women of older age, lower parity, and limited sexual activity based on number of sexual partners/lifetime and age at onset of sexual activity.

KEY POINTS: CURRENT APPROACH TO GBS

1. Screen all pregnant women between 35 and 37 weeks' gestation for GBS colonization.

2. Treat at-risk mothers at the time of delivery, including those who tested positive, women delivering a previously infected infant, and those with GBS-positive urine cultures.

3. Early-onset disease is decreasing in incidence as a consequence of these interventions, but late-onset disease is not.

51. **What are the patterns of GBS colonization during pregnancy?**
Although the prevalence of maternal colonization ranges from 15% to 40%, chronic, intermittent, or transient patterns of GBS colonization have been described. It is known that women can acquire the organism throughout pregnancy from sexual partners, so cultures remote from term are unlikely to be predictive of colonization status at delivery. Moreover, women who are chronically, heavily colonized have a significantly higher risk of delivering infants with early-onset GBS disease. The yield is greatest when GBS cultures are obtained during the last several weeks of pregnancy.

52. **How many serotypes of GBS have been identified? What is the clinical and immunologic significance of the serotypes?**
Seven serotypes have been identified: Ia, II, III, IV, V, VI, and VIII. Early studies of GBS disease in North America demonstrated a predominance of type III, thought also to be the most virulent serotype. It remains the most commonly isolated serotype to cause meningitis in the United States. Since the 1970s, there has been a progressive change in the predominance of serotypes, with type Ia now the leading cause of early-onset infection. During the last decade, several new serotypes have been identified.

Serotype V, initially isolated from nonpregnant HIV-positive adults in the United States, has become a common colonizing serotype among healthy, pregnant women.

Serotype IV is more commonly isolated in Europe, and serotypes VI and VIII predominate in Asia.

From an immunologic and public health perspective, the recognition of multiple new serotypes has confounded the efforts of investigators to develop an effective multivalent vaccine to prevent this disease in newborns.

53. **What are the major distinguishing characteristics of early-and late-onset GBS disease?**
See Table 12-9.

TABLE 12-9. DISTINGUISHING CHARACTERISTICS OF EARLY- AND LATE-ONSET DISEASES

	Early-Onset Disease	Late-Onset Disease
Age at onset*	First 7 days of life	Beyond day 7
Symptoms	Respiratory distress, apnea, PPHN, hypotension	Irritability, fever, poor feeding
Serotypes	All	All
Mode of transmission	Vertical transmission from mother to infant	Nosocomial acquisition
CDC IAP†	50–65% reduction in attack rate	No effect

PPHN = Persistent pulmonary hypertension of the newborn.
*Ages at onset were once (classically) defined as early onset occurring during the first 5 days of life and late onset occurring beyond day 10. Recent surveillance studies have redefined early onset as <day 7 and late onset as >day 7.
†CDC recommendations for intrapartum antibiotic prophylaxis (IAP) to prevent GBS disease.

54. **What is the optimal strategy for the identification of mothers who should receive intrapartum GBS prophylaxis?**
A recent population-based study compared the efficacy of screening cultures versus a risk factor (e.g., fever, prolonged rupture of membranes, preterm delivery) approach for the prevention of early-onset GBS disease. In this study, screening was more than 50% more effective than the risk factor approach; 18% of GBS-colonized mothers had a positive culture result in the absence of risk factors for disease. The efficacy of antibiotics in the screened group was 89%.

   Schrag SJ, Zell ER, Stat M, et al: A population-based comparison of strategies to prevent early-onset group B streptococcal disease in neonates. N Engl J Med 347:233–239, 2002.

55. **What are the CDC recommendations for IAP to prevent early-onset GBS disease?**
The 2002 CDC consensus guidelines (Fig. 12-3) recommend use of an antepartum screening strategy for the empiric management of newborns born to mothers who have received intrapartum antibiotic prophylaxis (IAP) or to treat suspected chorioamnionitis.

56. **What are the recommended regimens for intrapartum antimicrobial prophylaxis for GBS prevention?**
   - **Recommended:** Penicillin G, 5 million units loading dose given intravenously, followed by 2.5 million units every 4 hours until delivery

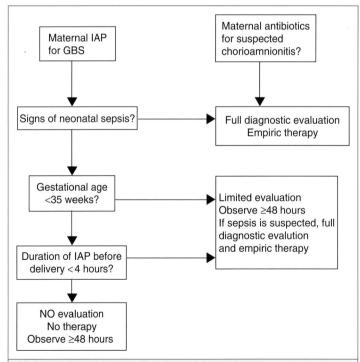

Figure 12-3. CDC recommendations for IAP to prevent early-onset GBS disease. (From Centers for Disease Control: Prevention of perinatal Group B streptococcal disease. Revised guidelines from CDC. MMWR 51:1–22, 2002.)

- **Alternative:** Ampicillin, 2-gm intravenous loading dose, followed by 1 gm every 4 hours until delivery
- **In cases of penicillin allergies:** *Low-risk for anaphylaxis,* cefazolin, 2-gm intravenous initial dose, then 1 gm intravenously every 8 hours until delivery; high-risk for anaphylaxis, clindamycin, 900 mg given intravenously every 8 hours until delivery or erythromycin, 500 gm given intravenously every 6 hours until delivery
- **Resistance to clindamycin, erythromycin, or susceptibility unknown:** Vancomycin, 1 gm given intravenously every 12 hours until delivery

57. **What is the optimal timing of maternal antibiotic prophylaxis for the prevention of GBS disease?**
    Current CDC guidelines indicate that 4 or more hours of intrapartum ampicillin or penicillin significantly reduces vertical transmission of GBS and early-onset disease. This reflects a change from previous guidelines, which suggested that two or more doses provided adequate therapy. In addition to efficacy, the duration of prophylaxis appears to be a more practical target for prevention.

58. **What are the pros and cons of IAP?**
    - **Pros:** IAP has resulted in a dramatic reduction in incidence of early-onset disease. Figure 12-4 illustrates the decline in incidence of early-onset GBS disease over the past decade as IAP programs were implemented. The graph is based on composite data from CDC surveillance centers, a National Institute of Child Health and Development (NICHD) multicenter study reviewing disease rates from 1992 to 1997, and ongoing surveillance at the author's center. The incidences of disease from 1990 to 1993 represent the pre-IAP era, whereas data from 1993 to 1996 followed the American College of Obstetrics and Gynecology (ACOG) and American Academy of Pediatrics (AAP) recommendations published in 1993. The third data set reflects the impact of the CDC recommendations published in 1996.

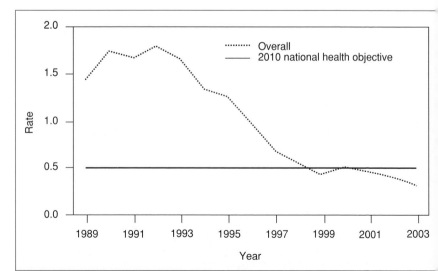

Figure 12-4. Rate per 1000 live births of early-onset invasive GBS disease by year—Active Bacterial Core surveillance, United States, 1989–2003. (Centers for Disease Control: Laboratory practices for prevental Group B streptococcal screening—seven states, 2003. MMWR 53:502–505, 2004.)

- **Cons:**
- Risk of maternal anaphylaxis
- IAP not 100% effective; 20% of cases occurred despite intrapartum antibiotics
- Screening-based strategy identifies only maximum of 85–90% of affected infants' mothers
- Emergence of resistant organisms in mothers and infants (e.g., *E. coli*, *Enterococcus* species)
- Increasing resistance of GBS to clindamycin and erythromycin
- Does not address other adverse outcomes of pregnancy (e.g., early fetal loss, preterm labor, premature rupture of fetal membranes)

59. What is the natural history of nosocomial acquisition of GBS in late-onset disease?

The majority of infants who present with late-onset disease acquire the organism outside the hospital. Mothers of these infants generally have no history of genital colonization with GBS during pregnancy.

STAPHYLOCOCCUS EPIDERMIDIS

60. Should vancomycin prophylaxis be used to prevent neonatal nosocomial CONS sepsis?

The answer is controversial. Selective use of vancomycin may prevent CONS bacteremia, but the risks of usage are high. These risks include an increased incidence of fungal or gram-negative infections in vancomycin-treated infants and the more general problem of emergence of vancomycin-resistant strains of CONS or enterococci in neonatal intensive care units (NICUs) on the whole. Because CONS are generally organisms of low virulence, one wonders about the risk-benefit ratio of such prevention strategies.

61. What are the risk factors for bloodstream infections with CONS?
- Prematurity
- Central venous catheters
- Lipid emulsions
- Mechanical ventilation

62. Does the I:T neutrophil ratio predict neonatal CONS infection?

The I:T neutrophil ratio is sensitive for the detection of nosocomial infection in infants. However, I:T neutrophil ratios may be normal in the presence of CONS disease, perhaps because of the relative avirulence of this organism.

63. Name the focal complications of persistent bacteremia with CONS.
- Infective endocarditis
- Necrotizing enterocolitis
- Pneumonia
- Meningitis

64. What is the recommended therapy for CONS infection?

The initial recommended therapy is vancomycin, which may be modified if the organism is sensitive to oxacillin and an aminoglycoside. In cases of persistent bacteremia, a combination of vancomycin and rifampin may be the best therapeutic regimen. In cases of an infected indwelling catheter, antibiotic therapy should be administered through the catheter. Removal of the catheter may be necessary if the culture result remains positive. The same is true for meningitis resulting from an infected CSF shunt.

CANDIDIASIS

65. **What are the most important risk factors for neonatal systemic candidiasis?**
    - Long-term use of broad-spectrum antibiotics suppresses normal GI flora and allows candidal overgrowth.
    - Prematurity and host immunosuppression are associated with abnormal skin barriers, humoral and cellular immune deficits, neutrophil dysfunction, and complement deficiencies.
    - Central intravenous catheterization and parenteral hyperalimentation allow a portal of entry for the organism into the bloodstream.
    - Prolonged steroid use may impair neutrophil function.

66. **Describe the spectrum of candidal disease in neonates.**
    Vertical transmission of *C. albicans* occurs in approximately 10% of term and 30% of preterm infants. Most commonly, acquisition leads to neonatal thrush or a perineal diaper rash with little associated morbidity. The more serious illnesses associated with *Candida* are shown in Table 12-10. Early-onset candidal disease, or *congenital candidiasis,* arises after exposure of the infant to organisms colonizing the maternal genital tract. Cutaneous findings are the hallmark of the disease, but the association with pulmonary disease conveys a grave prognosis despite systemic antifungal therapy. *Catheter-associated fungemia* generally arises from organisms within the GI tract. Affected infants have resolution of fungemia with prompt removal of the catheter and parenteral amphotericin therapy for 10–14 days. In contrast, infants with *disseminated candidiasis* have involvement of distant organs, including heart, kidney, bone, eyes, lungs, and meninges. Long-term therapy is recommended, and prognosis is guarded in these cases.

67. **Has late-onset candidal disease been described?**
    Recently, the recurrence of candidal disease has been described in four immunocompetent infants after a prolonged period of latency (up to 1 year). All of the infants presented with candidal arthritis and osteomyelitis, were born prematurely, had received parenteral nutrition through indwelling catheters, and had a history of systemic candidiasis during the newborn period. The pathogenesis of these latent infections is unknown.

    Harris MC, Pereira GR, Myers MD, et al: Candidal arthritis in infants previously treated for systemic candidiasis during the newborn period. Pediatr Emerg Care 16:249–251, 2000.

68. **Is there an association between *candida* sepsis and retinopathy of prematurity (ROP)?**
    One study has suggested an association between *Candida* sepsis and ROP in extremely-low-birth-weight infants. The study found increased severity of ROP and need for laser therapy after candidal infection. Although the mechanism is unknown, endothelial injury by the organism, elaboration of proinflammatory cytokines, and production of angiogenic substances may be involved. Another more recent study did not demonstrate this association. Rather, this data suggested that the lowest gestational ages predict the development of both threshold ROP as well as candidemia.

    Karlowicz MG, Giannone PJ, Pestian J, et al: Does candidemia predict threshold retinopathy of prematurity in extremely low birth weight (<1000 g) neonates? Pediatrics 105:1036–1040, 2000.

    Mittal M, Dhannireddy R, Higgins RD: Candida sepsis and association with retinopathy of prematurity. Pediatrics 101:654–657, 1998.

69. **What is the prevalence of end-organ damage after neonatal candidemia?**
    The medical literature concerning end-organ evaluation after neonatal candidemia is heterogeneous; however, a recent retrospective study suggested potential damage from the following sources: endophthalmitis (median, 3%), meningitis (15%), brain abscess or ventriculitis (4%), endocarditis (5%), positive renal ultrasound (5%), and positive urine culture (61%). Future prospective studies are needed to more accurately define this risk in neonates.

    Benjamin DK, Poole C, Steinbach WJ, et al: Neonatal candidemia and end-organ damage: A critical appraisal of the literature using meta-analytic techniques. Pediatrics 112:634–640, 2003.

TABLE 12-10. CANDIDAL DISEASE IN NEONATES

Clinical features	Congenital Candidiasis	Catheter-Related Fungemia	Systemic Candidiasis
Age at onset	Birth	>7 days	>7 days
Risk factors	None	Necessary	Necessary
Skin involvement	Hallmark	None	None
Respiratory involvement	Occasionally	Never	Frequent
Positive blood culture result	No	Yes	Yes
Multiorgan involvement	Never	Rare	Frequent
Treatment	Topical antifungals*	Catheter removal *and* parenteral amphotericin B	Parenteral amphotericin B
Prognosis	Excellent	Good	Fair/poor

*Death may occur in premature infants with pulmonary involvement, and parenteral amphotericin B should be used in these infants.
Adapted from Bendel CM, Hostetter MK: Systemic candidiasis and other fungal infections in the newborn. Semin Pediatr Infect Dis 5:34–41, 1994.

70. **How can systemic candidal disease be prevented in preterm infants?**
A recent prospective randomized double-blind clinical trial in preterm infants with birth weights <1000 gm demonstrated that prophylactic administration of fluconazole was effective in preventing fungal colonization and invasive fungal infection. In this study, fluconazole was administered intravenously for 6 weeks at a dose of 3 mg/kg every third day for the first 2 weeks, every other day during the third and fourth weeks, and daily during the day during the fifth and sixth weeks. Fluconazole resistance did not occur. Other strategies include the limitation of the use of broad-spectrum antibiotics, which may prevent fungal colonization of the GI tract in susceptible neonates. Alternatively, early introduction of enteral feedings may lessen the duration of parenteral nutrition and the need for intravascular catheters.

    Kaufman D, Boyle R, Hazen KC, et al: Fluconazole prophylaxis against fungal colonization and infection in preterm infants. N Engl J Med 345:1660–1666, 2001.

71. **What is the recommended treatment of neonatal systemic candidal infection?**
There is currently no consensus regarding the best approach to the treatment of systemic candidal infections in neonates because large, controlled studies of treatment strategies have not yet been performed. Amphotericin B remains the mainstay of therapy. The dose is 1 mg/kg/day administered for 14 days (catheter-associated fungemia: total dose 10–15 mg/kg) to 6 weeks (disseminated disease: total dose 25–30 mg/kg), depending on disease severity and site. Although side effects include nephrotoxicity, hypokalemia, hepatotoxicity, and bone marrow suppression, the drug appears to be well tolerated in neonates.

72. **Are there alternatives to amphotericin for treatment of neonatal systemic candidal infections?**
Amphotericin B lipid complex, which is incorporated into unilamellar liposomes, was developed to eliminate the severe adverse effects of conventional amphotericin with good central nervous

system (CNS) penetration. To date, randomized, clinical trials have not been performed to compare its efficacy to that of conventional amphotericin B, but several smaller studies have shown safety. 5-Flucytosine is a nucleoside analog that inhibits DNA replication in *Candida*. It may be used as adjunctive synergistic therapy for candidal meningitis or persistent fungemia because amphotericin B penetrates the spinal fluid poorly. Others have recommended combination therapy for all patients as optimal therapy. Fluconazole, another alternative agent, binds to fungal cytochrome P450 and affects fungal membrane integrity. There have been no controlled trials of this agent in neonatal candidiasis, so it is not recommended as first-line therapy in neonates. An additional therapeutic concern is the emergence of relative resistance of non-*albicans* species to conventional treatment with amphotericin B, necessitating susceptibility testing in cases refractory to therapy.

NEONATAL MENINGITIS

73. **What are the normal values for cells, protein, and glucose in the CSF of healthy term and preterm infants?**
    See Table 12-11.

TABLE 12-11.	NORMAL CSF VALUES IN HEALTHY INFANTS			
	WBC	PMN	Protein	Glucose
Term	$7 \pm 13^*$	$0.8 \pm 6^*$	$64 \pm 24^*$	$51 \pm 13^*$
	$4^\dagger$	$0^\dagger$		
Preterm (<1000 gm)	$4 \pm 3^*$	$6 \pm 15^*$	$160 \pm 56^*$	$61 \pm 34^*$
	$6^\dagger$			

WBC = white blood cell; PMN = polymorphonuclear neutrophil.
*Mean ± standard deviation.
†Median.
Term infant data from Ahmed A, Hickey SM, Ehrett S, et al: Cerebrospinal fluid values in the term infant. Pediatr Infect Dis J 15:298–303, 1996. Preterm infant data from Rodriguez AF, Kaplan SL, Mason EO: Cerebrospinal fluid values in the very low birth weight infant. J Pediatr 116:971–974, 1990.

74. **What is the likelihood of late-onset meningitis among VLBW infants?**
    Among VLBW infants who had a lumbar puncture performed, 5% had a diagnosis of late-onset meningitis. Furthermore, one third of the infants with meningitis had negative blood culture results. The pathogens associated with meningitis were similar to those associated with sepsis. In this population, meningitis may occur without the presence of a positive blood culture result and may be underdiagnosed.

    Stoll BJ, Hansen N, Fanaroff AA, et al: To tap or not to tap: High likelihood of meningitis without sepsis among very low birth weight infants. Pediatrics 113:1181–1185, 2004.

75. **What are the mechanisms of brain injury in meningitis?**
    - Vascular infarcts (vasospasm/thrombosis)
    - Reactive oxygen species
    - Excitotoxic amino acids
    - Alterations in cerebral blood flow

KEY POINTS: DIAGNOSIS OF NEONATAL INFECTION

1. The sensitivity of blood cultures increases with increasing volume.

2. Meningitis may occur in the absence of a positive blood culture result.

3. Urine culture specimens should be obtained if infection is evaluated after the first week of life.

4. No single laboratory test or combination of tests is 100% sensitive or specific for diagnosing infection.

76. **What factors influence antibiotic concentrations in CSF?**
    See Table 12-12.

TABLE 12-12.	FACTORS INFLUENCING ANTIBIOTIC CONCENTRATION IN CSF	
Variable	Effect on CNS Penetration	Example
High degree of protein binding	Reduced	Ceftriaxone
Lipid solubility	Enhanced	Rifampin
High degree of ionization	Reduced	β-lactams
Active transport system	Enhanced	Penicillin
Meningeal inflammation	Enhanced*	β-lactams, vancomycin

*Meningeal inflammation only influences penetration of hydrophilic antibiotics.

77. **What are the recommendations for initial empiric therapy of meningitis in the neonate?**
    - A regimen of ampicillin and cefotaxime or a combination of a penicillin (e.g., ampicillin) and an aminoglycoside is recommended for initial empiric therapy.
    - Ceftazidime is probably as efficacious as cefotaxime but should be reserved for *P. aeruginosa* infections.

78. **How should gram-positive and gram-negative meningitis be treated during the neonatal period?**
    - Treatment of meningitis caused by enteric organisms: There are no data demonstrating the superiority of cefotaxime or ceftriaxone over ampicillin plus an aminoglycoside. However, for gram-negative meningitis, cefotaxime is preferred and is often paired with an aminoglycoside. Gram-negative meningitis should be treated for at least 3 weeks.
    - **Treatment of meningitis due to gram-positive organisms:** Because there is synergism between ampicillin and aminoglycosides for most GBS, *L. monocytogenes*, and enterococci, combination therapy is recommended until the CSF is sterilized. If the GBS disease is shown to be tolerant to ampicillin (minimum bactericidal concentration [MBC]/minimum inhibitory concentration [MIC] = 30/1), combination therapy should be used for the duration of treatment (~14 days).

79. **What is the differential diagnosis for an infant with clinical signs of meningitis and sepsis whose culture results for bacteria are negative?**
    Two viral infections must be considered. The first is *disseminated HSV with CNS involvement*. One helpful diagnostic clue is the development of skin vesicles, which can also be used as a

source from which to isolate virus for diagnosis. However, about 20% of babies with this form of HSV never develop skin vesicles. Other sources of virus for culture include respiratory secretions, blood, and CSF. The CSF should be cultured for virus, although it is rare to isolate HSV from this source. If infection with HSV is strongly suspected, therapy with acyclovir can begin while viral cultures and other tests remain pending.

The other viral infection associated with such a severe neonatal syndrome is *enteroviral infection,* usually due to coxsackievirus or enteric cytopathic human orphan virus. Pleconaril, a new antiviral agent, has been used to treat life-threatening enteroviral infections.

INFECTION CONTROL

80. **What is the difference between incidence rate and prevalence rate?**
Incidence rate is the ratio of the number of new occurrences of a disease in a given period to the number of persons at risk (e.g., number of cases of bacteremia per 1000 catheter-days). *Prevalence rate* is the ratio of persons with a disease entity in a defined population at a specific time without regard to when the disease began.

81. **What is the difference between endemic and epidemic nosocomial infections?**
Sporadic (endemic) infections represent the bulk of nosocomial infections and are the usual level of infection expected during a given period for a given population. Epidemic infections are marked by an unusual increase in the incidence of disease entity. A knowledge of the endemic levels of a disease is needed to make this assessment.

82. **Which kinds of patients need to be isolated in negative-pressure rooms?**
Patients suspected of having tuberculosis, chickenpox, or measles need to be placed on respiratory isolation in negative-pressure rooms to prevent aerosol spread of their infection. It is important to assess the family members of such patients for infection or immune status as well.

83. **A nurse tells you that she has just been exposed to chickenpox, and she never had it as a child. What do you tell her about the period of isolation?**
Patients (or nonimmune staff or visitors) need to be isolated from day 10 to day 21 after documented exposure to a person with active varicella-zoster virus (VZV) infection. If a patient has received varicella-zoster immune globulin (VZIG), the incubation period is extended to 28 days.

84. **What is contact isolation?**
Contact isolation is a category of isolation for infectious entities that can be spread through direct contact with infectious secretions or fomites contaminated with infectious secretions. Patients undergoing contact isolation should be placed in a single room (when available), and health care workers should wash hands upon entering and leaving the room and wear gowns and gloves for contact with the patient or the patient's environment.

85. **Which diseases require contact isolation?**
- *Clostridium difficile*
- Rotavirus
- Respiratory syncytial virus
- Croup
- Herpes simplex
- Resistant organisms, including methicillin-resistant *S. aureus* and vancomycin-resistant enterococci

86. **What are droplet precautions?**
Droplet precautions are used to prevent transmission of diseases that are spread through large, aerosolized droplets containing infectious particles. Such particles are spread through sneezing and coughing and rapidly settle on horizontal surfaces within a few feet of the source patient.

Examples include influenza, adenovirus, *Parvovirus*, rubella, and meningitis caused by *H. influenzae* or *Neisseria meningitidis.*

87. **What is the best way to determine whether patient-to-patient transmission of a pathogen has occurred?**
   This possibility should be investigated in two ways:
   1. Epidemiologic investigation to determine whether there is a known epidemiologic link between the patients (e.g., sharing a hospital room or common health care workers)
   2. Further confirmation by molecular epidemiology (i.e., analysis of the DNA of the bacteria or fungus) to assess clonality of the patient's organisms

88. **What are the most frequently cited reasons that nursery personnel do not wash their hands?**
   - Handwashing takes too much time.
   - There is a lack of soap (54%) and lack of towels (65%).
   - One thorough wash per day is sufficient (26%).
   - Gloves can substitute for handwashing (25%, including 50% of physicians).
   - Handwashing is not important if an infant is receiving antibiotics (10%).

   Wharton KN, Karlowicz MG: Barriers to full compliance with handwashing in a neonatal intensive care unit. Pediatr Res 43:254A, 1998.

89. **What are the current recommendations for handwashing in the NICU?**
   - Removal of all rings; no nail polish or false nails
   - Initial 3-minute scrub to the elbow
   - A 10-second scrub before and after handling each infant
   - Use of alcohol-based hand gels before and after handling infant

90. **Do careful handwashing practices reduce the incidence of nosocomial infection?**
   Six of seven hospital-based studies (including two in NICUs) have demonstrated that improved handwashing techniques will reduce infection rates.

   Larson E: Skin hygiene and infection prevention: More of the same or different approaches? Clin Infect Dis 29:1287–1294, 1999.

91. **Is washing with soap and water an effective way to "de-germ" hands?**
   Handwashing with soap and water does not reliably prevent microbial transmission and may actually increase it by dispersing bacterial colonies.

92. **What is the disadvantage of frequent handwashing?**
   Frequent handwashing may actually transmit more bacteria by affecting skin health and raising pH.

   Ojajarvi J, Makela P, Rantasalo I: Failure of hand disinfection with frequent handwashing: A need for prolonged field studies. J Hyg (Lond) 79:107–119, 1977.

93. **What is the preferred method for hand disinfection in the NICU?**
   Hand disinfection with an alcohol-based hand rub is the preferred method because of its rapid action and effectiveness. In addition, alcohol-based rubs contain emollients that serve as dermal protectors and decrease bacterial dispersal. In contrast, antiseptic skin washes can damage the skin barrier and offer no advantages.

94. **What is the effect of prophylactic skin ointment on the rate of nosocomial infection in newborn infants?**
   In an initial small study whose primary outcome measure was transepidermal water loss, a lower incidence of nosocomial infection was found; however, in a recent report from the Vermont Oxford Network, the use of Aquaphor was associated with an increased incidence of nosocomial bacterial

sepsis in infants weighing 501–1000 gm. Another study has also found an association between the topical application of petrolatum ointment and systemic candidal infections in neonates weighing <1500 gm. At this time, the routine use of skin emollients is not recommended.

Campbell JR, Zaccaria E, Baker CJ: Systemic candidiasis in extremely low birth weight infants receiving topical petrolatum ointment for skin care: a case control study. Pediatrics 105:1041–1045, 2000.

Edwards WH, Conner JM, Soll RF: The effect of prophylactic ointment therapy on nosocomial sepsis rates and skin integrity in infants with birth weights of 501 to 1000 g. Pediatrics 113:1195–1201, 2004.

95. **Does gowning prevent infections in the NICU?**
There are very limited data to support the efficacy of gowning and much data to say that it is ineffective. The risk of transmitting infection through clothing is 2/10,000 encounters.

96. **Does gowning serve as a reminder for personnel to wash their hands?**
No!

Donowitz LG: Failure of the overgown to prevent nosocomial infection in a pediatric intensive care unit. Pediatrics 77:35–38, 1986.

97. **For which kinds of infants in the nursery should nursery personnel wear gown and gloves?**
- Infants colonized with a resistant microorganism or a bacterium known to cause infection in the nursery.
- Infants requiring contact isolation because of colonization with *C. difficile*, rotavirus, respiratory syncytial virus, or HSV.

CONJUNCTIVITIS

98. **What are the common causes of neonatal conjunctivitis? When do they present?**
The times of onset for infections caused by these organisms may overlap, particularly in the presence of prolonged rupture of membranes. In 10–46% of babies who present with conjunctivitis in the first month of life, *C. trachomatis* is the cause. The incidence of chlamydial conjunctivitis will probably decrease because pregnant women are now being screened and treated for chlamydia. *H. influenzae* and *S. pneumoniae* are frequently isolated in babies with lacrimal duct obstruction. Viral causes of conjunctivitis are rare during the first month; however, 70% of cases with viral etiology are due to HSV, which may also cause severe systemic disease. *Pseudomonas* is a rare cause of bacterial conjunctivitis in healthy term newborns, but the organism deserves mention because it is sometimes responsible for epidemic conjunctivitis in premature babies. *Pseudomonas* can be a dangerously virulent organism, and pseudomonas conjunctivitis requires systemic as well as local (even subconjunctival) antibiotic therapy (Table 12-13).

99. **A 5-day-old term baby presents in the emergency room with pus coming from one eye. What work-up should you do?**
You must do a Gram stain first. If the Gram stain shows gram-negative intracellular diplococci with abutting flattened sides, *Neisseria gonorrhoeae* should be assumed to be the cause of the eye discharge, and the baby should be admitted for systemic treatment. A bacterial culture should be performed, along with a culture specific for *N. gonorrhoeae*, to confirm the diagnosis. Note that the eye discharge seen in gonococcal ophthalmia is often thick, copious, and golden yellow in color. If the Gram stain is negative for intracellular diplococci, a culture for *C. trachomatis* and a rapid test for chlamydia (such as direct fluorescent antibody [DFA], enzyme immunoassay [EIA], or DNA probe) should be performed in addition to bacterial cultures. A combined DNA probe for the detection of both *N. gonorrhoeae* and *C. trachomatis* is commercially available. The chlamydia tests need to be done on conjunctival scrapings because *Chlamydia* organisms are obligate intracellular organisms. If herpes conjunctivitis is suspected, a rapid test for herpes simplex and culture should be sent to the lab.

TABLE 12-13. COMMON CAUSES OF NEONATAL CONJUNCTIVITIS	
Etiology	Usual Time of Onset After Birth
Chemical (with silver nitrate prophylaxis)	6–24 hours
C. trachomatis	5–14 days
Neisseria gonorrhoeae	2–5 days

Other bacterial etiology:
    Staphylococcus aureus
    Haemophilus species
    Streptococcus pneumoniae
    Enterococcus species
	>5 days

Herpes simplex	5–14 days

100. **What is the treatment for conjunctivitis?**

Conjunctivitis caused by gonorrhea should be treated with ceftriaxone, at a dose of 50 mg/kg administered intravenously or intramuscularly once a day for 7 days. Additional topical therapy is not needed when ceftriaxone is used, but the infant's eyes should be irrigated with normal saline frequently until the discharge is gone.

If gonococcal ophthalmia is not suspected, 0.5% erythromycin ointment can be applied to each eye four times a day for 7 days. If the chlamydia test result comes back positive, oral erythromycin (50 mg/kg/day divided into four equal doses) should be given for 14 days. Azithromycin is still undergoing clinical testing for use in newborns, but this drug at an oral dose of 20 mg/kg given once a day for 3 days may become the treatment of choice. After systemic antibiotics are started, topical treatment of the eye can be discontinued.

Herpes conjunctivitis is rare and is almost always accompanied by other systemic manifestations of neonatal herpes. The treatment for neonatal herpes conjunctivitis is acyclovir, 10 mg/kg given intravenously every 8 hours for 10 days, plus topical therapy with 1% trifluridine solution applied to the eye every 2 hours for 7 days or until the cornea has reepithelialized.

101. **Why doesn't conjunctivitis caused by *C. trachomatis* cause blindness in neonates when it causes so many cases of blindness in third-world countries?**

The visual loss from trachoma is caused by irreversible corneal damage from chronic folliculitis due to repeated chronic infection. Because of their immature immune systems, newborns lack the requisite lymphoid tissue in their conjunctiva to mount such a response. The length of infection also makes a difference. Even older children do not develop folliculitis until the infection has been present for at least 1–2 months; newborn conjunctivitis caused by *C. trachomatis* usually clears by 2 months even without antibiotic treatment, so no permanent scarring occurs. Another important factor may be that the serotypes of *C. trachomatis* that cause endocervical infections in women and conjunctivitis in neonates (types D–K) differ from the serotypes that cause blinding trachoma (types A–C).

102. **Does the use of antibiotic eye prophylaxis at birth decrease the incidence of neonatal conjunctivitis resulting from *C. trachomatis*?**

No. Topical silver nitrate, tetracycline, and erythromycin given at birth are equally effective in preventing gonococcal ophthalmia neonatorum, but none of these agents significantly decreases the incidence of chlamydial conjunctivitis.

CHLAMYDIAL INFECTIONS

103. **What is the risk of chlamydial infection in infants born to mothers whose endocervical culture result is positive for *C. trachomatis*?**
Neonatal acquisition usually occurs at the time of birth. In the absence of treatment during pregnancy, 50–75% of infants born to mothers with endocervical cultures positive for *C. trachomatis* become infected in at least one of the following anatomic sites: nasopharynx, conjunctiva, rectum, or vagina. Twenty to fifty percent develop conjunctivitis at 5–14 days of age that is generally not prevented by antibiotic eye prophylaxis at birth. Ten to twenty percent develop pneumonia between 4 and 12 weeks of life. The remaining infants develop an apparently asymptomatic colonization of the nasopharynx, rectum, or vagina. These infants can remain colonized for up to 3 years, although most clear the infection even without treatment by 1 year of age.
   Note that successful treatment of the mother during pregnancy with oral erythromycin or azithromycin prevents most cases of vertical transmission

104. **What procedures are used to diagnose *C. trachomatis* infection in infants?**
Chlamydia culture of the conjunctiva (for conjunctivitis) or nasopharynx (for pneumonia) is considered the gold standard for diagnosis, but there are disadvantages to this method. Culture specimens require special handling, which can make transport to the laboratory difficult. In addition, cultures generally require 3–7 days for processing, which may delay treatment.
   Since the mid-1980s, several commercial rapid tests have been developed. DFA tests and EIAs have been approved by the U.S. Food and Drug Administration (FDA) for detection of *C. trachomatis* in infants with conjunctivitis or pneumonia; these tests have a sensitivity of 93–100% and specificity of 94–97% compared with culture. Results are usually available in less than 24 hours. A DNA probe was marketed more recently. DNA probes have a detection sensitivity and specificity similar to that of the EIA test and, in the commercial version, have the additional advantage of being combined with a DNA probe for *N. gonorrhoeae*. This test has received clearance by the FDA for use with conjunctival specimens but not for use with nasopharyngeal specimens. Newly developed amplified DNA tests based on polymerase chain reaction (PCR) and ligase chain reaction appear to be even more sensitive than culture for chlamydia detection. However, these are expensive and are not yet FDA approved for infant conjunctival or nasopharyngeal specimens.
   Remember that *C. trachomatis* is an obligate intracellular organism, so the collection swab must be scraped across the conjunctiva or nasopharynx to ensure that there are adequate cells for detection. In the eye, the pus should be wiped away before the conjunctival scrapings are obtained.

105. **What is the proper treatment for *C. trachomatis* infections?**
Mothers with positive endocervical cultures should be treated during pregnancy. Maternal treatment consists of an erythromycin base, 500 mg administered orally four times a day for 7 days. Treatment for *C. trachomatis* is hampered by its long growth cycle and requires prolonged therapeutic levels of antibiotics. Compliance can be a problem with this erythromycin course. Azithromycin is a macrolide antibiotic that has a lower incidence of side effects and a much longer half-life, so once-a-day dosing for shorter periods is possible. Posttreatment follow-up cultures should be performed to determine whether treatment has been successful; if not, a second course of treatment may be indicated. Sexual partners of positive women must be treated as well. Chlamydia infection in both male and female genital tracts can be asymptomatic, which is why routine screening, especially in pregnancy, is warranted.
   Until recently, the AAP *Red Book* recommended that babies born to mothers with untreated chlamydial cervical infections receive oral erythromycin (50 mg/kg per day in four divided doses) for 14 days, starting on the first day of life. However, the efficacy of prophylactic treatment is unknown; moreover, reports of an association between the prophylactic use of oral erythromycin for pertussis and infantile hypertrophic pyloric stenosis have appeared. The AAP now recommends that treatment be reserved for infants with actual infection.

Neonates with chlamydial conjunctivitis should receive oral erythromycin, 50 mg/kg/day in four divided doses, for 14 days. Additional topical therapy is not needed. Erythromycin with the same dose given for 2–3 weeks is the treatment of choice for chlamydial pneumonia. Treatment failure requiring a second course of erythromycin occurs in about 20% of cases.

Azithromycin may soon be approved for use in neonates. Its shorter treatment course and less severe GI side effects should improve treatment compliance. Preliminary data indicate that azithromycin, in a dose of 20 mg/kg once a day for 3 days, successfully treats conjunctivitis caused by *C. trachomatis*.

106. What are the characteristics of *C. trachomatis* pneumonia?

The onset of *C. trachomatis* pneumonia usually occurs between 4 and 12 weeks of age (a few cases present as early as 2 weeks, but none has been reported beyond 4 months). Most infants have a prodrome of about 1 week's duration of a stuffy nose without fever and a persistent paroxysmal staccato cough that can lead to breathlessness. They may present with tachypnea and inspiratory rales. Expiratory wheezing occurs in less than 25% of infants with the disease; 60% have abnormal eardrum findings. Although a severe illness is relatively rare, affected infants appear irritable, eat poorly, and cough often. The chest x-ray shows hyperinflation with bilateral diffuse nonspecific infiltrates. Lab values are significant for eosinophilia (>300–$400/mm^3$), an elevated total serum IgG level (>500 mg/dL), and an elevated total IgM level (>110 mg/dL). Without treatment, symptoms last an average of 6 weeks. Treatment of any previous conjunctivitis with oral erythromycin seems to prevent this pneumonia, although there are case reports of treatment failures. Half of the infants with chlamydial pneumonia do not have a history of previous conjunctivitis.

107. Does *C. pneumoniae* cause disease in newborns?

C. pneumoniae, a recently discovered species of the genus *Chlamydia*, has not been isolated in any children younger than the age of 2 years. It is a common cause of pneumonia, bronchitis, and upper respiratory tract infections in older children between the ages of 5 and 15 years.

108. Does *C. trachomatis* infection in pregnant women cause complications other than neonatal infection?

Although studies are conflicting, *C. trachomatis* infection in pregnancy is weakly linked to premature rupture of membranes and premature delivery. Ten to thirty percent of women with chlamydial infections who undergo induced abortions develop late endometritis. Chronic salpingitis caused by *C. trachomatis* can lead to infertility and an increased risk for ectopic pregnancy.

OSTEOMYELITIS AND SEPTIC ARTHRITIS

109. What pathogens cause neonatal osteomyelitis?

- *S. aureus*
- GBS
- Gram-negative enteric bacilli (e.g., *E. coli, Klebsiella* species, *Pseudomonas* species)
- *Candida* species
- *Mycoplasma hominis*
- *Treponema pallidum*

110. What is the incidence of osteomyelitis in the neonate?

The overall rate of nosocomial bone and joint infections is 1–2/1000 admissions.

111. What is the pathogenesis of osteomyelitis in the newborn?

Hematogenous dissemination is responsible for most infections; however, skeletal infections can also result from:

- Extension from infection in surrounding tissues

- Direct inoculation
- Transplacental infection leading to fetal sepsis (e.g., syphilis)

112. **What distinct anatomic and physiologic features place the newborn at risk for osteomyelitis and septic arthritis?**
The metaphysis is usually the site of seeding caused by sluggish flow in the metaphyseal vessels (also referred to as *sinusoidal vessels*). In the newborn period, these transphyseal vessels form a conduit between the metaphysis and the epiphysis. Additionally, the relatively thin cortex and loosely applied periosteum are poor barriers against the spread of infection. The hip, shoulder, and knee can easily become infected because the epiphyseal-metaphyseal junction is entirely within the joint capsule.

113. **What are the manifestations of osteomyelitis in neonates?**
   - Systemic signs are usually absent in neonatal osteomyelitis but occasionally are present.
   - In most infants, the earliest presenting signs are pain (with pseudoparalysis), limitation of motion, and swelling. Discoloration and increased warmth may accompany the swelling.
   - Feeding and weight gain are usually undisturbed.
   - The distribution of bone involvement is as follows:
      - Femur (39%)
      - Humerus (18%)
      - Tibia (14%)
      - Fibula (10%)
      - Radius (5%)
      - Maxilla (4%)
      - Ulna (3%)
      - Clavicle (2%)
      - Tarsal bones (2%)
      - Ribs (2%)
      - Vertebrae (1%)

   Remington JS, Klein JO (eds): Infectious Diseases of the Fetus and Newborn Infant. Philadelphia, W.B. Saunders, 1995.

114. **How often are bacterial culture results positive in neonatal osteomyelitis?**
   - Sixty percent of blood cultures are positive.
   - Seventy percent of bone aspirates are positive.

115. **Is the erythrocyte sedimentation rate (ESR) or CRP more helpful in the management of osteomyelitis?**
In most studies, the ESR was significantly elevated on days 2–5. ESR values slowly returned to normal within 3 weeks of therapy. In contrast, CRP rises within 6–12 hours of a triggering stimulus and returns to normal within a week of therapy. A secondary rise in either ESR or CRP could be a sign of recrudescence.

116. **How common is fungal septic arthritis?**
Candida species cause 17% of septic arthritis in premature infants.

117. **What are the unique features of *Candida* bone infections?**
   - Unlike bacterial infections, inflammatory signs other than edema of the extremity are generally lacking.
   - Radiographs demonstrate "punched out" metaphyseal lucencies that appear less aggressive than staphylococcal osteomyelitis.

- Affected babies often have a history of central line–related fungemia.
- Fungal septic arthritis can appear as late as 1 year after a treated fungal infection.
- Fluconazole may be a good alternative to amphotericin B because of good joint penetration.

118. **What is the first line of management for a suspected septic arthritis in a newborn infant?**
Joint aspiration with incision and drainage whenever there is significant collection of pus in the soft tissues. Often, surgical drainage is indicated for relief of intra-articular pressure when the hip or shoulder is affected.

119. **What radiologic studies are helpful in the diagnosis of osteomyelitis?**
See Table 12-14.

TABLE 12-14.	RADIOLOGIC STUDIES FOR DIAGNOSIS OF OSTEOMYELITIS	
Test	**Pros**	**Cons**
Skeletal x-rays	Eventually, bony changes will be seen (i.e., punched-out lytic lesions, osseous lucencies, and periosteal elevation). Multiple sites of involvement can eventually be seen. Trauma (i.e., fracture) as a cause of swelling or pseudoparalysis can be ruled out.	X-ray changes do not occur for 7–12 days. Conventional radiographs are insensitive to the destruction of <30% of the bone matrix.
^{99m}Tc	Osteomyelitis can be detected earlier than on traditional skeletal surveys. With the higher-resolution gamma cameras used today, multiple sites of infection are often noted.	Patient is exposed to radiation. False-negative studies have been reported. False-positive results occur from increased metabolic bone activity.
Gallium bone scan	In equivocal ^{99m}Tc bone scans, gallium might be useful.	The radiation dose is significantly higher than in ^{99m}Tc bone scan.
Sonography	Most useful as a tool for guiding needle aspiration of fluid collections in joints or adjacent to bone. It is inexpensive. There is no radiation exposure.	An experienced sonographer is required. Accuracy is variable in neonates.
MRI	Detects inflammatory or destructive intramedullary disease in older children or adults.	Not helpful in neonates because the marrow compartment is rarely involved.

$^{99m}Tc = {}^{99m}$Technetium, MRI = magnetic resonance imaging.

120. **What is the presentation of maxillary osteomyelitis?**
   - Early edema and redness of the cheeks.
   - Unilateral nasal discharge.
   - Swelling of the eyelid with conjunctivitis.

KEY POINTS: FUNGAL DISEASE IN PREMATURE INFANTS

1. Invasive candidal disease should be considered in infants who have had prolonged exposure to broad-spectrum antibiotics.

2. Congenital candidal disease almost always involves the skin and may infect the respiratory tract leading to significant lung disease, but it rarely causes systemic candidemia.

3. Prophylactic fluconazole in infants weighing less than 1000 gm for several weeks may decrease the incidence of systemic candidiasis.

4. Infants with candidemia should be evaluated for involvement of end organs including eyes, kidneys, meninges, lungs, and heart.

5. Amphotericin is well tolerated in neonates, but liposomal amphotericin is available for infants with impaired kidney function.

6. 5-Flucytosine may be added as an adjunct treatment for candidal meningitis or persistent candidemia.

121. **What are the initial antibiotics used for the treatment of osteomyelitis?**
   Optimal coverage is provided by a penicillinase-resistant penicillin coupled with an aminoglycoside until an organism is identified and antibiotic sensitivities have been determined. Therapy should be continued for a minimum of 4–6 weeks. In the neonatal age group, orally administered antibiotics are not used because there are insufficient data regarding their absorption and efficacy.

PYELONEPHRITIS AND URINARY TRACT INFECTION

122. **A 10-day-old male infant presents with a 2-day history of fever, vomiting, lethargy, and jaundice. Examination reveals a temperature of 39°C, a blood pressure measurement of 65/40, and a pulse of 170 beats/min; there are no focal abnormal physical findings. Laboratory data include the following levels: bilirubin, 7 mg/dL (direct, 2 mg/dL); creatinine, 0.2 mg/dL; WBC count, 20,000 cells/mm³; and urinalysis 60 WBCs per high-power field. What is the most likely diagnosis?**
   The signs and symptoms indicate an acute infectious process. The urinalysis suggests a diagnosis of acute pyelonephritis. Symptomatic urinary tract infections (UTIs) occur in 1.4/1000 newborns.

123. **What is the incidence of asymptomatic bacteriuria in neonates?**
   Asymptomatic bacteriuria occurs in 2% of healthy term neonates and up to 10% of premature infants. Males are affected more often than females in the neonatal period, and uncircumcised males are even more susceptible.

124. **What is the pathogenesis of UTI in the neonate?**
   Unlike older infants, hematogenous spread of infection is more common than ascending infection. For this reason, some neonates may have associated meningitis and septicemia. Therefore,

in addition to urinalysis and urine culture, neonates older than 3 days of age should have blood and CSF culture specimens drawn before the initiation of antibiotics. The yield of urine culture in neonates younger than 3 days of age is poor. Unlike the distinction of cystitis and pyelonephritis in older infants and children, infection of the urinary tract in the neonate often includes that of the kidney.

125. What are the signs and symptoms of UTI in the neonate?

The symptoms of UTI are often nonspecific and include vomiting, diarrhea, failure to thrive, fever, lethargy, and jaundice, which is unconjugated if the UTI occurs in the first week of life and conjugated if UTI occurs later.

126. How is the diagnosis of a UTI in the neonate made?

The definitive diagnosis is made by positive culture of urine that is obtained using sterile precautions. Urinalysis is not very helpful; up to 25 leukocytes/mm^3 in males and up to 50 leukocytes/mm^3 in clean-catch specimens are considered normal. The absence of pyuria does not rule out UTI. However, enhanced urinalysis (leukocytes measured in unspun urine by a hemocytometer) has been shown to be a sensitive marker of UTI when >10 WBC/mm^3 are found. Although this laboratory test has demonstrated utility in the febrile neonate, it has not yet been evaluated in the NICU as part of a sepsis evaluation.

127. What are the common organisms responsible for UTI in newborn infants?

The most common organism causing UTI in neonates is *E. coli*, which accounts for 91% of community-acquired infection in children younger than 8 weeks of age. Other organisms include *Proteus*, *Pseudomonas*, *Klebsiella*, and *Enterococcus* species and *S. aureus*, which may be associated with suppurative lesions in the testis, epididymis, or kidneys. With prolonged hospitalization, coagulase-negative *Staphylococcus* and *Candida* organisms can also cause UTI. Candidiasis can be associated with fungal balls in the kidney and renal pelvis, which can lead to obstruction.

128. How should pyelonephritis be treated?

Treatment of pyelonephritis is similar to that of bacterial UTI and consists of parenteral antibiotics, usually a combination of a penicillin and an aminoglycoside, or, in older infants, a third-generation cephalosporin. For suspected staphylococcal infection, a penicillinase-resistant penicillin could be used. Amphotericin is used for *Candida* infection, and in premature neonates liposomal amphotericin can be used if there is impaired kidney function. The duration of therapy is 10–14 days, and it is advisable to repeat a urine culture after 48 hours to ensure clearance of the organisms from the urinary tract. Antibiotic prophylaxis is indicated for structural anomalies of the urinary tract or vesicoureteric reflux. Prophylaxis is used until spontaneous resolution or surgical correction of the underlying lesion has occurred.

129. In addition to urinalysis and urine culture, what other tests are indicated in the treatment of an infant with possible UTI?

In addition to diagnosing UTI, it is also important to evaluate the urinary tract for underlying structural or functional abnormalities that may predispose the infant to recurrent UTIs. Urinary tract anomalies have been detected in 30–55% of infants with UTI younger than 2 months of age.

Abdominal ultrasound is a safe and noninvasive method of evaluating structural abnormalities of the urinary tract and is the initial imaging test of choice. *Intravenous pyelography* can be useful in assessing the function of the kidneys. *Radionuclide scans* such as dimercaptosuccinic acid scans can be used to evaluate function and structural abnormalities, specifically renal scars following UTI. *Vesicoureterography* to evaluate the presence or absence of vesicoureteric reflux should be performed after completion of treatment of the UTI, because transient vesicoureteral reflux commonly occurs with the acute infection.

OMPHALITIS

130. **What are the presenting signs of omphalitis in neonates?**
   - Foul-smelling discharge
   - Periumbilical erythematous streaking, induration, and tenderness to palpation
   - Purulent or serosanguinous discharge
   - On rare occasions, signs of a systemic infection

131. **What is the incidence of omphalitis?**
   In hospitalized infants, the incidence is ~2%. In infants delivered at home, the incidence may be as high as 21%.

132. **What are the predisposing factors for omphalitis?**
   - Prematurity
   - Complicated delivery
   - Improper severing of the umbilical cord
   - Poor hygienic practices during the neonatal period

133. **Which bacteria cause omphalitis?**
   - *S. aureus*
   - *Streptococcus pyogenes* (infections with group A, β-hemolytic streptococci may result in a wet, malodorous stump with only mild evidence of inflammation)
   - Gram-negative organisms (e.g., *E. coli*, *Klebsiella* species)

134. **What are the noninfectious causes of increased umbilical drainage?**
   Serosanguinous drainage may be seen with a patent urachus or omphalomesenteric duct.

135. **What are the major complications of omphalitis?**
   - Septic umbilical arteritis
   - Suppurative thrombophlebitis of the umbilical or portal veins (resulting in portal vein thrombosis and portal hypertension)
   - Liver abscess
   - Endocarditis
   - Abdominal wall necrotizing fasciitis
   - Peritonitis

136. **How should infants with omphalitis be treated?**
   Infants with omphalitis should receive a penicillinase-resistant penicillin and an amino-glycoside antibiotic. Topical therapy can be used to eliminate surface colonization.

137. **What syndrome can be associated with chronic omphalitis or delayed separation of the umbilical cord?**
   Leukocyte adhesion deficiency is a life-threatening, autosomal-recessive inherited deficiency of cell adhesion molecules associated with chronic omphalitis or delayed separation of the umbilical cord. The hallmark of leukocyte adhesion deficiency is the absence of granulocytes at the site of infection.

138. **You are informed during sign-out rounds that a newborn is suspected to have funisitis. Where should you look for that infection?**
   Funisitis is no fun for the baby or the attending physician caring for the child! Funisitis is an inflammation of the umbilical cord vessels and Wharton's jelly and has been described as

either an acute exudative or subacute necrotizing process accompanying chorioamnionitis. The predominant organisms identified as etiologic agents are gram-negative bacteria, including *E. coli*, *Klebsiella* species, and *Pseudomonas* species. Gram-positive organisms (e.g., streptococci, staphylococci) and candidal species are less commonly responsible.

LISTERIOSIS

139. Is *L. monocytogenes* still a significant pathogen to consider when evaluating sepsis in neonates?
Yes. Although it is an uncommon infection in the United States (7.4 cases per million population, according to the CDC), an estimated 1850 cases per year result in 425 deaths. The largest affected groups are neonates and adults older than 60 years of age. Pregnant women account for about 27% of cases and have an increased tendency to develop listeriosis during the third trimester, often resulting in septic abortion. Vertical transmission from the colonized mother is the only human-to-human acquisition of the organism.

140. How do mothers acquire *L. monocytogenes*?
L. monocytogenes is acquired by susceptible adults (i.e., those with lower cellular immunity) through eating contaminated food. Surprisingly, the incidence of *L. monocytogenes* infection is low considering that food contamination is relatively common. The CDC sampled all refrigerator foods, 11% of which yielded the organism. *L. monocytogenes* loves refrigerator temperatures (4–10°C), which facilitates its growth. Additionally, it resists killing by routine pasteurization. Therefore, soft cheese products are the most common sources, along with delicatessen meats, fish, and poultry products. However, any undercooked food source is likely to contain this common organism (prevalent also in all soil and raw vegetable matter). One recent outbreak occurred with gravad-treated (cold-smoked) rainbow trout.

141. What are the signs and symptoms of clinical *L. monocytogenes* infection in a pregnant mother?
After ingestion of the microorganism, mothers may incubate *L. monocytogenes* for 11–70 days (mean, 31 days). Invasion of the intestinal mucosal barrier ensues with bacteremia, resulting in a flu-like illness with fever, chills, myalgias, arthralgias, headache, and backache. Symptoms may be mild and manifest most commonly between 26 and 30 weeks' gestation. Often the placenta becomes a reservoir for bacterial proliferation, resulting in amnionitis with persistence of symptoms until abortion or delivery occurs, with a 22% occurrence of either stillbirth or neonatal death. If cultured and recognized, the mother may be treated effectively, preserving the pregnancy.

142. How do *Listeria* infections present in neonates?
Neonatal infection may manifest at birth as disseminated listeriosis, termed *granulomatosis infantiseptica*, with microabscesses throughout the body, but particularly the liver and spleen. This entity may be accompanied by hemorrhagic amnionitis presenting as "chocolate syrup" meconium. Death usually occurs within a few hours. Vertical transmission from the mother may occur shortly before or at birth, resulting in either early-onset neonatal sepsis with pneumonia before 2 weeks of life (from organisms inhaled with amniotic fluid) or late-onset sepsis with meningitis within the first month. Papular rash (pinpoint, evanescent) and conjunctivitis are reported but are not specific for listeriosis. As with any virulent bacterial infection, disseminated intravascular coagulation and multiple organ system involvement are common. Mortality reports vary from 50% to 100%, with the highest death rates occurring in early-onset infections in premature infants.

143. **What is the pathogenesis of _L. monocytogenes_ infection, and why does insufficiency of cellular immunity in particular contribute to the development of disease?**

L. monocytogenes is an intracellular, facultative anaerobic parasite. Once phagocytized, _L. monocytogenes_ replicates rapidly within the cytosol, but it repels phagosome killing through its major virulence factor, listeriolysin O (characteristic of only this species of _Listeria_). Using the cell's own cytoskeletal actin polymerization mechanism, _L. monocytogenes_ pushes outward on the host cell's membrane forming filopods, which are then injected into neighboring cells. Cell-to-cell transmission spreads rapidly without exposure to circulating humoral antibodies or neutrophils. T-lymphocytes, therefore, provide the only natural recognition and immunity toward _L. monocytogenes_, although macrophage killing (probably using nitric oxide) may also occur. Because cellular immunity is suppressed during pregnancy and is naturally deficient during early neonatal life, _L. monocytogenes_ enjoys an advantage during these host-vulnerable periods. In the cellular immunocompetent host, significant infection is rare and self-limited.

144. **How should listeriosis be treated in a neonate?**

L. monocytogenes remains sensitive to ampicillin, and gentamicin may augment antimicrobial killing. Because of the organism's tendency to hide in tissue reservoirs, higher doses of ampicillin (200 mg/kg/day) are usually recommended for extended durations (2 weeks for bacteremia, 3 weeks for meningitis). Trimethoprim-sulfamethoxazole (TMP-SMX) is the best alternative for mothers who are penicillin sensitive, although erythromycin has been used in case reports (not currently recommended). Iron therapy for anemia should be withheld during treatment of listeriosis, because iron enhances the organism's growth in vitro and is therefore a virulence factor contributing to the host's susceptibility to infection.

SYPHILIS

145. **In 1987, the reported rate of congenital syphilis was 10.5 cases/100,000 live births. By 1991, this had risen to 107 cases/100,000 births. What factors account for these changes?**

- New surveillance case definition
- Substantial under-reporting of actual disease
- Coinfection with HIV
- Insufficient public health resources
- Promiscuity, failure to implement safer sexual practices, and drug use, particularly among adolescents and young adults

The last several years, however, have seen a reversal of this trend, perhaps because of public awareness, wider screening practices, and community-based prevention programs.

146. **What are the recommendations for syphilis screening in pregnancy?**

All women should have a Venereal Disease Research Laboratory test for syphilis (VDRL) performed at the first prenatal visit, with a second screen during the third trimester. If the nontreponemal test yields positive results, a treponemal serology specimen should be obtained. The CDC currently recommends that no infant be discharged from the hospital without a determination of maternal serology for syphilis.

147. **What are the effects of maternal coinfection with HIV on fetal infection with _T. pallidum_?**

Although the effects of maternal HIV infection on the transmission of syphilis are incompletely understood, the cellular immune abnormalities associated with HIV may allow greater treponemal proliferation and higher fetal infection. In addition, HIV-infected women may not respond adequately to benzathine penicillin, rendering their fetuses more susceptible to disease.

148. **What is the relationship between illicit drug use during pregnancy and congenital syphilis?**
Recent studies have found an increased risk of congenital syphilis among neonates following maternal illicit drug use, particularly cocaine. Reasons suggested include poor prenatal care among pregnant drug addicts and predisposing sexual behaviors in this population.

149. **Which infants should be evaluated for congenital syphilis?**
Asymptomatic infants born to successfully treated mothers do not need evaluation. Infants born to seropositive mothers (nontreponemal test confirmed by treponemal test) should be evaluated if mothers:
- Have untreated syphilis
- Were treated for syphilis <1 month before delivery
- Were treated for syphilis with a nonpenicillin regimen
- Did not have the expected decrease in nontreponemal antibody titers after treatment
- Were treated but had insufficient follow-up during pregnancy

150. **What is pneumonia alba?**
The pneumonia alba of congenital syphilis is characterized by yellow-white, heavy, grossly enlarged lungs. There is a marked increase in the amount of connective tissue in the interalveolar septa and interstitium histologically, with loss of alveolar spaces and obliterative fibrosis.

151. **What is Hutchinson's triad?**
The findings of Hutchinson's teeth, interstitial keratitis, and eighth nerve deafness comprise Hutchinson's triad and are virtually pathognomonic for late congenital syphilis. The stigmata represent scars induced by the lesions of early congenital syphilis or reactions to persistent inflammation.

152. **How useful are treponemal antibody tests in the diagnosis of congenital syphilis?**
Not very. Both treponemal and nontreponemal tests currently available detect maternal IgG antibody. Moreover, although treponemal antibody tests are more specific and sensitive for diagnosis, they remain reactive indefinitely, so active versus past infection cannot be distinguished. Therefore, treponemal antibody tests are not recommended screens for newborn infants.

153. **Which infants should be treated for congenital syphilis?**
Even if the evaluation is normal, all infants born to mothers who are untreated or who have evidence of relapse or reinfection should be assumed to be infected and treated.
Infants should be treated if they have:
- Any evidence of active disease (physical examination findings or x-ray)
- A reactive CSF VDRL
- An abnormal CSF finding, regardless of serology
- Quantitative nontreponemal antibody titers that are four times greater than maternal titers

154. **What is the derivation of the word *syphilis*?**
Syphilis is derived from the name of the shepherd Syphilus, the hero of a poem written by Frascatorius in 1530. Syphilus was afflicted with this disease as punishment for cursing the gods.

HUMAN IMMUNODEFICIENCY VIRUS

155. **What is the relative seroprevalence of HIV infection among pregnant women?**
It depends on location. Worldwide, the rate varies markedly. In the United States, the overall prevalence is estimated at 1.5/1000 women, with much higher rates reported from urban areas.

In Philadelphia, the rate is about 7.5/1000, whereas in New York City, the prevalence is around 25/1000 (or 1 in 40). These numbers pale in comparison to those found in sub-Saharan Africa, where rates as high as 25–33% (250–330/1000 pregnant women) are reported from several prenatal care centers.

156. **What is the risk of transmission of HIV infection to newborns?**
Untreated, the rate varies worldwide, from a high of 30–40% in Africa (confounded by breast-feeding and poor nutritional status) to 20–25% in the United States and 13–15% in Europe. With the use of perinatal zidovudine (AZT, ZDV) the rate of infant infection drops to 8%. When perinatal zidovudine is combined with elective cesarean section, the rate of infant infection is less than 5%. When pregnant women are treated with two to three drugs in combination therapy and maintain a low viral load, the risk to the infant is less than 3–4%.

157. **What risk factors are associated with increased risk of perinatal transmission of HIV infection?**
    - Maternal AIDS diagnosis
    - CD4 count <200/mm^3
    - High viral load
    - Vitamin A deficiency (?)
    - Breast-feeding
    - Preterm delivery
    - Chorioamnionitis
    - Prolonged rupture of membranes
    - Vaginal delivery
    - Untreated sexually transmitted diseases (?)

158. **When during the perinatal period is HIV transmitted?**
HIV infection may be transmitted in utero, intrapartum, or after birth through breast-feeding. In the absence of breast-feeding, it is believed that approximately 20–30% of perinatal infections occur in utero, with the remaining 70–80% occurring during the intrapartum period. In the event an infant escapes infection in utero and during delivery but is then breast-fed, the risk is approximately 15% when breast-feeding is continued for at least 6 months.

159. **Which pregnant women should be offered HIV testing?**
All of them. Because risk factor assessments fail to detect more than 40% of HIV-infected pregnant women, the AAP and ACOG both recommend routine HIV counseling to all pregnant women, with voluntary HIV testing.

160. **What percentage of HIV-exposed neonates will test positive for the virus by the enzyme-linked immunosorbent assay (ELISA) HIV antibody screening test?**
Virtually all of them. The ELISA measures IgG anti-HIV antibodies, which readily cross the placenta in the third trimester; hence, all infants born to antibody-positive women will be antibody positive themselves. These maternal antibodies will remain detectable in the infants' bloodstream until 12–18 months of age.

161. **What is the best diagnostic test for defining HIV infections in infants, and when should it be ordered?**
All HIV-exposed infants should have an HIV PCR-DNA assay (or HIV blood culture) performed at birth, at 1 month of age, and at 3–4 months of age. Any positive test result should be repeated immediately. If the test results at 1 month and 4 months of age are negative, the infant is considered HIV uninfected. Currently, quantitative RNA measurements (termed *viral load*) are not recommended for diagnostic purposes. In addition, the p24 antigen test is no longer used for diagnosis.

162. **What tests are used to monitor immune dysfunction related to HIV infection? How do the normal values differ from those in adults?**
The CD4 percentage and the absolute CD4 count are used to monitor immunogenic function in HIV infection. It should be remembered that normal CD4 counts for infants and children are much higher than those found in adults (normal infant CD4 count is 2500–3500/mL^3, and normal adult values are 700–1000/mL^3).

163. **What therapies are recommended for pregnant HIV-infected women?**
Close prenatal monitoring, attention to nutritional issues, antiretroviral therapy (at a minimum, prenatal and intrapartum AZT), and elective cesarean section are all recommended care for infected pregnant women.

KEY POINTS: PREVENTION OF AND TESTING FOR HIV TRANSMISSION

1. All pregnant women should be offered HIV testing.

2. Mothers and their infants should receive zidovudine to reduce the risk of transmission.

3. Exposed neonates should have HIV PCR-DNA testing at birth, 1 month, and 3–4 months of age.

4. Updates on recommendations for additional antiretroviral regimens are available at http://www.aidsinfo.nih.gov.

164. **Does therapy for a neonate change if the mother has a high viral load or has not received antiviral treatment?**
Zidovudine therapy alone remains the only therapy that has demonstrated efficacy in reducing HIV transmission in the exposed neonate in U.S. trials. Clinical trials in Africa have demonstrated a decrease in transmission by adding nevirapine or 3TC. Updated information and treatment recommendations are available online at http://www.aidsinfo.nih.gov.

165. **What are the major HIV-related complications seen in HIV-infected infants?**
Pneumocystis carinii pneumonia (PCP) is the most common serious HIV-related infection in infancy. The peak age of onset is 3–9 months, and it carries a 50% mortality rate. Fortunately, PCP can be prevented by thrice-weekly doses of TMP-SMX as prophylaxis. All exposed infants should be administered PCP prophylaxis at 6 weeks of age and should continue to be given the medicine until HIV infection is definitively ruled out (two negative HIV PCR-DNA test results, both after 1 month of age). Growth failure (i.e., failure to thrive) and a progressive encephalopathy are also common serious complications of HIV infection in the first year of life.

CYTOMEGALOVIRUS

166. **What is the most common congenital viral infection in the United States?**
Congenital cytomegalovirus (CMV) infection, occurring in 1–2% of all live births.

167. **What are the most common manifestations of congenital cytomegalovirus infection in neonates?**
- Petechiae
- Small-for-gestational-age birth weight

- Hepatosplenomegaly
- Jaundice at birth

Istas AS, Demmler GJ, Dobbins JG, Stewart JA: Surveillance for congenital cytomegalovirus disease: A report from the National Congenital Cytomegalovirus Disease Registry. J Infect Dis 20:665–670, 1995.

168. **What are the most reliable methods for diagnosing congenital cytomegalovirus infection?**
Isolation of cytomegalovirus from urine during the first 3 weeks of life is the most reliable method for diagnosing congenital infection. Detection of IgM antibodies to cytomegalovirus in serum obtained within the first few days after birth is highly suggestive of congenital infection. False-positive results may be reported by laboratories that do not use appropriate methods for detecting IgM antibodies to cytomegalovirus.

169. **What methods are available to prevent the transmission of cytomegalovirus to neonates through blood products?**
Transmission of cytomegalovirus to neonates by blood transfusion can be prevented by using blood that is obtained from seronegative donors, frozen in glycerol, or depleted of WBCs.

170. **What is the frequency of hearing loss in infants with congenital cytomegalovirus infection?**
See Table 12-15.

TABLE 12-15. FREQUENCY OF HEARING LOSS IN INFANTS WITH CONGENITAL CMV INFECTION

Type	Severity*	% Affected
Bilateral		11
	Mild	5
	Moderate to profound	6
Unilateral		8
	Mild	4
	Moderate to profound	4

*Mild hearing loss, 22–55 dB; moderate to profound ≥55 dB.
Adapted from Volpe JJ (ed): Neurology of the Newborn, 3rd ed. Philadelphia, W.B. Saunders, 1995.
Data from Hanshaw JB, Schneider AP, Moxley AW, et al: School failure and deafness after "silent" congenital cytomegalovirus infection. N Engl J Med 295:468–470, 1976; Kumar ML, Nankervis GA, Jacobs IB, et al: Congenital and postnatally acquired cytomegalovirus infections: Long-term follow-up. J Pediatr 104:674–679, 1984; Saigal S, Lunyk O, Larke RP, Chernesky MA: The outcome in children with congenital cytomegalovirus infection. A longitudinal follow-up study. Am J Dis Child 136:896–901, 1982; Stagno S, Pass RF, Dworsky ME, Alford CA: Congenital and perinatal cytomegalovirus infections. Semin Perinatol 7:31–42,1983.

171. **What is the relationship between neonatal clinical signs and neurologic outcome in congenital cytomegalovirus infection?**
See Table 12-16.

TABLE 12-16. RELATIONSHIP BETWEEN CLINICAL SIGNS AND NEUROLOGIC OUTCOME IN NEONATAL CMV INFECTION

Neonatal Signs	Neurologic Sequelae*			
	Normal	Major	Minor	Death
Neurologic				
Microcephaly, intracranial calcifications, chorioretinitis	7	79	0	14
Other	40	50	0	10
Systemic				
Jaundice, hepatosplenomegaly, or purpura, but no neurologic signs	48	12	36	4
No neurologic or systemic signs	81	3	16	0

Data from MacDonald and Tobin and based on 80 infants.
*Expressed as percentage of those with designated neonatal clinical signs.
Adapted from Volpe JJ (ed): Neurology of the Newborn, 3rd ed. Philadelphia, W.B. Saunders, 1995.

172. **Is there treatment available to improve neurologic outcome?**
Infants with symptomatic cytomegalovirus and signs of CNS involvement will have an improved chance of preserving hearing if treated with ganciclovir at 6 mg/kg/dose every 12 hours for 6 weeks. Unfortunately, there is no evidence of improvement in other neurologic outcomes with this or any other treatment.

Kimberlin DW, Lin C-Yu, Sanchez PJ, et al: Effect of ganciclovir therapy on hearing in symptomatic congenital cytomegalovirus disease involving the central nervous system: A randomized, controlled trial. J Pediatr 143:16–25, 2003.

173. **What are the side effects of ganciclovir treatment?**
Patients treated with ganciclovir need to have their absolute neutrophil count monitored closely, because as many as 60% of patients will have significant neutropenia. If neutropenia occurs, the dose should be cut in half. If neutropenia persists, the therapy should be discontinued.

HERPES SIMPLEX VIRUS

174. **What diagnostic approaches should be taken when a baby develops skin vesicles in the neonatal period?**
Newborns with skin vesicles should be rapidly worked up for the possibility of neonatal herpes simplex virus (HSV) infection. The most useful test for rapid diagnosis of HSV is a smear of material obtained from a skin vesicle that is fixed and stained with monoclonal antibodies to HSV, which are commercially available. This test is simple to perform and highly sensitive and accurate; results can be available within an hour and will indicate whether the virus is type 1 or type 2. Cultures for virus should also be performed, but this will often take as long as 48 hours to be completed. PCR, if available, can also be useful for diagnosis.

Babies in whom the diagnosis is established or who are strongly suspected of having neonatal HSV should be further tested for the possibility of disseminated infection and involvement of the CNS. Usually this means performing liver function tests, an ophthalmologic examination, lumbar puncture, and magnetic resonance imaging (MRI) or computed tomography (CT) scan. These tests usually need to be repeated after 1–2 weeks, with the first battery of tests serving as a baseline.

175. **How should women with a history of genital herpes be screened during pregnancy?**

Until fairly recently, it was thought that women with frequent reactivation episodes of genital HSV were at greatest risk to deliver an infected infant. Prospective studies, however, indicate that the infant at greatest risk to develop neonatal HSV is born to a woman with primary asymptomatic genital HSV at term. The risk of infection of the infant is only about 2% in mothers with recurrent HSV but 50% in those with primary HSV at term. Therefore, the women who should be screened at term, theoretically, are those who have no history of past HSV and who feel well. Unfortunately, however, there is still no good screening test for these women. Obtaining viral culture specimens on so many women is impractical and expensive. PCR does not necessarily indicate the presence of infectious HSV and in any case is not widely available. Examination to ensure no active lesions before a vaginal delivery is the only practical approach, but even this will miss asymptomatic primary infections. The best screening test for prevention of severe neonatal HSV is a high index of suspicion when an infant develops vesicular skin lesions.

176. **How is neonatal HSV classified? What is the importance of the classification with regard to prognosis?**

Clinically, the infection is divided into three categories: (1) skin, eye, or mouth (SEM) involvement; (2) disseminated infection that has extended to the viscera, especially the liver and lungs; and (3) CNS involvement. Even with appropriate antiviral therapy, the prognosis for infants with disseminated HSV and CNS disease is much poorer with regard to morbidity and mortality than infants who have infection confined to the SEM. It is believed that early therapy with acyclovir to infants with SEM disease can decrease the incidence of disseminated and CNS disease. Therefore, it is recommended that all infants with skin lesions due to HSV, even if they are otherwise well, be treated with acyclovir.

Typing of the infecting virus is also important because type 1 infections have a better prognosis than type 2 infections. Most infants with encephalitis due to type 1 HSV have a good long-term prognosis, whereas those with encephalitis due to type 2 HSV do not.

177. **What is the usual pathogenesis of HSV infections that present in the newborn?**

Most often, the virus multiplies on the mucosa of the maternal genital tract, and the baby is infected during the vaginal delivery. In only about 5% of infections does it appear that the virus crossed the placenta and caused congenital rather than neonatal infection. If the diagnosis of maternal primary HSV is known at delivery and the membranes are not ruptured, infections in infants can be prevented by performing a cesarean section. The chances of infection of the infant are increased if the skin is broken for any reason (e.g., from a scalp monitor).

Infants also can be infected with HSV type 1 if a mother has primary active HSV 1 infection, usually in the throat and mouth, at delivery. Presumably in this case, infection of the infant occurs from close maternal contact, such as kissing the baby, and aerosols.

178. **What is the treatment for neonatal HSV?**

The treatment is administration of intravenous acyclovir to all infants in whom the diagnosis of neonatal HSV is either established or pending diagnostic studies. Acyclovir is an antiviral drug that interferes with the replication of HSV DNA by acting as a chain terminator and interfering with the action of DNA polymerase. Because its action occurs mainly in infected cells, it is very well tolerated. Early therapy with acyclovir has decreased mortality and morbidity from serious HSV infections by 30–50%. Acyclovir is usually administered at a dosage of 60 mg/kg/day intravenously for 14–21 days, depending on the condition of the infant.

179. **How should infants with neonatal HSV be followed up after treatment?**

Follow-up is best individualized. Most asymptomatic infants should have a CT or MRI scan at some point after completion of therapy and discharge, usually after 4–6 weeks. Infants with symptoms such as recurrent skin vesicles, developmental delay, or seizures may have scans performed after a shorter interval. Infants who develop new or recurring symptoms should have a lumbar puncture for examination of the CSF. Those with CSF abnormalities or in whom the PCR remains positive should probably receive another course of intravenous acyclovir and be followed up closely. Infants suspected of having continued low-grade replication of HSV in the CNS may be given oral acyclovir on a long-term basis.

180. How safe is long-term therapy with acyclovir for an infant?
This therapy is considered an off-label use of acyclovir, and it needs to be discussed carefully with the parents. Long-term therapy is used by some physicians who suspect that low-grade multiplication of HSV in the CNS is ongoing. This form of therapy is not of proven use but intuitively makes sense. The dose is 300 mg/m^2, three times a day, taken orally. Monitoring for toxicity, particularly on the bone marrow, is important and should be performed every 1–2 weeks while the medication is being administered. The usual duration of long-term therapy is several months. The long-term safety of acyclovir is unknown.

181. How should infants born to women with active recurrent genital HSV infection be managed?
This remains somewhat controversial. Some obstetricians perform a cesarean section on any woman at term known to have active genital HSV. Others no longer recommend cesarean section in women with known recurrent HSV because the risk of infection to the infant is very low—about 2%.

182. Are antibody titers useful for diagnosis of HSV? What are their limitations?
Antibody titers are of little use for diagnosis of HSV because it takes at least several days after infection for antibodies to rise. Therefore, it is preferable to demonstrate the presence of virus or viral antigens or DNA in tissues for diagnosis. In instances when no virus can be demonstrated, antibody titers may be useful. Ideally, acute and convalescent sera (10–14 days apart) should be obtained from mother and baby. Practically speaking, however, by the time it becomes clear that antibody titers might be useful, the acute serum samples have already been discarded.
It is now possible to identify women who have not been infected with HSV 2 previously by measuring antibodies to an HSV antigen that is not shared between type 1 and type 2 (e.g., glycoprotein G).

VARICELLA-ZOSTER VIRUS

183. What is the congenital varicella syndrome?
This congenital syndrome is usually associated with maternal varicella between 8 and 20 weeks of pregnancy. Transmission of VZV from mother to infant occurs in 25–50% of cases of infected mothers. Fortunately, however, the syndrome is much less common than fetal infection. The syndrome in the infant occurs in only about 2% of cases of maternal chickenpox. Common manifestations of the syndrome include skin scarring (either generalized or localized in a dermatomal distribution), limb deformities (such as hypoplasia or missing digits), eye involvement (such as chorioretinitis, cataract, nystagmus, and hypoplasia), low birth weight, and mental retardation. Reactivation of VZV acquired in utero is a common event. Thus, zoster develops in about 20% of infants with the congenital syndrome in the first few years of life.

184. What is the appropriate management of an infant born to a woman with varicella at term delivery?
Infants whose mothers have the onset of the rash of varicella within 4 days before delivery and within 2 days postpartum have about a 50% chance of also developing varicella. In as many as 30% of infants who are untreated, the varicella may be disseminated and even fatal. This form of varicella resembles that seen in highly immunocompromised patients such as children with leukemia receiving chemotherapy. It is possible to prevent this severe form of infant varicella by

administering VZIG to the baby as soon as possible after birth. Rarely, VZIG may be ineffective in infants, so babies given this prophylaxis warrant close follow-up. Many will develop a mild form of clinical varicella with fewer than 100 skin vesicles despite VZIG. Indications for adding antiviral therapy (acyclovir) are extensive skin lesions and development of pneumonia, which suggests severe varicella. Infants whose mothers develop varicella more than 2 days postpartum are at significantly less risk from varicella and do not require VZIG, although some physicians may elect to administer it. In this case, infection of the infant would not be from exposure to VZV in utero, but from postpartum exposure. Infants whose mothers had the onset of varicella more than 5 days before delivery do not need to receive VZIG because they will have developed sufficient transplacental VZV antibodies by this time (as if nature provided them with a dose of VZIG). With regard to isolation of infants perinatally exposed to VZV, there are two points to consider:

1. The incubation period can be as short as 10 days and is counted from the time of onset of maternal rash.
2. Infants are contagious only around the time when rash is expected to occur.

185. What is the appropriate management of an infant born to a woman with zoster at term?

There is almost no chance that such an infant will develop varicella, and no special management is required. Women with zoster have high antibody titers to VZV, and their infants are well protected from the virus by transplacental antibodies.

186. When is it appropriate to administer acyclovir to a pregnant woman with chickenpox?

There is no question that varicella in adults tends to be more severe than in children. Although the data are far from conclusive, most experts believe that varicella in pregnant women is likely to be more severe than in nonpregnant women, especially in the third trimester of pregnancy. Therefore, pregnant women with varicella should be closely observed, particularly for development of primary pneumonia. Pneumonia usually presents with fever, cough, dyspnea, and bilateral fluffy interstitial infiltrates on chest x-ray. Pregnant women with varicella pneumonia or even suspected varicella pneumonia should be treated with intravenous acyclovir (30 mg/kg/day, divided into three doses). Usually treatment is continued for 7 days. Maternal acyclovir therapy has not been associated with fetal malformations; nevertheless, it is advisable to avoid its use if possible. Orally administered acyclovir is not well absorbed and has demonstrated only modest success against varicella in clinical trials. Therefore, it is preferable to monitor pregnant women with varicella closely and to intervene if necessary with intravenous acyclovir, which is known to be effective if given early in the course of illness.

187. Should children be immunized against varicella if their pregnant mother has never had varicella?

Each instance is best individualized, weighing the potential risks and benefits to the mother. For example, in a family with several young, varicella-susceptible children who attend school or day care, there is a very high likelihood (estimated at 9% per child) that they will introduce chickenpox into the household while their mother is pregnant. In such a situation, it is preferable to immunize the children against chickenpox. Only about 5% of immunized children develop rash after immunization, and the infectivity of these children to others is extremely low. Should the vaccine virus nevertheless infect the mother, the illness is predicted to be mild, and no cases of the congenital varicella syndrome have been associated with vaccine-type VZV. In contrast, the wild-type VZV is highly contagious, so if the children bring this virus home, maternal infection is inevitable, may be severe, and is known to be associated with a congenital syndrome. On the other hand, in a family in which there is only one child who is cared for at home and who has few visitors, it may be preferable to immunize the child after the mother is delivered. There would be no known risk to the newborn if a sibling developed a vaccine-associated rash.

TOXOPLASMOSIS

188. How is the infection acquired in the mother?

Toxoplasma gondii is a protozoan parasite that exists in three developmental stages: tachyzoite, tissue cyst, and oocyst. Once infected with the tachyzoite, the organism may encyst—commonly in the skeletal muscles. Ingestion of the oocyst, probably the most common route of infection, is found to occur only in the intestinal tract of cats and other felines. Oocysts must mature or sporulate in the soil (at least 24 hours) before they are infectious. Therefore, *Toxoplasma* infection is acquired through ingestion of undercooked or raw meat containing tissue cysts or if water or other foods become contaminated by oocysts that have been excreted in the feces of infected cats. It is possible to become infected through exposure to soil contaminated with cat feces.

The incidence of acute toxoplasmosis during pregnancy based on seroprevalence among women of child-bearing years is estimated at 0.2–1%. Transmission rates to the fetus depend on the stage of the pregnancy and treatment during pregnancy (Table 12-17). Treatment during pregnancy consists of spiramycin throughout the remainder of the pregnancy. Pyrimethamine-sulfadiazine is alternated with spiramycin if fetal infection was confirmed by prenatal testing.

Wong SY, Remington JS: Toxoplasmosis in pregnancy. Clin Infect Dis 18:853–862, 1994.

TABLE 12-17. INCIDENCE OF T. GONDII INFECTION		
	Without Maternal Treatment	With Maternal Treatment
First trimester	10–15%	5%
Second trimester	30%	17%
Third trimester	60%	29%

189. What are the clinical manifestations of congenital toxoplasmosis?

Congenital toxoplasmosis affects approximately 3500 newborns in the United States each year. Most infected newborns are born asymptomatic, and only on thorough evaluation is infection suspected. The clinical manifestations of congenital toxoplasmosis include:

- Intrauterine growth retardation
- Developmental delay
- Hydrocephalus
- CSF pleocytosis
- Seizures
- Deafness
- Blindness
- Cataracts
- Chorioretinal scars or chorioretinitis
- Nystagmus
- Strabismus
- Myocarditis
- Encephalitis
- Hydrops fetalis
- Thrombocytopenia
- Intracranial calcifications
- Eosinophilia

- Nephrotic syndrome
- Hepatomegaly with calcification and jaundice
- Metaphyseal bone lucencies
- Interstitial pneumonia
- Petechial purpura
- Maculopapular rash

190. **What is the treatment of congenital toxoplasmosis for neonates?**

The treatment is continued for approximately 12–14 months (consult an expert on infectious diseases for confirmation on a specific case). The dosage should be adjusted weekly. In addition, a CBC with differential should be performed by finger stick twice weekly to measure the absolute neutrophil count. Remember that pyrimethamine is a folic acid antagonist and therefore may cause thrombocytopenia, granulocytopenia, and anemia resulting from bone marrow suppression. The use of folinic acid can counteract this side effect (Table 12-18).

TABLE 12-18.	TREATMENT FOR NEONATAL TOXOPLASMOSIS
Medication	**Dosage**
Sulfadiazine	100 mg/mL; half of the infant's weight (kg) equals number of milliliters given in A.M. and P.M.
	100 mg/mL; 10 mg (two tablets) on Monday, Wednesday, and Friday. Crush and give with formula or apple juice.
Pyrimethamine	2 mg/mL; half of the infant's weight (kg) equals number of milliliters given once daily.
Leucovorin	10 mg three times a week during and for 1 week after pyrimethamine.
Prednisone	1 mg/kg divided twice a day when active chorioretinitis threatens vision.

191. **If maternal infection is suspected but full evaluation for toxoplasmosis in the newborn is negative except for *T. gondii*–specific IgG antibodies, what is the best management plan?**

In this case, transfer of maternal antibodies may be suspected if all other evaluations have negative results. A monthly Sabin-Feldman dye test should be obtained from the infant to observe a fall in antibody titers over time (50% per month). One may calculate *Toxoplasma* antibody load with the following formula:

Toxoplasma antibody load = (dye test titer × dye test sensitivity)/quantitative IgG

Table 12-19 gives an example of the expected fall in antibody titers in an infant without infection who has received maternal antibody.

UREAPLASMA UREALYTICUM

192. **What is the carriage rate of *Ureaplasma urealyticum* in the female lower genital tract?**

Seventy percent, with a range of 40–80%. Colonization in adults is related to the number of sexual exposures but occurs in 50% of men and 70% of women with three or more partners.

193. **What is the rate of vertical transmission for *U. urealyticum*, and what factors influence that rate?**

The vertical transmission rate ranges from 25% to 60%. Transmission occurs in utero by ascending infection or during delivery through an infected birth canal. Preterm and VLBW infants are more likely to acquire *U. urealyticum* in their lower respiratory tract. The mode of delivery does not influence the rate of transmission, but it is increased in the presence of clinical

TABLE 12-19. ANTIBODY TITERS

Age (days)	Dye Test Titer	Test Sensitivity*	Quantitative Immunoglobulins (mg/dL)	Antibody Load
10	1–16,000	0.2	886	3.61
28	1–8000	0.2	518	3.09
43	1–4096	0.2	427	1.92
67	1–2048	0.2	285	1.08
102	1–1024	0.2	255	0.80
132	1–256	0.2	119	0.43
189	1–64	0.2	209	0.06

*Value obtained from Research Institute, Palo Alto Foundation.

intra-amniotic infection and histologic chorioamnionitis and may be increased in the presence of prolonged rupture of membranes.

194. **What are the clinical manifestations of *U. urealyticum* infection?**
   - It is the most common agent isolated when there is chorioamnionitis and is the most frequent isolate from placentas after preterm delivery.
   - Several case reports suggest that *U. urealyticum* causes pneumonia in the newborn.
   - Surfactant-deficient respiratory distress syndrome is twice as frequent in premature infants of <34 weeks' gestation who have *U. urealyticum* isolated from the endotracheal aspirate. However, there is no association with superficial colonization.
   - In two meta-analyses, *U. urealyticum* colonization was associated with a relative risk of chronic lung disease (CLD) of approximately 1.8. It is hypothesized that infection causes a subacute pneumonia and chronic damage. This is supported by the finding of increased levels of cytokines, IL-1-β, and TNF-α in colonized VLBW infants.
   - *U. urealyticum* has been isolated from CSF. In the preterm population, it may be associated with hydrocephalus. There may be a pleocytosis, and it may persist for weeks. Several case reports describe a clinical response to treatment.

195. **How is *U. urealyticum* diagnosed?**
   Although usually limited to research settings, it is appropriate to sample endotracheal aspirates, blood, and CSF from the premature neonate. The organism is fastidious; it should be transported to the laboratory in special transport media and refrigerated if transport is not immediately possible.

196. **Does treatment of *U. urealyticum* prevent CLD?**
   Although numerous studies have demonstrated the association of colonization of the lower respiratory tract and CLD, several randomized, controlled trials have not demonstrated any decrease in the incidence of CLD after treating infants colonized with *U. urealyticum* with erythromycin.

INFECTIOUS HEPATITIS

197. **What are the common causes of infectious hepatitis in the neonate?**
   Several infectious agents can cause hepatitis in neonates, and infants, including the TORCH pathogens: *T. gondii*, **O**ther infectious etiologies (i.e., syphilis; hepatitis B, C, and D; and rarely hepatitis A virus), **R**ubella, **C**ytomegalovirus, and **H**erpes simplex types I and II. Additional

etiologies in this age group include generalized viral infections with adenovirus, coxsackievirus, enterovirus, Epstein-Barr virus, HIV, and varicella.

198. **How is hepatitis B virus (HBV) transmitted?**
HBV is transmitted by percutaneous or mucosal exposure to infectious body fluids, sexual contact, or perinatal transmission from an infected mother to her newborn. Women who are hepatitis B e antigen (HBeAg) positive are more likely to transmit hepatitis than women who are only hepatitis B surface antigen (HBsAg) positive and HBeAg negative (70–90% versus 5–20%).

199. **What are the best ways to prevent transmission of HBV from an infected mother to a newborn?**
  - Screen all pregnant women for hepatitis B.
  - Provide active immunization with hepatitis B vaccine and passive immunization with hepatitis B immunoglobulin within 12–24 hours of birth. Breast-feeding is not associated with increased risk.
  - Routinely immunize all infants.
  - Vaccinate all 11–12-year-olds and high-risk adolescents.

200. **What are the complications of HBV?**
Hepatic complications of hepatitis B include chronic active hepatitis and cirrhosis that can progress to liver failure and hepatocellular carcinoma. The risk of chronic infection is inversely related to age; as many as 90% of newborns, 30% of children 1–5 years of age, and 5–10% of older children may have persistence of HBsAg.

201. **How is hepatitis C virus (HCV) transmitted, and how are the clinical manifestations different from hepatitis A and B?**
Hepatitis C is transmitted by parenteral exposure to blood and blood products from a hepatitis C–infected person. Sexual transmission is less common. Approximately 5% of infected women transmit HCV to their neonates, and transmission only occurs if the mother is HCV RNA positive. Breast-feeding has not been shown to be a risk factor for transmission. Only 25% of patients have jaundice, and liver function abnormalities are frequently less severe than those seen with HBV. However, 85% of persons infected with HCV develop persistent infection, as many as 70% develop chronic hepatitis, 20% develop cirrhosis, and some may progress to hepatocellular carcinoma.

202. **How is hepatitis C infection diagnosed in a neonate after in utero exposure?**
The most sensitive test for HCV infection remains enzyme immunoassay for IgG antibody. Hepatitis C antibody can persist in a neonate for up to 18 months. Therefore, diagnosis can only be made early using reverse transcriptase PCR assays for hepatitis C RNA, which can be detected within 1 to 2 weeks of exposure. However, these tests have more false-positive and false-negative results than antibody testing. Furthermore, there are no FDA-approved treatments available for persons younger than 18 years of age. As a result, diagnosis is usually made through antibody testing after 18 months of age.

PARVOVIRUS

203. **What percentage of women of child-bearing age is immune to parvovirus B19 infection?**
Approximately 50%. This means that B19 infection in pregnancy is only a concern for about 50% of pregnant women because previous infection confers immunity. Immunity can be assessed by screening for parvovirus B19 IgG antibody. If exposure to parvovirus or clinical signs or symptoms suggestive of B19 infection occur during pregnancy in a woman with unknown B19 status, both IgG and IgM anti-B19 antibodies should be measured to determine whether recent infection has occurred.

204. **If B19 infection occurs during pregnancy, what is the risk for an adverse fetal outcome (i.e., nonimmune hydrops fetalis or fetal demise)?**
Less than 10%. When intrauterine B19 infection associated with hydrops was first described, a high risk for fetal complications after maternal infection was emphasized. With prospective follow-up of a large number of women with B19 infection in pregnancy, adverse fetal outcome appears to be the exception, not the rule. Harger et al. reported no fetal or neonatal deaths attributable to B19 infection in 52 IgM-positive women, and the calculated frequency of hydrops and death from B19 infection is 0–8.6% (95% confidence interval). These data are similar to data from other prospective studies.

   Obstetric follow-up of women with B19 infection usually relies on frequent ultrasound examinations in the weeks after infection. Based on the low risk for adverse outcomes, Harger et al. suggest brief "screening" ultrasound to detect fetal ascites or other early signs of nonimmune hydrops with full exams only if abnormalities are detected.

   Harger JH, Adler SP, Koch WC, Harger GF: Prospective evaluation of 618 pregnant women exposed to parvovirus B19: Risks and symptoms. Obstet Gynecol 91:413–420, 1998.

205. **You get a call from a worried mother of a 2-year-old patient. The family puppy was just diagnosed with parvovirus hemorrhagic colitis. She is concerned about possible transmission to her toddler or herself (she is 3 months pregnant). What advice do you give?**
Not to worry. Canine parvovirus is not a human pathogen!

206. **Parvovirus B19 is the cause of erythema infectiosum (EI). How often do children or adults infected with B19 develop classic EI?**
Classic EI with "slapped cheeks" appearance followed by a characteristic lacy or reticular rash on the trunk and limbs is fairly easy to diagnose clinically. Unfortunately, most persons infected with B19 do not develop classic signs. A nondiagnostic exanthem may be present in approximately one third to one half of infections. In the study by Harger et al., 38% of B19-infected women manifested rash; none were clinically diagnosed as having EI. In adults, especially women, joint symptoms occur in 60–80% of cases and may be helpful diagnostically. The clinical illness in adults—with fever, rash, and joint symptoms—mimics rubella.

   Harger JH, Adler SP, Koch WC, Harger GF: Prospective evaluation of 618 pregnant women exposed to parvovirus B19: Risks and symptoms. Obstet Gynecol 91:413–420, 1998.

207. **Why does B19 infection cause aplastic anemia in patients with hemolytic anemia?**
Parvoviruses require actively dividing cells to replicate, and B19 preferentially infects red blood cell (RBC) precursors. In patients with hemolytic anemia and a high RBC turnover, the viral cytopathic effect destroys bone marrow RBC precursors, resulting in reticulocytopenia. The transient arrest of erythrocyte production results in profound anemia in persons with a shortened RBC survival, such as patients with hemolytic anemia. In fetuses, shortened RBC survival (60–80 days versus 110–120 days in adults) also contributes to the severity of anemia in some cases.

BIBLIOGRAPHY

DEVELOPMENTAL IMMUNOLOGY

1. Erdman SH, Christensen RD, Bradley PP, Rothstein GJ: Supply and release of storage neutrophils: A developmental study. Biol Neonate 41:132–137, 1982.

2. Johnston RB: Function and cell biology of neutrophils and mononuclear phagocytes in the newborn infant. Vaccine 16:1363–1368, 1998.

3. Speer C, Johnston RB: Neutrophil function in newborn infants. In Polin RA, Fox WW (eds): Fetal and Neonatal Physiology, 2nd ed. Philadelphia, W.B. Saunders, 1997, pp 1954–1998.

4. Stiehm ER (ed): Immunologic Disorders in Infants and Children, 3rd ed. Philadelphia, W.B. Saunders, 1989.

5. Yoder MC, Polin RA: Developmental immunology. In Fanaroff AA, Martin RJ (eds): Neonatal-Perinatal Medicine, 7th ed. St. Louis, MO, Mosby, 1997, pp 676–705.

EARLY-ONSET NEONATAL SEPSIS

6. Eichenwald EC: Perinatally transmitted neonatal bacterial infections. Infect Dis Clin North Am 11:223–239, 1997.

7. Hickman ME, Rench MA, Ferrieri P, Baker CJ: Changing epidemiology of group B streptococcal colonization. Pediatrics 104:203–209, 1999.

8. Hyde TB, Hilger TM, Reingold A, et al: Trends in incidence and antimicrobial resistance of early-onset sepsis: Population-based surveillance in San Francisco and Atlanta. Pediatrics 110:690–695, 2002.

9. Schuchat A, Zywicki SS, Dinsmoor MJ, for the PENS Study Group: Risk factors and opportunities for prevention of early-onset neonatal sepsis: A multicenter case-control study. Pediatrics 105:21–26, 2000.

10. Stoll BJ, Gordon T, Korones SB, et al: Early-onset sepsis in very low birth weight neonates: A report from the National Institute of Child Health and Human Development Neonatal Research Network. J Pediatr 129:72–80, 1996.

11. Stoll BJ, Hansen N, Fanaroff AA, et al: Changes in pathogens causing early-onset sepsis in very-low-birth-weight infants. N Engl J Med 347:240–247, 2002.

NOSOCOMIAL SEPSIS

12. Kilbride HW, Powers R, Wirtschafter DD, et al: Evaluation and development of potentially better practices to prevent neonatal nosocomial bacteremia. Pediatrics 111:504–518, 2003.

13. Kilbride HW, Wirtschafter DD, Powers RJ, Sheehan MB: Implementation of evidence-based potentially better practices to decrease nosocomial infections. Pediatrics 111:e519–e533, 2003.

14. Schuchat A, Zywicki SS, Dinsmoor MJ, et al: Risk factors and opportunities for prevention of early-onset neonatal sepsis: A multicenter case-control study. Pediatrics 105:21–26, 2000.

15. Stoll BJ, Gordon T, Korones S, et al: Late-onset sepsis in very low birth weight neonates: A report from the NICHD Neonatal Research Network. J Pediatr 129:63–71, 1996.

16. Stoll BJ, Hansen N, Fanaroff AA, et al: Late-onset sepsis in very low birth weight neonates: The experience of the NICHD neonatal research network. Pediatrics 110:285–292, 2002.

17. Stoll BJ, Holman RC, Schuchat A, et al: Decline in sepsis-associated neonatal and infant deaths in the United States, 1979 through 1994. Pediatrics 102:e18, 1994.

18. Stoll BJ, Temprosa M, Tyson JE, et al: Dexamethasone therapy increases infection in very low birth weight infants. Pediatrics 104:e63, 1999.

DIAGNOSIS OF NEONATAL SEPSIS

19. Benitz WE, Han MY, Madan A, Ramachandra P: Serial serum C-reactive protein levels in the diagnosis of neonatal infection. Pediatrics 102:E41, 1998.

20. Gerdes JS: Clinicopathologic approach to the diagnosis of neonatal sepsis. Clin Perinatol 18:361–381, 1991.

21. Lieberman E, Lang J, Richardson DK, et al: Intrapartum maternal fever and neonatal outcome. Pediatrics 105:8–13, 2000.

22. Ng PC: Diagnostic markers of infection in neonates. Arch Dis Child Fetal Neonatal Ed 89:F229–F235, 2004.

23. Powell K, Marcy M: Laboratory aids in the diagnosis of neonatal sepsis. In Remington JS, Klein JO (eds): Infectious Diseases of the Fetus and Newborn Infant, 4th ed. Philadelphia, W.B. Saunders, 2001, pp 1327–1344.

ANTIMICROBIAL THERAPY

24. Edwards MS, Baker CJ: Nosocomial infections in the neonate. In Long SS, Pickering LK, Prober CG (eds): Principles and Practice of Pediatric Infectious Diseases. New York, Churchill Livingstone, 2003, pp 547–553.

25. Klein JO: Bacterial sepsis and meningitis. In Remington JS, Klein JO (eds): Infectious Diseases of the Fetus and Newborn Infant, 5th ed. Philadelphia, W.B. Saunders, 2001, pp 943–998.

GROUP B STREPTOCOCCAL INFECTIONS

26. de Cueto M, Sanchez M-J, Sampedro A, et al: Timing of intrapartum ampicillin and prevention of vertical transmission of group B streptococcus. Obstet Gynecol 91:112–114, 1998.
27. Lim K, Clemens J, Azimi P, et al: Capsular polysaccharide types of group B streptococcal isolates from neonates with early-onset systemic infection. J Infect Dis 177:790–792, 1998.
28. Lin FC, Weisman LE, Troendle J, Adams K: Prematurity is the major risk factor for late-onset group B streptococcus disease. J Infect Dis 188:267–271, 2003.
29. Schrag S, Gorwitz R, Fultz-Butts K, Schuchat A: Prevention of perinatal group B streptococcal disease. MMWR 51:1–22, 2002.
30. Schrag SJ, Phil D, Zell ER, et al: A population-based comparison of strategies to prevent early-onset group B streptococcal disease in neonates. N Engl J Med 347:233–239, 2002.
31. Schrag SJ, Zywicki S, Farley MM, et al: Group B streptococcal disease in the era of intrapartum antibiotic prophylaxis. N Engl J Med 342:15–20, 2000.
32. Schuchat A: Epidemiology of group B streptococcal disease in the United States: Shifting paradigms. Clin Microbiol Rev 11:497–513, 1998.

STAPHYLOCOCCUS EPIDERMIDIS

33. Baier RJ, Bocchini JA, Brown EG: Selective use of vancomycin to prevent coagulase-negative staphylococcal nosocomial bacteremia in high-risk very low birth weight infants. Pediatr Infect Dis J 17:179–183, 1998.
34. Baltimore RS: Neonatal nosocomial infections. Semin Perinatol 22:25–32, 1998.
35. Clark R, Powers R, White R, et al: Nosocomial infection in the NICU: A medical complication or unavoidable problem? J Perinatol 24:382–388, 2004.
36. Craft A, Finer N: Nosocomial coagulase negative staphylococcal (CoNS) catheter-related sepsis in preterm infants: Definition, diagnosis, prophylaxis, and prevention. J Perinatol 21:186–192, 2001.
37. Isaacs D: A ten year, multicentre study of coagulase negative staphylococcal infections in australasian neonatal units. Arch Dis Child Fetal Neonatal Ed 88:F89–F93, 2003.
38. Karlowicz MG, Buescher ES, Surka AE: Fulminant late-onset sepsis in a neonatal intensive care unit, 1988–1997, and the impact of avoiding empiric vancomycin therapy. Pediatrics 106:1387–1390, 2000.
39. Struthers S, Underhill H, Albersheim S, et al: A comparison of two versus one blood culture in the diagnosis and treatment of coagulase-negative staphylococcus in the neonatal intensive care unit. J Perinatol 22:547–549, 2002.

CANDIDA INFECTION

40. Benjamin DK, Poole C, Steinbach WJ, et al: Neonatal candidemia and end-organ damage: A critical appraisal of the literature using meta-analytic techniques. Pediatrics 112:634–640, 2003.
41. Butler KM, Baker CJ: *Candida:* An increasingly important pathogen in the nursery. Pediatr Clin North Am 35:543–563, 1988.
42. Harris MC, Bell LM, Pereira GR, et al: Candidal arthritis in infants previously treated for systemic candidiasis during the newborn period: Report of three cases. Pediatr Emerg Care 16:249–251, 2000.
43. Hughes WT, Flynn PM: Candidiasis. In Feigin RD, Cherry JD (eds): Textbook of Pediatric Infectious Diseases, 4th ed. Philadelphia, W.B. Saunders, 1998, pp 2303–2313.
44. Karlowicz MG, Giannone PJ, Pestian J, et al: Does candidemia predict threshold retinopathy of prematurity in extremely low birth weight (<1000 g) neonates? Pediatrics 105:1036–1040, 2000.
45. Kaufman D, Boyle R, Hazen KC, et al: Fluconazole prophylaxis against fungal colonization and infection in preterm births. N Engl J Med 345:1660–1666, 2001.
46. Mittal M, Dhanireddy R, Higgins RD: Candida sepsis and association with retinopathy of prematurity. Pediatrics 101:654–657, 1998.

NEONATAL MENINGITIS

47. Stoll BJ, Hansen N, Fanaroff AA, et al: To tap or not to tap: High likelihood of meningitis without sepsis among very low birth weight infants. Pediatrics 113:1181–1186, 2004.
48. Wiswell TE, Baumgart S, Gannon CM, Spitzer AR: No lumbar puncture in the evaluation for early neonatal sepsis: Will meningitis be missed? Pediatrics 95:803–806, 1995.

INFECTION CONTROL

49. American Academy of Pediatrics: 2003 Red Book: Report of the Committee on Infectious Diseases, 26th ed. Elk Grove Village, IL, AAP, 2003.

50. Bennett JV, Brachman PS: Hospital Infections. Boston, Little, Brown, 1992.

51. Campbell JR, Zaccaria E, Baker CJ: Systemic candidiasis in extremely low birth weight infants receiving topical petrolatum ointment for skin care: A case-control study. Pediatrics 105:1041–1046, 2000.

52. Edwards WH, Conner JM, Soll RF: The effect of prophylactic ointment therapy on nosocomial sepsis rates and skin integrity in infants with birth weights of 501 to 1000g. Pediatrics 113:1195–1202, 2004.

53. Mayhall CG: Hospital Epidemiology and Infection Control. Baltimore, MD, Williams & Wilkins, 1996.

CONJUNCTIVITIS

54. de Toledo AR, Chandler JW: Conjunctivitis of the newborn. Infect Dis Clin North Am 6:807–813, 1992.

55. Hammerschlag MR: Neonatal conjunctivitis. Pediatr Ann 22:346–351, 1993.

56. Hammerschlag MR, Cummings C, Roblin PM, et al: Efficacy of neonatal ocular prophylaxis for the prevention of chlamydial and gonococcal conjunctivitis. N Engl J Med 320:769–772, 1989.

CHLAMYDIAL INFECTIONS

57. American Academy of Pediatrics: Chlamydial infections. In Pickering LK (ed): 2000 Red Book: Report of the Committee on Infectious Diseases, 24th ed. Elk Grove Village, IL, AAP, 2000, pp 205–212.

58. Hammerschlag MR: *Chlamydia trachomatis* in children. Pediatr Ann 23:349–353, 1994.

59. Hammerschlag MR, Gelling M, Roblin PM, et al: Treatment of neonatal chlamydial conjunctivitis with azithromycin. Pediatr Infect Dis J 17:1049–1050, 1998.

60. Hammerschlag MR, Rawstron SA: Sexually transmitted infection. In Jenson HB, Baltimore RS (eds): Pediatric Infectious Diseases: Principles and Practice. Norwalk, CT, Appleton & Lange, 1995, pp 1249–1276.

61. Normann E, Gnarpe J, Gnarpe H, Wettergren B: *Chlamydia pneumoniae* in children with acute respiratory tract infections. Acta Paediatr 87:23–27, 1998.

OSTEOMYELITIS AND SEPTIC ARTHRITIS

62. Asmar BI: Osteomyelitis in the neonate. Infect Dis Clin North Am 6:124–125, 1992.

63. Jaramillo D, Treves ST, Kasser JR, et al: Osteomyelitis and septic arthritis in children: Appropriate use of imaging to guide treatment. AJR Am J Roentgenol 165:399–403, 1995.

64. Ogden J, Lister G: The pathology of neonatal osteomyelitis. Pediatrics 55:474–478, 1975.

65. Swanson H, Hughes P, Messer SA, et al: *Candida albicans* arthritis one year after successful treatment of fungemia in a healthy infant. J Pediatr 129:688–694, 1996.

66. Trujillo M, Nelson JD: Suppurative and reactive arthritis in children. Semin Pediatr Infect Dis 8:242–249, 1997.

67. Unkila-Kallio L, Kallio MJ, Eskola J, Peltola H: Serum C-reactive protein: Erythrocyte sedimentation rate and white blood cell count in acute hematogenous osteomyelitis of children. Pediatrics 93:59–61, 1994.

68. Wong M, Isaacs D, Howman-Giles R, Uren R: Clinical and diagnostic features of osteomyelitis occurring in the first three months of life. Pediatr Infect Dis J 14:1047–1053, 1995.

PYELONEPHRITIS AND URINARY TRACT INFECTION

69. Jakobsson B, Berg U, Svensson L: Renal scarring after acute pyelonephritis. Arch Dis Child 70:111–115, 1994.

70. Klein JO, Long SS: Bacterial infections of the urinary tract. In Remington JS, Klein JO (eds): Infectious Diseases of the Fetus and Newborn Infant, 4th ed. Philadelphia, W.B. Saunders, 1995, pp 925–934.

OMPHALITIS

71. Brook I: Microbiology of necrotizing fasciitis associated with omphalitis in the newborn infant. J Perinatol 18: 28–30, 1998.

72. Cushing AH: Omphalitis: A review. Pediatr Infect Dis 4:282–285, 1985.

73. Faridi MMA, Rattan A, Ahmed SH: Omphalitis neonatorum. J Ind Med Assoc 91:283–285, 1993.

74. Guvenc H, Aygun AD, Uysar P, et al: Omphalitis in term and preterm appropriate for gestational age and small for gestational age infants. J Trop Pediatr 43:368–372, 1997.

75. Hartman GE, Boyajian MJ, Choi SS, et al: General surgery. In Avery GB, Fletcher MA, MacDonald MG (eds): Neonatology: Pathophysiology and Management of the Newborn, 5th ed. Philadelphia, Lippincott Williams & Wilkins, 1999, pp 1036–1037.

76. Mason WH, Andrews R, Ross LA, Wright HT: Omphalitis in the newborn infant. Pediatr Infect Dis J 8:521–525, 1989.

77. Meberg A, Schoyen R: Hydrophobic material in routine umbilical cord care and prevention of infections in newborn infants. Scand J Infect Dis 22:729–733, 1990.

78. Monu JUV, Okola AA: Diffuse abdominal wall cellulitis in ascending omphalitis: A lethal association in neonatal necrotizing fasciitis. J Natl Med Assoc 85:457–459, 1993.

79. Nezelof C: Chronic omphalitis in a 4-month-old girl. Path Res Pract 187:334–337, 1991.

80. Oudesluys-Murphy AM, Eilers GAM, deGroot CJ: The time of separation of the umbilical cord. Eur J Pediatr 146:387–389, 1987.

81. Samuel M, Freeman NV, Vaishnav A, et al: Necrotizing fasciitis: A serious complication of omphalitis in neonates. J Pediatr Surg 29:1414–1416, 1994.

82. Sawin RS, Schaller RT, Tapper D, et al: Early recognition of neonatal abdominal wall necrotizing fasciitis. Am J Surg 167:481–484, 1994.

LISTERIOSIS

83. Bortolussi R, Schlech WF: Listeriosis. In Remington JS, Klein JO (eds): Infectious Diseases of the Fetus and Newborn Infant, 4th ed. Philadelphia, W.B. Saunders, 2001, pp 1157–1178.

SYPHILIS

84. Sanchez PJ, Wendel GD: Syphilis in pregnancy. Clin Perinatol 24:71–90, 1997.

85. Sison CG, Ostrea EM, Reyes MP, Salari V: The resurgency of congenital syphilis: A cocaine-related problem. J Pediatr 130:289–292, 1997.

HUMAN IMMUNODEFICIENCY VIRUS

86. American Academy of Pediatrics Committee on Pediatric AIDS: Evaluation and medical treatment of the HIV-exposed infant. Pediatrics 99:909–917, 1997.

87. Centers for Disease Control and Prevention: Public Health Service Task Force recommendations for the use of antiretroviral drugs in pregnant women infected with HIV-1 for maternal health and for reducing perinatal HIV-1 transmission in the United States. MMWR 47:RR2, 1998.

88. Centers for Disease Control and Prevention: U.S. Public Health Service Recommendations for Human Immunodeficiency Virus Counseling and Voluntary Testing for Pregnant Women. Atlanta, CDC, 2001.

89. Centers for Disease Control and Prevention: Working Group on Antiretroviral Therapy and Medical Management of HIV-Infected Children: Guidelines for the use of antiretroviral agents in pediatric HIV infection. MMWR 47:1–43, 1998.

90. Public Health Service Task Force. Recommendations for Use of Antiretroviral Drugs in Pregnant HIV-1-Infected Women for Maternal Health and Interventions to Reduce Perinatal HIV-1 Transmission in the United States February 24, 2005.

CYTOMEGALOVIRUS

91. Kimberlin DW, Chin-Yu L, Sanchez PJ, et al: Effect of ganciclovir therapy on hearing in symptomatic congenital cytomegalovirus disease involving the central nervous system: A randomized, controlled trial. J Pediatr 143:16–25, 2003.

92. Volpe JJ (ed): Neurology of the Newborn, 4th ed. Philadelphia, W.B. Saunders, 1995.

HERPES SIMPLEX VIRUS

93. Annunziato PW, Gershon A: Herpes simplex virus infections. Pediatr Rev 17:415–423, 1996.

94. Brown Z, Selke S, Zeh J, et al: The acquisition of herpes simplex during pregnancy. N Engl J Med 337:509–515, 1997.

95. Prober CG, Arvin AM: Perinatal herpes: Current status and obstetric management strategies. The pediatric perspective. Pediatr Infect Dis J 10:832–835, 1995.

VARICELLA-ZOSTER VIRUS

96. Enders G, Miller E, Cradock-Watson J, et al: Consequences of varicella and herpes zoster in pregnancy: Prospective study of 1739 cases. Lancet 343:1548–1551, 1994.

97. Gershon A: Chickenpox, measles, and mumps. In Remington JS, Klein JO (eds): Infectious Diseases of the Fetus and Newborn Infant, 5th ed. Philadelphia, W.B. Saunders, 2001, pp 638–732.

CONGENITAL TOXOPLASMOSIS

98. Montoya JG, Liesenfeld O. Toxoplasmosis. Lancet 363:1965–1976, 2004.

99. Wong SY, Remington JS: Toxoplasmosis in pregnancy. Clin Infect Dis 18:853–862, 1994.

UREAPLASMA UREALYTICUM

100. Wang EE, Matlow AG, Ohlsson A, Nelson SC: *Ureaplasma urealyticum* infections in the perinatal period. Clin Perinatol 24:91–105, 1997.

INFECTIOUS HEPATITIS

101. American Academy of Pediatrics Hepatitis C. In Pickering LK (ed): Red Book: 2003 Report of the Committee on Infectious Diseases, 26th ed. Elk Grove Village, IL, American Academy of Pediatrics, 2003, pp 336–340.

102. Fishman LN, Jonas MM, Lavine JE: Update on viral hepatitis in children. Pediatr Clin North Am 43:57–74, 1996.

103. Mahoney FJ: Hepatitis B virus. In Long SS, Pickering LK, Prober CG (eds): Principles and Practice of Pediatric Infectious Diseases. New York, Churchill Livingstone, 1997, pp 1194–1205.

104. Mahoney FJ: Update on diagnosis, management, and prevention of hepatitis B virus infection. Clin Microbiol Rev 12:351–366, 1999.

105. Snyder JD: Acute hepatitis. In Long SS, Pickering LK, Prober CG (eds): Principles and Practice of Pediatric Infectious Diseases. New York, Churchill Livingstone, 1997, pp 448–453.

PARVOVIRUS

106. Harger JH, Adler SP, Koch WC, Harger GF: Prospective evaluation of 618 pregnant women exposed to parvovirus B19: Risks and symptoms. Obstet Gynecol 91:413–420, 1998.

CHAPTER 13

NEUROLOGY

Kent R. Kelley, MD, and M. Richard Koenigsberger, MD

NEUROLOGIC EXAMINATION OF THE NEWBORN INFANT

1. **What is the object of the neurologic examination?**
   The object of the neurologic history and examination is to localize a process in time and space, that is, to determine what the lesion is and where it is located.

KEY POINTS: BASIC ELEMENTS OF THE NEONATAL NEUROLOGIC EXAMINATION ✔️

1. Mental status (level of alertness)

2. Eyes and other cranial nerves

3. Primitive (neonatal) reflexes

4. Motor and sensory function

5. Deep tendon reflexes

2. **What are a normal baby's states of alertness?**
   1. Crying, inconsolable
   2. Alert and irritable, possibly tremulous or jittery
   3. Awake, alert, calm
   4. Drowsy
   5. Sleeping
   The ideal state for an examination, state 3, is usually achieved 1–2 hours after feeding, or conversely, 1–2 hours before the next feed.

   Prechtl HFR: Continuity of Neonatal Function from Prenatal to Postnatal Life. Oxford, England, Spastics International Medical, 1984.

3. **What are the primitive reflexes, and when do they extinguish?**
   The Moro reflex is elicited by rapidly extending the head in relation to the body. A newborn will respond by opening the hands and abducting and extending the arms and legs followed by flexion. It is abnormal if asymmetric or depressed. The tonic neck reflex is elicited (imposed) by turning the head to the side with the newborn responding by extending one arm toward the side to which the head was rotated while the other flexes in a "fencing posture." It is present from 35 weeks' gestation and should not persist beyond 6 months of life. The palmar grasp reflex extinguishes when voluntary hand grasp appears at 2–3 months. A number of other reflexes, although fun to demonstrate, are more inconsistent and less useful.

4. **When does the Moro reflex appear and disappear?**
   The Moro reflex is one of the most fascinating of the primitive reflexes. It is thought to be an evolutionary remnant that relates to the way that humankind's ancestors carried their infants. Monkeys and apes carry their young in front, and the young animal typically wraps its arms and legs around the mother and with movement, the young animal extends these and tightens its grasp around the mother. In humans, the Moro reflex begins to appear at about 28–30 weeks' postconceptional age. It is strongly present at birth in a term infant and begins to extinguish at around 3 months of life; persistence beyond 4 months is worrisome.

5. **What is the scarf maneuver? How is it helpful?**
   The maneuver is performed by grasping the baby's hand and trying to bring the baby's elbow across the midline. In a healthy term infant, the elbow can be brought no further than the mid-clavicular line on the same side. In the case of an Erb's palsy (C5–C6) brachial plexus injury, the elbow is easily brought to the midline or farther.

6. **Is Babinski's sign (up-going toes) present in a normal neonate?**
   The plantar response is downgoing in more than 90% of normal neonates when examined properly. An asymmetry of response is abnormal.

7. **How are the eyes examined?**
   It is important to determine whether an infant can follow an object with the eyes. Some authors believe a high percentage of normal newborns can pursue when using a large red object, an optokinetic drum, or the examiner's face. Observing visual pursuit naturally leads one into noting spontaneous eye movements. Are the eye movements conjugate? A useful maneuver is to hold up the child facing the examiner with the head 30 degrees below horizontal, then rotate slowly two turns. The baby's eyes will turn in the direction of the rotation. Upon stopping, the baby's eyes will rotate or jerk for up to 10 seconds in the opposite direction. This tells the examiner about the ocular movements and intactness of the vestibular apparatus. Pupillary response to light develops after 30 weeks.

8. **How are the rest of the cranial nerves examined?**
   The glabellar tap, evident at 32 weeks' gestational age, is performed by tapping between the eyes to elicit bilateral blinking. It is a "poor man's" corneal reflex that tests the afferent loop (cranial nerve V) and the efferent loop (cranial nerve VII). Facial nerve function is noted with good bilateral eye closure and symmetry of the face during crying. Auditory function is tested by a startle response to a loud noise. A coordinated suck and swallow should develop by 35 weeks' gestation, and a poor suck should be of concern. Observe the tongue for fasciculations. Listen to the cry. An encephalopathic neonate has a characteristic cry that is shorter and higher pitched. One who has been intubated is hoarse. One with laryngeal palsy will be stridorous or hoarse.

9. **In newborns with facial paralysis, how is peripheral nerve involvement distinguished from central nerve involvement?**
   In both forms of paralysis, the mouth is drawn back on the normal side when crying, and the nasolabial fold is obliterated on the affected side. A central nerve lesion is distinguished by an associated hemiplegia. Is there also an asymmetry of movement on the same side of the body? The classical lack of wrinkling of the affected side noted in older children and adults is extremely difficult to discern in the newborn. A trap to this diagnosis is hypoplasia of the depressor angulus oris muscle that produces an apparent contralateral asymmetric face during crying. It is occasionally associated with congenital heart disease.

10. **How is the motor examination performed?**
    First, observe the position of the baby and the spontaneous movements. Observe the quality of the hand opening. Examine the tone by gentle flexion and extension of the limbs. Is there an associated paucity of movement of an arm or leg? Observe the rebound of the extremity; the rate at which a limb returns to its original position is helpful in gauging tone (see Ballard

Score, Fig. 13-1). Measuring the popliteal angle (which is 180 degrees at 28 weeks' gestation and decreases to less than 90 degrees at term) allows for objective interobserver comparison of lower extremity tone (see Ballard Score). Head control can be gauged by either sitting the infant in the neutral position or by pulling the baby off the surface of a bed (traction maneuver).

Ballard JL, Khoury JC, Wedig K, et al: New Ballard Score, expanded to include premature infants. J Pediatr 119:417–423, 1991.

11. When do the tendon stretch reflexes develop?

The deep tendon reflexes develop, as does tone, several weeks earlier in the legs than the arms, and the patellar and Achilles' responses are attainable by 33 weeks' gestation in almost all neonates. Note that when a knee jerk response is obtained, a crossed adductor response is also obtained up through 6 months of age.

Neuromuscular maturity

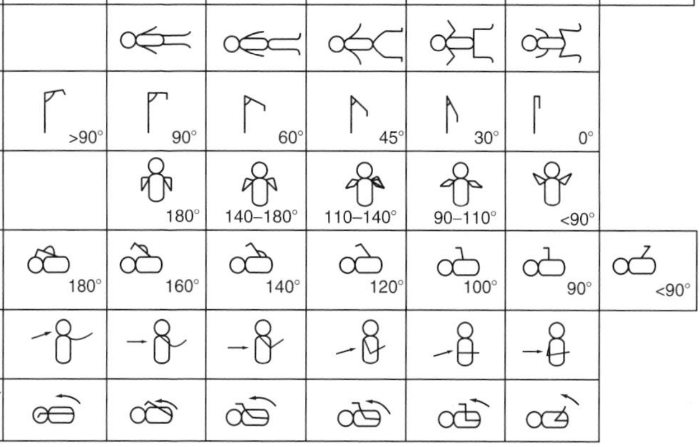

	−1	0	1	2	3	4	5
Posture							
Square window (wrist)	>90°	90°	60°	45°	30°	0°	
Arm recoil		180°	140–180°	110–140°	90–110°	<90°	
Popliteal angle	180°	160°	140°	120°	100°	90°	<90°
Scarf sign							
Heel to ear							

Physical maturity

Skin	Sticky friable, transparent	Gelatinous, red, translucent	Smooth, pink, visible veins	Superficial peeling &/or rash, few veins	Cracking, pale areas, rare veins	Parchment, deep cracking, no vessels	Leathery, cracked, wrikled
Lanugo	None	Sparse	Abundant	Thinning	Bald areas	Mostly bald	
Plantar surface	Heel–toe 40–50 mm: −1 <40 mm: −2	>50 mm no crease	Faint red marks	Anterior transverse crease only	Creases ant. 2/3	Creases over entire sole	
Breast	Imperceptible	Barely perceptible	Flat areola, no bud	Stippled areola, 1–2 mm bud	Raised areola, 3–4 mm bud	Full areola, 5–10 mm bud	
Eye/ear	Lids fused loosely: −1 tightly: −2	Lids open pinna flat stays folded	Sl.curved pinna: soft: slow recoil	Well-curve pinna: soft but ready recoil	Formed & firm, instant recoil	Thick cartllage, ear stiff	
Genitals male	Scrolum flat, smooth	Scrolum empty, faint rugae	Testes in upper canal, rare rugae	Testes descending, few rugae	Testes down, good rugae	Testes pendulous, deep rugae	
Genitals female	Clitoris prominent, labia flat	Prominent clitoris, small labia minora	Prominent clitoris, enlarging minora	Majora & minora equally prominent	Majora large, minora small	Majora cover clitoris & minora	

Maturity rating

Score	Weeks
−10	20
−5	22
0	24
5	26
10	28
15	30
20	32
25	34
30	36
35	38
40	40
45	42
50	44

Figure 13-1. The Ballard scoring system. (From Ballard JL. Khoury JC, Wedig K, et al: New Ballard Score, expanded to include extremely premature infants. J Pediatr 119:417–423, 1991, with permission.)

12. **Is ankle clonus normal in a newborn infant?**
Bilateral ankle clonus of 3–5 beats may be a normal finding, especially in infants who are crying, hungry, or jittery. Sustained ankle clonus is abnormal.

THE SKULL AND SPINE

13. **What is the normal head circumference in a term neonate?**
The 50th percentile for females is 34 cm, and for males it is 35 cm. Normal head circumference will grow approximately 2 cm per month for 3 months, 1 cm per month for 3 more months, and then roughly 0.5 cm per month for the next 6 months, being 46.5–47 cm at 1 year of age in males and 1 cm less for females. Premature infants should attain the head circumference of a healthy term infant, but illness and nutritional factors may slow the rate of growth. There are limited data for 24-week premature infants; many eventually show catch-up growth, but the smallest may not (Table 13-1).

TABLE 13-1. NORMAL HEAD CIRCUMFERENCE BY GESTATIONAL AGE	
Gestational Age (weeks)	Head Circumference (cm; boys/girls)
28	25/24
32	29/28
36	32/31
40	35/34

Adapted from Usher R, McLean F, Scott KE: Judgment of fetal age. II: Clinical significance of gestational age and an objective method for its assessment. Pediatr Clin North Am 13:835–862, 1966.

14. **Is the examination of the anterior fontanel useful?**
Yes, it is useful for evaluating intracranial pressure. The examination of the anterior fontanel is somewhat subjective, difficult, and inexact, but the anterior fontanel should be slightly depressed and pulsatile when a neonate is sleeping comfortably. Sitting the baby up should depress the fontanel further in a normal newborn.

15. **What is craniosynostosis? What are the different variations of this problem?**
Craniosynostosis is the result of premature closure of a cranial suture. Normal cranial sutures are shown in Fig. 13-2. Premature closure results in the arrest of growth perpendicular to the affected suture. Types of craniosynostosis and their appearance (Fig. 13-3) are:
- **Dolichocephaly:** Sagittal synostosis (long, narrow head)
- **Brachycephaly:** Coronal synostosis (wide head)
- **Acrocephaly:** Coronal, sagittal, and lambdoidal synostosis (tower head)
- **Trigonocephaly:** Metopic synostosis (pointed front of the head)

16. **What are the normal cerebrospinal fluid (CSF) values for healthy neonates?**
See Table 13-2.

17. **What are two devastating spinal cord injuries that can occur in the neonatal period?**
Spinal cord injury is fortunately an uncommon occurrence in neonates. One instance in which it can occur, however, is when excessive traction is applied to the neck during a difficult delivery, especially if there is shoulder dystocia. The resulting injury causes a flaccid quadriplegia with sparing of the face and CNs. An indwelling umbilical arterial catheter misplaced at T11 can obstruct Adamkiewicz' artery, which feeds the anterior spinal artery. The resulting cord ischemia causes an irreversible paraplegia.

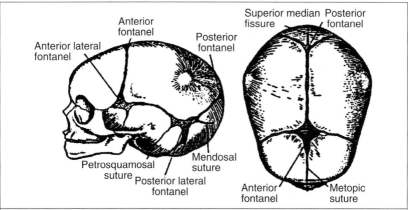

Figure 13-2. Normal cranial sutures. (From Silverman FN, Kuhn JP [eds]: Caffey's Pediatric X-Ray Diagnosis, 9th ed. St. Louis, MO, Mosby, 1993, p 5.)

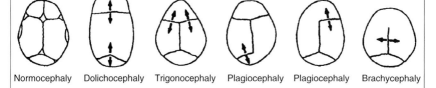

Normocephaly   Dolichocephaly   Trigonocephaly   Plagiocephaly   Plagiocephaly   Brachycephaly

Figure 13-3. Types of craniosynostosis. (From Gorlin JR: Craniofacial defects. In Oski FA, Deangelis CD, Feigin RD, Warshaw JB [eds]: Principles and Practice of Pediatrics, 2nd ed. Philadelphia, J.B. Lippincott, 1994, p 508, with permission.)

TABLE 13-2. NORMAL CSF VALUES		
	Term	Preterm
WBC count (cells/mm^3)	8.2 (0–32)	9.0 (0–29)
Protein (mg/dL)	90 (20–170)	115 (65–150)
Glucose (mg/dL)	52 (34–119)	50 (24–63)
CSF/blood glucose (%)	81 (44–248)	74 (55–105)
WBC = white blood cell.		

MALFORMATIONS OF THE CENTRAL NERVOUS SYSTEM

18. **Which neurologic conditions are associated with polyhydramnios?**
    In many cases of polyhydramnios, the cause is unknown. It is seen in 50% of cases of anencephaly, in neurologically impaired fetuses with poor swallowing, and in hypotonic neonates from diverse causes.

19. **What fetal conditions are associated with an elevated α-fetoprotein (AFP) level in maternal serum, and where is it produced?**
Elevated AFP is seen in open neural tube defects, esophageal or duodenal atresia, congenital nephrosis, and fetal demise. AFP is synthesized by the fetal liver and excreted by the kidney. It peaks at 10–13 weeks of gestational age.

20. **What is the difference between meningocele, meningomyelocele, and spina bifida occulta?**
A meningocele is the protrusion of only the meninges through a bony defect in the spine, whereas both meninges and spinal cord protrude through bone when a meningomyelocele is present. Spinal bifida occulta is a vertebral cleft in the absence of spinal cord and meningeal herniation and is a frequent incidental finding when neuroimaging the lumbar spinal region.

21. **What is the incidence of meningomyelocele, and what is the best way to prevent its occurrence?**
The incidence of meningomyelocele is approximately 0.5–1 per 1000 live births. Prophylaxis is accomplished in most cases by the intake of 0.4 mg of folic acid per day, starting, if possible, before the pregnancy begins. If there has been a previous child with spina bifida, 4 mg/day is recommended. With supplementation there has been a significant decrease in neural tube defects in the United States.

22. **If the diagnosis of meningomyelocele is made prenatally, should the delivery be done by cesarean section?**
In one study, infants delivered by cesarean section before the onset of labor had significantly less paralysis at the age of 2 years than did infants with comparable lesions who were delivered vaginally after a period of labor. However, later studies have not confirmed this finding.
   Lewis D, Tolosa JE, Kauffman M, et al: Elective cesarean delivery and long term motor function or ambulation status in infants with meningomyelocele. Obstet Gynecol 103:469–473, 2004.

23. **Which congenital cerebral disorders are associated with meningomyelocele?**
The Arnold-Chiari type II (ACTII) malformation is frequently associated with meningomyelocele. This consists of a low-lying cerebellar vermis and ventral medulla oblongata that often protrudes into the foramen magnum. By obstructing the flow of CSF, it leads to hydrocephalus. Aqueductal stenosis may be found with Arnold-Chiari type II malformation or in isolation, again leading to CSF flow obstruction. Agenesis of the corpus callosum can also be associated with meningomyelocele.

24. **What is the prognosis for mental normality in children with meningomyelocele?**
The answer is multifactorial. In general, the lower the level of the lesion, the better the prognosis. However, the degree of hydrocephalus present at birth and the complications inherent in

shunting procedures (e.g., infection) also play a part in determining the IQ of the patient. The associated central nervous system (CNS) malformations, including agenesis of the corpus callosum, are also important determinants. Thus, a child with a relatively low-lying lesion with an Arnold-Chiari type II lesion, who has hydrocephalus, is likely to be mentally normal if there are no complications related to the shunting procedure.

Fobe JL, Rizzo AM, Silva IM: IQ in hydrocephalus and meningomyelocele: Implications of surgical treatment. Arch Neuropsychiatr 57:44–50, 1999.

25. **In an infant born with meningomyelocele, how does the cord level of the lesion on initial evaluation predict long-term ambulation potential?**
This assessment is accomplished by determining motor level and reflex level. Sensory level assessment is tedious and inexact (Table 13-3).

26. **What is a tethered cord? Why is it clinically important?**
A tethered cord is a low-lying lumbosacral cord anchored posteriorly by a thickened filum terminale. It can occur in association with meningomyelocele or with other lumbosacral abnormalities such as lipomeningocele. It may be overlain by a dermal defect such as a hair tuft or sacral dimple. Ultrasound is a good screening procedure, but magnetic resonance imaging (MRI) provides a definitive diagnosis. The lesion may be asymptomatic, but with growth it may lead to problems with sphincter control and walking and may also cause lumbar back pain.

27. **What is the Dandy-Walker malformation? What are the associated abnormalities and treatment?**
The components of the Dandy-Walker malformation are cystic dilation of the fourth ventricle, partial or complete agenesis of the cerebellar vermis, and enlargement of the posterior fossa with a high attachment of the tentorium cerebelli. The Dandy-Walker malformation is frequently associated with hydrocephalus, which may not be present at birth but often develops in the first year of life. Agenesis of the corpus callosum (60%) and cortical migrational defects account for retardation in many of the cases (75–90%). Treatment consists of observation and shunting of the ventricles. Sometimes the cyst itself needs to be shunted.

28. **What is the distinction between porencephaly, schizencephaly, and lissencephaly?**
Porencephaly is an acquired abnormality that is seen as an outpouching from the ventricular system. It usually results from a parenchymal bleed, infarct, or infection. Schizencephaly, a

TABLE 13-3. SPINAL LEVELS: MOTOR, REFLEXES, AND AMBULATION*			
Level	Movement	Reflexes	Ambulation
Thoracic	No extremity	Increased	None
L1–L2	Hip flexion/adduction		Rarely
L3	Knee extension	Knee jerk present	Often-high leg braces
L4	Knee flexion/ankle extension		Lower leg braces, below the knee
L5	Toe extension		Less bracing
S1	Ankle dorsiflexion/ some toe flexion		May not need braces
S2–S4	Bowel and bladder only		

*S2–S4 levels have only bladder and bowel abnormalities, as do all higher levels.

"split brain," is a congenital migrational defect and is a cleft in one or both hemispheres from the surface of the brain down to the ventricular surface. *Lissencephaly* means "smooth brain," one in which there are few if any gyri formed on the brain's surface. This is a severe migrational disorder of two types. Type I involves the brain and can be part of the Miller-Dieker malformation. Type II is seen in association with severe muscle disease.

29. **What are the four types of holoprosencephaly and their common associations?**
Holoprosencephaly reflects an earlier failure of splitting of the forebrain, resulting in various kinds of single-ventricle anomalies. There are now four types of holoprosencephaly described: alobar, semilobar, lobar, and a middle hemispheric variant. The alobar form is particularly severe in terms of neurologic dysfunction, may show a wide spectrum of facial abnormalities, and may be observed in infants with trisomy 13 or 18 syndrome. The middle hemispheric variant and lobar holoprosencephaly may be quite mild, even asymptomatic.

Lewis AJ, Simon EM, Barkowich AJ, et al: Middle interhemispheric variant of holoprosencephaly—A distinct neuroradiologic subtype. Neurology 59:1860–1865, 2002.

Patterson MC: Holoprosencephaly: The face predicts the brain—the image predicts its function. Neurology 59:1833–1834, 2002.

30. **How is hydrocephalus classified?**
With one rare exception (choroid plexus papillomas), all hydrocephalus is obstructive. By convention, the obstruction can be "communicating," within the ventricular system itself, or "noncommunicating," in the subarachnoid space outside the ventricular system. Choroid plexus papillomas (90% benign) oversecrete CSF and lead to hydrocephalus that is often present at birth.

31. **What are main causes of intrauterine (fetal) hydrocephalus?**
Structural malformations, such as aqueductal stenosis and Arnold-Chiari type II malformation (usually associated with meningomyelocele and the Dandy-Walker malformation), account for 90% of noncommunicating hydrocephalus. Acquired causes (e.g., an intrauterine bleed) or an infection (e.g., toxoplasmosis) can cause communicating hydrocephalus.

32. **What are the principal causes of hydrocephalus acquired in the newborn period?**
Most are communicating, and posthemorrhagic hydrocephalus from intraventricular hemorrhage (IVH) is by far the most frequent cause. Other causes of hydrocephalus are subarachnoid hemorrhage and inflammation following meningitis or other infections.

33. **How does a malformation of Galen's vein usually present in the newborn period?**
The most common cranial arteriovenous malformation in the newborn is the malformation of Galen's vein, which typically presents as high-output congestive heart failure in the neonatal period. There may be a "bruit," sometimes quite loud, best heard over the posterior fossa. Sometimes there is head enlargement caused by an extrinsic aqueductal stenosis produced in the pons and midbrain by the bulk of the malformation. Only very rarely do these malformations present as bleeds at birth. The prognosis is variable.

NEUROCUTANEOUS SYNDROMES

34. **What is the derivation of the term *phakomatosis*?**
The term *phakomatosis* is derived from the Greek *phakos*, meaning "lentil" or "lens," and refers to patchy, circumscribed dermatologic lesions that are the hallmark of this group of disorders. In addition to dermatologic features, these syndromes have hamartomata (errors in development) with involvement of multiple tissues, especially the CNS and eye. More commonly, the term *neurocutaneous syndrome* is used when referring to this group of diseases.

KEY POINTS: DORSAL MIDLINE FEATURES SUGGESTING SPINAL DYSRAPHISM

1. An abnormal collection of hair is present.

2. Cutaneous abnormalities (e.g., hemangioma or pigmented nevi) occur.

3. Cutaneous dimples or tracts or a subcutaneous mass on the lower back appear.

4. In 80–90% of cases, there is an associated vertebral abnormality.

5. The diagnosis should also be suspected in patients with symptoms of progressive lower extremity weakness or sensory loss, gait abnormalities, foot deformities, or neurogenic bowel and bladder problems.

6. Spinal dysraphism is associated with Chiari hindbrain malformations, syringomyelia, and tethered cord.

---

35. **What are the two most common autosomal dominant neurocutaneous syndromes?**
    Neurofibromatosis (NF) and tuberous sclerosis complex (TSC) are both autosomal dominant conditions; the majority are sporadic. The prevalence of NF1 is about 3/10,000 live births, and the incidence of NF2 is 2/100,000 live births. The prevalence of TSC is 1/6000.

36. **How common are café au lait spots at birth?**
    Up to 2% of black infants will have three café au lait spots at birth; however, only one café au lait spot occurs in 0.3% of white infants. White infants with multiple café au lait spots at birth are more likely than black infants to develop NF. Because of the high spontaneous mutation rate for this autosomal dominant disease, only about 50% of newly diagnosed cases are associated with a positive family history.

    Hurwitz S: Neurofibromatosis. In Clinical Pediatric Dermatology, 2nd ed. Philadelphia, W.B. Saunders, 1993, pp 624–629.
    National NF Foundation: http://www.nf.org

37. **What is NF1?**
    NF1 is an autosomal dominant disorder of a tumor-suppressor gene located on chromosome 17q11.2 that encodes neurofibromin, a negative regulator of the *Ras* oncogene. Characteristic café au lait spots may appear at birth. Osseous lesions are usually apparent within the first year of life, and tumors of the optic chiasm present relatively early in life. Axillary freckling and peripheral, spinal, or central nerve NFs may develop in later childhood. Early ascertainment is difficult, and almost half of infants younger than 1 year of age do not fulfill the full criteria for this disorder.

    DeBella K, Szudek J, Friedman JM: Use of the National Institutes of Health criteria for diagnosis of neurofibromatosis 1 in children. Pediatrics 105:608–614, 2000.

38. **What is the spectrum of TSC?**
    TSC is characterized by multiple and variable organ involvement. Commonly recognized clinical features include hypomelanotic skin macules, facial angiofibromas, periungual fibromas, delayed development, epilepsy, and autism. The kidney, heart, and retina are among other commonly affected organs. Abnormalities on brain imaging include subependymal nodules, cortical tubers, and radial white matter lines.

KEY POINTS: PRIMARY CLINICAL DIAGNOSTIC FEATURES OF TSC IN THE NEONATAL PERIOD

1. Cardiac hamartomas (may be diagnosed in utero before developing neurologic and skin symptoms)

2. Subependymal nodules or giant cell astrocytomas

3. Multiple calcified subependymal nodules protruding into the ventricle

4. Multiple retinal astrocytomas

5. Skin lesions (uncommon in the neonate); hypopigmented macules and café au lait spots possibly observed

---

39. What is the significance of facial port-wine stains?

Port-wine stains can occur as isolated cutaneous birthmarks in association with structural abnormalities of choroidal vessels of the eye leading to glaucoma, and of the leptomeningeal vessels in the brain leading to seizures (Sturge-Weber syndrome). Almost invariably, the hemangioma involves the homolateral trigeminal V1 area or is bilaterally distributed. Ophthalmologic assessment and radiologic studies (computed tomography [CT] or MRI) are indicated for children who exhibit hemangiomas in the upper eyelid or forehead.

> The Sturge-Weber Foundation: http://www.sturge-weber.com

40. What sporadic neurocutaneous syndrome is associated with hemimegencephaly?

Epidermal nevi are hamartomatous lesions derived from ectodermal components that originate in pluripotential cell mutations during early embryonic stages. They reflect embryonic migration patterns of the skin and have been associated with dermal mosaicism. The incidence is approximately 1 in 1000 live newborns. Linear sebaceous nevus syndrome, or *epidermal nevus syndrome*, is characterized by a unilateral pigmented lesion around the eye, hemicrania (with an enlarged forehead), and hemimegencephaly. Whenever mosaicism affects the skin, the site may show patchy hypopigmentation or hyperpigmentation in a segmental or linear distortion.

41. What is incontinentia pigmenti?

Incontinentia pigmenti, or "*Bloch-Sulzberger syndrome*," is an X-linked dominant disorder characterized by abnormalities of skin, teeth, hair, and eyes; mental retardation; seizures; skewed X-inactivation; and recurrent miscarriages of male fetuses. The first stage (i.e., vesicular stage) is characterized by lines of blisters, particularly on the extremities in newborns, that disappear in weeks or months. This is followed by stage 2 (i.e., verrucous stage) in which lesions develop around age 3–7 months that are brown and hyperkeratotic, resembling warts. The final stage, stage 3 (i.e., pigmented stage), is characterized by whorled, swirling (marble cake–like) macular hyperpigmented lines that may fade with time.

42. What is hypomelanosis of Ito?

Hypomelanosis of Ito was originally described as a purely cutaneous disease with a swirling pigmentary pattern, but subsequent reports have included a frequent association with multiple extracutaneous manifestations, mostly of the central nervous and musculoskeletal systems. Neuro- logic complications include mental retardation, autism, brain malformations, microcephaly, and epilepsy. Miscellaneous chromosomal mosaicisms have been demonstrated in some but not all affected persons. Additional, associated abnormalities include limb length discrepancies, facial hemiatrophy, scoliosis, sternal abnormalities, dysmorphic facies, and genitourinary and cardiac abnormalities.

INTRACRANIAL HEMORRHAGE

43. **What are the three major forms of extracranial hemorrhage that can occur after a difficult delivery?**
    - **Caput succedaneum:** Involves hemorrhagic edema of the presenting portion of the scalp and is common in vacuum extractions.
    - **Cephalohematoma:** Involves hemorrhage that is confined by the periosteum and therefore respects the sutures. Cephalohematoma*s* sometimes calcify and may produce a cosmetic deformity.
    - **Subgaleal hemorrhage:** Involves the area under the epicranial aponeurosis and may become large and pitting, even dissecting into the neck. It is also associated with vacuum extractions (Fig. 13-4).

44. **What are the major forms of intracranial hemorrhage?**
    - **Subdural hemorrhage (SDH):** Occurs in term infants with difficult vaginal deliveries, more often with forceps or vacuum extraction, leading to bleeding in the subdural space where bridging veins can tear. Although more common supratentorially, SDH can occur beneath the tentorium cerebelli.
    - **Subarachnoid hemorrhage (SAH):** In premature infants, may be primary, often of cause unknown, or secondary to hypoxia-ischemia, whereas in term infants it may be the result of trauma or infarction.
    - **IVH:** Happens in very-low-birth-weight (VLBW) preterm babies due to the fragility of blood vessels in the germinal plate, adjacent to the lateral ventricle.
    - **Intraparenchymal hemorrhage:** Occurs in the brain substance of term infants as a result of trauma or arterial infarction, whereas in premature infants, venous infarction associated with IVH is the main cause.

45. **What are the three major clinical presentations of SAH?**
    - **Catastrophic deterioration:** In rare instances, newborn infants with large SAHs follow a rapidly fatal course characterized by coma, respiratory disturbances, seizures, loss of brain stem reflexes, and flaccidity.
    - **Well baby with seizures:** Convulsions resulting from SAH are often unifocal clonic and begin on the second day of life. In interictal periods, babies are alert and well, and the electroencephalogram (EEG) shows focal spikes. The diagnosis is suspected by the presence of blood in the CSF and is confirmed by CT or MRI. The prognosis is good.
    - **Asymptomatic:** In most cases, only small amounts of hemorrhage have occurred, and minimal or no clinical signs are present.

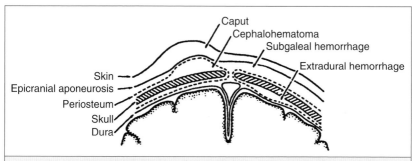

Figure 13-4. Types of traumatic external hemorrhage. (Adapted from Volpe JJ [ed]: Neurology of the Newborn, 4th ed. Philadelphia, W.B. Saunders, 2001, pp 813–838.)

46. **What are the symptoms, signs, diagnostic aids, and treatment of supratentorial SDH?**

Most SDHs are asymptomatic and are usually identified as incidental findings on CT and MRI scans. They may not be seen on ultrasound scans. When due to a tentorial or a falx tear, a newborn's condition can rapidly deteriorate and he or she can die due to blood loss and brain stem pressure. More often, an infant with symptomatic subdurals will be lethargic and may have seizures. Examination may reveal an enlarged head; bulging fontanel; excessive retinal hemorrhages; and focal weakness in the face, leg, or arm on one side of the body. Diagnosis is made by CT scan that shows a bright signal (i.e., blood) over one or both hemispheres. Treatment consists of watchful waiting the majority of the time. On occasion, sequential subdural taps may be necessary. Only rarely is surgical evacuation or subdural-peritoneal shunting required.

47. **What are the principal sites of origin of IVH in the newborn?**

The subependymal germinal matrix is the most common site for IVH in VLBW babies; venous hemorrhagic infarction of the white matter, which shares some of the pathogenesis with germinal matrix hemorrhage, may contribute. In term infants, bleeding originates in the choroid plexus of the lateral ventricle.

48. **What is the procedure of choice for the diagnosis of IVH?**

Cranial ultrasound is a reliable, portable, safe, and cost-effective method for evaluating infants for IVH and is able to visualize the subependymal germinal matrix, which is the most common site for IVH in VLBW babies. Cranial ultrasound can be performed at the bedside with minimal disturbance of the infant and has become the study of choice.

49. **What is the generally accepted classification of IVH?**

- **Grade I hemorrhage:** Hemorrhage into the subependymal germinal matrix only
- **Grade II hemorrhage:** Blood has spilled into the ventricle(s) with little or no ventricular enlargement
- **Grade III hemorrhage:** Ventricular dilatation in addition to ventricular blood
- **Grade IV hemorrhage:** Grade III hemorrhage accompanied by parenchymal hemorrhage

50. **What variables contribute to the development of IVH in a newborn?**

Many of the following factors may be simultaneously present and contribute to neonatal IVH:
- Prematurity, particularly very low or extremely-low-birth-weight infants
- Increased venous pressure during delivery or due to mechanical ventilation
- Increased cerebral blood flow associated with systemic hypertension or hypercarbia.
- Fluctuating cerebral blood flow due to mechanical ventilation or hypotension followed by reperfusion
- Coagulopathy due to thrombocytopenia and platelet dysfunction
- The immature, friable microvascular network in the germinal matrix
- An inflammatory response with cytokine production, most often from prenatal maternal infection or postnatal neonatal infection

51. **What are the major courses of progression of posthemorrhagic ventricular dilation and their rates of occurrence?**

- Slowly progressive ventricular dilatation (SPVD) with spontaneous arrest (<4 weeks)—65%
- Persistent SPVD (>4 weeks)—30%
- Rapidly progressive ventricular dilatation—5%

Of the persistent SPVD group, about 67% will have a spontaneous arrest, whereas 33% will continue to progress. In the spontaneous arrest group, 5% will have late progressive dilation.

Volpe JJ (ed): Neurology of the Newborn, 4th ed. Philadelphia, W.B. Saunders, 2001.

52. **What are some of the various treatment options for IVH and SVPD?**
- **Close observation:** This is the first step in managing the conditions. The infant's clinical condition and head circumference should be closely followed. Head growth >1 cm/week should be monitored with serial ultrasound scans.
- **Trial of serial lumbar punctures:** This is considered by some to be the initial procedure when progressive ventricular dilation does not resolve spontaneously. An ultrasound scan should be obtained after 10–15 mg of CSF are withdrawn to see whether the procedure has been helpful in reducing ventricular size. Recent studies, however, have suggested that this approach is not often helpful.
- **Carbonic anhydrase inhibitors:** Acetazolamide (up to a high dose 100 mg/kg/day) combined with furosemide (1–2 mg/kg/day) has no clear benefit and increases the risk of nephrocalcinosis.
- **Ventricular drainage:** This can be accomplished in a number of manners: direct external drainage, via an indwelling subcutaneous Ommaya reservoir, or by ventriculosubgaleal shunting. These are most often temporizing measures until an infant is able to undergo a more permanent procedure, usually a ventriculoperitoneal shunt. The smaller the infant, the greater likelihood of obstruction or infection (i.e., ventriculitis) by a shunting procedure.

de Vries LS, Liem KD, van Dikj K, et al: Early versus late treatment of posthemorrhagic ventricular dilatation: Results of a retrospective study from five neonatal studies in The Netherlands. Acta Pediatr 91:212–217, 2002.

Fulmer BB, Grabb PA, Oakew WJ, Mapstone TB: Neonatal ventriculosubgaleal shunts. Neurosurgery 47:80–84, 2000.

Kennedy CR, Ayers S, Campbell MJ, et al: Randomized, controlled trial of acetazolamide and furosemide in posthemorrhagic ventricular dilation in infancy: Follow-up at 1 year. Pediatrics 108:569–607, 2001.

53. **What is the incidence of long-term neurologic sequelae in children with IVH?**
The incidence of neurologic sequelae is linked not only to the grade of hemorrhage, but also to gestational age of the patient and the degree of parenchymal insult resulting from infarction and periventricular leukomalacia (PVL). Thus, although some series have shown a 5% incidence of hard neurologic sequelae (e.g., mental retardation, spastic diplegia, and seizures) for grade I IVH, 15% for grade II, 33% for grade III, and almost 90% for grade IV with large infarction, long-term studies have demonstrated that at least 50–70% of extremely-low-birth-weight (ELBW) and VLBW babies go on to have scholastic and behavioral abnormalities.

Hack M, Flannery DJ, Schluchter M, et al: Outcomes in young, very low-birth-weight infants. N Engl J Med 346:149–157, 2002.

Ment LR, Vohr B, Allan W: Change in cognitive function over time in very low-birth-weight infants. JAMA 289:705–711, 2003.

Roland EH, Hill A: Germinal matrix-intraventricular hemorrhage in the premature newborn: Management and outcome. Neurol Clin 21:833–851, 2003.

KEY POINTS: PERIVENTRICULAR LEUKOMALACIA

1. The definition of PVL has expanded over the past few decades as neuroimaging and neuropathologic techniques have evolved.

2. PVL was first described as punctate areas of necrosis and hemorrhage in the white matter dorsal and lateral to the lateral ventricles.

3. The term is now more broadly used to denote more extensive injury, including cystic change, scarring, hypomyelination/demyelination, and even hemorrhagic infarction of the white matter.

PERIVENTRICULAR LEUKOMALACIA

54. **Where is PVL localized?**
Although there can be extensive involvement by PVL throughout the white mater (WM), the anterior and posterior periventricular regions are most commonly affected. The former region is where WM fibers pass to the legs, accounting for subsequent leg spasticity, and the latter, posterior area is responsible for the visual abnormalities of PVL. Cystic changes in these areas can be seen on ultrasound scan. Underdevelopment of the WM and hypomyelinization are seen at term in 50% of VLBW survivors as diffuse excessive high signal intensity (DEHSI) in the centrum semiovale of the WM on T2 MRI sequences. Because of WM damage and dropout, there ensues ex vacuo ventriculomegaly that is visible on ultrasound, CT, and MRI scans. Even in the absence of marked ventriculomegaly, many premature infants will demonstrate loss of WM volume.

55. **What is the current thinking about the pathogenesis of PVL?**
Two mechanisms are thought to cause PVL:
1. **Anoxic/hypotensive:** The blood vessels supplying the WM are arrayed radially, thus creating vascular end zones. These vessels lack autoregulation and are susceptible to changes in systemic blood pressure. Hypotension then leads to brain tissue hypoxia followed by glutamate and free radical damage to the preoligodendrocytes, the precursor cells to the oligodendrocytes, which form the WM.
2. **Humoral/cytokine:** Maternal infection can produce cytokines that may cross the blood barrier in the fetus. The cytokines set off a free radical cascade that activates WM microglia that secrete products that damage those same preoligodendrocytes.

   Volpe JJ: Cerebral white matter injury of the premature infant: More common than you think. Pediatrics 112:176–180, 2003.

56. **What are the neuroimaging correlates of PVL in VLBW babies?**
In approximately 2–3 weeks after the hypoxic-ischemic insult, cystic changes can be detected on cranial ultrasound. Periventricular fluid-attenuated inversion recovery (FLAIR) WM densities, observed on ultrasound, may be significant but can also disappear. When VBLW babies reach term gestation, DEHSI and ventriculomegaly can be observed on T2 MRI images, in addition to the aforementioned cysts and infarcts. After 6 months to 2 years, the MRI will demonstrate periventricular demyelination and white matter scarring (particularly, but not exclusively, in the frontal and posterior periventricular areas) ventriculomegaly, ventricular wall irregularity (waviness), thinning of the corpus callosum, and brain atrophy, all of which can be seen on T2 and FLAIR sequences.

   Counsell SJ, Allsop JM, Harrison MC: Diffusion weighted imaging of the brain in preterm infants with focal and diffuse white matter abnormality. Pediatrics 112:1–7, 2003.

57. **What are the common neurologic sequelae of PVL?**
The long-term sequelae of PVL are still being established through follow-up studies. The principal sequelae include spastic diplegia and visual, auditory, and cognitive deficits.

58. **Name the primary visual deficits related to PVL.**
   - Poor visual acuity
   - Delayed visual maturation
   - Strabismus
   - Supranuclear disorders of eye movement

HYPOXIC ISCHEMIC ENCEPHALOPATHY (HIE) AND STROKE

59. **What is HIE?**
HIE is a neurologic syndrome in the newborn infant that results from asphyxia. For an intrapartum event to be the likely cause of neonatal brain injury, there should be (1) a history of

intrauterine distress, (2) depression at birth, and (3) an obvious neonatal neurologic syndrome in the immediate postnatal period.

American College of Obstetricians and Gynecologists and American Academy of Pediatrics (eds): Neonatal Encephalopathy and Cerebral Palsy: Defining the Pathogenesis and Pathophysiology. Washington, DC, ACOG and AAP, 2003.

60. **What are the American College of Obstetricians and Gynecologists (ACOG)/American Academy of Pediatrics (AAP) criteria to define an intrapartum event sufficient to cause cerebral palsy (CP)?**
Essential criteria (must meet all four):
1. Evidence of a metabolic acidosis in fetal umbilical cord arterial blood obtained at delivery (pH < 7 and base deficit $\geq$ 12 mmol/L)
2. Early onset of severe or moderate neonatal encephalopathy in infants born at 34 or more weeks of gestation
3. CP of the spastic quadriplegic or dyskinetic type
4. Exclusion of other identifiable etiologies such as trauma, coagulation disorders, infectious conditions, or genetic disorders

Criteria that collectively suggest an intrapartum timing (within close proximity to labor and delivery, [e.g., 0–48 hours]) but are nonspecific to asphyxial insults:
1. A sentinel (signal) hypoxic event occurring immediately before or during labor
2. A sudden and sustained fetal bradycardia or the absence of fetal heart rate variability in the presence of persistent, late, or variable decelerations, usually after a hypoxic sentinel event when the pattern was previously normal
3. Apgar scale score of 0–3 beyond 5 minutes
4. Onset of multisystem involvement within 72 hours of birth
5. Early imaging study showing evidence of acute nonfocal cerebral abnormality

61. **What are the Sarnat encephalopathy stages, and how are they clinically useful?**
   - **Stage 1:** Mild encephalopathy in a newborn infant who is hyperalert, irritable, and oversensitive to stimulation. There is evidence of sympathetic overstimulation with tachycardia, dilated pupils, and jitteriness. The EEG is normal.
   - **Stage 2:** Moderate encephalopathy with the newborn displaying lethargy, hypotonia, and proximal weakness. There is parasympathetic overstimulation with low resting heart rate, small pupils, and copious secretions. The EEG is abnormal, and 70% of infants will have seizures.
   - **Stage 3:** Severe encephalopathy with a stuporous, flaccid newborn and absent reflexes. The newborn may have seizures and has an abnormal EEG with decreased background activity and/or voltage suppression.

   Even without EEG availability, the use of the Sarnat scoring system gives clinicians a shorthand method to describe an infant's condition to one another.

62. **Which areas of the CNS are injured by HIE in a term newborn, and why?**
   There are areas of selective vulnerability to the injuries caused by HIE, the watershed areas of the cortex being most susceptible in subacute asphyxial injury, whereas most damage occurs in the basal ganglia and thalami after an acute ischemic insult. These areas of insult are not mutually exclusive, and some babies show both watershed and deep lesions. These areas may be most susceptible, because at or near 40 weeks' gestational age they are the richest in glutamate content, and this is thought to be the cause for their selective susceptibility. If the asphyxial insult is severe enough, these and other areas of the brain go on to cystic encephalomalacia, in which the brain appears to have holes in it resembling Swiss cheese.

63. **What is the pathogenesis of HIE at the cellular level?**
   The initial deprivation of oxygen causes swelling and necrotic cell death in the susceptible areas described above. Thus, early on, one finds an area of necrosis surrounded by a penumbral area

of brain in which reperfusion and reoxygenation takes place. In this area, further cellular damage is created by glutamate release, which in turns leads to free radical and calpain (apoptotic death factor) release that cause apoptotic (programmed cell) death. This is a process that may go on for days to weeks after the initial asphyxial insult.

64. **What are the four major neuropathologic varieties of neonatal HIE in the term newborn?**
    1. **Selective neuronal necrosis:** Usually occurs in a characteristic deep sulcal pattern.
    2. **Status marmoratus:** After neuronal loss, the development of gliosis and hypermyelination takes place in the basal ganglia
    3. **Parasagittal cerebral injury:** "Watershed infarcts" due to ischemia in the areas of overlapping supply; laterally by the middle cerebral artery and medially by both anterior and posterior cerebral arteries
    4. **Focal and multifocal ischemic brain necrosis:** Infarction due to ischemia, with large areas of necrosis in the distribution of major vessels

65. **What are currently the most useful clinical and laboratory tools in estimating prognosis in cases of HIE?**
    Clinically, judicious use of the Sarnat scoring method (previously discussed) is most helpful. Newborns with stage I generally do well. Surviving stage III newborns generally exhibit spastic quadriplegia, mental retardation, and seizures. The prognosis of stage II newborns is the most uncertain, and laboratory values may be very useful. Initial cord pH < 7.0, elevated serum and CSF lactate levels, evidence of multisystem involvement, and increased creatine kinase brain isoenzyme values in blood also have been correlated to guarded prognosis. Early evidence of infarction may be seen with diffusion-weighted MRI studies before there is anatomic change evident on standard T1 or T2 MRI.

66. **What are currently the most useful neurodiagnostic laboratory tools in estimating prognosis in cases of HIE?**
    EEG, especially when performed serially, may be very useful. Interictal EEG patterns of burst suppression and inactive low-voltage background have extremely guarded prognoses. Multifocal spikes and excessive discontinuity also bode poorly, with a 40–50% favorable outcome at best. MRI may also be useful. Abnormalities appear early on diffusion-weighted images within 3–6 hours, and then 2–3 days later, on T1- and T2-weighted sequences. An abnormal signal in the posterior limb of the internal capsule has a positive predictive value for bad outcome of nearly 100%, as long as the newborn is of more than 36 weeks' gestation and 3 days after birth. Magnetic resonance spectroscopy may also help define functional abnormality.

    Rutherford M, Ward P, Allsop J, et al: Magnetic resonance imaging in neonatal encephalopathy. Early Hum Dev 81:13–25, 2005.

67. **Are there objective markers of cerebral injury on MRI/MRS?**
    Apparent diffusion coefficient values from the posterior limb of the internal capsule are significantly greater in term infants with HIE who survive. Among survivors, a reduced apparent diffusion coefficient value in the posterior limb on the internal capsule is associated with a greater probability of an abnormal neuromotor outcome. In contrast, an elevated N-acetylaspartate to total creatine ratio is associated with a higher likelihood of a normal outcome at 18 months. Most important, the presence of a lactate peak predicts an abnormal outcome with a sensitivity of 100% and a specificity of 80%.

    Barkovich AJ, Baranski K, Vigneron D, et al: Proton MR spectroscopy for the evaluation of brain injury in asphyxiated, term neonates. AJNR Am J Neuroradiol 20:1399–1405, 1999.

    Hunt RW, Neil JJ, Coleman LT, et al: Apparent diffusion coefficient in the posterior limb of the internal capsule predicts outcome after perinatal asphyxia. Pediatrics 114:999–1003, 2004.

68. What is thought to be the most effective treatment for HIE?

The most effective therapy is a combination of supportive and specific therapies:

- **Supportive:** (1) Maintenance of vital signs and respiratory support, artificial ventilation when necessary; (2) careful fluid, glucose, electrolyte management, remembering that the asphyxial insult may involve myocardium, kidneys, liver, and gastrointestinal tract; (3) treatment of seizures, as indicated next.

- **Specific:** Recent trials have indicated that systemic cooling using a cooling blanket or cooling cap, for a 3-day period starting no later than 6 hours after delivery, is effective in reducing neurologic morbidity at 2 years in Sarnat stages I and II patients. There appears to be no effect in severely afflicted infants (i.e., Sarnat stage III).

  Eicher DJ, Wagner CL, Katikaneni LP: Moderate hypothermia in neonatal encephalopathy: Efficacy outcomes. Pediatric Neurol 32:11–17, 2005.

  Gluckman PD, Wyatt JS, Azzopardi D, et al: Selective head cooling with mild systemic hypothermia after neonatal encephalopathy: Multicentre randomised trial. Lancet 365:663–670, 2005.

69. After an asphyxial event, how long should feeding be delayed?

During an asphyxial event, vasoconstriction of the mesenteric vessels can result in intestinal ischemia. Because of the relationship between ischemia and the incidence of necrotizing enterocolitis, feedings should be delayed for 2–3 days to allow for repair of the intestinal mucosa.

70. What is the study of choice to diagnose neonatal strokes?

In any sick newborn with seizures or a focal neurologic abnormality, the suspicion for an underlying structural lesion should be high. Interestingly, 80% of neonatal strokes occur in the left hemisphere. Ultrasound examination is not very sensitive in detecting strokes, and although CT is superior to ultrasound in the acute setting, it also lacks the detail of MRI and exposes the infant to radiation. MRI is thus the diagnostic test of choice. Diffusion-weighted images can detect recent strokes from 1 day (as little as 6 hours) to 7 days after the event. Traditional MRI sequences T1 and T2 are adequate for older strokes.

  Cowan FM, Pennock JM, Hanrahan JD, et al: Early detection of cerebral infarction and hypoxic ischemic encephalopathy in neonates using diffusion-weighted magnetic resonance imaging. Neuropediatrics 25:172–175, 1994.

71. What is the further diagnostic work-up of perinatal stroke?

Once diagnosed, an etiologic work-up should be undertaken. A lumbar puncture to evaluate for treatable infection should be done. An EEG might demonstrate electrographic seizures, slowing, and attenuation. Magnetic resonance angiography helps to visualize the cerebral vessels. The placenta, if available, should be inspected as a possible source of emboli. An echocardiogram to rule out a cardiac source of emboli should also be done. Infants with stroke should undergo a complete blood count to rule out polycythemia, and protein C, protein S, and antithrombin III levels should be measured. Genetic tests looking for factor V Leiden mutation and prothrombin 20210G mutation are also in order. Finally, urinary toxicology should also be done, looking for substances of abuse.

  Nelson KB, Lynch KB: Stroke in newborn infants. Lancet Neurol 3:150–156, 2004.

72. What is the therapy and outcome of perinatal stroke?

Initial management includes general medical support and administration of antiepileptic medications if the child has seizures. Anticoagulation is controversial and is probably not indicated unless an active source of emboli is apparent. In a recent review of outcomes in infants with strokes in the perinatal period, 40% of infants were judged to be normal, 57% were neurologically or cognitively abnormal, and 3% died.

  Lynch JK, Nelson KB: Epidemiology of perinatal stroke. Curr Opin Pediatr 13:499–505, 2001.

  Mercuri E, Rutherford M, Cowan F, et al: Early prognostic indicators of outcome in infants with neonatal cerebral infarction: A clinical, electroencephalogram, and magnetic resonance imaging study. Pediatrics 103:39–46, 1999.

73. **How common is sagittal sinus thrombosis?**
Sinovenous thrombosis has been increasingly recognized, but it is relatively rare. Identifiable causes include extracorporeal membrane oxygenation (ECMO) and congenital heart disease in about half of cases. Additionally, more than half of infants tested had genetic thrombophilias. Evaluation is similar to stroke for etiology of hypercoagulability. Anticoagulation is controversial.

Wu YW, Miller SP, Chin K, et al: Multiple risk factors in neonatal sinovenous thrombosis. Neurology 3:438–440, 2002.

KEY POINTS: A HISTORICAL VIEW OF PERINATAL EVENTS

1. Since the orthopedic surgeon William Little wrote almost 150 years ago of the effect of "abnormal parturition, difficult labor, premature birth, and asphyxia neonatorum on the mental and physical condition of the child," the topic has been keenly debated.

2. Sigmund Freud contributed substantially to the discussion in 1897 and suggested that no adverse perinatal events were identified in about one third of children with CP.

CEREBRAL PALSY

74. **What is CP?**
CP is a nonprogressive disorder of motor function of central origin occurring usually in utero or early in life. Intellectual deficit is not implicit in CP, although it accompanies the process a high percentage of the time. The overall prevalence of CP is 1.7–2 per 1000 in survivors at the age of 1 year. Premature infants are at the highest risk. The lower the birth weight and gestational age, the greater the chance for the child to develop CP.

United Cerebral Palsy: http://www.ucp.org

75. **What is the etiology of CP, and what are its risk factors?**
   - Asphyxia (3–20%)
   - Intrauterine infection (28%)
   - Congenital malformations (30–50%)
   - Postnatal events (e.g., hyperbilirubinemia, hypoglycemia, hypotension, hypoxemia, sepsis)

KEY POINTS: FEATURES SUGGESTING A PROGRESSIVE CNS DISORDER RATHER THAN CP AS THE CAUSE OF A MOTOR DEFICIT

1. Plateau or regression of development

2. Abnormally increasing head circumference (possible hydrocephalus, tumor, or neurodegenerative disease)

3. Eye anomalies such as cataracts, retinal pigmentary degeneration, or optic atrophy (possible neurodegenerative disease)

4. Skin abnormalities such as vitiligo, café au lait spots, nevus flammeus (possible Sturge-Weber disease, NF)

5. Hepatomegaly or splenomegaly (possible storage disease)

6. Decreased or absent deep tendon reflexes

76. **What are the three major varieties of CP?**
The three types of CP are spastic, dyskinetic, and ataxic. The type of CP depends mainly on the location of the lesion(s). Furthermore, the site(s) affected depend on the etiology of the lesion. A child may have more than one type, and the movement abnormalities may change during development. CP is subdivided by abnormality of tone (i.e., spastic or hypotonic), location (i.e., hemiplegia, diplegia, or quadriplegia), and type of movement (i.e., athetotic or ataxic). Spastic variants are more common with injury to the corticospinal tracts. Basal ganglia lesions are associated with movement disorders and cerebellar lesions with ataxia.

77. **Why is CP difficult to diagnose clinically in the first year of life?**
- Hypotonia is more common than hypertonia and spasticity in the first year.
- Early abundance of primitive reflexes (with variable persistence) may be confusing.
- Infants have a limited variety of volitional movements for evaluation.
- Substantial myelination takes months to evolve and may delay the clinical picture of abnormal tone and increased deep tendon reflexes.
- Expected motor and developmental milestones are limited in the first year.
- Most infants who develop CP do not have identifiable risk factors, and most cases are not related to labor and delivery events.

78. **What percentage of cases of CP are caused by intrapartum asphyxia?**
Although obstetricians are frequently made to feel that they are responsible for CP, the fact is that spastic CP is the result of intrapartum asphyxia in only about 10–20% of children. Because so many children with spastic CP have no definable etiology for their problem, recent attention has focused on the possibility that in utero infection may be more important than previously thought in the etiology of CP.

79. **How does maternal infection affect the incidence of CP in term children of normal birth weight?**
Maternal temperature above 38°C (100.4°F) during labor or a clinical diagnosis of chorioamnionitis is associated with a marked (ninefold) increased risk of CP, especially spastic quadriplegic CP (19 fold increase). Remember that about 50% of maternal cases of chorioamnionitis are subclinical.

Neufeld MD, Frigon C, Graham AS, Mueller BA: Maternal infection and risk of cerebral palsy in term and preterm infants. J Perinatol 2:108–113, 2005.

Wu YW, Escobar GJ, Grether JK, et al: Chorioamnionitis and cerebral palsy in term and near-term infants. JAMA 290:2677–2684, 2003.

80. **What is the evidence to suggest that inflammatory cytokines have been found to be associated with prematurity and with development of CP?**
The inflammatory response to infection activates a number of cytokines and chemokines, which in turn may trigger preterm contractions, cervical ripening, rupture of the membranes, and prematurity. The levels of interleukin (IL) 1, IL-8, IL-9, and tumor necrosis factor α in dried neonatal blood specimens have been found to be significantly higher in infants who subsequently were diagnosed with CP than in control subjects. Moreover, experimental animal data and epidemiologic studies have shown that IL-6 and IL-8 are strong and independent risk factors for the subsequent development of CP at the age of 3 years.

Hagberg H, Mallard C, Jacobsson B: Role of cytokines in preterm labour and brain injury. BJOG 112 (Suppl 1):16–18, 2005.

Yoon BH, Park CW, Chaiworapongsa T: Intrauterine infection and the development of cerebral palsy. BJOG 110(Suppl 20):124–127, 2003.

81. **What problems are commonly associated with CP?**
- **Mental retardation:** Two thirds of all patients experience this, and it is most commonly observed in children with spastic quadriplegia.

- **Learning disabilities**
- **Ophthalmologic abnormalities:** Strabismus, amblyopia, nystagmus, refractive errors.
- **Hearing deficits**
- **Communication disorders**
- **Seizures:** One third of all patients have seizures. They are most commonly observed in children with spastic hemiplegia.
- **Failure to thrive**
- **Feeding problems**
- **Gastroesophageal reflux**
- **Behavioral and emotional problems:** Especially attention deficit hyperactivity disorder, depression.

Eicher PS, Batshaw ML: Cerebral palsy. Pediatric Clin North Am 40:537–551, 1993.

82. **How has the prevalence of CP changed since the advent of neonatal intensive care in the 1960s?**

The prevalence rose approximately 20% from the early 1960s to the late 1980s, almost entirely because of increased survival of low- and very-low-birth-weight infants.

83. **What is the neurodevelopmental outcome in ELBW infants?**

Fewer than half (41%) of children with a history of extreme prematurity (<26 weeks' gestation) when tested at age 6 years were cognitively impaired when compared with their classmates. The rates of severe, moderate, and mild disability were 22%, 24%, and 34%, respectively. Twelve percent had disabling CP (Fig. 13-5).

Marlow N, Wolke D, Bracewell MA, Samara M; EPICure Study Group: Neurologic and developmental disability at six years of age after extremely preterm birth. N Engl J Med 352:9–19, 2005.

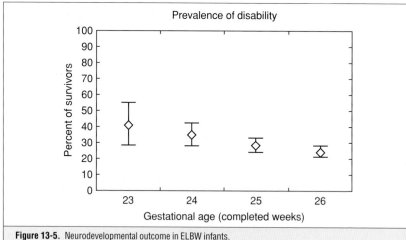

Figure 13-5. Neurodevelopmental outcome in ELBW infants.

NEONATAL SEIZURES

84. **What are neonatal seizures?**

Seizures are defined as sudden paroxysmal alterations in neurologic function (e.g., behavior, motor, autonomic function) due to abnormal, hypersynchronous discharges on the EEG. In other words, the clinical seizure is caused by an electrical seizure of the brain, demonstrated during an ictal EEG. It must be remembered that the clinical and EEG manifestations may be unusual, but not all paroxysmal behaviors in the neonate—especially the encephalopathic neonate—are accompanied by an EEG ictal discharge.

85. **What types of neonatal seizures usually have a consistent EEG correlate?**
   - **Clonic seizures:** These are characterized by sustained, repetitive, rhythmic jerking movements of a muscle group at 1–5 per second. Clonic seizures may be focal or multifocal, involving several body parts, often in a migrating fashion.
   - **Focal tonic seizures:** These are characterized by abrupt changes in muscle tone that produce sustained changes in muscle posture. Focal tonic seizures involve just an arm or leg or the extraocular muscles, producing sustained deviation of both eyes to one side.

86. **What types of neonatal "seizures" usually have inconsistent EEG correlates?**
   Generalized tonic seizures are rare in newborns. "Decerebrate" posturing is not uncommon and is often associated with severe intracranial disease. However, it is usually not epileptic (i.e., the simultaneous EEG is negative for electrographic seizure activity). Myoclonic seizures are rapid shock-like jerks of the muscle occurring as single or repetitive jolts of the affected muscles. The jerks are faster than clonic seizures and not rhythmic. Only rarely do myoclonic seizures have ictal accompaniments.

87. **What are "subtle seizures"?**
   Subtle seizure are repetitive, paroxysmal stereotyped alterations in motor activity or neonatal behavior, "automatisms" such as swimming movements in the arms, chewing, tongue thrusting, bicycling movements of the legs, autonomic changes, and apnea. These abnormal phenomena, often seen in encephalopathic neonates, are rarely linked to ictal EEG activity. Subtle seizures may result from injury to the basal ganglia or may represent brain stem "release phenomena." They may augur a guarded prognosis, but classifying them as *seizures* may lead to unwarranted treatment. Apnea is rarely the sole manifestation of a neonatal seizure.

88. **What is the incidence of neonatal seizures?**
   Seizures are the most common clinical sign of neonatal cerebral dysfunction and may occur in up to 1% of all newborns. The reported incidence of neonatal seizures, however, varies with the population studied, gestational age, and risk status. It also depends on whether subclinical seizures (i.e., seizures only seen on the EEG without any visible clinical signs) are included. Although some authors believe that the incidence of seizures is equal in term and preterm infants, our experience suggests that overt seizures are more common at or near term.

89. **What are the common causes of neonatal seizures?**
   Seizures occurring during the neonatal period are commonly symptomatic of an acute illness. Neonatal encephalopathy is the most frequent cause of neonatal seizures. Other common causes of brain injury include stroke, hemorrhage, infection, cerebral malformation, drug withdrawal, and metabolic causes. The latter include hypoglycemia and electrolyte abnormalities, hyponatremia, hypocalcemia, hypomagnesemia, and inborn errors of metabolism (e.g., urea cycle defects, phenylketonuria, maple syrup urine disease, lactic and organic acidurias, and nonketotic hyperglycinemia).

90. **What are the vitamin-responsive causes of neonatal seizures?**
   Vitamin-responsive neonatal seizures, especially vitamin B_6 dependency, should always be considered. Other vitamin and cofactor deficiencies with the potential to cause seizures include molybdenum, pyridoxal phosphate, and folinic acid.

91. **What are other causes of refractory or malignant neonatal seizures and epilepsy?**

    Two malignant epilepsy syndromes beginning in the neonatal period are characterized by refractory seizures, a suppression-burst EEG, and a poor prognosis. Early infantile epileptic encephalopathy (Ohtahara syndrome) is associated with tonic seizures and structural lesions, and early myoclonic epilepsy (Aicardi's syndrome) is associated with myoclonic seizures and metabolic etiologies.

92. **What are the more benign causes of neonatal seizures?**

    Seizures in a "well baby" may be due to simple hypocalcemia, primary supratentorial subarachnoid hemorrhage of venous origin, or epilepsy. Hypocalcemia and hypocalcemic tetany due to high phosphate-load milks are now rarely seen in the United States. Benign neonatal epilepsy syndromes have been described and have a good prognosis for seizure remission and development. The familial syndromes are associated with genetic abnormalities in sodium and potassium channels.

    Berkovic SF, Heron SE, Giordano L, et al: Benign familial neonatal-infantile seizures: Characterization of a new sodium channelopathy. Ann Neurol 55:550–557, 2004.

93. **How does one evaluate neonatal seizures?**

    The work-up should include a bedside glucose measurement followed by a laboratory glucose measurement and determination of calcium, magnesium, sodium, and acid-base status. A blood culture and lumbar puncture should be performed. A cranial ultrasound scan may confirm suspected hemorrhage and hydrocephalus, CT is particularly good at identification of blood and calcification, and MRI is best for evaluating for malformations of cortical development and the extent of hypoxic damage. Testing should not delay symptomatic treatment of seizures.

94. **Is the EEG helpful in the management of neonatal seizures?**

    Yes, it is useful in confirming electroclinical seizures and electrographic seizures and eliminating those movements without an electrical correlate. Furthermore, there is frequently a disconnect of the clinical appearance from the electrographic seizure. It is also useful in monitoring ongoing treatment. Finally, evaluation of the interictal background is most useful in predicting outcome.

95. **What is the treatment of neonatal seizures?**

    Current therapy is not very effective when used alone; phenobarbital or phenytoin are effective in suppressing seizures in a little fewer than half of neonates. When one drug fails, adding a second results in a 70% success rate. Nevertheless, our practice is to treat with intravenous phenobarbital (20 mg/kg) up to a total of 40 mg/kg. If clinical seizures persist, intravenous fosphenytoin (20 mg/kg) is slowly administered. Maintenance dosing of phenobarbital is 3–5 mg/kg/24h, and phenytoin is 6–10 mg/kg/24h, respectively. Third-line treatments are variable. The treatment of electrographic seizures is more controversial, but aggressive treatment should be tempered with the risk of cardiovascular depression and compromise of cerebral perfusion.

    Painter MJ, Scher MS, Stein AD, et al: Phenobarbital compared with phenytoin for the treatment of neonatal seizures. N Engl J Med 341:485–489, 1999.

96. **When is medication tapered?**

    In the well-appearing baby with a normal EEG, early discontinuation of medication is recommended while the neonate is still in the intensive care unit or upon discharge. In some cases, it is appropriate to allow the baby to self-taper by maintaining the dose without increasing it as the baby grows.

97. **What is the prognosis of neonates with seizures?**

    The ultimate prognosis is determined by the etiology of the seizures. EEG background activity and MRI/MRS are also useful in predicting prognosis. Fewer than one third of neonates with seizures later develop epilepsy; more than half of newborns with neonatal seizures will not be healthy (Table 13-4).

TABLE 13-4.   RELATIONSHIP OF NEUROLOGIC DISEASE TO PROGNOSIS IN NEONATAL SEIZURES

Disease	Children Who Survive and Become Healthy (%)	Comment
Perinatal asphyxia	50	
Subarachnoid hemorrhage	90	
Intraventricular hemorrhage	10	Seizures rare in premature infants
Hypoglycemia	50	Outcome may be related to early-onset therapy
Late hypocalcemia	90	Presents days 5–10
Early hypocalcemia	50	Presents days 1–3 in conjunction with other encephalopathies
Inborn metabolic errors	10	A few with phenylketonuria or pyridoxine dependency may do well
Bacterial meningitis	30	
Congenital anomalies	0	Defects include lissencephaly, polymicrogyria, pachygyria
Drug withdrawal	?	Good follow-up series unavailable; drugs include heroin, methadone
Cause unknown	67	10–20% of neonatal seizures, including benign familial epilepsy

Adapted from Koenigsberger MR, Kairam R: Merritt's Neurology. Philadelphia, Lippincott, Williams & Wilkins, 2000.

ADDICTION IN NEONATES

98. **When does withdrawal occur in infants of narcotic-addicted mothers?**
Most withdrawal occurs within 72 hours of birth; the range is from shortly after birth to as late as 2 weeks after delivery. In general, the closer to delivery the mother has used the drug, the greater the delay in onset of signs. Heroin-exposed infants with perinatal depression should not receive a narcotic antagonist, because it may precipitate seizures.

99. **Of cocaine, heroin, alcohol, marijuana, and cigarettes, which is considered usually compatible with breast-feeding by the AAP?**
The AAP states that maternal alcohol use is usually compatible with breast-feeding.

100. **Do most children with in utero cocaine exposure demonstrate significant neurologic damage?**
No. Although there is an early slowdown in head growth, controlled studies have found no clear-cut motor or cognitive deficits in toddlers.

Chiriboga CA: Neurological correlates of fetal cocaine exposure. Ann NY Acad Sci 846:109–125, 1998.

KEY POINTS: SIGNS AND SYMPTOMS OF DRUG WITHDRAWAL

1. **W** = Wakefulness

2. **I** = Irritability

3. **T** = Tremulousness, temperature variation, tachypnea

4. **H** = Hyperactivity, high-pitched cry, hyperacusis, hyperreflexia, hypertonus

5. **D** = Diarrhea, diaphoresis, disorganized suck

6. **R** = Rub marks, respiratory distress, rhinorrhea

7. **A** = Apneic attacks, autonomic dysfunction

8. **W** = Weight loss or poor weight gain

9. **A** = Alkalosis (respiratory)

10. **L** = Lacrimation

101. **What neonatal specimens should be obtained to detect intrauterine drug exposure?**
Urine is normally used, but meconium and particularly hair are most useful for detecting early exposure.

> Vinner E, Vignau J, Thibault D, et al: Hair analysis of opiates in mothers and newborns for evaluating opiate exposure during pregnancy newborns. Forensic Sci Int 133:57–62, 2003.

NEUROMUSCULAR DISORDERS

102. **When the process causing hypotonia is central, what neonatal conditions come to mind?**
Acute neonatal encephalopathy (now thought to be multifactorial) should be first. This process can result from asphyxia, but other important causes include birth trauma, maternal infection, neonatal sepsis, metabolic disease, and congenital abnormalities of the brain. Genetic syndromes, such as trisomy 21 and Prader-Willi syndromes, also cause central hypotonia and can be identified by associated dysmorphic features.

103. **What are the components of the lower motor neuron? Why is it useful to think in terms of these anatomic entities when evaluating a floppy newborn infant?**
It is useful to think anatomically because clinical localization is facilitated (Table 13-5). The components of the lower motor neuron from the spinal cord to most peripheral part are (with examples):
1. **Anterior horn cell:** Spinal muscular atrophy
2. **Peripheral nerve:** Congenital hypomyelinating neuropathy
3. **Neuromuscular junction:** Transient and congenital myasthenia gravis
4. **Muscle:** Congenital myopathy, such as "central core" disease and congenital muscular dystrophies

TABLE 13-5. ANATOMIC LOCALIZATION OF HYPOTONIC WEAKNESS IN NEWBORN

	CNS Lesion	Anterior Horn Cell	Nerve	NMJ	Muscle
Distribution	D (SA)	P > D	D	B (P)	P*
Symmetry	A	S	S	S	S
DTRs	Inc, N, Dim	0	0	N	Dim or 0
Face	N or A	N (F)	N	Ptosis 15%	Bifacial
Sensation	N or Dim	N	N or Dim	N	N

NMJ = neuromuscular junction, DTRs = deep tendon reflexes, D = distal, P = proximal, SA = shoulder-arm, B = bulbar, S = symmetric, A = asymmetric, N = normal, 0 = absent, F = tongue fasciculations, Inc = increased, Dim = diminished.
*Exception: myotonic dystrophy is D.

104. **What are the basic tests to confirm lower motor neuron disease?**
Blood creatine phosphokinase (CPK) measurement, serum carnitine measurement, an edrophonium or neostigmine test, motor nerve conduction velocities, needle electromyography (EMG), DNA testing, and muscle biopsy.
1. Elevated serum CPK values beyond the seventh postnatal day suggest active muscle disease, most commonly one of the congenital muscular dystrophies.
2. Low carnitine levels either suggest the very rare primary carnitine deficiency or result from fatty acid or organic acid abnormalities.
3. Abnormally low nerve conduction velocities suggest a neuropathy but are reported in 30–50% of cases of anterior horn cell disease. Needle EMG studies are helpful to distinguish a neuropathic from a myopathic process. Myotonia on insertion is rare in neonatal myotonic dystrophy but is invariably present in Pompe's disease (i.e., acid maltase deficiency).
4. In recent years, DNA analysis has been used to identify various entities; spinal muscular atrophy, myotonic dystrophy, and Prader-Willi syndrome are examples.
5. In some cases, muscle biopsy (with both histologic and biochemical analysis) is still the only way to make a precise diagnosis.

105. **Why do some clinicians prefer neostigmine testing to edrophonium testing?**
Edrophonium or neostigmine testing is done to rule out transient myasthenia gravis or congenital forms of myasthenia, not all of which are edrophonium positive. Some clinicians prefer neostigmine because the effect on the neuromuscular junction is more long-lived and more apparent to the observer. Because of cardiovascular and other cholinergic side effects, atropine and resuscitation equipment should be available at the time of testing.

106. **What entities cause ptosis is a newborn?**
Unilateral ptosis is most commonly familial and often dominant. Sometimes it is part of Horner's syndrome, which also includes meiosis of the pupil and decreased sweating on the same side of the face. Neck masses, iatrogenic injury during cardiac surgery, and birth injury to the lower brachial plexus are other causes. Facial trauma may cause a temporary pseudo-ptosis. Bilateral ptosis is seen in centronuclear (myotubular) myopathy, myotonic dystrophy, and myasthenic syndromes.

107. What is transient neonatal myasthenia, and how is it diagnosed?

Transient neonatal myasthenia occurs in 15% of deliveries to mothers with autoimmune myasthenia gravis due to the transplacental passage of maternal acetylcholine receptor (AChR) antibodies. Symptoms that affect respiration and deglutition usually predominate. There may be ptosis and generalized weakness with intact reflexes. AChR antibodies are present, but the diagnosis is more rapidly made by Tensilon or neostigmine testing. Repetitive stimulation on EMG shows a decrement in muscle amplitude potentials. Treatment is supportive, but supplementation with subcutaneous or oral pyridostigmine is often necessary. Symptoms may persist for 1–5 weeks.

108. What are the congenital myasthenic syndromes?

See Table 13-6.

TABLE 13-6. CONGENITAL MYASTHENIC SYNDROMES

Basic Abnormality	Usual Inheritance	Neonatal Onset Common	Extraocular Muscle Weakness	Response to AChE Inhibitor Common
Presynaptic abnormalities				
Defects in Ach synthesis or packaging (familial infantile myasthenia)	Recessive	+	−	+
Paucity of synaptic vesicles	Recessive	+	−	+
Synaptic abnormalities				
AChE deficiency	Recessive	+	+	−
Postsynaptic abnormalities				
ACh receptor deficiency	Recessive	+	+	+
Slow-channel syndrome	Dominant	−	+	−
Postchannel syndrome	Recessive	+	−	?

ACh = Acetylcholine, AChE = acetylcholinesterase, + = present, − = absent.

109. What are four characteristics of damage to the anterior horn cell?

1. Weakness
2. Fasciculations (in the newborn, only observed on the tongue) due to the neonatal fat pad
3. Atrophy; also difficult to see because of adipose tissue surrounding almost all muscles
4. Hyporeflexia or areflexia

110. Why is myotonic dystrophy an example of the phenomenon of "anticipation"?

Genetic studies have shown that the defect in myotonic dystrophy is an expansion of a trinucleotide (CTG) in a gene on the long arm of chromosome 19 that codes for a protein kinase. In successive generations, this repeating sequence has a tendency to increase, sometimes into the thousands (normal is <40 CTG repeats), and the extent of repetition correlates with the severity.

BRAIN DEATH

111. **What are the American Academy of Pediatrics Task Force recommendations to make the diagnosis of brain death?**
First, there must be an absence of a reversible etiology; that is, toxic-metabolic, medication, hypothermia, hypotension, or surgically remediable causes. Then, there must be an absence of neocortical function including spontaneous movements, response to stimuli, and awareness of the environment. Next, there must be a complete absence of brain stem function including non-responsive, midposition or fully dilated pupils, no spontaneous or reflexive eye movements on oculovestibular testing ("doll's eyes"), no bulbar muscle function (i.e., corneal, gag, cough, sucking and rooting reflexes), and no respirations on apnea testing. The patient, however, may have spinal cord reflexes or myoclonus of noncortical/brain stem origin. The examination must remain unchanged over time.

112. **What other supportive testing is recommended?**
The President's task force recommends an EEG, performed in accordance with a standardized protocol to document electrocerebral silence. Because hypotension, hypothermia (≤32.2°C for adults), and medications (including a phenobarbital level >25 µg/mL) may suppress the EEG, the patient must have a stable temperature, blood pressure, and appropriate metabolic/toxicology testing and drug levels. Absence of cerebral blood flow by four-vessel arteriography or radionuclide study is also supportive of electrocerebral silence.

113. **What are the task force recommendations for length of period of observation for neonates and infants?**
The task force recommends no determination of brain death be made in neonates younger than 7 days old. In infants 7 days to 2 months of age, two examinations and EEGs separated by at least 48 hours are recommended. In infants 2 months to 1 year of age, two examinations and EEGs separated by at least 24 hours are recommended.

114. **Why is there an exception for the first week of life?**
The most controversial group is the youngest, and the task force recommends that the determination of brain death not be made in neonates younger than 1 week of age. Very young infants are different because they have lower cerebral blood flow and oxygen requirements and greater cranial compliance. The lower blood flow requirements may explain why some neonates may transiently demonstrate EEG activity in the face of no discernible cerebral blood flow. Indeed, a retrospective review of preterm and term infants younger than 1 month of age showed that EEG or radionuclide study confirmed the clinical criteria for brain death in only one half to two thirds of patients. Even though the determination of brain death cannot be formally made in neonates younger than 7 days old, a retrospective review of the validity of brain death criteria suggests that if all clinical criteria are fulfilled, the chance of neurologic survival is nil.

115. **What are the ethical, moral, religious, and legal concerns about the formulation of brain death criteria for infants and children?**
The Ad Hoc Committee of the Harvard Medical School was asked to examine the definition of brain death and to define a new criterion for brain death. They perceived a conflict arising from the ability to indefinitely support the heart and lungs on the one hand and the potential for organ transplantation on the other. Individual and societal concerns regarding the determination of brain death include the possibility of diagnostic error and the conceptual difficulty of a definition of death—the "mind-body question." In a 1957 address, "The Prolongation of Life," Pope Pius XII stated that it was not "within the competence of the church," but was rather that of

the physician, to make the determination of death. Legislation and court rulings in the United States have concluded that it is lawful for the medical profession to diagnose brain death according to its own established criteria. It is the responsibility and right of the physician to make the determination of death by either the absence of cardiac or cerebral activity.

The Ad Hoc Committee of the Harvard Medical School to Examine the Definition of Brain Death: A definition of irreversible coma. JAMA 205:337–340, 1968.

Ashwal S: Brain death in the newborn. Pediatrics 84:429–437, 1989.

President's Commission for the Study of Ethical Problems in Medicine and Biomedical and Behavioral Research. Guidelines for the determination of death. JAMA 246:2184–2186, 1981.

CHAPTER 14

ORTHOPEDICS

Joshua E. Hyman, MD

1. **What are the components of the newborn orthopedic screening examination?**
   All newborn babies should be examined for evidence of hip dysplasia, spinal dysraphism, and lower and upper extremity deficiencies or deformities.

2. **A premature newborn infant receiving ventilator support in the neonatal intensive care unit (NICU) has decreased movement in the right lower extremity. What diagnostic tests may be appropriate?**
   Baseline laboratory testing should be considered (e.g., complete blood count, C-reactive protein, sedimentation rate) as part of the evaluation for possible joint infections, which are not uncommon in this setting. These tests may not be rewarding because infants may develop infection without abnormalities in their laboratory values. Plain radiographs of the entire extremity should be obtained to help detect subtle fracture that may not be apparent on clinical examination. Radiographs are often normal in the early phases of bone and joint infection. In this setting, bone and joint infections most often involve more than one site. Therefore, careful clinical assessment to detect subtle joint effusions or swelling over long bones is indicated. Often an ultrasound scan is helpful in confirming a joint effusion in the hip because overlying muscle may mask the usual clinical findings. A technetium-99 bone scan is very useful in detecting other sites of multicentric infection.

3. **The initial evaluation of a first-born infant reveals multiple stiff joints in both the upper and lower extremities and thin, tapered, and "shiny" fingers. What is the main diagnostic consideration?**
   Arthrogryposis multiplex congenita is a clinical syndrome characterized by poor development of the joints in utero leading to multiple contractures. This does not appear to be a hereditary condition, and there is no increased risk in siblings of the same family. Many mothers report decreased fetal movement in utero. On clinical examination, the limbs are usually symmetric. Joints may have either flexion or extension contractures. There is decreased active and passive motion of the affected joints. The normal skin creases are usually absent, and the skin is taut and glossy. Dimpling at the joints may be present. There is atrophy of the limbs. Often the hips are dislocated, and clubfoot (i.e., talipes equinovarus) or congenital vertical talus affects the feet. The upper extremities are usually internally rotated at the shoulder, with elbow flexion or extension contractures. There are often radial head dislocations. The forearms are pronated with adduction deformity of the thumbs. Delivery may be difficult as a consequence of the stiff elbow and knee joints. This may result in birth fractures of the humerus and the femur. General health is not affected by this syndrome, although patients often exhibit minor respiratory difficulties and failure to thrive as newborns.

4. **What congenital spine malformation is associated with maternal insulin-dependent diabetes?**
   Lumbosacral agenesis is more common in women with insulin-dependent diabetes. It is characterized by an absence of variable amounts of the sacrum and lumbar spine and the associated neural elements. There may also be concomitant anomalies of the genitourinary and

gastrointestinal tracts. The level of the lesion may vary, and this will influence the clinical picture. These lesions are classified into four types according to the Renshaw's classification:

- Type I is either partial or total sacral agenesis.
- Type II, the most common, is partial sacral agenesis with a symmetric defect but a stable sacroiliac joint.
- Type III is variable lumbar agenesis with total sacral agenesis. The ilia articulate with the lowest lumbar vertebra that is present.
- Type IV is similar to type III but with the end plate of the most caudal vertebra resting on a fused ilia.

Depending on the severity of the agenesis, the patient may have variable foot deformities and abnormalities of the hips and knees.

5. **A newborn infant is noted to have external rotation of the lower extremities at rest, with little spontaneous movement and bilateral foot deformities. What radiographs should be ordered?**
Both spine and pelvis radiographs. The abnormalities described can be due to anomalies of the spine or the lower extremities.

6. **A newborn child is suspected of having a genetic skeletal dysplasia. What is the most critical orthopedic radiographic examination?**
The most important radiograph is the lateral cervical spine. More than 150 distinct osteochondrodysplasias have been identified. Each has distinctive features, but many also have similar radiographic findings. One of the most common is agenesis or hypoplasia of the upper cervical spine elements. This can lead to instability and places the child at great risk of spinal cord injury during ordinary handling. Detection of cervical instability is mandatory to allow proper stabilization and protection.

7. **What is developmental dysplasia of the hip (DDH)?**
DDH is a maldevelopment of the hip joint characterized by a spectrum of pathology ranging from instability of the hip to irreducible dislocation.

8. **Why has the term *developmental dysplasia of the hips* replaced the term *congenital hip dislocation*?**
DDH is now preferred over *congenital hip dislocation* to reflect the evolutionary nature of hip problems in infants in the first months of life. About 2.5–6.5 infants per 1000 live births develop problems, and a significant percentage of these problems are not present on neonatal screening examinations. Clearly, the overt pathologic process may not be present at birth, and periodic examination of the infant's hip is recommended at each routine well-baby exam until the age of 1 year.

9. **How is the newborn hip exam performed?**
All newborn hips should be put through the Ortolani, Barlow, and Galeazzi maneuvers.

- The **Ortolani** exam is a reduction maneuver. It is performed with the child in the supine position. Beginning with the hips flexed 90 degrees and adducted to the midline, the examiner gently abducts the hip and lifts up on the greater trochanter. If the hip is dislocated and reducible, a palpable sensation will be felt as the hip reduces into the acetabulum (an Ortolani-positive hip).
- The **Barlow** exam is a provocative maneuver that identifies a dislocatable (unstable) hip. It is performed with the child supine on the exam table. The hip is flexed 90 degrees and adducted just beyond midline. Gentle downward pressure is then applied to the hip through the knee. The sensation of the femoral head sliding out of the acetabulum indicates a Barlow-positive hip. A normal hip will not subluxate.

- The **Galeazzi** exam is performed to identify apparent or real shortening of the femur. It is performed with the child supine. The hips and knees are flexed such that the feet are lying flat on the table. The examiner then looks at the heights of the knees. If there is a difference, there may be a dislocated hip.

KEY POINTS: DEVELOPMENTAL DYSPLASIA OF THE HIP IN NEWBORNS

1. Every newborn should have a hip examination.

2. The examination consists of the Ortolani, Barlow, and Galeazzi maneuvers.

3. The three main risk factors for DDH are first-born status, female sex, and breech presentation.

10. **What radiographic studies are helpful to make the diagnosis of DDH?**
    Ultrasound of the hip is the study of choice for suspected DDH in children younger than 4 months of age. In children of this age, the ossific nucleus of the femoral head is completely cartilaginous and therefore will not be seen on x-ray. After 4 months of age, radiographs should be obtained.

11. **What are the risk factors for DDH?**
    First-born female infants who present in the breech position and have a positive family history of DDH are at a significantly increased risk.

12. **What other conditions are associated with DDH?**
    Torticollis, congenital hyperextension of the knee, metatarsus adductus, and clubfoot.

13. **How is DDH treated in newborns?**
    In a newborn child, DDH can be very effectively treated with dynamic splinting in a brace such as a Pavlik harness. A child in a Pavlik harness will lie with her hips and knees flexed approximately 90 degrees and her hips abducted to 60 degrees. This position is quite comfortable and natural for the infant. In this position, the femoral head is deeply seated within the acetabulum. The soft tissue structures around the hip will then stabilize with the hip in this reduced position.

KEY POINTS: CLUBFOOT

1. The majority of clubfeet can be treated effectively with manipulation and casting.

2. Treatment should begin as soon as possible after birth.

3. Clubfoot may be associated with other congenital conditions; therefore, a thorough evaluation of the entire infant is necessary.

14. **What is clubfoot?**
    Clubfoot, or talipes equinovarus, is a congenital condition in which the foot points downward and inward. More specifically, the hind foot is in equinus and varus and the forefoot is in adduction and supination.

15. **What is the epidemiology of clubfoot?**
The incidence of clubfoot is 1.2 per 1000 live births. Boys are affected nearly twice as often as girls, and 50% of the patients have bilateral involvement.

16. **What are the causes of clubfoot?**
The etiology of clubfoot is unknown. It is seen in conjunction with cerebral palsy, myelomeningocele, arthrogryposis, and other neuromuscular conditions. Most often, however, it occurs as an isolated deformity in an otherwise healthy infant.

17. **What is the treatment for clubfoot?**
The initial treatment for clubfoot is weekly manipulation and casting. Approximately 6–10 casts are required. A brace is worn for 3–4 years to maintain the correct position. With this technique, approximately 80–90% of idiopathic clubfeet with be successfully treated. Those feet that cannot be corrected with this method will require surgical correction.

18. **When should clubfoot treatment be initiated?**
As soon as the deformity is recognized, treatment should be started. This can frequently occur in the newborn nursery.

19. **What is Klippel-Feil syndrome?**
A congenital condition characterized by the triad of a short neck, a low posterior hairline, and fusion of elements of the cervical spine. It results in decreased cervical spine motion.

20. **What is the general clinical significance of Klippel-Feil syndrome?**
The cervical spine develops embryologically at the same time as the genitourinary and cardiovascular systems. As a result, patients with cervical spine anomalies may also have genitourinary and cardiovascular anomalies. In addition, other fusions and malformations of the spinal column may occur. There may also be abnormalities within the spinal cord such as syringomyelia and cord tethering.

21. **What does the evaluation of a child with Klippel-Feil syndrome entail?**
These children must undergo an abdominal ultrasound scan to evaluate possible genitourinary anomalies. They should have a careful clinical cardiac examination. If the results of this exam are thought to be abnormal, an echocardiogram should be considered. Complete radiographs of the entire spinal column must be obtained to look for other vertebral anomalies. Finally, a thorough neurologic evaluation, including magnetic resonance imaging from the base of the brain to the cauda equina, should be performed.

KEY POINTS: NEONATAL INFECTIONS

1. Newborn children with a bone or joint infection may present with pseudoparalysis of the affected extremity.

2. A fever is not a prerequisite for a bone or joint infection.

3. Treatment of joint infections requires aspiration and antibiotics.

22. **What are the clinical findings of septic arthritis of the hip in the newborn?**
The inability of the newborn to communicate makes this diagnosis quite difficult; however, there are some hallmark signs to be aware of. These children will appear lethargic and irritable. They will have difficulty feeding and will exhibit pseudoparalysis, or decreased movement, of the affected limb. A fever is not obligatory. The diagnosis is made by joint aspiration and microscopic examination of the fluid.

23. **What are the consequences of a missed joint infection?**
Bacteria within the joint will lead to an inflammatory response by the host immune system. The enzymes released (e.g., collagenases, proteases, elastases) by both the leukocytes and bacterial cells cause cartilage damage. Initially, glycosaminoglycans are removed from the cartilage. Over time, there is eventual collagen destruction. This damage is irreversible. In addition, if sufficient pressure develops within the joint, blood flow to the epiphysis will be compromised and may lead to avascular necrosis.

24. **What are the most common bacterial agents in neonatal osteomyelitis?**
Staphylococcus aureus, group B streptococci, *Escherichia coli, Klebsiella, Salmonella*, and *Pseudomonas* species. As opposed to osteomyelitis (which is not very common), septic arthritis is extremely rare. Staphylococci are the most common organisms, but one should always think of gonococci as well with early septic arthritis.

25. **Which bone is most frequently fractured in newborns?**
The clavicle. This injury, which stems from excessive traction during delivery, generally results in a greenstick fracture. This fracture usually heals quite nicely without any therapy, although the callus formation may be notable.

26. **How long should fractures in neonates be immobilized?**
Neonatal fractures generally heal more quickly than their counterparts in children or adults. Because of this, and because of the difficulty in casting neonates, some fractures that would be severely problematic in an adult are barely treated in a neonate. A clavicular fracture will heal within 3 weeks in a newborn infant, as opposed to 6–8 weeks in an adult, and does not need to be immobilized in most cases. Femoral fractures, common in premature infants with rickets, are usually well healed within 3 weeks, compared with the 6–10 weeks in an older child or adult with this fracture. Femoral fractures usually are splinted to help healing, but not always if there is minimal displacement.

27. **Discuss the features of constriction ring syndrome (i.e., Streeter's dysplasia).**
Constriction ring syndrome is a rare syndrome that is characterized by ring-like constriction bands around the upper and lower extremities or the trunk. The etiology is unknown, and it is not hereditary. The extent and depth of the rings vary. The bands may be subcutaneous or may extend down to bone. These bands may interfere with lymphatic and venous return. This causes edema and enlargement of the distal part with decreased capillary refill. If there is great disruption to the local circulation, the part may undergo autoamputation in utero. Often there are other concomitant anomalies of the hand including syndactyly, acrodactyly, hypoplasia, camptodactyly, and symphalangia. Other associated anomalies include cleft palate and lip and talipes equinovarus deformity of the foot.

28. **The foot of a newborn appears to be dorsiflexed such that the top of the foot lies directly against the anterior portion of the lower leg. What are the two diagnostic considerations, and how would you differentiate between the two?**
Calcaneovalgus foot deformity is the most likely diagnosis. It is believed that there is no intrinsic problem with bone or joint development and that the deformity results from intrauterine positioning. The natural history of the untreated condition is one of spontaneous correction with no long-term sequelae. The second possibility is posteromedial bowing of the distal tibia. The foot

is folded on the anterior surface of the leg, but the flexibility of the foot and ankle are normal. There is significant shortening of the affected side and decreased soft tissue. Because the physical findings may be difficult to distinguish from calcaneovalgus foot deformity in the newborn, anteroposterior and lateral radiographs of the leg should be obtained. This condition improves with time, usually during the first 3 years of life. However, long-term orthopedic care is required because the affected limb always shows significant growth discrepancy and internal tibial torsion at maturity.

29. **Discuss the orthopedic manifestations of thrombocytopenia with absent radius (TAR) syndrome.**
TAR syndrome presents with several orthopedic findings. In the upper extremity, there is bilateral absence of the radius, usually with all five fingers present. The thumbs may be hypoplastic. Abnormalities of the fingers may include absence of the middle phalanx of the fifth finger, clinodactyly, or partial syndactyly. In almost one half of the patients, shortening or bowing of the ulna with deficiency of the extensor tendons may occur. In addition, the humerus may be short or absent. In almost 40% of patients, there are associated lower extremity anomalies. These mainly involve the knee and include subluxation or dislocation of the patella and hypoplasia of the knee. The most common deformity of the lower extremities is genu varum with a flexion contracture and internal tibial torsion. These patients also may have hip dislocations, varus or valgus deformities of the hips, and shortening of the legs with hypoplastic or absent tibiae or fibulae.

30. **A newborn exhibits swelling over the midshaft of the right clavicle. What are the two most common diagnostic considerations?**
Birth fractures of the clavicle are extremely common but most often are accompanied by pseudoparalysis of the extremity (caused by "splinting" from pain) for at least 3–5 days. There is pain with passive movement. Radiographs show the fracture, which usually heals with a massive callus. In the absence of pain, one must consider congenital pseudarthrosis of the clavicle. The pseudarthrosis is fully present at birth. There is no history of birth injury or other trauma. The right clavicle is almost always affected. At the pseudarthrosis, the clavicular ends are enlarged, and there is painless motion between the two fragments. The etiology remains unknown, but several theories have been proposed including exaggerated arterial pulsations and pressure on the clavicle by the subclavian artery that is normally more cranial on the right side. In bilateral cases, it is thought that there is an abnormally high subclavian artery on both sides. With growth, the deformity increases, and the overlying skin becomes thin and atrophic. The affected shoulder often droops, and there is asymmetry between the two shoulders. No functional impairment is noted. Treatment involves resection of the nonunion and internal fixation with bone grafting.

BIBLIOGRAPHY

1. Blasco PA: Pathology of cerebral palsy. In Sussman MD (ed): The Diplegic Child. Rosemont, IL, American Academy of Orthopaedic Surgeons, 1992, pp 3–20.
2. Drennan JC: Current concepts in myelomeningocele. Am Acad Orthop Surg Instr Course Lect. 48:543–550, 1999.
3. Guille JT, Pizzutillo PD, MacEwen GD: Development dysplasia of the hip from birth to six months. J Am Acad Orthop Surg 8:232–242, 2000.
4. Hyman JE, Roye DP Jr: Torticollis. In Burg FD, Ingelfinger JR, Polin RA, Gershon AA (eds): Gellis and Kagan's Current Pediatric Therapy. Philadelphia, W.B. Saunders, 2002, pp 849–850.
5. Roye BD, Hyman JE, Roye DP Jr: Congenital idiopathic talipes equinovarus. Pediatr Rev 25:124–130, 2004.
6. Shaw BA, Kasser JR: Acute septic arthritis in infancy and childhood. Clin Orthop Relat Res 257:212–225, 1990.
7. Simon SR: Orthopaedic Basic Science. Rosemont, IL, American Academy of Orthopaedic Surgeons.
8. Tracy MR, Dormans JP, Kusumi K: Klippel-Feil syndrome: Clinical features and current understanding of etiology. Clin Orthop Relat Res 424:183–190, 2004.

CHAPTER 15

PAIN MANAGEMENT IN THE NEONATE

K.J.S. Anand, MBBS, DPhil, and Richard W. Hall, MD

1. **An obstetrician is about to do a circumcision without using analgesia. When you question this practice, he replies that neonates cannot perceive pain. Is this correct?**
He is not correct. A traditional and common misconception assumed that neonatal responses to pain represented only physiologic or neuroendocrine reflexes. Multiple lines of evidence prove that the pain system is intact and functional in preterm and term neonates. Acute pain is processed in the somatosensory cortex (which suggests conscious perception); behavioral responses to pain are complex and nuanced forms of "self-expression," and effective mechanisms of hyperalgesia, allodynia, and referred pain occur in preterm and term neonates. Neonates exhibit flexion and adduction of the affected limb, distinct facial expressions, and specific features of a pain "cry" that has unique spectrographic characteristics to distinguish it from other types of crying.

2. **When does pain perception develop in the human fetus?**
Cutaneous sensory receptors first appear in the perioral area during the eighth week of gestation. They are present in all cutaneous and mucous surfaces by the twentieth week of gestation. Synapses between peripheral sensory afferents and dorsal horn neurons in the spinal cord first appear at 6 weeks of gestation. By 16–18 weeks of development, fetuses show specific hemodynamic and neuroendocrine responses to noxious stimuli. By 20 weeks of gestation, the thalamocortical connections are made that would allow painful stimuli to reach the somatosensory cortex. A current theory of pain processing postulates that pain perception occurs at the level of the thalamus, which is consistent with the fetal responses to pain (at 16 weeks) and accumulating data from adult pain patients and experimental studies.

3. **Are neonates less sensitive to pain than older children or adults?**
No! Developmentally regulated processes and behavioral reflexes suggest that pain thresholds increase progressively during late gestation and in the postnatal period. Preterm neonates have much greater sensitivity to pain than term neonates, and they manifest prolonged hyperalgesia after tissue injury. These phenomena have been further substantiated using experimental models for different types of pain in the newborn and infant rat.

4. **What kind of painful experiences are neonates exposed to in the neonatal intensive care unit (NICU)?**
Neonates admitted to a modern-day NICU are often exposed to pain or noxious stimulation from a variety of sources. These include postoperative pain resulting from surgery to repair a hernia or to ligate a patent ductus arteriosus; acute pain caused by circumcision, repeated heelsticks, venipunctures, tracheal suctioning, lumbar punctures, or chest tubes; and prolonged or chronic pain from necrotizing enterocolitis, meningitis, birth trauma, or ventilation. Even routine care such as diaper changes, daily weights, removal of adhesive tape, burns from transcutaneous probes, and rectal stimulation are not "gestationally appropriate" in term or preterm infants and will cause noxious stimulation.

5. **Even if neonates do feel pain, will they ever remember it?**

   Neonatal pain experiences are not accessed by conscious recall but lead to long-term or permanent alterations in brain development that are expressed in unique ways during different stages of development, depending on the type, duration, and severity of neonatal painful stimuli; the neurologic maturity at which pain occurs; and the use of analgesia. Tissue damage in the early neonatal period causes profound and lasting dendritic sprouting of sensory nerve terminals, resulting in hyperinnervation that continues into childhood and adolescence. Thus, repeated heelsticks may lead to an abnormal gait in childhood, perioral and nasal suctioning may promote an oral aversion syndrome, surgical sites maintain an increased sensitivity to pain, and gastric suctioning at birth can lead to an increased likelihood of developing irritable bowel syndrome. Nerve injury in infants, however, does not lead to neuropathic pain, as it does in adults.

6. **What are the long-term effects of pain in term neonates?**

   Term neonates exposed to acute, short-term pain develop significant degrees of hyperalgesia after tissue injury, which includes the areas where the injury occurred (i.e., primary hyperalgesia) as well as areas remote from the original injury (i.e., secondary hyperalgesia). Recent data indicate that primary and secondary hyperalgesia last for several months after neonatal surgery or circumcision, and that visceral hyperalgesia may last for months or years after noxious visceral stimulation at birth. Twin pairs that were discordant only for the experience of surgery in infancy showed greater signs of attention-deficit/hyperactivity disorder, impulsivity, and socialization problems during early school years in the twin who was exposed to surgical and postoperative pain. These persons may be at significant risk for developing chronic pain syndromes during their adult life.

7. **What are the long-term effects of pain in preterm neonates?**

   It is difficult to separate the long-term effects of repetitive pain in preterm neonates from the causes and consequences of premature birth and those of fetal brain development occurring *ex utero*. Similar to term neonates, pain/stress in the NICU leads to short-term heightened pain reactivity, noted as increased responses to heelstick pain after physical handling, tracheal suctioning after a higher number of skin-breaking procedures in the previous 24 hours, and routine nursing care if exposed to a heelstick in the previous hour. Conversely, cumulative pain since birth was significantly correlated with a dampened reactivity to heelstick pain and lower cortisol responses to stress at 32 weeks' postconceptional age, less pain reactivity at 4 months, faster recovery at 8 months, decreased everyday pain behavior at 18 months, increased somatization at 4.5 years, and increased affective responses to depicted pain at 8–10 years, compared with matched term control subjects at each of these corrected ages. Other cognitive and behavioral outcomes of preterm neonates have been correlated with their cumulative pain experiences or length of NICU stay, but the relative contributions of repetitive pain or severity of illness or effects of prematurity remain undefined.

8. **Are there any validated methods for pain assessment in neonates?**

   Many methods for measuring the intensity of acute pain in neonates have been validated, but other aspects of painful experiences (e.g., character, location, rhythmicity, duration of pain) cannot be assessed in neonates. Few methods are available for the assessment of postoperative pain and none for prolonged or chronic pain. The most commonly used methods include the Premature Infant Pain Profile, the Neonatal Infant Pain Scale, the CRIES score, and the Neonatal Pain, Agitation, and Sedation Scale (NPASS). The greatest challenge facing clinicians is to develop objective measures of prolonged pain in preterm and term neonates.

9. **What are the clinical effects of continuous morphine or fentanyl infusions in ventilated preterm neonates?**

   There have been relatively few randomized clinical trials comparing the efficacy and safety of intravenous fentanyl or morphine in ventilated preterm neonates. In infants treated with fentanyl, two trials reported lower behavioral stress scores at 16, 24, 48, and 72 hours, a third trial showed reduced pain scores compared with the placebo group. Infants receiving fentanyl had statistically lower heart rate values than the placebo group but required more ventilatory support. In infants receiving morphine infusions, three randomized controlled trials showed lower pain scores but no differences in intraventricular hemorrhage (IVH) (relative risk [RR] 1.13; 95% confidence interval [CI], 0.80–1.61), periventricular leukomalacia (RR, 0.81; 95% CI, 0.51–1.29), or mortality (RR, 1.14; 95% CI, 0.81–1.60) between the morphine and placebo groups. Infants receiving morphine spent more days on mechanical ventilation (weight mean difference [WMD], 0.24; 95% CI, 0.11–0.36). Thus, morphine and fentanyl appear to reduce pain and stress in ventilated preterm neonates but may increase their duration of ventilation.

10. **What are the side effects of using morphine or fentanyl in neonates?**
Opiates have numerous side effects, including respiratory depression, nausea, vomiting, urinary retention, decreased gut motility, and histamine release causing hypotension, itching, or bronchospasm. Histamine release occurs more commonly with morphine than with fentanyl. In addition, morphine is associated with greater effects on gut motility, and high doses may cause biliary tract spasm or seizures. Chest wall rigidity or laryngospasm are unique side effects of fentanyl and occur more frequently with the rapid administration of large intravenous doses. Fentanyl produces less sedation than morphine but has been associated with greater opioid tolerance because of its shorter duration of action. Despite these adverse effects, long-term outcomes of ex-preterm children at 5–6 years of age showed no differences in their cognitive, neuromotor, or behavioral outcomes but trends toward better performance in those receiving morphine (as opposed to no opioids) during the neonatal period.

11. **What are clinical signs of opioid withdrawal in neonates?**
Many of these signs were included in scoring systems designed to quantify opioid withdrawal in neonates and infants born from heroin-addicted mothers. Their applicability to iatrogenic opioid tolerance and withdrawal resulting from prolonged use in the NICU has not been tested.
- **Neurologic:** High-pitched crying, irritability, increased wakefulness, hyperactive deep tendon reflexes, increased muscle tone, tremors, exaggerated Moro reflex, generalized seizures
- **Gastrointestinal:** Poor feeding, uncoordinated and constant sucking, vomiting, diarrhea, dehydration
- **Autonomic signs:** Increased sweating, nasal congestion, fever, mottling
- **Other:** Poor weight gain, disorganized sleep states, skin excoriation

KEY POINTS: PAIN MANAGEMENT IN NEONATES

1. All neonates feel pain, and one must effectively deal with the potential for pain during any procedure performed during the neonatal period.

2. Premature infants have a greater sensitivity to pain than term infants.

3. Although children may not directly recall painful experiences from their NICU stay, they may demonstrate altered behavioral states from painful experiences that were not well managed.

4. Morphine and fentanyl appear to be equally effective for pain relief in neonates and appear to have similar outcomes in follow-up studies.

5. Methadone and some of the newer narcotic agonists (e.g., buprenorphine), as well as a number of other agents, appear to be optimal treatments for narcotic withdrawal in neonates. Paregoric and phenobarbital are no longer drugs of choice.

12. **Can we prevent opioid tolerance in neonates requiring prolonged opioid analgesia?**

    Preventing or delaying the onset of opioid tolerance may allow the rapid weaning of opioids, thus reducing the costs and complications of prolonged opioid weaning. *Although listed here, the safety and efficacy of these approaches have not been tested in neonates.*

    ■ Concomitant infusion of opioid agonists and *N-methyl-D-aspartate* (NMDA) antagonists such as low-dose ketamine (0.2–0.3 mg/kg/h) can delay the development of opioid tolerance. Opioid drugs such as ketobemidone and methadone also block NMDA receptors and produce less tolerance than morphine or fentanyl.

    ■ Continuous infusion of low-dose naloxone (0.1–0.5 µg/kg/h) selectively blocks the opioid receptors coupled with stimulatory G_s-proteins, thus blocking the mechanisms for superactivation of the cAMP pathway and inhibiting opioid tolerance.

    ■ Inhibition of inducible nitrous oxide (iNOS) induction decreases the neuroadaptive changes associated with opioid dependence, suggesting the use of an iNOS inhibitor, 7-nitroindazole, in clinical trials for opioid addiction.

    ■ Fluoxetine also suppresses tolerance to the analgesic effects of morphine, further accentuated by concomitant L-arginine and N- or G-nitro-L-arginine methyl ester (L-NAME) treatment.

    ■ Procedural changes in adult patients such as the daily interruption of sedatives, nurse-controlled sedation, sequential rotation of analgesics, or the use of neuraxial opioids may decrease the incidence of opioid tolerance and withdrawal.

13. **How can we treat opioid withdrawal syndrome in newborn infants?**

    In addition to supportive therapy and the slow weaning of opioids, some pharmacologic agents with a relatively long half-life can be used to manage opioid withdrawal. Drugs such as paregoric, camphorated tincture of opium, phenobarbital, and chlorpromazine are not used anymore because of significant side effects and lack of standardization. Therapeutic goals are to decrease the severity of symptoms to a tolerable degree, to enable regular cycles of sleeping and feeding, and to decrease the agitation caused by medical interventions or nursing care.

    ■ **Methadone:** This opioid agonist and NMDA antagonist has a long half-life (25–44 hours in neonates), can be given intravenously or enterally (bioavailability, 90%), and reverses the tolerance produced by morphine or other drugs. In one clinical study, a methadone dose equivalent to 2.5 times the total daily fentanyl dose was effective in minimizing symptoms of opioid withdrawal.

    ■ **Buprenorphine:** This is a partial µ-opioid agonist, a nociception/orphanin receptor agonist, and a κ-opioid antagonist with analgesic effects similar to morphine in preterm neonates. Buprenorphine was as potent as high-dose methadone for adult opioid addiction, and its clinical use in opioid-addicted mothers induced less opioid withdrawal in their infants.

    ■ **Clonidine:** This α_2-adrenergic receptor agonist has analgesic effects when administered intravenously, intramuscularly, intrathecally, orally, epidurally, or topically. Because α_2-adrenergic and opioid receptors activate the same K^+ channel via inhibitory G_i-proteins, clonidine has been used to treat opioid withdrawal in neonates.

    ■ **Gabapentin:** Gabapentin is an anticonvulsant but reduces neuropathic pain via effects on α_2-Δ calcium channels and reduces the severity of opioid withdrawal in adults.

    ■ **Benzodiazepines:** Benzodiazepines, such as diazepam or lorazepam, may be used for treating the seizures associated with opioid withdrawal, but they are not cross-tolerant with opioids and cannot be used as sole therapy.

14. **What are the methods for treating procedural pain in neonates?**

    A combination of topical anesthetics (e.g., EMLA, Ametop, LMX4, S-Caine), infiltration of local anesthetics (e.g., lidocaine, bupivacaine, ropivacaine), nonpharmacologic therapies (e.g., sucrose, dextrose, breast milk), and behavioral and environmental approaches (e.g., rocking, swaddling, skin-to-skin contact) can usually treat the acute pain associated with invasive procedures. The most effective approach is to limit the number of invasive procedures and the duration of acute pain only to instances when it is absolutely necessary. The use of systemic analgesia using opioids (e.g., morphine, fentanyl, alfentanil), non-opioids (e.g., acetaminophen, ibuprofen, ketorolac), or anesthetics (e.g., ketamine, propofol, thiopental) has been investigated but is rarely necessary for treating the pain associated with invasive procedures.

15. **Why should EMLA be used with caution in infants?**
EMLA is an acronym for *eutectic mixture of local anesthetics,* containing lidocaine (2.5%) and prilocaine (2.5%). Prilocaine is metabolized to orthotolidine, which can oxidize significant amounts of hemoglobin to methemoglobin in preterm neonates. This occurs because their stratum corneum is thinner, causing increased absorption and higher serum levels. Furthermore, the activity of the reduced nicotinamide adenine dinucleotide (NADH)-dependent methemoglobin reductase enzyme is 40% lower in neonates than in adults. Other factors that can contribute to systemic prilocaine toxicity include sepsis, metabolic acidosis, anemia, hypoxia, glucose-6-phosphate dehydrogenase deficiency, and co-treatment with other drugs leading to oxidative stress such as sulfonamides, phenobarbital, phenytoin, and acetaminophen. This appears to be a theoretical concern because the incidence of clinically significant methemoglobinemia is strikingly low, even among preterm neonates exposed to repeated daily doses of EMLA.

16. **What are the major goals for postoperative analgesia in neonates?**
The management of postoperative pain must ideally start before the operative procedure, considering the size and alignment of the surgical incision, the choice of anesthetic agents, infiltration of the surgical site with lidocaine or bupivacaine, and, if possible, the placement of an epidural catheter during surgery. The goals of perioperative analgesic approaches are the relief of pain, the maintenance of physiologic stability, and the prevention of adverse events including hypoventilation or shallow respiration due to diaphragmatic splinting, paralytic ileus, protein catabolism, and pulmonary hypertension. Use of analgesics may improve postoperative outcomes with fewer adverse events, shorter duration of mechanical ventilation, rapid return of gastrointestinal function, and reduced urinary retention or apnea.

17. **What are the options for safe and effective analgesia in neonates undergoing surgery?**
Postoperative analgesia is usually provided with opioids (e.g., morphine, fentanyl, methadone, alfentanil, remifentanil) or antipyretic analgesics, which include acetaminophen or its intravenous analog propacetamol, the nonspecific cyclooxygenase (COX) inhibitors (e.g., ibuprofen, ketorolac, diclofenac, and indomethacin), and the newer COX-2 inhibitors (e.g., parecoxib, valdecoxib, celecoxib, and meloxicam). Other options include epidural or caudal anesthesia with infusions continued into the postoperative period. The use of nurse-controlled analgesia with a patient-controlled analgesia pump is also under investigation.

18. **Are the doses of morphine and fentanyl for postoperative analgesia in neonates similar to the doses used for older children?**
Several studies suggest that neonates should receive lower morphine infusion rates than older children after surgery, starting as low as 0.005 mg/kg/h for preterm neonates and 0.01 mg/kg/h for term neonates. Neonates with cyanotic congenital heart defects require lower morphine infusion rates than neonates undergoing noncardiac surgery. Depending on the dose and other patient characteristics, fentanyl and sufentanil provide variable degrees of suppression of autonomic and hormonal/metabolic responses to major surgery in neonates, although fentanyl may promote postoperative hypothermia. Critically ill neonates, whose vascular tone depends on sympathetic outflow, may become hypotensive after bolus doses of fentanyl or morphine. Randomized controlled trials show no differences in the postoperative analgesia produced by bolus doses versus continuous infusions of fentanyl or morphine, although apnea and other complications were greater in the bolus-dosing groups. Intravenous boluses of opioids should be given slowly over 30–60 minutes in postoperative neonates.

BIBLIOGRAPHY

1. Anand KJS: Clinical importance of pain and stress in preterm neonates. Biol Neonate 73:1–9, 1998.

2. Anand KJS: International Evidence-Based Group for Neonatal Pain: Consensus statement for the prevention and management of pain in newborns. Arch Pediatr Adoles Med 155:173–180, 2001.

3. Anand KJS: Pain, plasticity, and premature birth: a prescription for permanent suffering? Nature Med 6:971–973, 2000.

4. Anand KJS: Relationships between stress responses and clinical outcome in newborns, infants, and children. Crit Care Med 21:S358–S359, 1993.

5. Anand KJS, Aranda JV, Berde CB, et al: Analgesia for neonates: Study design and ethical issues. Clin Therapeut 27:814–843, 2005.

6. Anand KJS, Arnold JH: Opioid tolerance and dependence in infants and children. Crit Care Med 22:334–342, 1994.

7. Anand KJS, Hall RW, Desai NS, et al: Effects of pre-emptive morphine analgesia in ventilated preterm neonates: Primary outcomes from the NEOPAIN trial. Lancet 363:1673–1682, 2004.

8. Anand KJS, Hickey PR: Halothane-morphine compared with high-dose sufentanil for anesthesia and postoperative analgesia in neonatal cardiac surgery. N Engl J Med 326:1–9, 1992.

9. Anand KJS, Hickey PR: Pain and its effects in the human neonate and fetus. N Engl J Med 317:1321–1329, 1987.

10. Anand KJS, Jacobson B, Hall RW: Gastric suction at birth: Not an innocent bystander. J Pediatr 145:714–715, 2004.

11. Anand KJS, Johnston CC, Oberlander T, et al: Analgesia and local anesthesia during invasive procedures in the neonate. Clinical Therapeut 27:844–876, 2005.

12. Anand KJS, McIntosh N, Lagercrantz H, et al: Analgesia and sedation in ventilated preterm neonates: Results from the pilot N.O.P.A.I.N. trial. Arch Pediatr Adolesc Med 153:331–333, 1999.

13. Anand KJS, Runeson B, Jacobson B: Gastric suction at birth associated with long-term risk for functional intestinal disorders in later life. J Pediatr 144:449–454, 2004.

14. Anand KJS, Scalzo FM: Can adverse neonatal experiences alter brain development and subsequent behavior? Biol Neonate 77:69–82, 2000.

15. Anand KJS, Sippell WG, Aynsley-Green A: Randomised trial of fentanyl anaesthesia in preterm babies undergoing surgery: Effects on the stress response. Lancet 1:243–248, 1987.

16. Anand KJS, Suresh S: Opioid tolerance in neonates: A state-of-the-art review. Paediatr Anaesth 11:511–521, 2001.

17. Andrews K, Fitzgerald M: Cutaneous flexion reflex in human neonates: A quantitative study of threshold and stimulus-response characteristics after single and repeated stimuli. Dev Med Child Neurol 41:696–703, 1999.

18. Andrews K, Fitzgerald M: The cutaneous withdrawal reflex in human neonates: Sensitisation, receptive fields and the effects of contralateral stimulation. Pain 56:95–101, 1994

19. Andrews K, Fitzgerald M: Wound sensitivity as a measure of analgesic effects following surgery in human neonates and infants. Pain 99:185–195, 2002.

20. Andrews KA, Desai D, Dhillon HK, et al: Abdominal sensitivity in the first year of life: Comparison of infants with and without prenatally diagnosed unilateral hydronephrosis. Pain 100:35–46, 2002.

21. Aretz S, Licht C, Roth B: Endogenous distress in ventilated full-term newborns with acute respiratory failure. Biol Neonate 85:243–248, 2004.

22. Backonja MM: Use of anticonvulsants for treatment of neuropathic pain. Neurology 59:S14–S17, 2002.

23. Barrett DA, Simpson J, Rutter N, et al: The pharmacokinetics and physiological effects of buprenorphine infusion in premature neonates. Br J Clin Pharmacol 36:215–219, 1993.

24. Bartocci M, Bergqvist LL, Lagercrantz H, Anand KJS: Pain activates cortical areas in the preterm newborn brain. Pain 2006 [in press].

25. Beacham PS: Behavioral and physiological indicators of procedural and postoperative pain in high-risk infants. J Obstet Gynecol Neonatal Nurs 33:246–255, 2004.

26. Berde CB, Sethna NF: Analgesics for the treatment of pain in children. N Engl J Med 347:1094–1103, 2002.

27. Bhutta AT, Anand KJS: Vulnerability of the developing brain: Neuronal mechanisms. Clin Perinatol 29:357–372, 2002.

28. Bouwmeester NJ, Anand KJS, van Dijk M, et al: Hormonal and metabolic stress responses after major surgery in children aged 0–3 years: A double-blind, randomized trial comparing the effects of continuous versus intermittent morphine. Br J Anaesth 87:390–339, 2001.

29. Bouwmeester NJ, Hop WC, Van Dijk M, et al: Postoperative pain in the neonate: Age-related differences in morphine requirements and metabolism. Intens Care Med 29:2009–2015, 2003.

30. Bouwmeester NJ, van den Anker JN, Hop WC, et al: Age- and therapy-related effects on morphine requirements and plasma concentrations of morphine and its metabolites in postoperative infants. Br J Anaesth 90:642–652, 2003.

31. Brook AD, Ahrens TS, Schaiff R, et al: Effect of a nursing-implemented sedation protocol on the duration of mechanical ventilation. Crit Care Med 27:2609–2615, 1999.

32. Chana SK, Anand KJS: Can we use methadone for analgesia in neonates? Arch Dis Child (Fetal Neonatal Edition) 85:F79–F81, 2001.

33. Craig AD: A new view of pain as a homeostatic emotion. Trends Neurosc 26:303–307, 2003.

34. Crain SM, Shen KF: Antagonists of excitatory opioid receptor functions enhance morphine's analgesic potency and attenuate opioid tolerance/dependence liability. Pain 84:121–131, 2000.

35. da Silva O, Alexandrou D, Knoppert D, Young GB: Seizure and electroencephalographic changes in the newborn period induced by opiates and corrected by naloxone infusion. J Perinatol 19:120–123, 1999.

36. Davis AM, Inturrisi CE: d-Methadone blocks morphine tolerance and N-methyl-D-aspartate–induced hyperalgesia. J Pharmacol Exp Therapeut 289:1048–1053, 1999.

37. Duhn LJ, Medves JM: A systematic integrative review of infant pain assessment tools. Adv Neonatal Care 4:126–140, 2004.

38. Fahnenstich H, Steffan J, Kau N, Bartmann P: Fentanyl-induced chest wall rigidity and laryngospasm in preterm and term infants. Crit Care Med 28:836–839, 2000.

39. Falcon M, Guendellman D, Stolberg A, et al: Development of thermal nociception in rats. Pain 67:203–208, 1996.

40. Fitzgerald M, Millard C, McIntosh N: Cutaneous hypersensitivity following peripheral tissue damage in newborn infants and its reversal with topical anaesthesia. Pain 39:31–36, 1989.

41. Fitzgerald M, Shaw A, MacIntosh N: The postnatal development of the cutaneous flexor reflex: A comparative study in premature infants and newborn rat pups. Dev Med Child Neurol 30:520–526, 1988.

42. Franck LS, Vilardi J, Durand D, Powers R: Opioid withdrawal in neonates after continuous infusions of morphine or fentanyl during extracorporeal membrane oxygenation. Am J Crit Care 7:364–369, 1998.

43. Frey B, Kehrer B: Toxic methemoglobin concentrations in premature infants after application of a prilocaine-containing cream and peridural prilocaine. Eur J Pediatr 158:785–788, 1999.

44. Furdon SA, Eastman M, Benjamin K, Horgan MJ: Outcome measures after standardized pain management strategies in postoperative patients in the neonatal intensive care unit. J Perinatal Neonatal Nurs 12:58–69, 1998.

45. Gale G, Franck LS, Kool S, Lynch M: Parents' perceptions of their infant's pain experience in the NICU. Int J Nurs Studies 41:51–58, 2004.

46. Gan TJ, Ginsberg B, Glass PS, et al: Opioid-sparing effects of a low-dose infusion of naloxone in patient-administered morphine sulfate. Anesthesiology 87:1075–1081, 1997.

47. Giannakoulopoulos X, Sepulveda W, Kourtis P, et al: Fetal plasma cortisol and beta-endorphin response to intrauterine needling. Lancet 344:77–78, 1994.

48. Gitau R, Fisk NM, Teixeira JM, et al: Fetal hypothalamic-pituitary-adrenal stress responses to invasive procedures are independent of maternal responses. J Clin Endocrinol Metab 86:104–109, 2001.

49. Grunau RE, Holsti L, Haley DW, et al: Neonatal procedural pain exposure predicts lower cortisol and behavioral reactivity in preterm infants in the NICU. Pain 113:293–300, 2005.

50. Grunau RE, Holsti L, Whitfield MF, Ling E: Are twitches, startles, and body movements pain indicators in extremely low birth weight infants? Clin J Pain 16:37–45, 2000.

51. Grunau RE, Oberlander TF, Whitfield MF, et al: Demographic and therapeutic determinants of pain reactivity in very low birth neonates at 32 weeks' postconceptional age. Pediatrics 107:105–112, 2001.

52. Grunau RE, Oberlander TF, Whitfield MF, et al: Pain reactivity in former extremely low birth weight infant at corrected age 8 months compared with term born controls. Infant Behav Dev 24:41–55, 2001.

53. Grunau RE, Whitfield MF, Petrie J: Children's judgments about pain at age 8–10 years: Do extremely low birth weight (< or = 1000 g) children differ from full birth weight peers? J Child Psychol Psychiatry Allied Disc 39:587–559, 1998.

54. Grunau RV, Whitfield MF, Petrie JH: Pain sensitivity and temperament in extremely low-birth-weight premature toddlers and preterm and full-term controls. Pain 58:341–346, 1994.

55. Grunau RV, Whitfield MF, Petrie JH, Fryer EL: Early pain experience, child and family factors, as precursors of somatization: a prospective study of extremely premature and full term children. Pain 56:353–359, 1994.

56. Guinsburg R, Kopelman BI, Anand KJS, et al: Physiological, hormonal, and behavioral responses to a single fentanyl dose in intubated and ventilated preterm neonates. J Pediatr 132:954–959, 1998.

57. Gustorff B, Kozek-Langenecker S, Kress HG: Gabapentin: The first preemptive anti-hyperalgesic for opioid withdrawal hyperalgesia? Anesthesiology 98:1520–1521, 2003.

58. Guy ER, Abbott FV: The behavioral response to formalin in preweanling rats. Pain 51:81–90, 1992.

59. Haberkern CM, Lynn AM, Geiduschek JM, et al: Epidural and intravenous bolus morphine for postoperative analgesia in infants. Can J Anaesth 43:1203–1210, 1996.

60. Hall RW, Kronsberg SS, Barton BA, et al: Morphine, hypotension and adverse outcomes in preterm neonates: Who's to blame? Pediatrics 115:1351–1359, 2005.

61. Harrison D, Evans C, Johnston L, Loughnan P: Bedside assessment of heel lance pain in the hospitalized infant. J Obstet Gynecol Neonatal Nurs 31:551–557, 2002.

62. Hoder EL, Leckman JF, Ehrenkranz R, et al: Clonidine in neonatal narcotic-abstinence syndrome. N Engl J Med 305:1284, 1981.

63. Hoder EL, Leckman JF, Poulsen J, et al: Clonidine treatment of neonatal narcotic abstinence syndrome. Psychiatry Res 13:243–251, 1984.

64. Hu D, Hu R, Berde CB: Neurologic evaluation of infant and adult rats before and after sciatic nerve blockade. Anesthesiology 86:957–965, 1997.

65. Hudson-Barr D, Capper-Michel B, et al: Validation of the Pain Assessment in Neonates (PAIN) scale with the Neonatal Infant Pain Scale (NIPS). J Neonatal Nurs 21:15–21, 2002.

66. Johnson RE, Chutuape MA, Strain EC, et al: A comparison of levomethadyl acetate, buprenorphine, and methadone for opioid dependence. N Engl J Med 343:1290–1297, 2000.

67. Johnston CC, Collinge JM, Henderson SJ, Anand KJS: A cross-sectional survey of pain and pharmacological analgesia in Canadian neonatal intensive care units. Clin J Pain 13:308–312, 1997.

68. Johnston CC, Stevens BJ: Experience in a neonatal intensive care unit affects pain response. Pediatrics 98:925–930, 1996.

69. Kostovic I, Judas M: Correlation between the sequential ingrowth of afferents and transient patterns of cortical lamination in preterm infants. Anat Rec 267:1–6, 2002.

70. Kostovic I, Judas M: Transient patterns of organization of the human fetal brain. Croatian Med J 39:107–114, 1998.

71. Kress JP, Pohlman AS, O'Connor MF, Hall JB: Daily interruption of sedative infusions in critically ill patients undergoing mechanical ventilation. N Engl J Med 342:1471–1477, 2000.

72. Kumar P, Jain MK: Gabapentin in the management of pentazocine dependence: A potent analgesic-anticraving agent. J Assoc Physicians India 51:673–676, 2003.

73. Lacroix I, Berrebi A, Chaumerliac C, et al: Buprenorphine in pregnant opioid-dependent women: First results of a prospective study. Addiction 99:209–214, 2004.

74. Lago P, Benini F, Agosto C, Zacchello F: Randomised controlled trial of low dose fentanyl infusion in preterm infants with hyaline membrane disease. Arch Dis Child (Fetal Neonatal Edition) 79:F194–F197, 1998.

75. Law RM, Halpern S, Martins RF, et al: Measurement of methemoglobin after EMLA analgesia for newborn circumcision. Biol Neonate 70:213–217, 1996.

76. Lehmann KA, Reichling U, Wirtz R: Influence of naloxone on the postoperative analgesic and respiratory effects of buprenorphine. Eur J Clin Pharmacol 34:343–352, 1988.

77. Levine JD, Gordon NC, Taiwo YO, Coderre TJ: Potentiation of pentazocine analgesia by low-dose naloxone. J Clin Invest 82:1574–1577, 1988.

78. Liu JG, Rovnaghi CR, Garg S, Anand KJS: Hyperalgesia in young rats associated with opioid receptor desensitization in the forebrain. Eur J Pharmacol 491:127–136, 2004.

79. Lynn A, Nespeca MK, Bratton SL, et al: Clearance of morphine in postoperative infants during intravenous infusion: the influence of age and surgery. Anesth Analg 86:958–963, 1998.

80. Lynn AM, Nespeca MK, Bratton SL, Shen DD: Intravenous morphine in postoperative infants: Intermittent bolus dosing versus targeted continuous infusions. Pain 88:89–95, 2000.

81. Lynn AM, Nespeca MK, Bratton SL, Shen DD: Ventilatory effects of morphine infusions in cyanotic versus acyanotic infants after thoracotomy. Paediatr Anaesth 13:12–17, 2003.

82. Lynn AM, Nespeca MK, Opheim KE, Slattery JT: Respiratory effects of intravenous morphine infusions in neonates, infants, and children after cardiac surgery. Anesth Analg 77:695–701, 1993.

83. MacGregor R, Evans D, Sugden D, et al: Outcome at 5-6 years of prematurely born children who received morphine as neonates. Arch Dis Child (Fetal Neonatal Edition) 79:F40–F43, 1998.

84. Mathew PJ, Mathew JL: Assessment and management of pain in infants. Postgrad Med J 79:438–443, 2003.

85. McClain BC, Probst LA, Pinter E, Hartmannsgruber M: Intravenous clonidine use in a neonate experiencing opioid-induced myoclonus. Anesthesiology 95:549–550, 2001.

86. McNair C, Ballantyne M, Dionne K, et al: Postoperative pain assessment in the neonatal intensive care unit. Arch Dis Child (Fetal Neonatal Edition) 89:F537–F541, 2004.

87. Menon G, Anand KJS, McIntosh N: Practical approach to analgesia and sedation in the neonatal intensive care unit. Semin Perinatol 22:417–424, 1998.

88. Mercadante S: Opioid rotation for cancer pain: Rationale and clinical aspects. Cancer 86:1856–1866, 1999.

89. Merkel SI, Voepel-Lewis T, Shayevitz JR, Malviya S: The FLACC: A behavioral scale for scoring postoperative pain in young children. Pediatr Nurs 23:293–297, 1997.

90. Moriarty A: In praise of the epidural space for analgesia in neonates. Paediatr Anaesth 12:836–883, 2002.

91. Oberlander TF, Grunau RE, Whitfield MF, et al: Biobehavioral pain responses in former extremely low birth weight infants at four months' corrected age. Pediatrics 105:e6, 2000.

92. Okada Y, Powis M, McEwan A, Pierro A: Fentanyl analgesia increases the incidence of postoperative hypothermia in neonates. Pediatr Surg Int 13:508–511, 1998.

93. Orsini AJ, Leef KH, Costarino A, et al: Routine use of fentanyl infusions for pain and stress reduction in infants with respiratory distress syndrome. J Pediatr 129:140–145, 1996.

94. Peters JW, Koot HM, Grunau RE, et al: Neonatal Facial Coding System for assessing postoperative pain in infants: Item reduction is valid and feasible. Clin J Pain 19:353–363, 2003.

95. Peters JW, Schouw R, Anand KJS, et al: Does neonatal surgery lead to increased pain sensitivity in later childhood? Pain 114:444–454, 2005.

96. Porter FL, Anand KJS: Epidemiology of pain in neonates. Res Clin For 20:9–16, 1998.

97. Porter FL, Wolf CM, Miller JP: The effect of handling and immobilization on the response to acute pain in newborn infants. Pediatrics 102:1383–1389, 1998.

98. Reynolds ML, Fitzgerald M: Long-term sensory hyperinnervation following neonatal skin wounds. J Compar Neurol 358:487–498, 1995.

99. Robinson S, Gregory GA: Fentanyl-air-oxygen anesthesia for ligation of patent ductus arteriosus in preterm infants. Anesth Analg 60:331–334, 1981.

100. Rossi AF, Seiden HS, Sadeghi AM, et al: The outcome of cardiac operations in infants weighing two kilograms or less. J Thorac Cardiovasc Sur 116:28–35, 1998.

101. Russell CT, Chaseling J: Topical anaesthesia in neonatal circumcision: A study of 208 consecutive cases. Austr Fam Physician Suppl 1:S30–S34, 1996.

102. Saarenmaa E, Huttunen P, Leppaluoto J, et al: Advantages of fentanyl over morphine in analgesia for ventilated newborn infants after birth: A randomized trial. J Pediatr 134:144–150, 1999.

103. Sharek PJ, Powers R, Koehn A, Anand KJS: Evaluation and development of potentially better practices to improve pain management of neonates. Pediatrics 2006 [in press].

104. Siddappa R, Fletcher JE, Heard AM, et al: Methadone dosage for prevention of opioid withdrawal in children. Paediatr Anaesth 13:805–810, 2003.

105. Simons SHP, van Dijk M, Anand KJS, et al: Do we still hurt newborn babies? A prospective study of procedural pain and analgesia in neonates. Arch Pediatr Adolesc Med 157:1058–1064, 2003.

106. Simons SHP, van Dijk M, van Lingen RA, et al: Routine morphine infusion in preterm newborns who received ventilatory support: A randomized controlled trial. JAMA 290:2419–2427, 2003.

107. Singh VP, Jain NK, Kulkarni SK: Fluoxetine suppresses morphine tolerance and dependence: modulation of NO-cGMP/DA/serotoninergic pathways. Meth Find Exp Clinical Pharmacol 25:273–280, 2003.

108. Stevens B, Johnston C, Taddio A, et al: Management of pain from heel lance with lidocaine-prilocaine (EMLA) cream: Is it safe and efficacious in preterm infants? J Dev Behav Pediatr 20:216–221, 1999.

109. Stevens B, McGrath P, Gibbins S, et al: Procedural pain in newborns at risk for neurologic impairment. Pain 105:27–35, 2003.

110. Stevenson J, Aynsley-Green A: The long term behavioural sequelae of surgery in infancy and early childhood studied in twins. Proc Br Psychol Soc 3:59, 1995.

111. Taddio A, Goldbach M, Ipp M, et al: Effect of neonatal circumcision on pain responses during vaccination in boys. Lancet 345:291–292, 1995.

112. Taddio A, Katz J, Ilersich AL, Koren G: Effect of neonatal circumcision on pain response during subsequent routine vaccination. Lancet 349:599–603, 1997.

113. Taddio A, Ohlsson A, Einarson TR, et al: A systematic review of lidocaine-prilocaine cream (EMLA) in the treatment of acute pain in neonates. Pediatrics 101:e1, 1998.

114. Taddio A, Shah V, Gilbert-MacLeod C, Katz J: Conditioning and hyperalgesia in newborns exposed to repeated heel lances. JAMA 288:857–861, 2002.

115. Teixeira J, Fogliani R, Giannakoulopoulos X, et al: Fetal hemodynamic stress response to invasive procedures. Lancet 347:624, 1996.

116. Teixeira JM, Glover V, Fisk NM: Acute cerebral redistribution in response to invasive procedures in the human fetus. Am J Obstet Gynecol 181:1018–1025, 1999.

117. Tobias JD, Schleien CL, Haun SE: Methadone as treatment for iatrogenic narcotic dependency in pediatric intensive care unit patients. Crit Care Med 18:1292–1293, 1990.

118. van Dijk M, Peters JW, Bouwmeester NJ, Tibboel D: Are postoperative pain instruments useful for specific groups of vulnerable infants? Clin Perinatol 29:469–491, 2002.

119. Vaughn PR, Townsend SF, Thilo EH, et al: Comparison of continuous infusion of fentanyl to bolus dosing in neonates after surgery. J Pediatr Surg 31:1616–1623, 1996.

120. Vaupel DB, Kimes AS, London ED: Nitric oxide synthase inhibitors. Preclinical studies of potential use for treatment of opioid withdrawal. Neuropsychopharmacology 13:315–322, 1995.

121. Wells S, Williamson M, Hooker D: Fentanyl-induced chest wall rigidity in a neonate: A case report. Heart Lung 23:196–198, 1994.

122. Whitfield MF, Grunau RE: Behavior, pain perception, and the extremely low-birth-weight survivor. Clin Perinatol 27:363–379, 2000.

CHAPTER 16

PULMONOLOGY

Reese H. Clark, MD

DIFFERENTIAL DIAGNOSIS OF NEONATAL PULMONARY DISORDERS

1. **Although apnea in premature infants is often due to the degree of immaturity (so-called *apnea of prematurity*), what are other causes of apnea in this population?**
   See Table 16-1.

TABLE 16-1.	CAUSES OF APNEA IN PREMATURE INFANTS
System	**Perturbation**
Central nervous	Intracranial hemorrhage, hypoxic-ischemic encephalopathy, seizures, congenital anomalies, maternal drugs, drugs used to treat the infant
Respiratory	Pneumonia, airway obstruction with lesions, anatomic obstruction (e.g., pharynx or tongue blocking airway), upper airway collapse (e.g., tracheal or laryngomalacia), severe respiratory distress syndrome, atelectasis
Infectious	Septicemia or meningitis due to bacterial, fungal, or viral agents
Gastrointestinal	Necrotizing enterocolitis, gastroesophageal reflux, positive result to Valsalva's test during bowel movements
Metabolic	Hypoglycemia, hypocalcemia, hyponatremia or hypernatremia, inborn errors of metabolism, increased or decreased ambient temperature, hypothermia
Cardiovascular	Hypotension, congestive heart failure, hypovolemia, patent ductus arteriosus
Hematologic	Anemia

2. **Is apnea of prematurity correlated with an increased incidence of sudden infant death syndrome (SIDS)?**
   No. Although apnea is often believed to be a provocative factor for SIDS, this relationship has never been causally established. It appears that premature infants with apnea of prematurity are no more likely to die from SIDS than those of comparable gestational age who do not have apnea of prematurity. Premature infants do, however, have a higher SIDS rate than do term infants, suggesting that immaturity of respiratory control may be a component of SIDS. Furthermore, several studies have indicated that unless one records respiratory patterns of premature infants, apnea will not be detected because the respiratory abnormalities in these babies are very difficult to see clinically.

3. **Of all newborn infants who die from culture-proven bacteremia, what proportion has pneumonia?**
   Ninety percent of infants dying from bacteremia have evidence of pneumonia on postmortem examination. Many of these infants, however, will not have positive blood cultures during life,

making the bacteriologic diagnosis of pneumonia a very difficult one in newborns. If pneumonia is suspected from clinical examination or chest x-ray, it should be treated aggressively until it has clinically resolved or until the child has been treated for a minimum of 10 days.

4. **What are the most common radiographic features of Group B streptococcal (GBS) pneumonia in premature infants? In term infants?**
   In premature infants, GBS often mimics respiratory distress syndrome (RDS) with a diffuse reticulogranular pattern and air bronchograms. It is unclear whether this is an indication of simultaneous disease processes (RDS and GBS) or whether the GBS disease causes a secondary surfactant deficiency that produces a radiographic appearance similar to RDS when a premature infant is infected.

   In term-gestation neonates, the most common GBS appearance mimics that of transient tachypnea of the newborn, with increased perihilar interstitial markings, hyperexpanded lung fields, and small pleural effusions.

5. **In a neonate who is breathing normally, is a low partial pressure of oxygen (PaO$_2$) and normal partial pressure of carbon dioxide (PaCO$_2$) most consistent with cyanotic heart disease or severe lung disease?**
   Neonates who have low oxygen saturations or arterial oxygen levels (PaO$_2$), normal carbon dioxide levels (PaCO$_2$), and no signs of respiratory distress most often have cyanotic congenital heart disease. Low PaO$_2$ and a rising PaCO$_2$ in a neonate with labored breathing (e.g., grunting, retractions, tachypnea) suggest intrinsic lung disease and its attendant intrapulmonary shunt. A high level of PaCO$_2$ in association with severe retractions, normal PaO$_2$ in minimal oxygen support, and signs of gas trapping on chest radiograph is most consistent with upper airway obstruction. Therefore, if an infant is easy to oxygenate and impossible to ventilate, think airway; if the infant is easy to ventilate and impossible to oxygenate, think heart; and if both oxygenation and ventilation are problems, think lung disease.

KEY POINTS: DIFFERENTIAL DIAGNOSIS OF NEONATAL PULMONARY DISORDERS

1. If a patient is easy to oxygenate but impossible to ventilate, airway disease should be considered the most likely pulmonary problem.

2. If a patient is easy to ventilate but impossible to oxygenate, cyanotic congenital heart disease is the most likely cause for the gas exchange problem.

3. If both oxygenation and ventilation are problems, intrinsic lung disease is the most likely problem.

NEONATAL RESUSCITATION

6. **What is the most important aspect of neonatal resuscitation?**
   Airway, airway, airway—managing the airway is always the most critical aspect of resuscitation! Most neonates who require support in the delivery room will respond to stimulation, opening of the airway, and gentle ventilation with a bag and mask.

7. **What is the maximum concentration of oxygen that a self-inflating anesthesia bag not connected to an oxygen reservoir can deliver?**
   Only about 40% oxygen can be delivered without a reservoir. Each time a self-inflating bag is squeezed, room air is drawn into the bag, diluting any oxygen that is connected. When a

reservoir is connected, concentrations up to 90% or more of oxygen may be delivered. One of the limitations of the self-inflating bag is that the desired concentration of oxygen cannot be altered easily.

8. **What are the approximate endotracheal (ET) tube sizes that would be appropriate for premature infants of varying birth weights?**
   - 2.5-mm internal diameter (ID) for infants weighing <1000 gm.
   - 3.0-mm ID for infants 1000–2000 gm.
   - 3.5-mm ID for infants 2000–3500 gm.
   - 4.0-mm ID for infants >3500 gm.

   These sizes are reasonable approximations for most infants, but attention should be paid to the ease of introduction of the ET tube into the airway. A 2.5-mm ET tube may be too small for some babies weighing <1000 gm, and it may be too large for a few infants with birth weights >1000 gm. The ET tube should slide easily into the airway, and a small leak should be audible around the ET tube when pressures of 25–30 cm H_2O are exceeded. An ET tube that is too snug may lead to tracheal inflammation and stenosis, whereas too small an ET tube simply may not allow adequate gas delivery to the lungs.

9. **Before radiographic verification, how far should an ET tube be inserted to be in the appropriate position for infants of varying birth weight?**
   The "tip-to-lip" rule for placement is the distance from the ET tube tip to the centimeter marking on the tube itself (Fig. 16-1). Good approximations are:
   - 7 cm for a child of 1000-gm birth weight
   - 8 cm for a child of 2000-gm birth weight
   - 9 cm for a child of 3000-gm birth weight
   - 10 cm for a child of 4000-gm birth weight

10. **Does the vigorous neonate born with thick meconium amniotic fluid need to have the trachea suctioned to remove meconium that may have been aspirated?**
    No. Compared with expectant management, intubation and suctioning of the apparently vigorous meconium-stained infant does not result in a decreased incidence of meconium aspiration

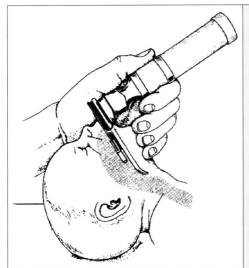

Figure 16-1. Appropriate position for ET tube insertion. (From Goldsmith JP, Karotkin EH [eds]: Assisted Ventilation of the Neonate, 3rd ed. Philadelphia, W.B. Saunders, 1996, p. 108.)

syndrome (MAS) or other respiratory disorders. In addition, it may provoke airway injury, especially if the child is active and moving after delivery.

Wiswell TE, Gannon CM, Jacob J, et al: Delivery room management of the apparently vigorous meconium-stained neonate: Results of the multicenter, international collaborative trial. Pediatrics 105(1 Pt 1):1–7, 2000.

11. **Which of the following is currently recommended by the neonatal resuscitation program: (A) calcium chloride for asystole, (B) atropine for bradycardia, (C) epinephrine for heart rate <60 beats/min, (D) 5% albumin for hypovolemia, or (E) room air ventilation instead of 100% oxygen ventilation?**
Only (C), epinephrine for heart rate <60 beats/min is currently recommended by the Neonatal Resuscitation Program. The other therapies have their advocates, but most studies have not shown them to be effective adjuncts for neonatal resuscitation. Room air resuscitation, in particular, has been suggested recently as an alternative to oxygen resuscitation to reduce free oxygen radical exposure, but no large-scale, prospective studies have demonstrated its safety and efficacy.

12. **Name some important historical figures who needed resuscitation after birth.**
Voltaire, Samuel Johnson, Johann Wolfgang von Goethe, Thomas Hardy, Pablo Picasso, and Franklin D. Roosevelt. The world would have been a very different place had these individuals not had the benefit of resuscitation, rudimentary as it was. Remember, there were no board-certified neonatologists until the mid 1970s!

KEY POINTS: NEONATAL RESUSCITATION

1. Airway, airway, airway—the most important aspect of neonatal resuscitation is managing the airway!

2. Most neonates who require support in the delivery room will respond to stimulation, opening of the airway, and gentle ventilation with a bag and mask.

13. **Who was the first to use a mechanical device for intubation and resuscitation of neonates?**
James Blundell (1790–1878), a Scottish obstetrician, used a "silver tracheal pipe" that had a blunt distal end with two side holes. He would slide his fingers over the tongue to feel the epiglottis and guide the tube into the trachea. Blundell would blow air into the tube approximately 30 times a minute to ventilate the baby.

14. **Name the three initial steps in neonatal resuscitation.**
    1. Thermal management—the infant should be dried and kept warm.
    2. The airway should be cleared of fluid and birth debris.
    3. The baby should receive tactile stimulation. One does not spank the baby's bottom. Gentle stroking and rubbing of the skin of the legs and buttocks should suffice. The thorax should not be rubbed because it may interrupt a respiratory effort.

15. **What is primary apnea? How is it distinguished from secondary apnea?**
A regular sequence of events occurs when an infant becomes hypoxemic and acidemic. Initially, gasping respiratory efforts increase in depth and frequency for up to 3 minutes, followed by approximately 1 minute of primary apnea (Fig. 16-2). If oxygen (along with stimulation) is provided during the apneic period, respiratory function spontaneously returns. If asphyxia continues, gasping then resumes for a variable period of time, terminating with the "last gasp" and

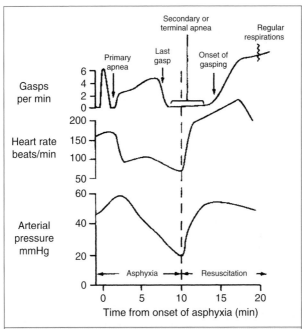

Figure 16-2. Asphyxial changes and the effects of resuscitation. (From Goldmsith JP, Karotkin EH [eds]: Assisted Ventilation of the Neonate, 4th ed. Philadelphia, W.B. Saunders, 2003, p. 62.)

followed by secondary apnea. During secondary apnea, the only way to restore respiratory function is with positive pressure ventilation and high concentrations of oxygen. Thus, a linear relationship exists between the duration of asphyxia and the recovery of respiratory function after resuscitation. The longer that artificial ventilation is delayed after the last gasp, the longer it will take to resuscitate the infant. Clinically, however, the two conditions are indistinguishable, although an infant's cyanosis will become progressively worse over time.

16. **How much pressure does it take to inflate the lungs of a healthy infant at the moment of birth?**
The first breath of an infant has been measured in the delivery room and is reported to be between −30 and −140 cm H_2O. These pressures are needed to overcome the substantial fluid and elastic forces present in the airway at the time of delivery. As surfactant is deposited, however, subsequent breaths rapidly decrease to −4 to −10 cm H_2O. If surfactant is decreased, as is the case in RDS, the baby must continue to exert the original very high effort to continue to inflate the lung. With limited energy reserves, this effort soon deteriorates, and respiratory failure ensues.

17. **Should infants be intubated nasally or orally?**
Studies support both routes of intubation for newborn infants. The oral intubation school argues that, because neonates are obligate nose breathers, they will demonstrate increased work of breathing and atelectasis after removal of nasotracheal tubes. On the other hand, nasal intubation proponents assert that orotracheal intubation results in grooving of the palate with subsequent orthodontic problems. Nasal tubes, however, have been associated with injury to the nasal cartilage. Therefore, operator skill and institutional tradition are primary considerations in this clinical decision. After extubation, however, there does appear to be a higher incidence of atelectasis with nasal ET tubes.

TRANSITIONAL PHYSIOLOGY AND THE ASPHYXIATED FETUS

18. **Asphyxia is a condition of impaired gas exchange characterized by what blood gas abnormalities: (A) hypoxemia, (B) hypercapnia, or (C) metabolic acidosis?**
C. Metabolic acidosis. Asphyxia has become a controversial subject because so much litigation has been initiated over difficult deliveries of babies. *Asphyxia* often is used inappropriately to describe infants who experience transient depression or delayed transition, much to the dismay of obstetricians, because of the medicolegal problems associated with birth asphyxia. In general, it is better not to label infants as "asphyxiated," but simply to describe numerically the metabolic derangements in the blood gases that are present after birth.

19. **A child is depressed and requires vigorous resuscitation in the delivery room. Subsequently, he demonstrates labile oxygenation and right-to-left shunting. A heart murmur is auscultated. What is the most likely anatomic or physiologic basis for the murmur?**
Tricuspid regurgitation is the most likely source of the murmur. Tricuspid regurgitation is due to increased pulmonary pressure and the backflow of blood into the right atrium. Although two fetal channels often remain open in this situation of transitional circulation (i.e., the foramen ovale and the ductus arteriosus), the source of heart murmurs is most likely from the associated tricuspid regurgitation.

20. **In the American Academy of Pediatrics–American College of Obstetricians and Gynecologists' guidelines regarding intrapartum asphyxia as a cause of brain injury, what criteria must be present?**
A neonate who has had severe enough hypoxia proximal to delivery to result in hypoxic-ischemic encephalopathy should show evidence of all of the following:
- Profound metabolic or mixed acidemia (pH < 7.00) on an umbilical cord arterial blood sample
- Early onset of neonatal encephalopathy
- Cerebral palsy (CP) of the spastic quadriplegic or dyskinetic type and no evidence of other potential causes for neonatal encephalopathy, such as trauma, coagulation or genetic disorders, or infectious conditions

American Academy of Pediatrics, American College of Obstetricians and Gynecologists: Neonatal Encephalopathy and Cerebral Palsy. Elk Grove Village, IL, AAP/ACOG, 2003.

KEY POINTS: TRANSITION AND ASPHYXIA

1. Most infants with CP do not have a history to suggest an intrapartum event as the cause for their CP.

2. The use of the term *asphyxia* should be avoided. Instead, it is much more useful and appropriate to describe the events and symptoms and assign more definitive diagnoses.

21. **What are the established relationships between Apgar scores and subsequently diagnosed CP?**
- Seventy-three percent of children who develop CP have 5-minute Apgar scores of 7–10.
- A child with a 1-minute Apgar Score of 0–3, but a 10-minute Apgar score of ≥4 has a 1% chance of subsequently developing CP.
- Of children with a 15-minute Apgar score of 0–3, 53% die, and 38% of survivors will subsequently develop CP.
- Of children with a 20-minute Apgar score of 0–3, 59% die, and 57% of survivors will subsequently develop CP.

22. **True or false? Mental retardation or seizures that are not associated with CP are not likely to be due to asphyxia or other intrapartum events.**
    True. The etiology of mental retardation and seizures is not known in most cases.

23. **In 1862, William John Little concluded that "spastic rigidity" (i.e., CP) was due exclusively to perinatal events. This led to the general belief for the next 100 years that CP was a preventable disorder due to obstetric events. What was Dr. Little's medical specialty?**
    Dr. Little was an orthopedic surgeon. He saw children with the spasticity and mobility problems associated with CP. Only in the past two decades has it been recognized that only 4–10% of CP can be attributed to intrapartum events. That understanding has not, however, prevented the initiation of litigation in many cases of CP, even when no obstetric or neonatal malpractice exists!

24. **What prominent neurologist in 1897 came to the conclusion that most CP was not due to intrapartum events?**
    Sigmund Freud. Although he is most well known for his work in psychiatry, Freud was a prominent neurologist who made many astute observations in the field.

25. **True or False? Electronic fetal monitoring of the fetal heart rate has resulted in decreased deaths and a decrease in the incidence of CP.**
    False. Electronic fetal monitoring has not been shown to be any better than intermittent auscultation of the fetal heart rate. There are no well-controlled trials that show any decline in deaths or CP rates that can be attributed to electronic fetal heart rate monitoring. Although the use of fetal heart rate monitoring has become a standard practice, its prognostic value remains unclear at the present time.

26. **What are the arterial PO_2 levels in a fetus?**
    If one were to obtain arterial blood gases in a fetus, the PaO_2 would be in the range of 25–35 mmHg. Although seemingly low, the high affinity of fetal hemoglobin for oxygen results in a highly saturated blood that is sufficient to meet the metabolic needs of the fetus. There is, however, little additional room for the PO_2 to decrease, and the fetus who begins to decrease his or her oxygen level even a small amount may develop problems quickly.

27. **Isn't fetal distress the same thing as "asphyxia" of the fetus?**
    No. Fetal distress will often manifest as nonreassuring fetal heart rate patterns, meconium staining of the amniotic fluid, or a low 1-minute Apgar score. None of these have any predictive value for long-term neurologic outcome. However, the presence of signs of fetal distress is a good predictor of the need for resuscitation after delivery.

28. **Is asphyxia reversible?**
    Shorter and less severe periods of asphyxia often reverse spontaneously and may not lead to any long-term damage unless they occur repeatedly. However, complete failure of gas exchange can cause death in as little as 10 minutes.
    The outcome of infants with asphyxia depends on several factors:
    - Speed of onset of asphyxia
    - Duration and extent of asphyxia
    - Presence of ischemia in addition to hypoxia
    - Resuscitative efforts
    The significance of ischemia, in particular, cannot be overstated. Unless circulation is restored, the administration of oxygen will not be effective, and acidemia will increase. The ABCs of resuscitation—airway, breathing, and circulation—remain the key to successful outcome in resuscitation.

29. **Who was Virginia Apgar?**

   Virginia Apgar, an anesthesiologist at Columbia Presbyterian Medical Center in New York City, introduced the Apgar scoring system in 1953 to assess newborn infants' responses to the stress of labor and delivery.

30. **If Apgar scores are not useful in predicting long-term outcome, why do we even bother recording them?**

   Apgar scores are useful for assessing and describing the condition of neonates after birth and their subsequent transition to an extrauterine state (Table 16-2). The Apgar scores are generally obtained and totaled at 1 minute and 5 minutes after birth; however, scores should be recorded for longer periods (at 10, 15, and even 20 minutes) if they are low (until the score is ≥7).

   Low Apgar scores are useful in identifying neonates who are depressed, and the change in score at 1 minute, 5 minutes, and subsequent time intervals is helpful in assessing the efficacy of resuscitation. Low Apgar scores (<3) that persist beyond 5 minutes have a better correlation with a poor long-term outcome than Apgar scores at 1 minute.

TABLE 16-2. APGAR SCORE			
Assessment	**0**	**1**	**2**
Breathing	No spontaneous respirations	Weak respiratory effort	Vigorous respiratory effort
Heart rate	No heart rate (HR)	HR < 100 beats/min	HR > 100 beats/min
Color	Generalized cyanosis	Acrocyanosis	Pink, including extremities
Reflex irritability	None	Weakly responsive	Vigorously responsive
Tone	Flaccid	Weak tone	Good tone

31. **What is the long-term outcome of infants who are severely asphyxiated?**

   The mortality among severely asphyxiated infants is high and can vary from 50% to 75%. Among survivors, long-term neurodevelopmental sequelae are common and occur in approximately one third of infants. Currently, there are no dependable predictors of long-term outcome. The presence and extent of neurologic abnormalities in the early postasphyxial phase and the persistence of abnormal neurologic findings at the time of discharge are the simplest and most effective predictors of long-term outcome. One measure of the severity of early neurologic dysfunction is the clinical staging system developed by Sarnat. Infants with Sarnat stage I encephalopathy are the ones who have mild asphyxia and recover without any significant neurologic sequelae. However, among infants with Sarnat stages II and III encephalopathy, the incidence of long-term neurodevelopmental handicaps can range anywhere from 50% to 100%. In one study of infants who had no detectable heart rate at birth and at 1 minute of age, two thirds died before discharge, and 33% of the survivors had severe neurologic handicaps (Table 16-3).

32. **Are newborn brains more resistant to perinatal hypoxic and ischemic injury?**

   Younger animals have been shown to have greater resistance to hypoxic-ischemic injury than older animals. However, certain areas of the brain appear to be more vulnerable to injury in neonates than in adults and in preterm compared with term infants. The neonatal brain is often described as having some degree of "plasticity," in which some areas may assume function of other areas of the brain after injury. To what degree this phenomenon actually takes place is not known, but it may explain why prediction of outcome after neurologic injury in neonates is so fraught with error.

TABLE 16-3.   SARNAT CLASSIFICATION OF POSTANOXIC ENCEPHALOPATHY

Sarnat Stage	Signs/Symptoms	EEG Results	Outcome
I	Lasts <24 hours; hyperalert; uninhibited Moro and stretch reflexes; sympathetic effects	Normal	Normal
II	Obtundation; hypotonia; strong distal flexion	Periodic EEG pattern, occasionally preceded by multifocal seizures	Normal if <5 days; abnormal if continuous delta activity >7 days
III	Stuporous; flaccid; suppressed autonomic and brainstem functions	Isopotential EEG or burst suppression	Probable neurologic impairment or death

EEG = Electroencephalography.
From Sarnat HB, Sarnat MS: Neonatal encephalopathy following fetal distress: A clinical and electroencephalographic study. Arch Neurol 33:696–705, 1976; and Jain L, Ferre C, Vidyasagar D, et al: Cardiopulmonary resuscitation of apparently stillborn infants. J Pediatr 118:778–782, 1991.

33. **What are the differences in the pattern of neurologic injury after hypoxic-ischemic insult in preterm and term infants?**
In preterm infants who survive with hypoxic-ischemic injury, periventricular leukomalacia is the most common (and most devastating) neuropathologic lesion. A large percentage of infants with periventricular leukomalacia develop spastic diplegia later in life. In term infants, patterns of neuropathologic injury commonly seen are "watershed infarcts" and diffuse cortical necrosis. These infants are at high risk for developing spastic monoplegia, hemiplegia, or quadriplegia.

34. **Asphyxiated infants who are successfully resuscitated often show signs of injury to multiple organ systems. What other organs are involved? Is the injury permanent?**
In asphyxiated infants who have been successfully resuscitated, the central nervous system (CNS) is the most frequently involved site (72%), followed by the kidneys (62%), heart (29%), intestines (29%), and lungs (26%). Multiple organ involvement occurs even as an asphyxiated fetus or neonate tries to redistribute blood to vital organs as a part of the "diving reflex." Fortunately, injury to these organs (except the CNS) is not permanent, and complete recovery of function can be expected in most infants who survive. However, the presence of multiorgan failure can seriously jeopardize chances of survival in the immediate postnatal period.

   Martin-Ancel A, Garcia-Mix A, Gaya F, et al: Multiple organ involvement in perinatal asphyxia. J Pediatr 127:786–793, 1995.

35. **What is the cause of oliguria in infants with hypoxic-ischemic perinatal injury?**
Oliguria is commonly seen in asphyxiated infants and can result from one or more of the following causes:
- Acute renal failure (either acute tubular necrosis or acute cortical necrosis)
- Asphyxiated bladder syndrome
- Syndrome of inappropriate antidiuretic hormone secretion (SIADH)

Although recovery from acute tubular necrosis is common, acute cortical necrosis is usually fatal. Infants with asphyxiated bladder syndrome, with marked distention, usually recover within a few days, as do most infants with SIADH, unless there has been a pituitary infarct.

36. **Prolonged resuscitation in the delivery room often makes resuscitated infants very cold. Is hypothermia harmful to these infants?**

Until recently, the presence of hypothermia in resuscitated infants was thought to correlate with poor survival and a higher occurrence of complications. However, recent studies have shown that selective cooling of the brain in infants suspected of having severe hypoxic-ischemic brain damage can improve long-term outcome. Initial studies from several nurseries around the world have been very promising in this regard. Randomized clinical trials evaluating the efficacy of hypothermia have been hampered by small sample sizes and an inability to predict who is most likely to benefit from this therapy. It appears, however, that the primary beneficiary is a child with mild to moderate perinatal asphyxia. Infants with more severe forms of injury do not appear to benefit as much.

37. **What is the outcome of infants receiving various forms of resuscitation?**

The outcome of depressed infants is usually determined by the degree of resuscitative efforts that are necessary. In one study, infants who required chest compressions and epinephrine had the worst outcome, with up to 56% dying in the neonatal period and 21% having an intracranial hemorrhage. Other complications noted in recipients of chest compressions included seizures (18%), respiratory distress (68%), and pneumothorax (24%).

Jain L, Vidyasagar D: Cardiopulmonary resuscitation of newborns: Its application to transport medicine. Pediatr Clin North Am 40:287–301, 1993.

38. **How is the outcome of resuscitation affected by prematurity and birth weight?**

Very-low-birth-weight (VLBW) infants have the greatest need for resuscitation at birth, with up to two thirds of infants weighing <1500 gm requiring some form of resuscitation. The morbidity and mortality in VLBW infants requiring cardiopulmonary resuscitation are inversely related to their birth weight. Recent data indicate that VLBW infants do better if they are delivered and cared for at tertiary care centers. The speed of an in-house response team to the delivery room for resuscitation unquestionably is a great advantage of the tertiary care center compared with a community hospital.

39. **What are the absolute indications for initiating positive pressure ventilation through a bag-and-mask apparatus in a newborn?**
   - Apnea
   - Bradycardia (heart rate < 100 beats/min)
   - Ineffective or gasping respirations
   - Intractable cyanosis

40. **What are two contraindications to immediate bag-mask ventilation?**

Immediate bag-and-mask ventilation is contraindicated when there is thick meconium in the hypopharynx and trachea or if a congenital diaphragmatic hernia is known or suspected. In all instances, however, the resuscitator must weigh the advantages of bag-and-mask therapy with the risks. At times, immediate intubation for suctioning or to avoid abdominal distention may be required.

41. **What are some indications for ET intubation during the resuscitation of a newborn?**
   - Need for prolonged bag-and-mask ventilation
   - Prolonged chest compressions (>1 minute)
   - Ineffective bag-mask ventilation
   - Delivery through thick or particulate meconium-stained amniotic fluid
   - Congenital diaphragmatic hernia (avoid insufflating the bowel with bag-mask ventilation, if possible)

42. **What causes persistent bradycardia or cyanosis in an infant who is receiving bag-mask ventilation?**
    - Improper mask size or fit (the mask should fit snugly from the bridge of the baby's nose to the base of the chin)
    - Poor seal of mask over the baby's face
    - Improper positioning of the infant (remember to place the baby in the "sniffing" position, with the neck slightly extended and the chin up)
    - Airway obstruction or need for suctioning
    - Ineffective manual ventilation (remember to watch for that chest rise and to use just enough positive pressure ventilation—about 15–20 cm H_2O pressure for an average term infant—to see good chest rise)
    - Make sure the oxygen source is turned on to the bag apparatus: "The heart and lungs can't run if there's no gas"

43. **What are the appropriate steps for the intubation of a neonate?**
    1. Always check the equipment to ensure proper functioning (e.g., laryngoscope blade bulb works, suction is on, 100% free-flow oxygen is turned on, tape for ET tube is available).
    2. Be sure that the warmer bed is flattened and not at an angle; the latter will distort landmarks.
    3. Choose the appropriately sized ET tube.
    4. Position the baby with the neck slightly extended and the chin up (use a roll under the shoulders to achieve proper extension if necessary). Do not hyperextend the neck! (*See* Fig. 16-3.)
    5. Make sure the hypopharynx has been suctioned to clear debris.
    6. Using the laryngoscope blade to visualize the vocal cords, insert the ET tube to the appropriate depth. (Limit intubation attempts to approximately 20 seconds to avoid reflex bradycardia.)
    7. Institute manual ventilation while holding the tube in a secure position.
    8. Listen for equal breath sounds on both sides of the chest.
    9. Auscultate over the stomach to make sure there is not an esophageal intubation.
    10. Watch for symmetric chest rise. Give just enough positive pressure to initiate chest rise.

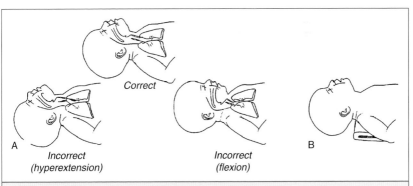

Correct

A   Incorrect
    (hyperextension)

Incorrect
(flexion)

B

Figure 16-3. *A,* Correct and incorrect head positions for resuscitation. *B,* Optimal shoulder roll use for maintaining correct head position. (From Goldmsith JP, Karotkin EH [eds]: Assisted Ventilation of the Neonate, 4th ed. Philadelphia, W.B. Saunders, 2003, p. 68.)

44. **When should epinephrine be given during a resuscitation in the delivery room?**
    In a depressed infant with gasping or absent respirations, 100% oxygen should be given via positive pressure ventilation. Depending on the extent of asphyxia (and depression of heart rate), cardiac compressions are usually initiated within 30 seconds. If there is no response (i.e., increased heart rate) after at least 30 seconds of positive pressure ventilation with 100%

oxygen and chest compressions, epinephrine is indicated. Epinephrine 1:10,000 can be given through an intravenous tube, umbilical vein, or into the ET tube at a dose of 0.1–0.3 mL/kg.

45. **When is sodium bicarbonate administered in a resuscitation?**
If there is no response to epinephrine in a severely asphyxiated infant (with continued apnea and a heart rate <100 beats/min), the administration of sodium bicarbonate (and/or a volume expander) should be considered. If an infant is being adequately ventilated, the partial correction of metabolic acidosis may improve pulmonary blood flow and improve oxygenation. Half-strength (4.2% solution or 0.5 mEq/mL) bicarbonate is preferable, given in a dose of 2 mEq/kg slowly over 2–5 minutes.

46. **Why is sodium bicarbonate not administered to treat respiratory acidosis?**
Unless ventilation is adequate, the carbon dioxide produced by the buffering reaction will not be eliminated and will act as a weak acid, further reducing the pH ("closed flask" phenomenon). It is therefore inappropriate and even dangerous to give bicarbonate until ventilation has been established and is found to be adequate.

47. **Are there complications of sodium bicarbonate therapy in infants?**
The relative risks of sodium bicarbonate therapy in infants are related to dosage (higher > lower), rapidity of administration (faster > slower), and osmolality (higher > lower). Physiologic complications include a transient increase in $PaCO_2$ and fall in PaO_2. The sudden expansion of blood volume and increase in cerebral blood flow may increase the risk of periventricular and intraventricular hemorrhage in preterm infants. Other potential complications include the development of hypernatremia and metabolic alkalosis.

48. **If a newborn is stabilized and the extent of acidosis is determined by an arterial blood gas, how is the therapeutic correction calculated?**

$$\text{dose of NaHCO}_3 \text{ (mEq)} = \text{base deficit (mEq/L)} \times \text{body weight (kg)} \times 0.3 \text{ (bicarbonate space)} \times 0.5 \text{ (half correction)}$$

Generally, it is safest to correct half the base deficit initially and then reassess acid-base status to determine whether further correction is necessary. Under optimal circumstances, sodium bicarbonate should be infused in small doses over 10–20 minutes as a dilute solution (0.5 mEq/mL). It is sometimes not possible to take that long to administer bicarbonate. The authors have not found that more rapid infusion (over 5 minutes) in a hypoxemic, acidemic baby is especially deleterious.

49. **What are the side effects of naloxone?**
Naloxone has a history of being remarkably free of adverse effects, except for the possible precipitation of sudden drug withdrawal in infants born to drug-addicted mothers. Other reported side effects relate to the sudden release of catecholamines, which can cause hypertension, sudden cardiac arrest, and cardiac dysrhythmias. It is important to remember that the half-life of naloxone is significantly shorter than that of opioids.

50. **Should umbilical arterial catheters be kept in a "low" or "high" position?**
Umbilical catheters kept in a low position (L3–L5) have a somewhat higher incidence of lower limb blanching and cyanosis compared with high lines (T6–T10). However, it may be preferable to see a lower limb blanch and be able to remove a catheter than to have a renal or mesenteric vessel blanch about which no one is aware! Also, high lines may be associated with a slightly increased risk of periventricular or intraventricular hemorrhage and embolization of clots to arterial vessels distal to the catheter site. No differences in the development of sepsis or necrotizing enterocolitis have been noted between infants with low or high umbilical catheters.

51. **What is the primary way by which an infant regulates cardiac output?**
Heart rate is the main variable through which an infant can increase cardiac output. A baby cannot significantly change stroke volume. Bradycardia will therefore significantly reduce a newborn's cardiac output.

52. **What are the indications for chest compressions in an infant, and how should they be done?**
If an infant's heart rate is <60, or 60–80 and not rising after 30 seconds of positive pressure ventilation, external cardiac massage should be initiated. Compressions are stopped when the heart rate rises above 80 beats/min. To do compressions on an infant correctly, place the hands around the chest, compress the mid to lower sternum with the thumbs, and press down firmly by one fourth to three fourths of an inch. Compression should continue at 1/4-second intervals with ventilation interposed after every third compression in a 3:1 ratio (i.e., 90 compressions and 30 ventilations per minute).

53. **What is a good source of emergent venous access in the newborn?**
An umbilical venous catheter (UVC). A UVC can be placed quickly by trimming the umbilicus to approximately 1 cm in length and inserting the catheter just far enough to obtain blood flow (usually about 4–5 cm in term infants). All medications (including vasopressor agents) and fluids can be given through this line. This source of access is often available for many days after birth with appropriate preparation of the cord.

54. **What are the common medications used for newborn resuscitation? How are they given, and in what doses?**
See Table 16-4.

TABLE 16-4.	NEONATAL RESUSCITATIVE DRUGS		
Drug	Concentration	Dose	Route(s)
Epinephrine	1:10,000	0.10–0.3 mL	Intratracheally Intravenously Intracardiac
Naloxone	0.4 mg/mL	0.25–0.5 mL/kg	Intravenously Intramuscularly Subcutaneously ET tube (dilute)

55. **What fluids are appropriate to use in newborn resuscitation?**
Crystalloids: normal saline and lactated Ringer's solution. Avoid the use of glucose solutions for acute volume expansion if possible. It is not necessary to use albumin or fresh frozen plasma in this situation.

56. **Why is it important to check blood glucose concentration during resuscitation?**
Hypoglycemia can be very damaging to the developing nervous system. It can result when hepatic glycogen stores are depleted from stress. A blood glucose level <45 mg/dL warrants immediate treatment. Ten percent dextrose in water should be infused at a dose of 2–4 mL/kg over 10–15 minutes in an attempt to correct hypoglycemia. It is not necessary to use higher concentrations of glucose in such circumstances, such as $D_{25}W$. After correction of

hypoglycemia has been achieved, normoglycemia can usually be maintained by an infusion rate of 4–8 mg/kg/min. In some circumstances, hypoglycemia may not be corrected until the infusion rate is 8–12 mg/kg/min.

57. **Why is measurement of hematocrit after acute blood loss not a good indicator of blood volume?**
The immediate response to acute blood loss is vasoconstriction to maintain blood pressure. The blood that has been lost contains the same percentage of red blood cells as the blood that is retained. The hematocrit will not drop until fluid repletion of the intravascular volume occurs.

58. **List the important clinical signs used to assess tissue perfusion.**
Pulse rate and quality, capillary refill time, and urine output.

KEY POINTS: RESPIRATORY DISTRESS SYNDROME

1. Prevention is better than rescue treatment in promoting a healthy outcome of a neonate with RDS.

2. The most studied and effective way to improve outcomes of neonates with RDS is instilling surfactant into the trachea.

59. **After a traumatic delivery, what are the most commonly injured systems?**
   - **Cranial injuries**: Caput succedaneum, subconjunctival hemorrhage, cephalohematoma, subgaleal hemorrhage, skull fractures, intracranial hemorrhage, cerebral edema
   - **Spinal injuries**: Spinal cord transection
   - **Peripheral nerve injuries**: Brachial palsy (Erb-Duchenne paralysis, Klumpke's paralysis), phrenic nerve, and facial nerve paralysis
   - **Visceral injuries**: Liver rupture or hematoma, splenic rupture, adrenal hemorrhage
   - **Skeletal injuries**: Fractures of the clavicle, femur, and humerus

60. **When should neonatal resuscitation be stopped?**
No precise answer is possible because clinical circumstances and responses are variable. However, in one study of 58 newborns with an Apgar score of 0 at 10 minutes despite appropriate resuscitative efforts, only 1 of 58 survived, and that infant had profound CP. Currently, a study is underway that is examining the effects of hypothermia and brain cooling on posthypoxic cerebral injury. It is hoped that this technique may alter outcome in such cases.
   Prolonged resuscitation has a very high risk of ischemic injury to the brain, resulting in cystic encephalomalacia, CP, severe microcephaly, and developmental delay. Failure of response after >10–15 minutes should prompt consideration of cessation.

   Jain L: Cardiopulmonary resuscitation of apparently stillborn infants: Survival and long-term outcome. J Pediatr 118:778–782, 1991.

61. **An infant who requires an extensive resuscitation should be observed closely for the development of hypoxic-ischemic encephalopathy. What are the acute neurologic components of this syndrome?**
   - Persistent and prolonged hypotonia
   - Depressed reflexes
   - Altered level of consciousness
   - Convulsions

RADIOLOGY OF PULMONARY DISORDERS OF THE NEONATE

62. **Where should the tip of an umbilical arterial catheter in satisfactory position project on an anteroposterior (AP) radiograph of the chest and abdomen?**

    There are two major schools of thought on this subject. For many years, the preferred position was between the third and fourth lumbar vertebrae, as projected on an AP radiograph. The tip lies below the take-off points for the renal and mesenteric arteries, theoretically reducing the risk of injecting fluids or drugs directly into those vessels. With this catheter placement, however, it has been shown that, even with relatively low pressure, injectable material can ascend retrograde into the aorta for quite some distance. Other neonatologists prefer a higher placement, in the thoracic aorta at approximately T10–T12, again avoiding placement of the catheter near the major tributaries off of the descending aorta. Positioning the tip there, however, means that anything injected will flow past major vessels. Several papers have argued for one placement versus the other, but both are probably safe as long as one takes the following precautions:

    - Careful placement under sterile conditions
    - Daily evaluation of ease of injection and withdrawal of blood
    - Assessment of the pressure waveform on the monitor screen
    - Inspection of the site for erythema and induration
    - Daily evaluation of urine output and blood pressure
    - Prompt removal of the line as soon as it is no longer needed

    Umbilical catheters may be left in place for many days as long as the above conditions are satisfactorily met. In extremes, a catheter can be kept in place for 3 weeks without complication.

63. **Where should the tip of an umbilical venous catheter (UVC) be placed for satisfactory projection on an AP radiograph of the chest and abdomen?**

    The UVC should be kept at the lower margin of the cardiac silhouette, approximately at the level of the right diaphragm, which would correspond to the junction of the inferior vena cava and right atrium of the heart. UVCs should not be allowed to remain below this level or within any of the branches of the portal system of the liver. Infusion of calcium or hyperalimentation into catheters in these incorrect positions may lead to liver toxicity, portal necrosis, cirrhosis, and cavernous transformation of the portal vein. Umbilical venous lines may also inadvertently cross the foramen ovale and enter the left heart. Catheters in this location occasionally will cause rhythm disturbances of the heart. This incorrect placement can be detected by the high levels of PO_2 obtained on a venous sample of blood.

64. **What is the best position, as seen on an AP radiograph of the chest, for the tip of an ET tube in an intubated neonate?**

    The optimal position for an ET tube is approximately halfway between the thoracic inlet (look for the medial ends of the baby's clavicles to get a good approximation) and the carina or level of tracheal bifurcation. In small neonates, ET tubes often enter the right mainstem bronchus and produce left-sided atelectasis. They may also exert vagal effects and cause bradycardia or irritation if they strike the carina. Tubes that are excessively high also may produce vagal effects and loss of effective ventilation.

65. **What is the most common radiographic appearance of the lungs in a premature neonate with RDS?**

    The classic RDS picture in a premature neonate has a diffuse increase in lung density (opacity) with a fine, reticulogranular (grainy) or ground-glass appearance, air bronchograms (a darker appearance to the branching central airway as contrasted with the opacity of the lungs), and low lung volumes (Fig. 16-4).

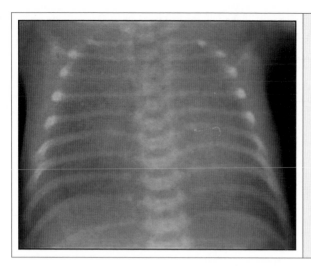

Figure 16-4. Radiograph of a baby with severe RDS. Note the generalized haziness from atelectasis and the air bronchograms throughout the lung.

66. **What disease process can produce a radiographic appearance to the lungs that is identical to RDS?**

GBS pneumonia in a premature infant is reported to have an appearance similar to RDS. It may be, however, that premature babies with GBS disease can also have surfactant inactivation or deficiency with true RDS as well as GBS septicemia. Although Sir William Osler might not like the concept of two diagnoses in one little patient, it probably happens more often than not!

KEY POINTS: MECONIUM-STAINED AMNIOTIC FLUID AND MECONIUM ASPIRATION SYNDROME

1. Vigorous meconium-stained infants do not need to be intubated and suctioned in the delivery room.

2. Those who have an initial heart rate >100 beats/min, good respiratory effort, and reasonable tone will not benefit from intubation and suctioning.

3. In fact, some vigorous infants may be injured in the process of suctioning because they are so difficult to restrain.

67. **What would be a typical appearance of the lungs in a newborn with significant meconium aspiration?**

These babies often have a coarse, irregular increase in lung markings accompanied by hyperinflation of the lungs. The pneumonic process here is one of patchy atelectasis and overdistention (Fig. 16-5). Pneumomediastinum and pneumothorax are frequent accompanying abnormalities as well.

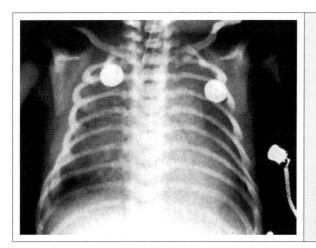

Figure 16-5. Radiograph of an infant with severe MAS, marked by hazy densities throughout the lung.

68. **In a newborn with suspected transient tachypnea of the newborn (e.g., wet lung syndrome, transient respiratory distress of the newborn, delayed reabsorption of fetal lung fluid), about how long should it take for the chest radiograph to return to a normal appearance in order to be consistent with this diagnosis?**
The textbook description of this clinical condition is a hazy-appearing lung, often with fluid in the right horizontal fissure and increased perihilar markings. The babies have rapid, shallow breathing, in contrast to the retractions of RDS or MAS. It usually is reported to last approximately 24 hours, with 48–72 hours considered the maximum. Some infants, however, seem to have this clinical problem for many more days, with subsequent uneventful recovery. What turns off fetal lung fluid production at birth has not been established. One theory is that some babies may continue to produce a low level of lung fluid for a period of time after they are born.

69. **What should one look for on the chest radiograph of a newborn in whom congenital diaphragmatic hernia is suspected (usually by antenatal sonography of the fetus)?**
A patient with congenital diaphragmatic hernia rarely presents at birth as the diagnostic dilemma in the delivery room that it once was. With fetal ultrasound, most of these infants are diagnosed before birth. Radiographically, they have a complex pattern of lucency in one hemithorax (usually the left side, and reflecting air-containing loops of intestine), contralateral shift of the heart and other mediastinal structures, and a lack of expected air-containing intestine in the abdomen.

70. **If a unilateral pneumothorax is suspected in a newborn, what is the best projection of the chest to confirm or exclude this diagnosis?**
Early air leaks are often difficult to diagnose. The most obvious finding, however, is a separation of the edge or margin of the lung from the inner margin of the chest wall, with no lung markings definable in that space. An AP decubitus view of the chest with the side of suspected pneumothorax to the top (nondependent) is also helpful. For example, if you suspect a left-sided pneumothorax, you should order a "right decubitus AP chest radiograph," which means the right side of the patient will be dependent and the left side nondependent. If a pneumothorax is present, look for a zone of lucency representing pleural air collecting between the lateral chest margin and the adjacent lung (Fig. 16-6).

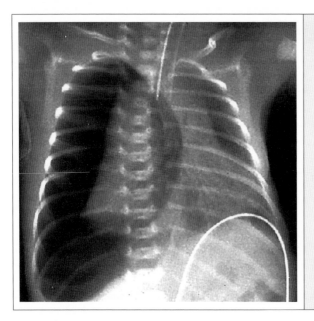

Figure 16-6. Radiograph of a child with a tension pneumothorax on the right.

RESPIRATORY DISTRESS SYNDROME

71. **Which collapses faster—a small bubble or a larger one?**
    The small one, because of surface tension. The LaPlace relationship states P =2T/R, where P is the pressure across the wall of the sphere, T is surface tension of the substance forming the bubble (i.e., its tendency to collapse), and R is the radius of the sphere. The smaller the radius, the greater the collapsing pressure (Fig. 16-7).

    When the bubbles are alveoli without surfactant, pressure on the alveolar surface is quite high because the surface tension is high. As the alveolus collapses without surfactant during exhalation, pressure increases as the radius of the alveolus decreases.

    Avery and Mead described the absence of a surface tension-reducing substance in the alveolar fluid of infants who died of hyaline membrane disease. The substance turned out to be surfactant, which greatly lowers the alveolar surface tension and, therefore, the alveolus's tendency to collapse. Surfactant also lowers surface tension as the diameter of the alveolus decreases, allowing for stable alveoli at end expiratory volumes.

72. **What are the physiologic, physical, and biochemical factors that result in pulmonary vasodilatation at the time of birth?**
    Within minutes after delivery, pulmonary artery pressure falls, and blood flow increases in response to birth-related stimuli, such as ventilation, increased PO_2, and shear stress. Physical stimuli, including increased shear stress, lung inflation, ventilation, and increased oxygen, cause pulmonary vasodilation in part by increasing production of vasodilators, nitric oxide, and prostacyclin. Pretreatment with the nitric oxide synthase inhibitor, nitro-L-arginine, attenuates pulmonary vasodilation after delivery by 50% in near-term fetal lambs. These findings suggest that a significant part of the rise in pulmonary blood flow at birth may be related directly to the acute release of nitric oxide. Each of the birth-related stimuli can stimulate nitric oxide release independently, followed by vasodilation through cyclic guanosine monophosphate kinase-mediated stimulation of K+ channels. Although the endothelial isoform of nitric oxide synthase

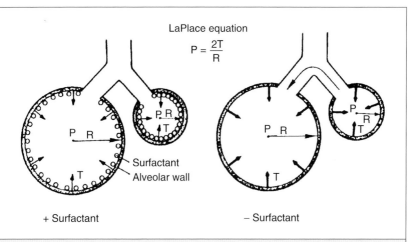

Figure 16-7. The LaPlace relationship. In the absence of surfactant, the smaller alveolus has a greater surface tension and tends to empty into the larger alveolus. In the presence of surfactant, the compacting of surface-tension reducing surfactant acts to "splint" the lung against further collapse. (Courtesy of F. Netter, CIBA-Geigy Corp., Ardsley, NY.)

III has been presumed to be the major contributor of nitric oxide at birth, recent studies suggest that other isoforms (neuronal type I and inducible type II) may be important sources of nitric oxide release in utero and at birth. Other vasodilators, especially prostacyclin, also modulate changes in pulmonary vascular tone. Rhythmic lung distention and shear stress stimulate both prostacyclin and nitric oxide production in late gestation. Increasing oxygen tension also triggers nitric oxide activity and overcomes the effects of prostacyclin inhibition at birth. Thus, although nitric oxide does not account for the entire fall in pulmonary vascular resistance at birth, nitric oxide synthase activity appears important in achieving postnatal adaptation of lung circulation.

Abman SH, Stevens T: Perinatal pulmonary vasoregulation: Implications for the pathophysiology and treatment of neonatal pulmonary hypertension. In Haddad G, Lister G (eds): Tissue Oxygen Deprivation: Developmental, Molecular, and Integrative Functions. New York, Marcel Dekker, 1996, pp 367–432.

73. **What is the composition of surfactant?**
Surfactant, from "surface active material," is 80% phospholipids and 8% neutral lipids. The phospholipid most responsible for surface tension reduction is dipalmitoyl phosphatidylcholine. Twelve percent of surfactant is protein, half of which most likely comprises serum contaminants. Surfactant proteins A, B, C, and D (SP-A, SP-B, SP-C, SP-D) are active in surfactant's surface tension reduction, secretion, absorption, and immune function. SP-A works with other proteins and lipids to improve surface actions and regulate secretion and reuptake. It also works with host defense in the alveolus. Lipophilic SP-B and SP-C facilitate adsorption and spread of lipid across the alveolar surface. SP-D is known to be a ligand for pathogens.

74. **Where is surfactant manufactured in the lung?**
Surfactant is made in alveolar type II cells. The endoplasmic reticulum and Golgi apparatus package the lipid and protein precursors. Lamellar bodies are formed, including more protein with increasing gestational age. Catecholamines, corticosteroids, and other hormones stimulate the type II cell's secretion of lamellar bodies. These unravel to form tubular myelin. Tubular

myelin then adsorbs as a lipid-protein monolayer on the alveolar surface, giving maximum surface support to the alveolus. The interaction between intact protein and phospholipid allows optimal surfactant functioning.

Surfactant is inactivated in the alveolar space without large changes in amounts of its components. The monolayer does break down as protein and lipid dissociate. Surfactant changes to a small aggregate form that minimally reduces surface tension. These aggregates are then absorbed by macrophages and type II cells, which recycle lipid and protein components.

75. **When should surfactant be given?**
Most agree that earlier is better. Prophylactic surfactant (versus treatment) results in lower mortality, fewer pneumothoraces, less pulmonary interstitial emphysema, and perhaps less bronchopulmonary dysplasia, especially for infants of <29 weeks' gestation. By prophylaxis, most agree that for babies of <27–29 weeks' gestation, treatment should be given soon after birth (within 20 minutes), after initial stabilization. It is better not to wait for radiographs to show the ground-glass appearance or other markers for definite RDS.

76. **What are the advantages of prophylactic surfactant?**
Four major randomized trials have addressed the issue of preventive versus rescue treatment strategies for exogenous surfactant administration in VLBW infants. In studies using synthetic surfactant, there were significant reductions in pneumothorax and pulmonary interstitial emphysema when surfactant was administered at or soon after birth compared with selective administration in infants with established RDS. Infants randomly selected to receive early selective surfactant administration demonstrated a decreased risk of neonatal mortality, chronic lung disease, and death at 36 weeks. No differences in other complications of RDS or prematurity were noted. In the meta-analysis of Soll, prophylactic rather than delayed administration of surfactant to all infants deemed at high risk for RDS reduced the risk of pneumothorax, pulmonary interstitial emphysema, bronchopulmonary dysplasia, and death. Similar benefits are associated with early selective rather than delayed surfactant administration in premature infants intubated for respiratory distress within the first 2 hours of life. Although no randomized trials compare prophylactic surfactant treatment with early selective surfactant treatment, studies suggest that the greatest benefit may come from the earliest care. Kendig and colleagues demonstrated that the benefits of prophylactic treatment remain even if initial surfactant therapy is delayed until 10–15 minutes after birth. This distinction is important in that attention to neonatal resuscitation, ET tube positioning, and adequate oxygen saturation can be assessed before intratracheal bolus surfactant administration.

OSIRIS Collaborative Group: Early versus delayed neonatal administration of a synthetic surfactant: The judgment of OSIRIS. Lancet 340:1363–1369, 1992.

Soll RF, Morley CJ: Prophylactic versus selective use of surfactant in preventing morbidity and mortality in preterm infants. Cochrane Database Syst Rev 2:CD000510, 2001.

77. **What other therapies are effective in infants with RDS?**
The goal of therapy is to maintain minute volume by maintaining functional, open alveoli for gas exchange. When atelectasis occurs in infants with RDS, CO_2 cannot get out, and O_2 cannot get in. To maintain alveolar volume and, therefore, gas exchange, positive end-expiratory pressure (PEEP) is essential. Continuous positive airway pressure (CPAP) can be used to maintain alveolar volume during exhalation despite inadequate surfactant. It works if the pressure delivered to the alveoli prevents closing pressure (remember $P = 2T/R$) from completely collapsing alveoli, but it should not be so great that it hinders adequate exhalation. Early institution of CPAP appears to avoid the need for intubation in a percentage of VLBW infants.

When alveolar collapse is too rapid or widespread, positive pressure ventilation is the best tool. Positive pressure opens the alveoli for inhalation. End-expiratory pressure maintains alveolar volume during exhalation. Positive pressure ventilation will be necessary until adequate surfactant reduces surface tension and enough alveoli are inflated for adequate minute ventilation.

Should infants with RDS receive high-frequency ventilation? The primary pathology of RDS comes from an inability to maintain lung inflation and fluid leak into the alveolar space. Secondary pathology originates from positive pressure reexpansion of collapsed alveoli. A ventilation strategy that maintains lung volume and avoids large distending pressure seems ideal. That is the idea behind high-frequency ventilation for RDS. The lung is inflated, and lung volumes are maintained while gas exchange occurs, using tidal volumes less than dead space. High-frequency ventilator technology is improving, and its applicability as the first-line treatment for RDS continues to be evaluated. The jury is still out, however.

Courtney SE, Durand DJ, Asselin JM, et al: High-frequency oscillatory ventilation versus conventional mechanical ventilation for very-low-birth-weight infants. N Engl J Med 347:643–652, 2002.

Henderson-Smart DJ, Bhuta T, Cools F, Offringa M. Elective high frequency oscillatory ventilation versus conventional ventilation for acute pulmonary dysfunction in preterm infants (Cochrane Review). Cochrane Database Syst Rev 1:CD000104, 2003.

Johnson AH, Peacock JL, Greenough A, et al: High-frequency oscillatory ventilation for the prevention of chronic lung disease of prematurity. N Engl J Med 347:633–642, 2002.

78. **Are there complications and problems with surfactant therapy?**
U.S. mortality from RDS and prematurity declined significantly with the introduction of exogenous surfactant. By 1994, the combination of congenital and chromosomal defects had become the leading cause of infant mortality, and RDS with prematurity fell, for the first time, to number two on the list. Although bronchopulmonary dysplasia (BPD) has not significantly decreased in numbers, the severity of chronic lung disease has declined for most surviving premature infants with RDS.

The only pulmonary complication that has increased with therapy is a small but noticeable increase in pulmonary hemorrhage. Other nonpulmonary complications have not been significantly affected.

79. **What is CPAP?**
CPAP can be applied to an infant's airway using a variety of devices to maintain positive pressure in the airway during spontaneous breathing. These devices include a head hood, face chamber, face mask, several types of nasal cannulae, nasopharyngeal tube, and ET tube. Nasal cannulae inserted into the nares are used most often. Not all CPAP devices are equal, and they have varying degrees of success. They have been associated with a number of problems such as difficulty with access to the baby, maintaining connection to the airway, increase in dead space, and increase in airway resistance.

80. **What is the effect of CPAP?**
Like many things in life, the right amount is beneficial, and too much is detrimental. When the proper amount of positive pressure is used, CPAP will:
- Increase transpulmonary pressure and functional residual capacity
- Prevent alveolar collapse and decrease intrapulmonary shunting
- Increase compliance
- Conserve surfactant
- Increase airway diameter and splint the airway
- Splint the diaphragm

However, if too much CPAP is applied, it can cause overdistention of the alveoli, worsen ventilation-perfusion match, increase pulmonary vascular resistance, decrease compliance, and impede venous return to the right side of the heart, thereby decreasing cardiac output.

81. **What are the indications for using CPAP in neonates?**
These include but are not limited to the following:
- Diseases with a low functional residual capacity (e.g., RDS)
- Apnea and bradycardia of prematurity

- MAS
- Airway closure disease (e.g., bronchiolitis, BPD)
- Tracheomalacia
- Partial paralysis of the diaphragm
- Respiratory support after extubation

82. **What are the complications of nasal CPAP?**
    - **Pneumothorax** (<2%): Usually occurs in the acute phase and is usually more benign than when it occurs during mechanical ventilation. Pneumothorax is *not* a contraindication for CPAP therapy.
    - **Nasal obstruction:** Obstruction from secretions or improper positioning of CPAP prongs. Secretions in nasal cavities should be suctioned every 4 hours or as needed.
    - **Abdominal distention from swallowed air:** This is usually benign and occurs more commonly in the chronic than acute phase, especially in infants treated with aminophylline. Abdominal distention can be treated by intermittent aspiration of the stomach. For severe distention, an indwelling orogastric tube may be required.
    - **Nasal or septal erosion or necrosis:** This is a concern in a VLBW premature infant with sensitive skin, who may need CPAP therapy for weeks. However, this can be prevented by choosing a properly sized CPAP cannula and avoiding compression of the septum. A snug cap is used to hold the tubings securely in place, and self-adhesive Velcro is used to keep the cannulae away from the septum.

83. **What is the OI?**
    The OI is not the name of a television show about teenagers in Orange County, California. The OI stands for the *oxygen index*. It is used to express the severity of the respiratory disease.

    $$OI = MAP \times FiO_2 / PaO_2 \text{ and } MAP = (PIP - PEEP) \times T_I / (T_I + T_E) + PEEP,$$

    where MAP = mean arterial pressure, FiO_2 = fractional concentration of oxygen in inspired gas, PaO_2 = partial pressure of oxygen in arterial blood, PIP = peak inspiratory pressure, PEEP = positive end-expiratory pressure, T_I = inspiration time, and T_E = expiration time.

    Note that the MAP is influenced by all respirator controls except the FiO_2. However, without a uniform ventilation strategy, the OI cannot be universally applied as an expression of severity of respiratory disease. This is especially true in the neonatal intensive care unit, where patients may be hyperventilated; in these patients, the MAP, and thus the OI, is elevated regardless of the severity of disease.

MECONIUM-STAINED AMNIOTIC FLUID AND MECONIUM ASPIRATION SYNDROME

84. **Do vigorous meconium-stained infants need to be intubated and suctioned in the delivery room?**
    No. Those who have an initial heart rate >100 beats/min, good respiratory effort, and reasonable tone will not benefit from intubation and suctioning. In fact, some vigorous infants may be injured in the process of suctioning because they are so difficult to restrain.

85. **How long has meconium been present in the amniotic fluid if an infant has evidence of meconium staining?**
    Gross staining of the infant is a surface phenomenon proportional to the length of exposure and meconium concentration. With heavy meconium, staining of the umbilical cord begins in as little as 15 minutes, and with light meconium, after 1 hour. Yellow staining of the newborn's nails requires 4–6 hours. Yellow staining of the vernix caseosa takes about 12–14 hours.

86. **Is meconium staining a good marker for neonatal asphyxia?**
Because 10–20% of all deliveries have in utero passage of meconium, meconium staining alone is not a good marker for neonatal asphyxia. For an infant to pass meconium, however, there does need to be a period of hypoxemia that initiates increased bowel contractility before birth. Simply having hypoxemia, however, is not the same thing as having perinatal asphyxia.

87. **What pulmonary disorder is most frequently associated with persistent pulmonary hypertension of the newborn (PPHN)?**
MAS is associated with the majority of cases of PPHN. Other associated disorders include RDS, sepsis or pneumonia, idiopathic PPHN, and lung hypoplasia (including congenital diaphragmatic hernia). In all instances, the pulmonary artery pressure remains near systemic levels and results in right-to-left shunting of blood.

88. **What factors are involved in the pathophysiology of MAS?**
Aspirated meconium causes:
- Airway obstruction
- Alveolar and parenchymal inflammation
- Alveolar and parenchymal edema
- Altered pulmonary vasoreactivity leading to pulmonary vasoconstriction, increased pulmonary resistance, and right-to-left shunting
- Direct toxicity of meconium constituents on pulmonary parenchyma leading to ischemia and necrosis
- Surfactant dysfunction (inactivation and decreased production of SP-A and SP-B)
- Pulmonary vascular remodeling
- Altered lung elastic forces (increased resistance, decreased compliance) (Fig. 16-8)

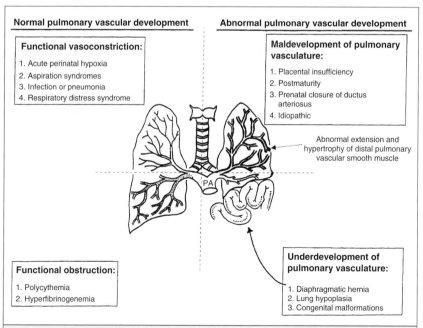

Figure 16-8. Classification of persistent pulmonary hypertension of the newborn (PPHN) based on the primary abnormality involved. PA = pulmonary artery.

KEY POINTS: PPHN AND CONGENITAL DIAPHRAGMATIC HERNIA

1. The most studied and effective therapy for neonates with pulmonary hypertension is inhaled nitric oxide.

2. Ventilator-induced alkalosis, bicarbonate infusions, and prostaglandin products have not been adequately studied and should be avoided.

3. Inhaled nitric oxide does not reduce the need for ECMO in neonates with congenital diaphragmatic hernia.

89. **What disorder makes up the largest proportion of neonates who are treated with extracorporeal membrane oxygenation (ECMO)?**
Infants with MAS make up 30–40% of infants who are treated with ECMO. Unfortunately, the circumstances that lead to MAS in many cases are precipitous and unavoidable. As a result, by the time therapy can be started, the pathophysiology is sufficiently far advanced and can be halted only by the use of ECMO. Other disorders that are managed with ECMO include sepsis, pneumonia, pulmonary hypoplasia (most often due to congenital diaphragmatic hernia), and RDS. Patients with MAS tend to have the shortest ECMO courses and the highest survival rates, approaching 97% in the most experienced ECMO centers.

90. **Meconium happens! Meconium-stained amniotic fluid (MSAF) is found across all races and socioeconomic strata in humans. Additionally, MSAF and MAS are noted frequently in domestic animals. How do farmers and veterinarians manage MSAF in an effort to prevent MAS?**
Farmers and veterinarians grab newborn animals by their hindquarters and swing them in a circular motion. Centrifugal forces move MSAF outward into the upper airway and oropharynx. Caretakers then manually remove the material. But it is not suggested that infants be swung by the legs to remove meconium from the airway!

91. **Is thin-consistency MSAF more likely to enter the airways and cause MAS or other respiratory distress compared with thick-consistency MSAF?**
No. The thicker the consistency of MSAF, the greater the likelihood of MAS or other respiratory distress. There is at least a sevenfold increase in the incidence of respiratory disorders among infants born through "pea-soup" MSAF compared with those born through watery-consistency MSAF.

92. **What mechanisms of meconium aspiration into the lungs contribute to ventilatory failure, and what is the role of surfactant therapy in the treatment of this condition?**
Meconium-induced lung injury is associated with many pulmonary changes that contribute to respiratory failure. These include airway obstruction, inflammation with release of vasoactive substances, and surfactant dysfunction. Meconium has the ability to inactivate surfactant both in vivo and in vitro and has direct effects on type II pneumocyte function. In both animal models and human infants who have aspirated meconium and who are undergoing pulmonary fluid analysis, inflammatory cell numbers and total protein are significantly elevated compared with control infants. Various inflammatory mediators, including myeloperoxidase and interleukin-8, are increased. Maximal influx of inflammatory cells occurs by 16 hours of age with some recovery by 72 hours. These findings support the role of surfactant replacement in infants with

MAS that requires ventilatory support. The optimal method of surfactant treatment is currently under refinement, however, with some preliminary evidence supporting a surfactant lavage of the airways that is distinct from bolus administration of surfactant as used in preterm infants with RDS.

PERSISTENT PULMONARY HYPERTENSION OF THE NEWBORN

93. **What is PPHN?**

Successful transition from intrauterine to extrauterine life requires that the pulmonary vascular resistance decreases precipitously at birth. In infants with PPHN, this decrease does not occur. Pulmonary arterial pressure remains elevated, and blood continues to shunt right to left across the ductus arteriosus and foramen ovale, resulting in significant hypoxemia.

94. **When was PPHN first described? Why is *persistent fetal circulation* not an accurate term to describe PPHN?**

Gersony and coworkers (1969) described a group of term infants without structural heart disease who became cyanotic shortly after birth and who had only mild respiratory distress. These infants all had suprasystemic pulmonary arterial pressures with right-to-left shunting across persistent fetal pathways (ductus arteriosus and foramen ovale). Hence, this condition was called *persistent fetal circulation.*

The shunting across the foramen ovale and ductus arteriosus as a result of suprasystemic pulmonary arterial pressure seen in PPHN is very similar to fetal circulation. However, the exclusion of placental circulation and the fact that ductus venosus may or may not be patent preclude the use of the term *persistent fetal circulation* to describe this condition. The term *persistent pulmonary hypertension of the newborn* describes the pathophysiology of the disease more accurately, indicating that the critical problem in this situation is the failure of the pulmonary circulation to decrease to normal pressures.

Gersony WM, Due GV, Sinclair JC: "PFC" syndrome (persistence of fetal circulation). Circulation 40:3–9, 1969.

95. **What are the clinical features of PPHN?**

Infants with PPHN are usually delivered at term or post-term. Often they are born through MSAF. The typical clinical manifestations of a neonate with PPHN are as follows:

- Labile hypoxemia or cyanosis disproportionate to the level of respiratory distress may be present. These infants are extremely sensitive to environmental stimuli.
- Infants with significant ductal shunting have higher oxygen saturation in the right hand (preductal) than in the legs (postductal). Similarly, PaO_2 in the right radial artery is significantly greater than that obtained from the umbilical artery. Infants with predominant shunting at the level of foramen ovale have similar preductal and postductal oxygen levels.
- Cardiac murmur compatible with tricuspid insufficiency is present.
- Chest radiograph may reveal cardiomegaly. The underlying disease (such as congenital diaphragmatic hernia or RDS) alters the radiologic picture. Infants with idiopathic PPHN have clear and undervascularized lung fields ("black-lung" PPHN).
- Echocardiography is important to rule out cyanotic congenital heart disease and to establish the diagnosis. In infants with PPHN, shunting at the atrial and ductal level can be demonstrated. Tricuspid insufficiency, right ventricular hypertrophy, septal deviation to the left, and prolonged right ventricular systolic intervals support the diagnosis of PPHN.

96. **What are the common causes of PPHN?**

The common causes of PPHN are summarized in the mnemonic **DIAPHRAGMATIC:**

- **D**iaphragmatic hernia (hypoplastic lungs)
- **I**nfection (including pneumonia), especially GBS
- **A**spiration syndromes (e.g., meconium, amniotic fluid)
- **P**ostmaturity

- **H**yperviscosity (polycythemia, hyperfibrinogenemia)
- **R**espiratory distress syndrome (i.e., hyaline membrane disease)
- **A**sphyxia
- **G**rowth retardation (placental insufficiency)
- **M**aternal nonsteroidal anti-inflammatory drug ingestion
- **A**ir leak
- **T**ransient tachypnea of newborn
- **I**diopathic ("black lung" PPHN)
- **C**ongenital anomalies of the lung, alveolar-capillary dysplasia

The causes of PPHN can also be classified depending on the predominant abnormality involved (*see* Fig. 16-2).

97. Why is the right hand a preferred site to obtain preductal pulse oximetry readings?

In some infants, the left subclavian artery arises from the arch of the aorta just distal to the level of the insertion of the ductus arteriosus. In these infants, a pulse oximetry probe applied to the left hand indicates postductal saturations. Hence, it is always better to obtain preductal oxygen saturation from the right upper limb, a site that indicates preductal saturation.

98. What is the pathophysiology of PPHN?

Persistent elevation of pulmonary arterial pressure in PPHN results from active constriction of pulmonary vessels (as in pneumonia), underdevelopment of the pulmonary vessels (as in congenital diaphragmatic hernia), or maldevelopment of the pulmonary vasculature (as in prenatal ductal closure from maternal ingestion of nonsteroidal anti-inflammatory drugs and idiopathic PPHN).

Vascular remodeling: In infants dying from PPHN caused by maldevelopment of the pulmonary vessels, pulmonary arterial smooth muscle hypertrophies and extends from pre-acinar arteries into normally nonmuscular intra-acinar arteries, even to the level of the alveolus. This thickened muscle encroaches on the vessel lumen and results in mechanical obstruction to blood flow.

Functional abnormalities in the pulmonary vessels (e.g., reduced nitric oxide synthase, reduced soluble guanylyl cyclase, and increased levels of vasoconstrictors such as endothelin) have been described.

Persistently elevated pulmonary vascular resistance increases right ventricular afterload and oxygen demand and impairs oxygen delivery to cardiac muscle. Ischemic damage to the myocardium, papillary muscle necrosis, and tricuspid regurgitation can occur. Increased right ventricular pressure displaces the septum into the left ventricle, impairs left ventricular filling, and decreases cardiac output. Myocardial dysfunction is an important cause for mortality in PPHN (Fig. 16-9).

99. How are infants with a cyanotic congenital heart disease differentiated from those with PPHN?

It is often very difficult clinically to differentiate between these two conditions. Patients with PPHN are more labile and exhibit wide swings in oxygen saturations. A significant difference between the preductal and postductal oxygen saturations is also a clinical finding in favor of PPHN. An additional test that is sometimes used in this clinical situation is the *hyperoxia test*. The child to be tested is placed on an inspired oxygen level of 100%. On an arterial blood gas determination, if the PaO_2 level rises above 100 mmHg, it is unlikely that the infant has significant cyanotic heart disease and more likely has pulmonary hypertension or pulmonary parenchymal disease. This test, however, is not infallible, and some children with PPHN may not be able to increase their PaO_2 above 100 mmHg. In addition, it may be necessary to give positive pressure ventilation to a baby to be sure that one is ventilating the lungs of a child with pulmonary disease adequately to maximize the arterial oxygen levels. The best way to differentiate between these two entities is by echocardiography.

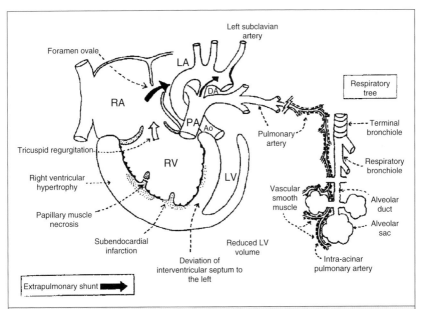

Figure 16-9. Pathophysiology of PPHN. Suprasystemic pulmonary arterial pressure results in right ventricular (RV) hypertrophy and deviation of the intraventricular septum to the left. This reduces the left ventricular (LV) volume and decreases systemic output. Extrapulmonary right-to-left shunting occurs at the foramen ovale from the right atrium (RA) to the left atrium (LA) and at the level of the ductus arteriosus (DA) from the pulmonary artery (PA) to the aorta (Ao). Normally, PAs distal to the level of terminal bronchioles are not muscular. Abnormal extension and hypertrophy of distal pulmonary vascular smooth muscle (shown as interrupted lines), sometimes to the level of intra-acinar arteries, is seen in severe PPHN.

100. What is the long-term outcome of infants treated for PPHN?

In the past, the mortality for infants with PPHN ranged from 20% to 40%, and the incidence of neurologic handicap ranged from 12% to 25%. With recent advances in conservative management, survival and neurodevelopmental outcome have improved considerably. In most centers, inhaled nitric oxide and ECMO have further reduced mortality from severe PPHN. Survival rates between 76% and 93% have been reported for infants with pneumonia, meconium aspiration, and idiopathic PPHN who require ECMO. The outlook for infants with diaphragmatic hernia requiring ECMO has not been as dramatic, and survival is still only about 60%.

Most infants treated for PPHN have few respiratory symptoms or neurologic or developmental sequelae by 1 year of age. However:

- Infants presenting with more severe parenchymal disease may have persistent tachypnea and bronchospasm.
- Neurologic development may be impaired in children with PPHN, especially if they are severely asphyxiated.
- An increased incidence of sensorineural hearing loss among infants with PPHN treated with hyperventilation and alkalization has been reported.

101. What are the future prospects for treating infants with PPHN?

Although ECMO has considerably reduced the mortality from PPHN, it is an invasive procedure limited to a few tertiary care centers. Inhaled nitric oxide has reduced the use of ECMO. Unfortunately, this reduction has not been associated with an improvement in long-term outcome. Two possibilities for enhancing the effect of inhaled nitric oxide are being currently investigated:

1. Nitric oxide acts by stimulating soluble guanylyl cyclase and producing cyclic guanosine mono-phosphate (GMP) in vascular smooth muscle. Cyclic GMP induces smooth muscle relaxation but is rapidly broken down by phosphodiesterase-5 (PDE-5) enzyme. PDE-5 inhibition should increase the level of cyclic GMP in vascular smooth muscle and enhance nitric oxide–induced relaxation. An inhibitor of this enzyme, sildenafil (Viagra), is currently used in the treatment of impotence. Several other PDE-5 inhibitors (Zaprinast, dipyridamole, and E4021) have been used successfully in animal models of PPHN. None of these therapies are approved by the U.S. Food and Drug Administration (FDA), and all should be considered experimental.

2. High levels of oxygen free radicals are present in many disease states that cause PPHN. Superoxide anion combines nitric oxide to produce the toxic free radical peroxynitrite. Antioxidants such as superoxide dismutase remove these toxic free radicals and enhance nitric oxide-mediated vasorelaxation in isolated pulmonary vessels. Similar results might be obtainable in vivo.

INHALED NITRIC OXIDE

102. What is inhaled nitric oxide?

Nitric oxide is an important regulator of vascular muscle tone at the cellular level. Nitric oxide is generated enzymatically by nitric oxide synthases from L-arginine. Nitric oxide activates guany-lyl cyclase by binding to its heme component, leading to the production of cyclic GMP. The mechanism by which cyclic GMP relaxes vascular smooth muscle is not clear. It appears to involve inhibition of activation-induced elevation in cytosolic calcium concentration.

Several randomized control trials indicate that inhaled nitric oxide reduces the incidence of the combined end point of death or need for ECMO compared with patients not offered treat-ment with inhaled nitric oxide. This reduction seems to be entirely due to a reduction in the use of ECMO since mortality is not reduced.

Finer NN, Barrington KJ: Nitric oxide for respiratory failure in infants born at or near term. Cochrane Database Syst Rev 2:CD000399, 2001.

KEY POINTS: MAJOR ANOMALIES THAT ALTER PULMONARY FUNCTION

1. Both intrinsic defects in the larynx or trachea and extrinsic compression of the trachea can cause airway obstruction syndrome.

2. Lung function is normal in most of these disorders so that airway management, which relieves the obstruction, usually normalizes gas exchange.

103. Inhaled nitric oxide acts like an endothelium-relaxing factor and is a major regulator of vascular smooth muscle tone. Why doesn't it also dilate the systemic vascular system?

Nitric oxide has a high affinity for the iron of all heme proteins, including reduced hemoglobin, with which it forms nitrosyl-hemoglobin (NOHb). The NOHb is then oxidized to methemoglobin with the production of nitrate. As a result, when given by inhalation, nitric oxide is inactivated before acting on any systemic vascular bed, while relaxing the pulmonary vascular smooth mus-cle through the cyclic GMP production. In normal development, endogenous nitric oxide pro-duced in endothelial cells from oxygen and L-arginine diffuses into smooth cells in the vascular wall and causes vasodilatation. Nitric oxide that diffuses into the blood vessel lumen is avidly bound by hemoglobin and does not cause systemic vasodilatation.

104. **Does inhaled nitric oxide reduce the use of ECMO in neonates with congenital diaphragmatic hernia?**

Meta-analysis showed that infants with diaphragmatic hernia do not appear to share the benefits of inhaled nitric oxide that infants with other causes of hypoxemic respiratory failure experience. Indeed, there are suggestions that outcomes may be worse in infants with congenital diaphragmatic hernia who received inhaled nitric oxide compared with control subjects. This analysis showed that the incidence of death or requiring ECMO was 40 of 46 among control patients and 36 of 38 among patients treated with nitric oxide (relative risk, 1.09; 95% confidence interval [CI], 0.95–1.26). Mortality rates were similar in control and treatment patients (18 of 46 in the control group compared with 18 of 38 in the treatment group; relative risk of death, 1.20; 95% CI, 0.74–1.96), but there was a significant increase in the requirement for ECMO in infants treated with inhaled nitric oxide (31 of 46 in the control group compared with 32 of 38 in the treatment group; relative risk, 1.27; 95% CI, 1.00–1.62).

Finer NN, Barrington KJ: Nitric oxide for respiratory failure in infants born at or near term. Cochrane Database Syst Rev 2:CD000399, 2001.

105. **What are the major concerns regarding the weaning of nitric oxide and oxygen in infants with PPHN?**

When nitric oxide and O_2 come into contact, peroxynitrite (ONO), a potent oxidant, is formed. The relative amount of nitric oxide, O_2^-, ONO^-, and antioxidants in the airway will determine whether nitric oxide will be beneficial or potentially toxic. These oxidants can contribute to lung injury by enhancing lung inflammation, producing pulmonary edema, and reducing surfactant function. Furthermore, recent findings have shown that abrupt withdrawal of inhaled nitric oxide, even in infants with minimal or no response, can induce worsening pulmonary hypertension. Thus, many infants with pulmonary hypertension continue to require inhaled nitric oxide at less than 5 ppm for a considerable time. The potential for pulmonary inflammatory injury can be decreased as the concentrations of inhaled nitric oxide and O_2 are lowered, although many infants will continue to require several days of inhaled nitric oxide to prevent recurrence of pulmonary hypertension.

106. **What are the indications and the risks associated with the use of inhaled nitric oxide for the treatment of ventilatory failure in preterm infants?**

Three randomized controlled trials of inhaled nitric oxide therapy in preterm infants have been reported, and several are ongoing. In a meta-analysis of these studies, there is no evidence of significant effect of inhaled nitric oxide on mortality or bronchopulmonary dysplasia. One study showed a reduction in days receiving assisted ventilation in the nitric oxide group, which was a secondary outcome.

In the meta-analysis, there was no evidence that inhaled nitric oxide increased the risk of intraventricular hemorrhage. There are no data on long-term neurodevelopmental outcomes. Evidence from randomized trials does not support the use of inhaled nitric oxide in preterm infants with hypoxic respiratory failure. Further studies are ongoing.

Barrington KJ, Finer NN: Inhaled nitric oxide for respiratory failure in preterm infants. Cochrane Database Syst Rev 4:CD000509, 2001.

Kinsella JP, Walsh WF, Bose CL, et al: Inhaled nitric oxide in premature neonates with severe hypoxaemic respiratory failure: A randomised controlled trial. Lancet 354:1061–1065, 1999.

MAJOR ANOMALIES THAT ALTER PULMONARY FUNCTION

107. **Infants with fetal akinesia syndrome (Pena-Shokeir phenotype) frequently have pulmonary anomalies. Describe the pulmonary anomalies in this disorder.**

Infants with Pena-Shokeir phenotype (also termed *arthrogryposis multiplex congenita with pulmonary hypoplasia*) have gracile ribs and reduced thoracic volume. Also present are a lack of fetal breathing activity, polyhydramnios resulting from a lack of fetal swallowing, and intrauterine constraint, resulting in muscular hypoplasia involving both intercostal and diaphragmatic musculature. Thoracic wall weakness, hypotonia of the muscles of respiration, and anterior horn cell atrophy or deficiency lead to reduced ventilatory drive, which may improve over time in selected infants.

108. **Fetal airway obstruction can be the direct result of intrinsic defects in the larynx or trachea, resulting in congenital high airway obstruction syndrome. What is the differential diagnosis of extrinsic fetal obstruction?**
   - Cervical teratoma
   - Lymphangioma
   - Vascular rings
   - Occipital encephalocele
   - Cervical myelomeningocele
   - Thyroglossal duct cyst
   - Thyroid cyst or tumor
   - Congenital goiter
   - Branchial cleft cysts

   The major causes of extrinsic fetal airway obstruction are cervical lymphangioma, teratoma, and vascular rings (e.g., double aortic arch, pulmonary vascular sling).

109. **What precautions should be taken for a child with suspected fetal airway obstructive syndromes during pregnancy and at the time of delivery?**
   As fetuses with fetal airway obstruction reach viability, they should be monitored closely for development or progression of hydrops (for intrinsic obstruction cases) or polyhydramnios (when extrinsic obstruction is present). The fetus should be delivered by using the ex utero intrapartum treatment procedure, with maintenance of uteroplacental circulation and gas exchange. This approach provides time to perform procedures such as direct laryngoscopy, bronchoscopy, or tracheostomy to secure the fetal airway, thereby converting an emergent airway crisis into a controlled situation.

MECHANICAL VENTILATION OF THE NEONATE

110. **What are the two basic ways of cycling conventional mechanical ventilators?**
   1. Time-cycled, pressure-limited ventilators have become the standard in neonatal mechanical ventilation because of the problems associated with volume-cycled ventilators. Time-cycled, pressure-limited ventilators have the advantage of providing continuous flow through the circuit, which allows the infant to take spontaneous breaths of fresh gas between mechanical breaths (the mechanical breaths are referred to as *intermittent mandatory ventilation* [IMV]). The system gives the operator direct control over the delivered peak inspiratory pressure (PIP) and allows easy compensation for leakage around ET tubes, and the decelerating flow pattern allows better gas distribution within the lungs.
   2. Volume-cycled ventilators deliver a preset tidal volume, usually in a constant flow fashion, generating whatever pressure is necessary to deliver the gas into the lungs. This results in a triangular pressure and volume waveforms with maximum volume and pressure being reached just before the onset of exhalation.

111. **What are the disadvantages of time-cycled, pressure-limited ventilators?**
   The chief disadvantage is the fact that tidal volume is not directly controlled. The delivered tidal volume is determined by the interaction between PIP and lung compliance. Consequently, as compliance changes, so will the delivered tidal volume. Improving lung compliance can lead to

excessive tidal volume and can cause lung injury. Conversely, worsening compliance can lead to hypoventilation and loss of lung volume. In addition, if an infant is breathing asynchronously with the ventilator, peak pressures are reached quickly, and volume is reduced. This situation may result in a serious deterioration of blood gases.

112. **What unique problems make volume-cycled ventilation difficult in newborn infants?**

Uncuffed ET tubes that are used in newborn infants result in a variable degree of air leak around the tube, causing variable loss of tidal volume. Additional tidal volume is lost through gas compression within the relatively large volume of gas in the ventilator circuit and humidifier, and to stretching of the relatively compliant circuit during inspiration. As a result, the tiny premature infant with poorly compliant lungs receives only a small and variable fraction of the tidal volume generated by the ventilator. In essence, one ends up ventilating the circuit rather than the baby!

113. **What are the ways to increase ventilation (improve CO_2 removal) in an infant on time-cycled, pressure-limited ventilation?**

- Increase IMV.
- Decrease PEEP.
- Increase PIP.
- Decrease dead space (e.g., by shortening the ET tube).

There is an upper limit to the effective respiratory rate. An excessively rapid IMV rate may lead to inadequate expiratory time with incomplete exhalation and air trapping. Thus, paradoxically, when the IMV is >90–120 breaths/min, further increases in rate may lead to CO_2 retention. This situation is most likely to occur in infants with increased airway resistance and prolonged time constants. In such infants, the best way to improve ventilation is to *decrease* the IMV rate.

Tidal volume is proportional to the difference between PIP and PEEP. This is referred to as ΔP. Thus, lowering PEEP will increase ΔP and improve ventilation (although it can lead to loss of lung volume with deterioration of oxygenation). Occasionally, excessively high PEEP in a patient with relatively compliant lungs can lead to incomplete exhalation and CO_2 retention. This is not a common problem but should be considered in a patient with improving oxygenation and a worsening respiratory acidosis.

114. **Name the two major factors that affect oxygenation in neonatal mechanical ventilation.**

- Mean airway pressure (Paw)
- FiO_2

Mean airway pressure has been shown to be a major determinant of oxygenation. Adequate distending pressure is needed to maintain lung volume and avoid the diffuse microatelectasis that leads to ventilation-perfusion imbalance with consequent hypoxemia.

115. **List the key ventilator variables that affect mean airway pressure in conventional time-cycled, pressure-limited ventilation.**

- PIP
- Inspiratory to expiratory ratio
- PEEP
- Inspiratory flow

Mean airway pressure is the area under the pressure curve (Fig. 16-10). Increasing the PEEP is usually the most effective means of increasing the Paw. The least recognized factor affecting the area under the curve is the slope of the upstroke of pressure, which determines the shape of the pressure waveform. Higher flow leads to more rapid upstroke and a more square-shaped curve, which has a larger area than one with a gradual upstroke and a more triangular shape.

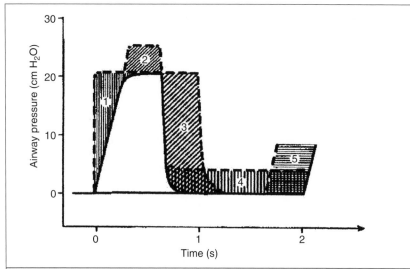

Figure 16-10. Effects of changes in airway pressures and timing on the respiratory waveform and mean airway pressure (MAP). Different waveforms will have different associated blood gases in many instances. (From Reynolds EOM: Pressure waveform and ventilator settings for mechanical ventilation in severe hyaline membrane disease. Int Anesthesiol Clin 12:259, 1974.)

116. **When placing an infant on conventional time-cycled, pressure-limited ventilation, how do you choose the initial PIP?**

For any given PIP, the delivered tidal volume will be determined by the compliance of the baby's lungs. Select a pressure based on the best estimate of what the infant will need, and observe the result. If there is adequate chest rise, good breath sounds, and oxygenation, the pressure is appropriate. If the chest rise is excessive, reduce the PIP, and if the chest movement is inadequate, higher PIP is needed (assuming the ET tube is correctly positioned).

Most modern infant ventilators now have the means to directly measure tidal volume (V_T), eliminating the dependence on subjective assessment of adequacy of chest wall movement and allowing more accurate determination of optimal PIP. The target V_T measured at the airway opening should be 4–6 mL/kg in the acute phase of the disease.

Note: Some devices measure V_T at the point where the circuit attaches to the ventilator. This position is undesirable because it will give an artificially large V_T measurement, ignoring the loss of V_T to compression of gas in the circuit and circuit stretching. Furthermore, gadgets do malfunction, so continue to use your eyes and ears to verify that the "numbers" are believable!

117. **List as many possible causes of acute CO_2 retention in an infant on mechanical ventilation as you can. (There are many more than you may think!)**
   - The ET tube is dislodged.
   - The ET tube is occluded with secretions.
   - The ET tube is up against the carina.
   - There is an accumulation of secretions in the airways (patient needs suctioning).
   - The patient has a pneumothorax and some other condition that acutely decreased lung compliance.
   - Acute bronchospasm is present.
   - Oversedation with suppression of spontaneous respiratory effort is occurring.
   - The ventilator is malfunctioning (e.g., leak in circuit, partial disconnection).

- There has been an acute onset of sepsis with loss of spontaneous respiratory effort.
- Acute abdominal distention or the presence of a large abdominal mass is leading to decreased diaphragmatic excursion.

Most of these should be readily recognizable clinically. If the chest is not moving, the first priority is to make sure that the airway is patent, the ET tube is in place, and the ventilator is cycling. Many modern infant ventilators have the ability to display flow and pressure waveforms, which should help diagnose or confirm the problem. *When in doubt, reintubate.* Manual ventilation may be appropriate if a circuit or ventilator problem is suspected, but be careful to avoid using excessive pressure that may cause lung injury.

118. **What are some adverse effects associated with mechanical ventilation?**
- Acute lung injury (barotrauma or volutrauma, such as pneumothorax, pneumomediastinum, pneumopericardium, pulmonary interstitial emphysema)
- Chronic lung injury (chronic lung disease, bronchopulmonary dysplasia)
- Hemodynamic impairment due to increased intrathoracic pressure
- Intraventricular hemorrhage and periventricular leukomalacia
- Tracheitis or pneumonia
- Tracheal damage with subglottic stenosis
- Palatal groove and damage to tooth buds of the upper incisors

Some degree of impairment of venous return to the heart is inevitable because, unlike spontaneous breathing, intrathoracic pressure rises above ambient pressure during positive pressure ventilation. The problem becomes more severe when high or excessive pressures are used. Intraventricular hemorrhage can be triggered by hemodynamic instability, elevated venous pressure, and sudden increases in cerebral blood flow (as might occur with retention of CO_2). Periventricular leukomalacia is associated with hypotension and with marked respiratory alkalosis.

119. **Which of the following scenarios is more likely to lead to acute air leak, such as a pneumothorax: (A) PIP of 25 cm H_2O in a 3.5-kg infant with normal lungs who is ventilated because of neurologic dysfunction or (B) PIP of 32 in a 1.2-kg, 28-week premature infant with "white-out" lungs on chest radiograph resulting from severe RDS?**
A. Normal lungs are quite compliant, and a PIP of 12–14 cm H_2O is usually sufficient to produce normal tidal volume. A pressure of 25 cm H_2O would produce an excessively large tidal volume in this infant, leading to overstretching of the tissues and air leak. Excessive tidal volume has been shown to be more important than pressure in the genesis of lung injury. The term *volutrauma* is increasingly used in place of *barotrauma* for this reason. On the other hand, the high PIP in scenario B is most commonly necessary to achieve an adequate tidal volume, given the disease severity, and is less likely to cause pneumothorax.

KEY POINTS: MOST EFFECTIVE WAYS TO AVOID INJURY IN NEONATES WHO REQUIRE MECHANICAL VENTILATION

1. Optimize oxygen delivery and avoid hyperoxia and hypoxia (by carefully adjusting FiO_2 levels).

2. Normalize functional residual capacity to prevent lung collapse (by giving surfactant to patients with RDS and using end-expiratory pressure to maintain lung volume).

3. Avoid volutrauma (by limiting the tidal volume used to support ventilation).

120. Which of the following infants, each ventilated and with PIP of 25 cm H_2O, PEEP of 5 cm H_2O, IMV of 90 breaths/min, and an inspiratory time of 0.3 seconds, is *least* likely to experience hypercarbia, hemodynamic impairment, and air leak resulting from incomplete exhalation (air-trapping): (a) A 12-hour-old, 760-gm premature infant of 26 weeks' gestation who has RDS; (b) A 2-hour-old, 3.8-kg infant of 41 weeks' gestation who has MAS; or (c) A 6-week-old, 1420-gm, former 25 weeks' gestation premature infant with severe chronic lung disease?

A. Hypercarbia, hemodynamic impairment, and air leak caused by incomplete exhalation occur when the expiratory time is too short to allow complete exhalation before the next mechanical breath occurs. This situation is most likely to occur in infants who have increased airway resistance, such as is seen in meconium aspiration with acute airway obstruction or in chronic lung disease in which airway edema, copious secretions, and bronchospasm are present.

121. What is a "time constant," and why is it important to consider when venting a newborn infant?

A time constant is the product of lung compliance and airway resistance ($Tc = R \times C$). Conceptually, time constants reflect the time it takes for gas flow to cease and pressure to be fully equilibrated between the large airways and the alveoli when a sudden pressure change is applied to the airway opening (three time constants are needed for 95% equilibration) (Fig. 16-11).

In acute RDS, compliance is low, and airway resistance is also low, (normal). Therefore, short inspiratory times can be used. In addition, time constants are

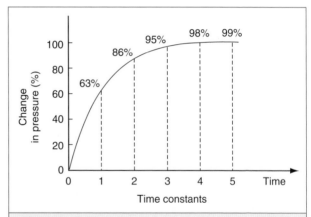

Figure 16-11. Time constants in the lung. A percentage change in pressure in relation to the time (in time constants) allowed for equilibration. As a longer time is allowed for equilibration, a higher percentage change in pressure occurs. (From Carlo WA, Martin RJ: Principles of assisted ventilation. Pediatr Clin North Am 33:321, 1986.)

also a function of size (total compliance, not compliance per kilogram, is used). Consequently, large subjects such as adults or horses have long time constants, and small premature infants and hummingbirds have short time constants. Time constants are a major determinant of resting respiratory rate, which turns out to fall exactly where work of breathing is lowest. This is why, at rest, adults breathe at a rate of 14 breaths/min, term infants breathe at 40 breaths/min, and small premature infants at about 60 breaths/min. Mice and hummingbirds breathe a lot faster than that! In infants with acute respiratory distress, tachypnea is a reflection of shorter time constants as lung compliance decreases because of various causes. Asthmatics, on the other hand, prefer to breathe rather slowly because of their prolonged expiratory phase. The bottom line is this: Consider the underlying disease process and its pathophysiology before making decisions about ventilator settings.

122. What are some of the advantages of synchronized mechanical ventilation?
- Avoidance of asynchrony (baby "bucking" or "fighting" the ventilator)
- Less need for sedation and/or neuromuscular blockade
- Lower airway pressures, because the baby and the ventilator work in tandem
- Decreased risk of barotrauma/volutrauma and intraventricular hemorrhage
- Preservation of respiratory muscle training (compared with muscle paralysis)
- Greater ease of weaning from mechanical ventilation

123. What is assist-controlled (A/C) ventilation? How does it differ from synchronized intermittent mandatory ventilation (SIMV)? When should it be used?

A/C ventilation is a form of mechanical ventilation in which the infant triggers the ventilator to cycle with each breath (Fig. 16-12). With a small triggering effort, therefore, the baby can

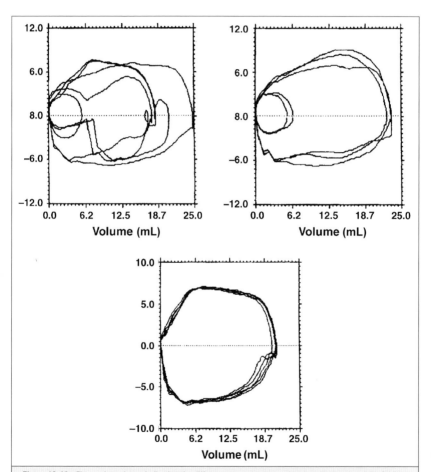

Figure 16-12. Flow-volume loops indicating the differences among conventional ventilation *(top left)*, SIMV *(top right)*, and A/C ventilation *(bottom)*. The loops are erratic with conventional ventilation. With SIMV, the loops are either triggered by the patient or the ventilator. In A/C mode, all loops are ventilator generated, either triggered by the patient (if breathing above the set rate) or by the ventilator (if the infant's respiratory rate falls below the set level). (From Goldsmith JP, Karotkin EH [eds]: Assisted Ventilation of the Neonate, 4th ed. Philadelphia, W.B. Saunders, 2003, p. 208.)

achieve a much higher level of ventilatory support than with spontaneous breathing. In general, A/C ventilation can be used very successfully to treat VLBW babies with RDS or pulmonary insufficiency of prematurity. It has become the most common way to initiate mechanical ventilation therapy in these clinical situations. It often enables patients to be ventilated at lower PIP levels than with conventional mechanical ventilation or SIMV. It differs from SIMV in that, with A/C, the baby will trigger a ventilator breath with each respiratory effort. In SIMV, the ventilator is synchronized to the baby's respiratory cycle so as to avoid stacking of the ventilator and infant breaths, but the baby is only given a preset amount of synchronized breaths. With modern ventilators, if the baby becomes apneic during either A/C ventilation or SIMV, the machine will deliver a preset number of breaths per minute.

124. **An infant is now on PIP of 18 cm H_2O, IMV rate of 30 breaths/min, and FIO_2 of 0.3. Which is the correct way of weaning the infant from mechanical ventilation in A/C mode: (A) progressively decrease the PIP and IMV; (B) progressively lower the IMV, leaving the PIP unchanged; or (C) progressively lower the PIP, leaving the IMV unchanged?**

    C. In A/C mode, every breath that the infant takes triggers a ventilator breath—every breath is supported. As a result, the baby is in control of the ventilatory rate. The IMV rate is only a backup rate in case the infant is apneic or the triggering mechanism is not functioning. Decreasing the IMV rate does not actually decrease the level of support the infant is receiving. Weaning occurs by lowering the degree of support for each breath (i.e., the PIP). Ultimately, when the PIP is down to where the ventilator is generating only enough pressure to overcome the resistance of the ET tube and circuit, the baby is ready for extubation (usually about 10 cm H_2O).

125. **Why does hand ventilation with a bag often work when mechanical ventilation is failing?**

    With manual ventilation, we commonly use much higher PIP levels than that we would dare to set on the ventilator! It is easy to inadvertently generate pressures >40 cm H_2O with all the adrenaline flowing in a crisis. Beware of the risk of pneumothorax! Using a manometer may be helpful, but most of the mechanical gauges grossly underestimate the actual PIP and the actual duration of inspiration, especially when the ventilatory rate is rapid. This explains, in part, why it is that when you place the baby back on the ventilator, ostensibly on the same settings as the pressures that were used with hand ventilation, the saturation usually drifts down again (because the ventilator PIP is actually lower than that with which you were bagging). It is sometimes preferable to maintain the infant on the ventilator and simply increase the level of support (PIP and IMV) as needed to achieve the desired result. This approach allows you to continue to use the monitoring function of the ventilator to provide feedback regarding the tidal volume and other parameters, and it provides controlled and accurate pressure delivery. However, if the baby is still doing poorly, hand ventilation is an acceptable alternative.

126. **What do you do when an infant's condition seems to deteriorate on a ventilator?**

    When a baby is doing poorly on a ventilator, one should remove the baby from the machine and hand ventilate with an anesthesia (preferably) or self-inflating bag. The chest excursion should be carefully examined and breath sounds auscultated to be sure that the ET tube is still well positioned and not plugged. If there is any question about the tube, it should be replaced promptly. A chest radiograph is often helpful to be certain about position of the tube and to make sure no air leak is present. If the tube seems fine and there are no radiologic changes, the ventilator itself must be carefully checked for malfunction. Respiratory therapists should be available around the clock in any intensive care nursery in which infants are ventilated.

127. How does one prepare to extubate a baby?

Although there is a great deal of literature on neonatal intubation, few articles describe the risks of extubation. Nothing is more frustrating than successfully completing a course of neonatal mechanical ventilation on a sick baby, only to have a serious setback from a poor effort at extubation. When a child has reached the predetermined levels for extubation, the following should be done:

- A chest radiograph should be obtained as a baseline so that postextubation changes can be compared.
- The child should be NPO for at least 4 hours before extubation and should be given intravenous fluids during that time.
- A CPAP setup or oxygen should be available to help the child's transition to spontaneous breathing.
- A laryngoscope and a new ET tube should be at hand in case the child does poorly.
- It is not necessary to initiate steroids or methylxanthines before extubation in all children. These adjuncts, however, may be useful if a child has failed one or two prior attempts at extubation. The evidence for the value of steroids, however, is mostly anecdotal.

128. How does one proceed to extubate the infant after these preparations?

When the child is ready to be extubated, the tube should be untaped from the face carefully to avoid causing any abrasions. An anesthesia bag should be attached to the ET tube, and a long, slow, low-level (15 cm H_2O), positive-pressure breath should be administered as the ET tube is withdrawn from the airway. This breath overcomes the natural negative pressure created as the tube is withdrawn from the airway. The child should be given CPAP or oxygen and observed closely. Stridor or hoarseness is common and typically indicates upper airway edema. Marked retractions also may be seen and are worrisome, indicating either volume loss in the lung or upper airway obstruction. If the child has difficulty, the tube should be replaced immediately and another extubation attempt made in 2–3 days. Adequate humidification of inspired gas is essential after extubation. Because of the initial inability to oppose the vocal cords, feeding should not be resumed for at least 6–12 hours postextubation. Clinical deterioration that occurs 24–48 hours after extubation may be due to a number of factors: increased atelectasis, upper airway edema and obstruction, or muscular fatigue. If reintubation is deemed necessary, it should be carried out promptly. "Cheerleading" the child to recovery rarely works, and occasionally significant pulmonary hypertension appears when the work of breathing leads to increased acidosis after a trial of extubation. This setback can be extremely difficult to manage.

NEONATAL HIGH-FREQUENCY VENTILATION

129. What is neonatal high-frequency ventilation?

Neonatal high-frequency ventilation uses devices that provide respiratory support for critically ill neonates with the use of small tidal volume, rapid rate assisted ventilation. Generally, this means rates >150 breaths/min and tidal volumes <2–3 mL/kg.

130. Name the three different types of high-frequency ventilation and what makes each distinct.

1. High-frequency oscillation (Sensormedics)
2. High-frequency jet ventilation (Bunnell, Inc.)
3. High-frequency flow interruption (Infant Star)

Oscillation exchanges gas by producing positive and negative flow in the ventilator circuit through the use of a vibrating diaphragm. Jet ventilation delivers high-frequency breaths through the interruption of a continuous gas flow directly into the airway through a unique ET tube located in the airway. The interruption takes place in a patient box located close to the baby, by a pincher valve that opens and closes on a piece of plastic tubing. With jet ventilation, inspiration is active; exhalation is passive. High-frequency flow interruption generates the signal by interrupting the flow of gas. It is similar to the jet ventilator except that the interruption of the gas flow occurs at a site much farther from the infant.

KEY POINTS: HIGH-FREQUENCY VENTILATION IN NEONATES

1. There are several different types of high-frequency ventilation, but the device used may be less important than the ventilatory strategy with which the device is used.

2. If the lung is poorly inflated, a strategy of lung recruitment (increased mean airway pressure compared with that being used on a conventional ventilator) is appropriate.

3. If air leak is present or the lung is overinflated, a strategy that minimizes intrathoracic pressure is important, and a lower mean airway pressure may be the most appropriate approach.

131. **Have the three types of high-frequency ventilation been compared in clinical trials?**
No. Because there have been no comparison trials, each type has its advocates and critics.

132. **What happens to tidal volume delivery to the alveolus when frequency is increased during high-frequency oscillation?**
It decreases. Impedance of the airway and ET tube are frequency dependent. As rate is increased, impedance to transmission of pressure swings increases. Thus, tidal volume decreases as frequency is increased.

133. **How is minute ventilation estimated on high-frequency ventilation?**
With standard mechanical ventilation or spontaneous breathing, minute ventilation = frequency $\times$ tidal volume. In high-frequency ventilation, minute ventilation = (frequency) $\times$ (tidal volume)^2.
These questions emphasize the importance of understanding the differences between high-frequency oscillation and conventional ventilation. In conventional ventilation, increasing the rate will increase carbon dioxide elimination in most cases. With high-frequency ventilation, turning up the rate generally causes a decrease in minute ventilation due to the loss of tidal volume delivery. When ventilation is inadequate during high-frequency ventilation, turning the rate down can increase carbon dioxide elimination.

134. **How does high-frequency ventilation work?**
No one really knows. Modeling of the wave flow in high-frequency ventilation is exceedingly complex. Several theories have been proposed, however, to explain high-frequency ventilation:
1. **Spike theory:** This theory postulates that the resistance along the periphery of the airway is higher than in the center so that a spike is produced that extends far down the center of the airway, bypassing much of the lung's dead space.
2. **Pendelluft:** The rapid to-and-fro movement of air between lungs or between lung segments may be enhanced at higher frequencies.
3. **Brownian diffusion:** This may increase at higher frequencies.
4. **Coaxial flow:** This theory speculates that gas flow in the airway is not simply a to-and-fro movement. Rather, inhaled gas spikes down the center of the airway, whereas the exhaled carbon dioxide moves along the periphery in a circuitous fashion. As frequencies increase, a whirlpool may actually arise within the airway that literally pulls the small-volume puffs of gas to a very deep region of the lung (Fig. 16-13).

135. **What factors affect ventilation during high-frequency ventilation?**

Just as in conventional ventilation, changes in respiratory system impedance affect carbon dioxide elimination during high-frequency ventilation. The important distinction is that high-frequency ventilation is more sensitive to changes in impedance than conventional modes of ventilation. Changes in ET tube size, respiratory system compliance, airway patency, and mucus plugging can all have a profound effect on tidal volume delivery and therefore ventilation. Because of the frequencies used and the small tidal volumes, these changes seem to be significantly magnified with high-frequency ventilation compared with conventional ventilation.

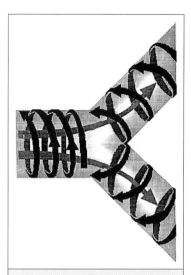

Figure 16-13. Coaxial flow during high-frequency ventilation. Fresh air moves down the center of the airway, while exhaled CO_2 is removed along the periphery. (From Spitzer AR [ed]: Intensive Care of the Fetus and Neonate, 2nd ed. Philadelphia, Elsevier, 2005.)

136. **In neonates with poor lung inflation, should high-frequency oscillation be used at lower, the same, or higher mean airway pressure than that being used on conventional ventilation?**

The strategy with which high-frequency oscillation is used is important. Patients with diffuse loss of lung volume (i.e., atelectasis) should be treated with a lung recruitment strategy. High-frequency oscillation allows the use of higher mean airway pressures than conventional ventilation because the small tidal volumes promote ventilation without causing lung overinflation. This approach has been studied in animal models of hyaline membrane disease and has been shown to improve lung inflation, decrease acute lung injury, decrease pulmonary air leaks, and promote survival. Often referred to as a "high mean airway pressure strategy," the real goal is not a high mean airway pressure, but rather optimal lung inflation. Unfortunately, measures of optimal lung inflation are not available. Clinically, the goal is to promote lung recruitment while avoiding lung overinflation, cardiac compromise, and lung atelectasis.

137. **When high-frequency ventilation is used, what measurements help guide choice of ventilation settings?**

The chest radiograph and the PaO_2/FiO_2 ratio can be used to help guide therapy. If the chest radiograph shows more than nine posterior ribs of inflation, flattened diaphragms, a small heart, or very clear lung fields, the lung may be overinflated. Similarly, if the mean airway pressure is high and the FiO_2 is low, then mean airway pressure should be decreased before FiO_2. If the chest radiograph shows fewer than seven posterior ribs of inflation, domed diaphragms, a normal heart size, or diffuse radiopacification, the lung may be underinflated. Therefore, if the mean airway pressure is low and the FiO_2 is high, the mean airway pressure should be increased. The assessment of cardiac function is also important for the safe use of high-frequency ventilation. Monitoring heart rate, blood pressure, urine output, and capillary refill can help to alert the care provider to changes in cardiac output.

138. **What adverse events have been reported with the use of high-frequency ventilation?**

Several studies have shown evidence of increased brain injury (i.e., periventricular leukomalacia and intraventricular hemorrhage) associated with high-frequency ventilation, particularly when initiated as an initial treatment modality in a VLBW baby. Although meta-analysis does not confirm this finding, the concern remains, and further studies are needed in this regard. Necrotizing tracheobronchitis was a complication reported with early models of high-frequency ventilation. This complication has disappeared with the development of improved humidification systems.

139. **What are the variables used to alter oxygenation during high-frequency ventilation?**
Altering mean airway pressure to optimal levels will change lung volume, improve ventilation-perfusion matching, and decrease intrapulmonary shunt. FiO_2 is used to change the alveolar oxygen concentration.

   In oscillatory ventilation, mean airway pressure can be altered directly by changing that setting on the ventilator. With jet ventilation, mean airway pressure is a measured value that is a combination of several factors: PIP, PEEP, duration of inspiratory phase (jet valve on time), and background sigh rate.

140. **Has high-frequency ventilation been conclusively shown to reduce the use of ECMO in neonates with MAS?**
No. Only anecdotal evidence exists to support the efficacy of high-frequency ventilation in neonates with MAS. In fact, in neonates with MAS and signs of air trapping, high-frequency ventilation may be dangerous. Reported success in MAS with high-frequency ventilation is about 30–40%.

141. **Theoretically, how does high-frequency ventilation prevent acute lung injury in hyaline membrane disease?**
Volutrauma occurs most rapidly when the lung is repeatedly cycled from a low volume to a high volume. Use of zero end-expiratory pressure and excessive tidal volumes can create acute lung injury within minutes. Application of end-expiratory pressure reduces "atelectotrauma" by preserving functional residual capacity at the end of each assisted breath. Lung overinflation is avoided by using small tidal volumes. Thus, the extremes of low and high lung volumes are avoided with high-frequency ventilation.

142. **What other tools are used in neonatology to promote better lung inflation and to reduce the injury associated with ventilating a collapsed lung?**
The use of end-expiratory pressure, surfactant, prone positioning, and liquid ventilation all promote lung recruitment over time. They work by stabilizing recruited alveoli at the end of exhalation.

143. **To use high-frequency ventilation safely, what factors must be carefully monitored?**
Hyperventilation must be avoided. Data on brain injury in neonates suggest that hyperventilation may cause brain injury through ischemia as CO_2 is lowered. This finding has been observed in a number of published studies, both with conventional and high-frequency ventilation.

   Lung over- or underinflation also may have adverse affects on the baby. Currently, no good methods are available for defining optimal lung volume during high-frequency ventilation. Evaluating cardiac performance, chest radiographs, and PaO_2/FiO_2 ratio can help the clinician avoid extremes, but the Holy Grail of high-frequency ventilation is defining when the lung is optimally inflated.

144. **In what pulmonary disease states has high-frequency ventilation been shown to promote improved oxygenation compared with conventional modes of ventilation?**
The most dramatic improvements in oxygenation have been reported in patients with poor lung inflation. In general, this means neonates with RDS or pneumonia. Lung disease in which there

is a significant amount of airway debris or resistance does not seem to respond as well to high-frequency ventilation.

NEONATAL EXTRACORPOREAL MEMBRANE OXYGENATION

145. What is ECMO?

ECMO is a modification of standard cardiopulmonary bypass techniques used in the operating room during open heart surgery. It was adapted in a simplified circuit to provide artificial life support to pulmonary patients in an intensive care unit setting. Neonatal ECMO was the first clinically successful application of this technology to treat severe and progressive cardio-respiratory failure caused by MAS and complicated by persistent pulmonary artery hypertension occurring in the first week of life. At the core of ECMO technology are the heart-lung pump (a semiocclusive roller device) and the innovative Kolobow polycarbonate-spooled, silicone membrane oxygenator (Fig. 16-14). Both devices are powerful enough to completely support cardiac output and lung function in neonates.

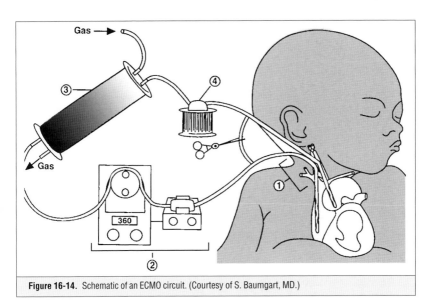

Figure 16-14. Schematic of an ECMO circuit. (Courtesy of S. Baumgart, MD.)

146. What is ECLS?

Extracorporeal life support (ECLS) includes ECMO, hemofiltration, hemodialysis, and indwelling oxygenator filaments (i.e., intravenous oxygenator). Many of these other techniques can be incorporated with an ECMO circuit or can be applied separately.

147. What evidence suggests that ECMO actually works?

The definitive randomized trial establishing the effectiveness of neonatal ECMO was conducted by the National Health Service in the United Kingdom. Thirty of 93 infants (32%) referred to ECMO centers died compared with 54 of 92 (59%) receiving conventional care. The relative risk for reduced mortality with ECMO was 0.55 (95% CI, 0.39–0.77; P < 0.0005). Of survivors, 1 child in each group was severely disabled at 1 year, and 10 ECMO patients (compared with 6 conventionally treated infants) were disabled to a lesser degree. The UK Collaborative ECMO

Trial Group concluded that ECMO support should be actively considered for mature neonates with severe but potentially reversible respiratory failure.

UK Collaborative ECMO Trial Group: UK collaborative randomised trial of neonatal extracorporeal membrane oxygenation. Lancet 348:75–82, 1996.

148. Who is a neonatal ECMO candidate?

ECMO's success relies on the physician's ability to recognize, within the first week of illness, those near-term or term newborn infants with reversible pulmonary disease and to exclude infants with irreversible pulmonary disease. The ECLS Organization's Registry data estimate that only 1 in about 1700 infants can benefit from ECMO. Criteria for ECMO patient selection have been widely debated during the past decade, and two controversial questions have arisen: (1) Is less invasive therapy likely to succeed? (2) With constantly improving neonatal ventilatory and pharmacologic techniques, must physicians continually reassess ECMO criteria? In general, the earlier the ECMO physician can identify the infant with a high probability of dying from his or her disease (before iatrogenic consequences of conventional therapy), the better the patient selection and outcome will be. The following inclusion and exclusion criteria provide general neonatal ECMO guidelines that are currently widely accepted:

- \>34 weeks' gestational age
- \>2.0 kg birth weight
- <2 weeks' postnatal age (or ≤10 days' high-pressure mechanical ventilation, relative age)
- Reversible cardiopulmonary condition
- No major cardiac malformation
- No syndromes with unsurvivable prognosis
- No uncontrollable bleeding diathesis (e.g., disseminated intravascular coagulation with bleeding uncontrolled despite multiple component transfusions or progressive parenchymal brain hemorrhage)
- No irrecoverable brain injury

149. What pulmonary indices are used to identify ECMO candidates?

Once the above inclusion and exclusion criteria have been considered, one of several pulmonary indices is used to assess the severity of respiratory illness and the likelihood of death if the infant is treated conventionally. The simplest and most popular index is the oxygenation index (OI) (Fig. 16-15). Briefly, the OI is equivalent to the mean airway pressure generated during mechanical ventilation multiplied by the FiO_2 (both of these values indicate the level of conventional ventilatory support) divided by the postductal arterial oxygen tension in the blood (a sensitive indicator of both ventilation and perfusion of the baby's lung). The resulting value is multiplied by 100. The relative importance of the ratio between mean airway pressure and arterial oxygen tension in the calculation of OI performed at 1.00 (FiO_2) is further demonstrated graphically in Fig. 16-15. Once the PaO_2 is below 40 mmHg in the denominator

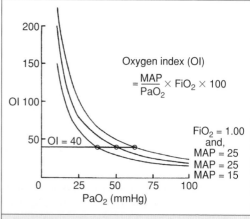

Figure 16-15. Oxygenation index versus PaO_2 and mean airway pressure (MAP).

of the OI equation, a geometric rise in OI occurs. This rise parallels increased pulmonary vascular resistance with increased right-to-left shunting in the patient with severe pulmonary arterial hypertension.

150. **How may vascular access for ECMO be achieved, and what are the benefits and liabilities of venoarterial (VA) versus venovenous (VV) bypass?**

VA bypass

The gold standard for ECMO therapy is VA bypass. An internal jugular drainage cannula and a second common carotid arterial infusion cannula are placed surgically through a right neck incision performed at the bedside. VA ECMO provides complete cardiopulmonary support to an infant's native heart and lungs when either or both are failing.

Advantages:

- Complete cardiopulmonary support
- Used for heart and lung failure
- Cardiac function not essential

Disadvantages:

- Carotid artery ligation
- Embolism (clot, air) infused into arterial circulation
- Potential hyperoxic reperfusion injury

VV bypass

A less invasive technique for augmenting systemic oxygenation using ECMO is VV bypass. In neonates, a novel double-lumen cannula (12 or 14 French) is surgically inserted into the internal jugular vein and positioned within the right atrium. Blood is withdrawn from the lateral lumen, reoxygenated, and infused back into the medial lumen. The right atrial admixture of oxygenated and deoxygenated blood then crosses through fetal channels (the foramen ovale and the ductus arteriosus) in the infant with severe pulmonary arterial hypertension to supply systemic oxygenation via shunt flow. Because systemic blood supply is delivered entirely by the infant's native left ventricle, sufficient ventricular force must be available to circulate this oxygenated admixture against systemic vascular resistance, which is usually increased in critically ill patients. Frequently, both cardiotonic pressors and generous volume infusions of saline, albumin, or plasma along with blood transfusions are required to maintain an infant's circulation on VV ECMO. VV access avoids invasion of the carotid artery; therefore, systemic embolism is less risky, and the right common carotid artery is left intact following decannulation from bypass.

Advantages:

- Spares carotid artery
- Embolism less risky
- One double-lumen cannula sufficient

Disadvantages:

- Less effective cardiac support
- Lower PaO_2 with mixing in right atrium
- Recirculation into double-lumen cannula
- Mixed venous saturation (SvO_2) and SaO_2 monitors unreliable; must follow PaO_2, pH to judge oxygen sufficiency

151. **What is the single most important parameter for monitoring the effectiveness of ECMO?**

SvO_2 from the jugular venous cannula drain is monitored continuously during bypass using a fiberoptic device inserted directly into the blood path coming out of the patient. SvO_2 does not so much reflect pulmonary function (as does the systemic arterial saturation) but represents the adequacy of tissue oxygen delivery from the native heart and the ECMO circuit combined. If the oxygen delivered by ECMO is enough to meet tissue oxygen demand, then the SvO_2 is generally >70%. Failure to meet tissue oxygen demand results in the progressive desaturation of venous

KEY POINTS: NEONATAL EXTRACORPOREAL MEMBRANE OXYGENATION

1. A definitive randomized trial established the effectiveness of neonatal ECMO. It showed that survival in neonates offered ECMO was better than in neonates receiving conventional care.

2. The relative risk reduction in mortality with ECMO was 0.55 (95% CI, 0.39–0.77; P < 0.0005). ECMO is one of the few therapies that has been shown to save the lives of critically ill neonates.

3. We should be careful not to place children at unnecessary risk by using therapies that have not been established to improve outcome.

blood returning from the capillary beds into the right atrium. An SvO_2 <65–70% indicates marginal oxygen delivery, and an SvO_2 <60% may be associated with lactic acid production through anaerobic metabolism. Therefore, the single most important parameter monitored during ECMO and used to assess the adequacy of bypass is the SvO_2. Notably, during VV ECMO, the SvO_2 may be artificially elevated because of recirculation of arterialized blood back into the drainage side of the double-lumen cannula; however, trends in SvO_2 may still be useful, and the patient may be taken off bypass briefly to assess a true SvO_2.

152. **How long do babies stay on bypass? How do you know when to wean ECMO flow?**

The average ECMO course typically proceeds over 3–7 days, awaiting spontaneous lung recovery. Cardiac recovery and mobilization of capillary leak edema usually precede lung recovery and weaning the ECMO pump flow rate. As the tissue edema is mobilized, fluid is transferred back into the intravascular space, increasing the baby's native cardiac output. Therefore, the infant's systemic arterial saturation and PaO_2 may actually decrease during recovery (as ECMO support is weaned and the infant's native cardiac output drives right-to-left shunting of deoxygenated blood through fetal channels in an accelerated fashion). During this early improvement phase on ECMO, diuretic therapy (e.g., furosemide, mannitol) or hemofiltration may assist in reducing this native circulation of desaturated blood. Thereafter, as the mixed venous saturation improves in the jugular venous cannula (above 80%), the ECMO pump flow is reduced in 10 mL/min decrements until a pump idle rate is reached of approximately 100-mL/min minimum flow (to prevent stasis and clotting within the circuit). Frequent arterial *and* venous blood gas assessments are important during the weaning process. Recent reports have suggested that pulmonary function testing demonstrating increased functional residual capacity (>15 mL/kg) and improved dynamic lung compliance may be useful in determining more exactly when lung recovery is sufficient to warrant coming off bypass.

NEONATAL LIQUID VENTILATION

153. **What is liquid ventilation?**

Liquid ventilation refers to the process of filling the lung with a "breathable" liquid through which gas exchange can take place. Perfluorochemicals are nontoxic, poorly absorbed, and capable of carrying respiratory gases. It is possible to breathe a perfluorochemical liquid, but because of the density and viscosity of the fluid, support from a ventilator is required.

The two forms of liquid ventilation generally discussed are partial liquid ventilation, in which a conventional ventilator is used on the liquid-filled lung, and total liquid ventilation, which uses a special liquid ventilator to push and pull tidal volumes of liquid.

154. **What is the effect of filling the lung with a liquid on lung compliance?**
Compliance markedly increases as surface tension is reduced to near zero. *Compliance* refers to the change in volume divided by the change in pressure ($C_L = \Delta V/\Delta P$). When the air-liquid interface is eliminated and replaced with a liquid-liquid interface, virtually all surface tension is eliminated, and the lung becomes significantly more compliant.

155. **Name some diseases that might benefit from liquid ventilation.**
   - RDS (improves compliance and recruits lung volume)
   - MAS (removes debris and recruits lung volume)
   - Pneumonia (removes debris, may be a vehicle to deliver drugs such as antibiotics)
   - Congenital malformations (may act as a good contrast medium for radiographs and magnetic nuclear imaging)

156. **How long has the technique of liquid ventilation been studied?**
Breathing liquids was introduced into the medical literature in the 1920s as a way to cleanse the lung after poisonous gas inhalation. Later, liquid ventilation was evaluated in animals to reduce surface tension in surfactant-deficient lungs and as a means to improve underwater diving for adults. In the last three decades, animal studies have been specifically directed at the clinical applications in the pathologic lung. Clinical trials began in 1989. Concerns over safety led to the FDA stopping all trials in neonates and children in the late 1990s, and there has not been any clinical research progress in the past 7 years.

157. **When will liquid ventilation be clinically available?**
A lot of work still needs to be done before this technique can be used widely to treat neonatal lung diseases. At present, there is little active clinical work because of safety concerns.

AIR LEAK SYNDROMES

158. **Which respiratory conditions in newborn infants have the highest incidence of air leak?**
Air leak occurs in 41% of babies with MAS, 27% with RDS, 10% with transient tachypnea, and 1–2% of all newborns. The reason for the increase with MAS is the viscosity of meconium, which results in a ball-valve mechanism that leads to air trapping. Newborns in general have a higher incidence of air leaks than the general population because of the high transpulmonary pressure (–30 to –150 cm H_2O) associated with the onset of breathing.

159. **What is the least common form of neonatal air leak syndrome?**
Fortunately, pneumopericardium is the least common, occurring in 2% of babies with air leak. Pneumopericardium must be recognized promptly because of its high morbidity and mortality. Interstitial emphysema is quite common (35%) and in many cases precedes other forms of air leak. Pneumothorax accounts for 20% of neonatal air leaks, and 3% of babies have a pneumo-mediastinum.

160. **Why has the incidence of neonatal air leak syndromes declined?**
One of the major factors has to be the "kinder, gentler" approach to neonatal ventilation. Permissive hypercapnia was all the rage of the 1990s and has led to more conservative ventilatory management strategies.

A second important change was the introduction of surfactant replacement therapy in the later 1980s. Most of the early surfactant trials documented about a 30–50% reduction in the rate of neonatal air leaks.

161. **You are called to the bedside of a baby who has suddenly become cyanotic while on a ventilator. You listen to the chest, and you hear better breath sounds on the right side. You call for a chest radiograph, but the x-ray technician is on a break. Neither the senior resident nor the neonatologist is available, and you are on your own. What do you suspect, and how do you tell whether you are correct?**

    Your suspicion should be high for a tension pneumothorax in this clinical situation. Before you place a needle into the chest, however, consider the following:

    You could transilluminate the chest with a high-intensity fiberoptic light. If a pneumothorax is present, the left side should "light up," whereas the right will transilluminate less.

    Also, check the position of the ET tube. Make sure it is in good position and has not changed (look at the numeric value of the ET tube and compare with where it is supposed to be). If there is evidence that the position of the ET tube has changed and it is out or has been pushed in too far, secure the airway and make sure it is in appropriate position. If the acute deterioration is due to ET tube malposition, repositioning of the tube should lead to rapid improvement in gas exchange. Repositioning that does not lead to improvement supports the diagnosis of air leak as a possible cause for the deterioration.

162. **A baby is breathing asynchronously on a conventional ventilator, and you are concerned that she is at risk for a pneumothorax. Name some things you can do to decrease the risk of air leak in this patient.**

    - Increasing the gas temperature may slightly decrease the incidence of air leak.
    - Decreasing the inspiratory time will decrease mean airway pressure and could decrease the risk of pneumothorax, but it may reduce oxygenation.
    - Increasing the ventilatory rate may allow you to take over ventilation and decrease the baby's effort, but you need to watch for air trapping.
    - Use of a synchronized mode of ventilation (SIMV or A/C) will help the baby to breathe with the ventilator breaths.
    - Sedation and pain relief may help significantly.
    - Paralytic agents such as pancuronium prevent pneumothorax in premature babies who are actively expiring against positive pressure ventilation, but these should be used as a last resort.

163. **Name several possible ways to treat unilateral pulmonary interstitial emphysema.**

    The primary goal of treatment of unilateral pulmonary interstitial emphysema is to allow the affected lung to deflate. Selective bronchial intubation will allow the contralateral lung to deflate (of course, selective left mainstem intubation may be technically difficult), but it may pose problems because the perfusion to the ventilated lung may not be sufficient for gas exchange in all cases. A randomized trial of high-frequency jet ventilation did show effectiveness in treating pulmonary interstitial emphysema by lowering the mean airway pressure, which may allow the emphysema to resolve. In infants, the lung in the superior position will receive more of the ventilation. Placing the affected lung in the downward position may be helpful in deflating that lung.

164. **What important sign distinguishes a tension pneumothorax from one without tension?**

    There is no specific sign. In a tension pneumothorax, an ongoing air leak contributes to a progressive increase in intrathoracic pressure. Shift of the trachea or the point of maximal impulse, decreased breath sounds, pallor, or cyanosis and retractions may occur in either tension or nontension pneumothorax. In a tension pneumothorax, the critical factor is the ongoing increase in cardiopulmonary embarrassment to the patient. In most instances, when a pneumothorax is first detected, it is very difficult to tell whether a pneumothorax is under tension. If the child appears clinically stable for the moment, one can wait for a period of time (30–60 minutes) and repeat a chest radiograph before a chest tube is inserted. In some cases, however, one cannot wait, and a thoracentesis must be done immediately.

165. **Why do neonates have an increased susceptibility to alveolar rupture?**
Neonates are subject to air leaks because of uneven alveolar ventilation in RDS or MAS. Air trapping also frequently occurs because of small airway plugs. The areas that are more distensible receive more ventilation, which leads to high transpulmonary pressure that, in turn, increases the likelihood of alveolar rupture. An additional factor is that the neonate has fewer alveolar connecting channels (pores of Kohn), which allow air to redistribute between ventilated and nonventilated alveolar spaces. Lastly, resuscitation by an overzealous, inexperienced practitioner also increases the newborn's susceptibility to air leaks.

166. **Where do you place a chest tube for best drainage of an air leak?**
Ideally, one wants to place a chest tube in the thoracic cavity where it will do the most good with the least risk to the infant. Positioning of the infant is the key to the entire procedure. All too commonly, the baby is allowed to remain supine. When one enters the chest in that position, the catheter hits the lung and moves posteriorly (Fig. 16-16). If the child, however, is placed nearly vertical to start the procedure, it is easy to angle the catheter anteriorly for optimal placement. The thoracostomy tube is inserted through an incision made in the fifth interspace in the midaxillary line. After the incision is made, one tunnels up an interspace with a hemostat, which is used to pop through the strong muscular wall of the chest (yes, it is tough even in a tiny premature infant!). If a pneumothorax is present, a gush of air should be seen when the chest is opened. The catheter should be advanced so that no end holes lie outside the chest wall. If the catheter is inserted too far, it must be pulled back. The chest tube is then connected to a suction apparatus. The suction rarely needs to be greater than −10 to −15 cm H_2O. Noisy bubbling from the drainage apparatus at the bedside from high wall suction is also unnecessary.

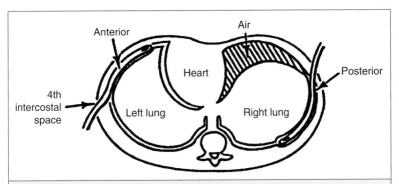

Figure 16-16. Appropriate chest tube placement is shown of the left side of the figure, with the chest tube in the proper position to reach the air that sits in the superior part of the thorax. On the right side of the figure, the chest tube has migrated to a posterior position, preventing it from evacuating the air lying superiorly.

167. **Why should the second intercostal space be avoided for chest tube placement?**
The use of anterior catheter insertions in the second interspace is not advocated, except in rare circumstances. It is too easy to hit the breast bud, which may damage future breast development or leave unsightly scars in any patient.

168. **How can renal malformations increase the likelihood of pneumothorax in newborns?**

Obstructive uropathies lead to oligohydramnios. Insufficient amniotic fluid volume leads to pulmonary hypoplasia. The mechanism is not completely understood but in part is due to external compression of the neonate's thorax that impedes fetal lung growth. It is also believed that fetal breathing movements against an intrauterine fluid volume may be critical for normal lung development.

169. **A term infant with a nontension air leak may be treated by placing him/her in 100% oxygen. Explain how this works.**

The air in a spontaneous or nontension pneumothorax will have the same nitrogen concentration as room air. By allowing the baby to breathe pure oxygen, a gradient for nitrogen is created from the extrapulmonary to the intrapulmonary spaces. Nitrogen will naturally diffuse across this gradient, allowing the pneumothorax to reabsorb more rapidly. Caution should be used when considering this approach in preterm infants, who are more subject to oxidant injury.

BRONCHOPULMONARY DYSPLASIA

170. **What is BPD?**

BPD is the chronic lung disease that often follows RDS in VLBW babies. First described by Northway in 1967, it has become the greatest foe of all neonatologists and the focal point of perhaps more studies than any other clinical syndrome in neonatology. BPD was not a disease until the neonate became a patient. Once people attempted to save critically ill neonates with lung disease, a certain percentage developed BPD. In most nurseries, the BPD rate is about 30% in infants <1500 gm. The more immature the infant, the more likely it is that BPD will develop. BPD is defined as a need for oxygen at either 28 days of life or, more recently, at 36 weeks postconception, with radiographic changes consistent with chronic lung disease. Recent studies have also emphasized the fact that the rate of BPD can be influenced by the degree of hypoxemia one is willing to tolerate. If a child's saturation in room air is only 90%, a nursery staff that decides to supplement the inspired oxygen in that situation will have a higher BPD rate than one that tolerates saturations of 90%.

Northway WH Jr, Rosan RC, Porter DY: Pulmonary disease following respirator therapy of hyaline membrane disease. N Engl J Med 276:357–368, 1967.

171. **What are the histopathologic features of BPD in the lungs of newborn infants?**

In a series of open lung biopsies from VLBW infants aged 14 days to 7 weeks who were receiving ventilatory support with radiographic changes consistent with chronic lung disease, Coalson and colleagues described a consistent lack of alveolarization with variably widened alveolar septae and minimal changes in the airways. Mild to moderate septal fibrosis was also apparent. These widened alveolar septae were hypercellular with disordered capillary growth. Typically, the alveolar spaces were laden with numerous alveolar macrophages and neutrophils.

Transmission electron microscopy demonstrated poor differentiation of type I and type II lung epithelial cells. These epithelial cells had relatively abundant cytoplasm and extensive glycogen stores; however, lamellar bodies were extremely rare to totally absent. There was no progression of alveolarization with enlarged simplified terminal airspaces or minimal and focal saccular fibroplasia. The interstitium of the lung contained myofibroblasts, and there was focal deposition of elastin and collagen fibers. Most saccular walls showed blunted "outpouchings" or secondary crest formation.

Coalson I, Kuehl T, Prihoda T, et al: Diffuse alveolar damage in the evolution of bronchopulmonary dysplasia in the baboon. Pediatr Res 24:357–366, 1988.

Coalson JJ, Winter VT, Siler KT, et al: Neonatal chronic lung disease in extremely immature baboons. Am J Respir Crit Care Med 160:1333–1346, 1999.

172. **How does BPD develop?**
The etiology of BPD is not clear, but several factors likely contribute to its development (the six Ps of BPD):
1. Prematurity
2. Positive pressure ventilation
3. Prolonged oxygen exposure
4. Protracted use of ET tubes
5. Pulmonary edema (from a patent ductus arteriosus, overhydration, or delayed diuresis)
6. Pulmonary air leak (e.g., interstitial emphysema, pneumothorax)

Other factors, such as free oxygen radical exposure and sepsis, also seem to be contributory in many instances. Sepsis, in particular, has recently become an increasingly important piece of the puzzle of BPD. The key to this disease, however, appears to be the chronic exposure that babies have to the six Ps.

In extremely-low-birth-weight infants, BPD appears to be due to a combination of nutritional failure and failure of alveolarization, resulting in both diminished somatic and lung growth. These factors lead to oxygen and ventilator dependency in a manner different from the original etiology of BPD.

173. **One of your patients is now being treated with dexamethasone for BPD. The child is receiving a 6-week course of therapy. Should you be concerned about adrenal suppression when treatment is discontinued?**
Adrenal suppression in newborns usually does not seem to pose as many problems as it does in older children or adults. After 30 days, however, there is a high likelihood of some adrenal insufficiency. It may therefore be better to try to limit steroid use to less than 14 days, which seems to have a lesser effect on adrenal suppression. If longer courses are used, however, some of the effects can be minimized by giving every-other-day treatment for the last week or two.

174. **Do steroids administered postnatally have an adverse effect on the nervous system?**
Both animal and human studies indicate that chronic steroid use may result in reduced amounts of neural tissue mass. Neurologic handicap rates are higher in infants treated with dexamethasone. Somatic growth may also be adversely affected.

Yeh TF, Lin YJ, Lin HC, et al: Outcomes at school age after postnatal dexamethasone therapy for lung disease of prematurity. N Engl J Med 350:1304–1313, 2004.

175. **Why can a child recover from BPD, but an adult cannot repair the lung injury seen in emphysema?**
Children continue to add new alveoli until approximately 8 years of age. After that time, surface area and volume within the lung continue to increase with growth, but new alveoli are no longer added. Although scarring does occur in the lungs of patients with BPD, there appears to be sufficient healthy tissue to regenerate an adequate new alveolar volume.

176. **What other treatments besides steroids help in the treatment of BPD?**
The key to recovery from BPD is growth of alveoli and overall growth. As a result, optimal nutritional support is critical in BPD, perhaps more than anything else. Other therapeutic adjuncts that help are:
- Optimal ventilator management
- Provision of optimal PEEP for tracheobronchomalacia
- Bronchodilators
- Fluid restriction (it is difficult in neonates to give many calories and restrict fluids at the same time!)
- Diuretic therapy
- Chloride supplementation to prevent metabolic alkalosis from diuretics

- Prompt closure of a patent ductus arteriosus, if present
- Methylxanthines (both caffeine and theophylline decrease work of breathing and apnea)
- Sedation and pain relief

177. What are BPD spells? How should they be treated?

BPD spells are acute episodes of deterioration encountered during the course of treatment of a child with BPD. The baby typically becomes increasingly cyanotic, agitated, and inconsolable, with a marked deterioration in overall pulmonary status. Oxygen and ventilatory assistance often need to be increased during these episodes. They may, at times, be very acute and severe and occasionally result in sudden death.

BPD spells frustrate even the best of neonatologists with respect to their management. Bronchospasm is often cited as the cause of this deterioration, but our personal experience suggests that many such episodes, especially the more acute, severe forms, are more commonly the result of airway collapse from tracheobronchomalacia. Increasing the PEEP to stabilize an airway (assuming the child is intubated) can be beneficial in such cases. Computerized pulmonary function testing readily allows determination of optimal PEEP in this clinical situation. If one does suspect bronchospasm, prebronchodilator and postbronchodilator therapy can be evaluated with pulmonary function testing. Flexible fiberoptic bronchoscopy is also valuable to detect granulomas that might be causing airway obstruction.

178. Why are chlorothiazide and spironolactone preferred as diuretics in BPD as opposed to furosemide? Isn't furosemide a more powerful diuretic?

There is no question that furosemide is a more potent diuretic than either chlorothiazide or spironolactone. In chronic situations such as BPD in a neonate, however, calcium sparing is important to prevent rickets, and thiazide diuretics are thought to be more effective in this regard. Spironolactone helps prevent potassium loss and reduces the severity of metabolic alkalosis from diuretics. It is always a good idea, however, to initiate potassium chloride supplementation whenever diuretics are initiated for BPD, because so many of these children develop a significant metabolic alkalosis. Furosemide also has a greater tendency to produce nephrocalcinosis when used on a chronic basis, which is less likely to occur with thiazide diuretics.

APNEA OF PREMATURITY

179. What is apnea of prematurity?

Apnea is the cessation of breathing. Although this problem affects people of all ages in many different forms, it is most prevalent in premature infants of <36 weeks' gestation. *Pathologic apnea* refers to cessation of breathing for >20 seconds; cessation of breathing for <20 seconds and accompanied by bradycardia 20% below the baseline heart rate; or cessation of breathing for <20 seconds with oxygen desaturation below 80%. Apnea in a newborn is classified as central, obstructive, or mixed. Most apnea of prematurity is classified as central apnea (Fig. 16-17), in which there is complete absence of respiratory effort. Obstructive apnea occurs when an infant makes a respiratory effort but no airflow is present because of the presence of obstruction (*see* Fig. 16-17, bottom). Obstructive apnea can be associated with gastroesophageal reflux. Mixed apnea is a combination of central and obstructive apnea.

180. What is periodic breathing?

Periodic breathing is a type of central apnea characterized by brief pauses in breathing of <10 seconds, followed by periods of regular respiration of <20 seconds' duration. This pattern repeats itself for at least three cycles and often many more times (Fig. 16-18). The significance of this form of breathing is unknown at present. Many prematurely born infants demonstrate periodic breathing for as much as 20–30% of total sleep time. Because of the frequency of this finding, some neonatologists consider periodic breathing to be a normal maturational process.

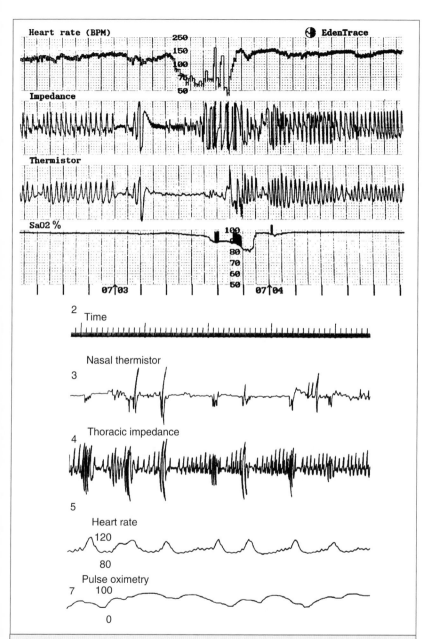

Figure 16-17. An episode of central apnea, with bradycardia and oxygen desaturation *(top)*. An episode of obstructive apnea with recurring desaturation *(bottom)*.

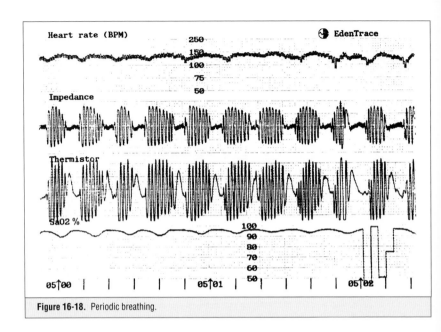

Figure 16-18. Periodic breathing.

On the other hand, it also may be a reflection of significant immaturity of respiratory control and a variant of apnea.

181. What is the incidence of apnea of prematurity?

Virtually all premature infants have some degree of apnea. At 34–35 weeks' postconceptional age, about 65% of infants have demonstrable apnea. About two thirds of these children have central apnea or periodic breathing, and one third have obstructive or mixed apnea.

182. What is the significance of apnea of prematurity?

In the short term, particularly in the intensive care nursery, extremely premature infants can have prolonged apneic episodes that may be fatal. As they mature, most infants will have more self-limited episodes. Less clear are the long-term effects on infants who have had a history of severe apnea of prematurity. New studies suggest apnea of prematurity, particularly with oxygen desaturation, may affect learning and other aspects of childhood development.

Hunt CE, Corwin MJ, Baird T, et al: Cardiorespiratory events detected by home memory monitoring and one-year neurodevelopmental outcome. J Pediatr 145:465–471, 2004.

Mattia FR, deRegnier RA: Chronic physiologic instability is associated with neurodevelopmental morbidity at one and two years in extremely premature infants. Pediatrics 102:E35, 1998.

183. When does apnea of prematurity resolve?

Although the majority of apnea of prematurity is gone by 37 weeks' postconceptional age, in many cases it can persist even beyond 45 weeks' postconceptional age (and occasionally longer). Recent evidence indicates that apnea persists longest in the most immature infants.

184. Does apnea of prematurity need treatment?

In the most severe cases, infants with severe apnea of prematurity may need ET intubation and mechanical ventilation, CPAP, or oxygen therapy. Some infants may require methylxanthines (caffeine or theophylline) to control apnea. Caffeine is the preferred treatment because of its once-a-day dosing and fewer side effects. Patients are typically loaded with 20 mg/kg of caffeine citrate and maintained on 7–8 mg/kg/day. The therapeutic range is between 12 and 20 μg/mL. Some patients may be controlled at very low serum levels (under 5 μg/mL), whereas others need to be near or above 20 μg/mL. At our institution, caffeine is maintained until the infant weighs >1500 gm and stays apnea free for 5 days. At that point, the medication is discontinued. The half-life of caffeine is over 100 hours, and the level drops slowly. In rare instances, infants develop apnea after caffeine discontinuation, and it may need to be restarted.

185. Do premature infants with apnea need to be discharged with home monitors?
Home cardiorespiratory monitoring is a technology developed in the 1970s after several studies suggested a possible relationship between apnea and SIDS. Since that time, hundreds of thousands of premature infants have been discharged with these monitors. Although anecdotal evidence has shown that these devices are effective in decreasing SIDS, no large, controlled study has demonstrated this conclusively.

SUDDEN INFANT DEATH SYNDROME

186. What is SIDS?
SIDS is unexpected death of an infant younger than 1 year that remains unexplained after a thorough autopsy, history, and investigation of the scene of the death. It was given the name *SIDS* in 1969. Although people of all ages die suddenly, the rate of sudden death is highest under 1 year of age. The 1-year cutoff has been arbitrarily assigned; in actuality, the overwhelming majority of SIDS deaths occur before 6 months of life.

187. How many infants die of SIDS each year?
In the United States, there were about 3000 deaths from SIDS in 1998. This represents a rate of approximately 0.75 deaths from SIDS per 1000 live births. The peak age of SIDS is 2–5 months. The rate is substantially higher in urban areas, particularly among African-American infants. Interestingly, the SIDS rates in the Hispanic and Asian populations are equal to or lower than that of the white population in the United States. In the developed nations of Europe and Asia, SIDS rates are slightly lower than in the United States. SIDS rates are also lower in Australia and New Zealand.

188. Has the rate of SIDS changed since 30 years ago, when it was first recognized as an entity?
The SIDS rate slowly declined from 1985 to 1994, then it began to drop precipitously from about 2 deaths per 1000 births in 1992 to the present 0.55 per 1000 births. This rapid decline paralleled the institution of the "Back to Sleep" campaign, sponsored by the National Institutes of Health, the SIDS Alliance, and the American Academy of Pediatrics. This initiative followed the discovery that the simple act of changing infants' sleeping positions from the stomach to the back in England and Australia was responsible for a dramatic reduction in the SIDS rate. The rate of infants sleeping on their backs has risen from 15% to over 70% in the past 5 years in the United States. It is likely that the SIDS rate will decrease even lower as more and more infants sleep on their backs.

189. How did such a simple change have such a great effect?
Good question! In medicine, as in all aspects of life, uncomplicated and elegant observations can make great differences. Although the exact physiology is unclear, it is likely that sleeping on the back reduces the re-breathing of carbon dioxide, adjusts the position of the airway, thus reducing obstruction, or reduces the possibility of poor oxygenation-ventilation through the

mattress. The effects on the baby's thermal environment and the ability to eliminate heat may also be important.

190. **Is SIDS a form of child abuse?**
There has been a great deal of publicity about infants originally diagnosed with SIDS who were ultimately found to be the victims of a homicidal parent. These children included the case that established the supposed link between SIDS and apnea. Again, like many things in the news, this represents an extremely small number of cases and is the exception rather than the rule. Although it is impossible to quantify, it is thought that less than 2% of SIDS cases are probable homicides.

KEY POINTS: SUDDEN INFANT DEATH SYNDROME

1. The SIDS rate in the United States has dropped precipitously from about 2 deaths per 1000 births in 1992 to the present 0.55 per 1000 births.

2. This rapid decline paralleled the institution of the "Back to Sleep" campaign, sponsored by the National Institutes of Health, the SIDS Alliance, and the American Academy of Pediatrics.

3. This initiative followed the discovery (in England and Australia) that the simple act of changing infants' sleeping positions from the stomach to the back was responsible for a dramatic reduction in the SIDS rate.

191. **What are the risk factors for SIDS?**
The greatest known risks for SIDS appear to be prone sleeping and maternal smoking, both prenatally and postnatally. The American Academy of Pediatrics' "Back to Sleep" program, which encourages parents to put their infants to sleep lying on their backs, has led to a decrease in the number of SIDS cases reported in the United States. Other apparent risk factors include African-American race, low socioeconomic status, young maternal age, winter season, and prematurity. More recently, some evidence has suggested that there are genetic markers for SIDS in some families. The SIDS rate for premature infants is about 2.25 times that for term infants. Infants with apnea of prematurity are at no greater risk for SIDS than premature infants without apnea of prematurity.

LUNG ABNORMALITIES

192. **What are the different types of congenital cystic lesions of the lung?**
Congenital cystic lesions of the lung generally include those diseases that result from a problem in the formation of mesodermal and ectodermal tissue during lung development. These lesions include pulmonary sequestrations, congenital cystic adenomatoid malformations, congenital lobar emphysema, and bronchogenic pulmonary cysts.

193. **What is the most common congenital lung malformation?**
Pulmonary sequestration is thought to be the most common congenital lung malformation. A pulmonary sequestration is an area of nonfunctioning lung tissue with no connection to the tracheobronchial tree but with a systemic arterial supply. Pulmonary sequestrations can be diagnosed antenatally. They can be asymptomatic in the newborn or can cause respiratory distress caused by lung compression or congestive heart failure. Resection is generally recommended, even if asymptomatic, to reduce secondary risk of recurrent infection.

194. **How are pulmonary sequestrations classified?**

Pulmonary sequestrations are either extralobar or intrapulmonary. Extralobar pulmonary sequestrations include lesions with lung tissue surrounded by its own pleura. Intrapulmonary sequestrations, also known as *intralobar sequestrations*, have no discernible pleural tissue.

195. **What is a congenital cystic adenomatoid malformation of the lung? How does it generally present?**

Congenital cystic adenomatoid malformation originates as an adenomatous growth in the terminal bronchioles early in gestation. In most cases, there is a connection with the tracheobronchial tree that causes these lesions to increase in size. Only one lobe of the lung is usually involved. Congenital cystic adenomatoid malformations are now frequently diagnosed in the antenatal period by sonography. The most common presentation in the postnatal period is respiratory distress. Surgical removal of the affected lobe is the treatment of choice.

196. **What is the most common cause of mortality from congenital lung malformations?**

PPHN. Lung malformations such as congenital diaphragmatic hernia and congenital cystic adenomatoid malformation can lead to lung hypoplasia and concomitant PPHN. Recent efforts have been made to identify infants at greatest risk of mortality who might be candidates for fetal surgical intervention.

197. **When are congenital lung malformations diagnosed in the antenatal period? What are some poor prognostic signs?**

The presence of nonimmune hydrops fetalis, shift of the mediastinum, bilateral lesions, and the presence of other associated congenital abnormalities all portend a poor prognosis for infants with congenital lung lesions.

198. **Are there any congenital lung malformations that have been successfully treated antenatally?**

Congenital cystic adenomatoid malformation has been treated with some success in the antenatal period. Antenatal surgical repair of congenital cystic adenomatoid malformations is generally limited to infants with fetal hydrops. One series of 13 infants had 8 survivors; 5 infants died in the intraoperative or perioperative period. In all survivors, resection of the malformation led to resolution of fetal hydrops and increased lung growth. The principal operative concern is the initiation of maternal labor. Antenatal treatment of congenital diaphragmatic hernia has been ineffective.

199. **What is the cause of congenital lobar emphysema?**

Congenital lobar emphysema is caused by antenatal bronchial obstruction. This obstruction can be either intrinsic or extrinsic to the bronchiole and causes an overinflation of the pulmonary lobe. Intraluminal obstruction can result from a cartilaginous deficiency or inflammatory changes. Extrinsic causes include compression from an adjacent vascular structure or mass. Infants can present with respiratory distress or be asymptomatic in the newborn period. This lesion is more common in males, is usually seen in the left upper lobe, and is frequently associated with other congenital abnormalities of the heart and kidney. The treatment of congenital lobar emphysema is usually lobectomy.

200. **What is a bronchogenic cyst?**

A bronchogenic cyst results from abnormal budding of bronchial tissue during development. Bronchogenic cysts are single unilocular lesions of 2–10 cm in diameter. The cysts may or may not communicate with the remainder of the tracheobronchial tree. Bronchogenic cysts can be found in the mediastinum or in the peripheral lung tissue. Mediastinal cysts are thought to arise earlier in the development than those found in the periphery. Bronchogenic cysts can be asymptomatic at birth and may not present until adulthood. Other lesions are symptomatic from compression or infection. Surgical resection is generally recommended.

BIBLIOGRAPHY

NEONATAL RESUSCITATION

1. American Heart Association/American Academy of Pediatrics Neonatal Resuscitation Program Steering Committee: Textbook of Neonatal Resuscitation. Elk Grove Village, IL, AAP, 2003.
2. Jain L, Keenan W (eds): Resuscitation of the fetus and newborn. Clin Perinatol 26:549–792, 1999.
3. Saugstad OD, Ramji S, Irani SF, et al: Resuscitation of newborn infants with 21% or 100% oxygen: Follow-up at 18 to 24 months. Pediatrics 112:296–300, 2003.

TRANSITIONAL PHYSIOLOGY AND THE ASPHYXIATED FETUS

4. Donn SM, Faix RG: Delivery room resuscitation. In Spitzer AR (ed): Intensive Care of the Fetus and Neonate. St. Louis, Mosby, 1996, pp 326–336.
5. Donn SM, Faix RG: Special procedures used in resuscitation. In Donn SM (ed): The Michigan Manual: A Guide to Neonatal Intensive Care, 2nd ed. Armonk, NY, Futura Publishing, 1997, pp 10–17.
6. Faix RG, Donn SM: General principles. In Donn SM (ed): The Michigan Manual: A Guide to Neonatal Intensive Care, 2nd ed. Armonk, NY, Futura Publishing, 1997, pp 5–9.
7. Rennie JM: Neonatal resuscitation. In Sinha SK, Donn SM (eds): Manual of Neonatal Respiratory Care. Armonk, NY, Futura Publishing, 2000, pp 101–105.

RESPIRATORY DISTRESS SYNDROME

8. American Academy of Pediatrics Committee on the Fetus and Newborn: Surfactant replacement therapy for respiratory distress syndrome. Pediatrics 103:684–685, 1999.
9. Kendig JW, Ryan RM, Sinkin RA, et al: Comparison of two strategies for surfactant prophylaxis in very premature infants: A multicenter, randomized trial. Pediatrics 101:1006–1012, 1998.

MECONIUM–STAINED AMNIOTIC FLUID AND MECONIUM ASPIRATION SYNDROME

10. Cleary GM, Wiswell TE: Meconium-stained fluid and the meconium aspiration syndrome: An update. Pediatr Clin North Am 45:511–529, 1998.
11. Cochrane CG, Revak S, Merritt TA, et al: Bronchoalveolar lavage with KL4-surfactant in models of meconium aspiration syndrome. Pediatr Res 44:705–715, 1998.
12. Findaly RD, Taeusch HW, Walther FJ: Surfactant replacement therapy for meconium aspiration syndrome. Pediatrics 97:48–52, 1996.
13. Lam BCC, Yeung CY: Surfactant lavage for meconium aspiration syndrome: A pilot study. Pediatrics 103:1014–1018, 1999.
14. Miller PW, Coen RW, Benirschke K: Dating the time interval from meconium passage to birth. Obstet Gynecol 66:459–462, 1985.
15. Moses D, Holm B, Spitale P, et al: Inhibition of pulmonary surfactant function by meconium. Am J Obstet Gynecol 164:477–481, 1991.
16. Wiswell TE, Fuloria M: Resuscitation of the meconium-stained infant. Clin Perinatol 26:659–668, 1999.
17. Wiswell TE, Knight GR, Finer NN, et al: A multicenter, randomized, controlled trial comparing Surfaxin lavage with standard care for treatment of meconium aspiration syndrome. Pediatrics 109:1081–1087, 2002.
18. Vain NE, Szyld EG, Prudent LM, et al: Oropharyngeal and nasopharyngeal suctioning of meconium-stained neonates before delivery of their shoulders: Multicentre, randomised controlled trial. Lancet 364:597–602, 2004.

PULMONARY HYPERTENSION AND INHALED NITRIC OXIDE

19. Clark RH, Kueser TJ, Walker MW, et al: Low-dose nitric oxide therapy for persistent pulmonary hypertension of the newborn. Clinical Inhaled Nitric Oxide Research Group. N Engl J Med 342:469–474, 2000.

20. Fineman J, Heymann MM, Morin FC 3rd: Persistent pulmonary hypertension in the newborn. In Allen HD, Gutgesell HP, Clark EB, Driscoll DJ (eds): Moss and Adams' Heart Disease in Infants, Children, and Adolescents. Baltimore, MD, Lippincott Williams & Wilkins, 2000.

21. Finer NN, Barrington KJ: Nitric oxide for respiratory failure in infants born at or near term. Cochrane Database Syst Rev 2:CD000399, 2001.

22. Hallman M, Waffarin F, Bry K, et al: Surfactant dysfunction after inhalation of nitric oxide. J Appl Physiol 30:2026–2034, 1996.

23. Hansen T, Corbet A: Disorders of transition. In Taeusch HW, Ballard RA (eds): Avery's Diseases of the Newborn, 7th ed. Philadelphia, W.B. Saunders, 1998, pp 498–514.

24. Hedrick MH, Ferro MM, Filly RA, et al: Congenital high airway obstruction syndrome (CHAOS): A potential for perinatal intervention. J Pediatr Surg 29:271–274, 1994.

25. Kinsella JP, Abman SH: Inhaled nitric oxide: Current and future uses in neonates. Semin Perinatol 24:387–395, 2000.

26. Kinsella JP, Shaffer F, Neish SR, et al: Low-dose inhalational nitric oxide in persistent pulmonary hypertension of the newborn. Lancet 340:8819–8820, 1992.

27. Liechty KW, Crumbleholme TM: Management of fetal airway obstruction. Semin Perinatol 23:496–506, 1999.

28. Moerman P, Fryns JP, Goddeeris P, Lauweryns JM: Multiple ankyloses, facial anomalies, and pulmonary hypoplasia associated with severe antenatal spinal muscular atrophy. J Pediatr 103:238–241, 1983.

29. Neonatal Inhaled Nitric Oxide Study Group: Inhaled nitric oxide and hypoxic respiratory failure in infants with congenital diaphragmatic hernia. Pediatrics 99:838–845, 1997.

30. NINOS Study Group: Inhaled nitric oxide for near-term infants with respiratory failure. N Engl J Med 336:602–605, 1997.

31. Robbins CG, Davis JM, Merritt TA, et al: Combined effects of nitric oxide and hyperoxia on surfactant function and pulmonary inflammation. Am J Physiol 269:L545–L550, 1995.

32. Roberts JD Jr, Fineman JR, Morin FC 3rd, et al: Inhaled nitric oxide and persistent pulmonary hypertension of the newborn. The Inhaled Nitric Oxide Study Group. N Engl J Med 336:605–610, 1997.

33. Roberts JD, Zapol WM: Inhaled nitric oxide. Semin Perinatol 24:55–58, 2000.

34. Shokeir MHK: Multiple ankyloses, camptodactyly, facial anomalies, and pulmonary hypoplasia (Pena-Shokeir syndrome). In Vinken PJ, Bruyn GW (eds): Handbook of Clinical Neurology. Amsterdam, North Holland Publishers, 1982, pp 437–439.

35. Van Meurs KP, Rhine WD, Asselin JM, Durand DJ: Response of premature infants with severe respiratory distress to inhaled nitric oxide. Pediatr Pulmonol 24:319–332, 1997.

36. Whitsett JA, Pryhuber OS, Rice WR, et al: Acute respiratory disorders. In Avery GB, Fletcher MA, MacDonald MG (eds): Neonatology: Pathophysiology and Management of the Newborn, 4th ed. Philadelphia, Lippincott Williams & Wilkins, 1999, pp 405–508.

CONVENTIONAL MECHANICAL VENTILATION OF THE NEONATE

37. Carlo WA, Martin RJ: Principles of assisted ventilation. Pediatr Clin North Am 33:221–327, 1986.

38. Clark RH, Gerstmann DR, Jobe AH, et al: Lung injury in neonates: Causes, strategies for prevention, and long-term consequences. J Pediatr 139:478–486, 2001.

39. Goldsmith JP, Karotkin EH (eds): Assisted Ventilation of the Neonate. Philadelphia, W.B. Saunders, 2004.

NEONATAL HIGH-FREQUENCY VENTILATION

40. Clark RH: High-frequency ventilation. J Pediatr 124:661–670, 1994.

41. Clark RH, Dykes FD, Bachman TE, Ashurst JT: Intraventricular hemorrhage and high-frequency ventilation: A meta-analysis of prospective clinical trials. Pediatrics 98:1058–1061, 1996.

42. Courtney SE, Durand DJ, Asselin JM, et al: High-frequency oscillatory ventilation versus conventional mechanical ventilation for very-low-birth-weight infants. N Engl J Med 347:643–652, 2002.

43. Dreyfuss O, Saumon G: Role of tidal volume, FRC, and end-inspiratory volume in the development of pulmonary edema following mechanical ventilation. Am Rev Respir Dis 148:1194–1203, 1993.

44. Froese AB, Bryan AC: High-frequency ventilation. Am Rev Respir Dis 135:1363–1374, 1987.

45. Froese AB, McCulloch PR, Sugiura M, et al: Optimizing alveolar expansion prolongs the effectiveness of exogenous surfactant therapy in the adult rabbit. Am Rev Respir Dis 148:569–577, 1993.

46. Gerstmann DR, Fouke JM, Winter DC, et al: Proximal, tracheal, and alveolar pressures during high-frequency oscillatory ventilation in a normal rabbit model. Pediatr Res 28:367–373, 1990.

47. Johnson AH, Peacock JL, Greenough A, et al: High-frequency oscillatory ventilation for the prevention of chronic lung disease of prematurity. N Engl J Med 347:633–642, 2002.

48. Meredith KS, deLemos IRA, Coalson JJ, et al: Role of lung injury in the pathogenesis of hyaline membrane disease in premature baboons. J Appl Physiol 66:2150–2158, 1989.

49. Michna J, Jobe AH, Ikegami M: Positive end-expiratory pressure preserves surfactant function in preterm lambs. Am J Respir Crit Care Med 160:634–639, 1999.

50. Spitzer AR: High-frequency jet ventilation. In Spitzer AR (ed): Intensive Care of the Fetus and Neonate. St. Louis, Mosby, 1996.

51. Stark AR: High-frequency oscillatory ventilation to prevent bronchopulmonary dysplasia—Are we there yet? N Engl J Med 347:682–684, 2002.

52. Vannucci RC, Brucklacher RM, Vannucci SJ: Effect of carbon dioxide on cerebral metabolism during hypoxia-ischemia in the immature rat. Pediatr Res 42:24–28, 1997.

53. Wiswell TE, Graziani LI, Kornhauser MS, et al: High-frequency jet ventilation in the early management of respiratory distress syndrome is associated with a greater risk for adverse outcomes. Pediatrics 98:1035–1043, 1996.

AIR LEAK SYNDROMES

54. Cotton CM, Goldberg RN: Air leak syndrome. In Spitzer AR (ed): Intensive Care of the Fetus and Neonate. Philadelphia, Elsevier, 2005, pp 715–728.

55. Miller MJ, Fanaroff AA, Martin RJ: The respiratory system: Other problems. In Fanaroff AA, Martin RJ (eds): Neonatal-Perinatal Medicine: Diseases of the Fetus and Infant, 5th ed. St. Louis, Mosby, 1992, pp 834–860.

56. Soll RE, McQueen ME: Respiratory distress syndrome. In Sinclair JC, Bracken MB (eds): Effective Care of the Newborn Infant. Oxford, Oxford University Press, 1992.

57. Tarnow-Mordi WO, Reid E, Griffiths P, Wilkinson AR: Low inspired gas temperature and respiratory complications in very low birth weight infants. J Pediatr 114:438–442, 1989.

58. Yu VYH, Wong PY, Bayuk B, Szymonowicz W: Pulmonary air leak in extremely low birth weight infants. Arch Dis Child 61:239, 1986.

BRONCHOPULMONARY DYSPLASIA

59. Husain A, Siddiqui N, Stocker J: Pathology of arrested acinar development in postsurfactant bronchopulmonary dysplasia. Hum Pathol 29:710–717, 1998.

60. Jobe AH, Bancalari E. Bronchopulmonary dysplasia. Am J Respir Crit Care Med 163:1723–1729, 2001.

61. Jobe AH, Ikegami M. Prevention of bronchopulmonary dysplasia. Curr Opin Pediatr 13:124–129, 2001.

62. Rojas M, Gonzalez A, Bancalari E: Changing trends in the epidemiology and pathogenesis of neonatal chronic lung disease. J Pediatr 126:605–610, 1995.

63. Van Lierde S, Cornelis A, Devlieger H, et al: Different patterns of pulmonary sequelae after hyaline membrane disease: Heterogeneity of bronchopulmonary dysplasia. Biol Neonate 60:152–162, 1991.

64. Van Marter LJ, Allred EN, Pagano M, et al: Do clinical markers of barotrauma and oxygen toxicity explain interhospital variation in rates of chronic lung disease? The Neonatology Committee for the Developmental Network. Pediatrics 105:1194–1201, 2000.

65. Van Marter LJ, Dammann O, Allred EN, et al: Chorioamnionitis, mechanical ventilation, and postnatal sepsis as modulators of chronic lung disease in preterm infants. J Pediatr 140:171–176, 2002.

LUNG ABNORMALITIES

66. Adzick NS, Harrison MR, Crombleholme TM, et al: Fetal lung lesions: Management and outcome. Am J Obstet Gynecol 179:884–889, 1998.
67. Kravitz RM: Congenital malformations of the lung. Pediatr Clin North Am 41:453–472, 1994.
68. Miller MJ, Fanaroff AA, Martin RJ: Respiratory disorders in preterm and term infants. In Fanaroff AA, Martin RJ (eds): Neonatal-Perinatal Medicine: Diseases of the Fetus and Infant, 5th ed. St. Louis, Mosby, 1992, pp 1040–1065.
69. Pilling D: Fetal lung abnormalities: What do they mean? Clin Radiol 53:789–795, 1998.
70. Ribet ME, Copin M, Gosselin BH: Bronchogenic cysts of the lung. Ann Thorac Surg 61:1636–1640, 1996.
71. Schwartz MZ, Ramachandran P: Congenital malformations of the lung and mediastinum: A quarter century of experience from a single institution. J Pediatr Surg 32:44–47, 1997.
72. Takeda S, Miyoshi S, Inoue M, et al: Clinical spectrum of congenital cystic disease of the lung in children. Eur J Cardio Thorac Surg 15:11–17, 1999.

CHAPTER 17

SURGERY

Philip J. Wolfson, MD, and T. Ernesto Figueroa, MD

1. **Is the etiology of most congenital malformations known? Are they likely due to genetic factors, environmental factors, or both?**
   The etiology of most birth defects is not known, but the majority most likely result from a combination of genetic and environmental factors.

CONGENITAL DIAPHRAGMATIC HERNIA (CDH)

2. **What are the embryologic events that lead to the development of a CDH?**
   The posterolateral portion of the diaphragm is the last to form, when the pleuroperitoneal canal closes. If it has remained open by the time the extruded midgut returns to the peritoneal cavity between the ninth and tenth weeks of gestation, the viscera will pass into the chest, and a CDH will result.

3. **What are three causes of respiratory distress in a baby born with a CDH?**
   1. Mechanical compression of the lungs from the herniated viscera
   2. Pulmonary hypoplasia from compression of the developing lungs in utero
   3. Pulmonary hypertension from abnormally high pulmonary vascular resistance caused by the paucity of pulmonary arterioles and their abnormal vascular reactivity

4. **Describe the common clinical presentation of a baby with a CDH.**
   Although affected infants will occasionally be asymptomatic, they usually present with moderate to severe respiratory distress. There are diminished breath sounds on the side of the hernia and usually a shift of the heart and trachea to the opposite side. The abdomen is characteristically scaphoid. Increasingly, CDH is being diagnosed in utero by antenatal ultrasound.

KEY POINTS: MOST COMMON CHARACTERISTICS OF A NEWBORN INFANT WITH CDH

1. Dyspnea

2. Cyanosis

3. Scaphoid abdomen

4. Diminished breath sounds on the side of the hernia (usually the left)

5. **If a baby is suspected of having a CDH, which study is most useful?**
   A chest x-ray, which will usually demonstrate air-filled intestinal loops in the chest (once the baby has had time to swallow air); the diaphragmatic contour on the affected side is obliterated, and the mediastinum is often shifted to the opposite side (Fig. 17-1). In babies with the less common right-sided CDH, the findings may be more confusing, with opacification of the right lower chest from the herniated liver; in these cases, ultrasonography will provide clarification.

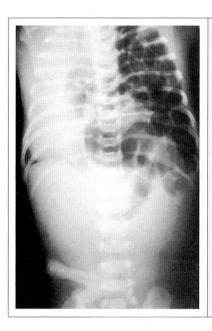

Figure 17-1. Left-sided diaphragmatic hernia with air-filled loops of intestine in the left chest and deviation of the mediastinum to the right.

6. **What is the initial management strategy for an infant with a CDH?**
Supplemental oxygen and endotracheal intubation with mechanical ventilation are used immediately in the presence of respiratory distress. Under no circumstance should positive pressure ventilation be administered through a face mask, because gas will enter the gastrointestinal tract and further compress the lungs. A nasogastric tube should be placed to suction. Exogenous surfactant, high-frequency ventilation, and inhaled nitric oxide are often instituted, but their value has not been definitively established. Barotrauma to the lungs from aggressive ventilation MUST be avoided, and the PCO_2 may be allowed to rise to 50–60 mmHg (permissive hypercapnia), so long as the arterial pH remains in the normal range.

Congenital Diaphragmatic Hernia Study Group: Surfactant does not improve survival rate in preterm infants with congenital diaphragmatic hernia. J Pediatr Surg 39:829–833, 2004.

7. **What is the role of extracorporeal membrane oxygenation (ECMO) in babies with CDH?**
ECMO, the use of a modified heart-lung machine to provide cardiorespiratory support independent of the lungs, may be used before or after corrective surgery if the baby does not respond to the ventilatory therapy outlined above. ECMO allows time for pulmonary hypertension to improve while avoiding lung damage caused by barotrauma and excessive oxygen concentrations from the ventilator. It is not clear, however, whether ECMO makes a significant difference in the outcome for many babies with a CDH.

8. **What is the optimal timing for the surgical repair of a CDH?**
There is no universal agreement, although immediate surgical repair of the defect is no longer considered to be necessary nor advisable. Instead, resuscitation followed by a period of stabilization until the neonate's clinical condition is more optimal, which may require days, is preferable. If the baby requires ECMO preoperatively, surgical repair is usually delayed until the ECMO settings have been lowered and the patient is considered ready to come off ECMO, but before decannulation.

Rozmiarek AJ, Qureshi FG, Cassidy L, et al: Factors influencing survival in newborns with congenital diaphragmatic hernia: The relative role of timing of surgery. J Pediatr Surg 39:821–824, 2004.

9. **What is the current survival rate for infants with CDH? Which factors are most responsible for the recent improvements?**
Several institutions are now reporting survival rates of 80–90% (compared with historical survival rates of 50–60%) for infants with CDH, with most of the improvement thought to be due to referral to high-volume tertiary care centers for management of these babies as well as minimization of iatrogenic pulmonary injury through the avoidance of high ventilatory settings.

Downard CD, Jaksic T, Garza JJ, et al: Analysis of an improved survival rate for congenital diaphragmatic hernia. J Pediatr Surg 38:729–732, 2003.

Javid PJ, Jaksic TG, Skarsgard ED, et al: Survival rate in congenital diaphragmatic hernia: The experience of the Canadian Neonatal Network. J Pediatr Surg 39:657–660, 2004.

Kays DW, Langham MR Jr, Ledbetter DJ, Talbert JL: Detrimental effects of standard medical therapy in congenital diaphragmatic hernia. Ann Surg 230:340–351, 1999.

Sakurai Y, Azarow K, Cutz E, et al: Pulmonary barotraumas in congenital diaphragmatic hernia: A clinico-pathological correlation. J Pediatr Surg 34:1813–1817, 1999.

10. **Explain what is meant by the term _hidden mortality_ in association with CDH.**
Michael Harrison coined this term to account for a large group of patients with CDH who succumb in utero or shortly after birth, before they can reach a tertiary care center. As a result, they may not be included in that center's statistics. Geographically, defined survival data may therefore be considerably lower than institution-based figures due to this selection bias.

Harrison MR, Adzick S, Estes JM, et al: A prospective study of the outcome for fetuses with diaphragmatic hernia. JAMA 271:382–384, 1994.

Harrison MR Bjordal RI, Langmark F, et al: Congenital diaphragmatic hernia: The hidden mortality. J Pediatr Surg 13:227–230, 1978.

Toronto Congenital Anomalies Study Group: Apparent truth about congenital diaphragmatic hernia: A population-based database is needed to establish benchmarking for clinical outcomes for CDH. J Pediatr Surg 39:661–665, 2004.

CONGENITAL MASS LESIONS OF THE CHEST

11. **Describe the various types of congenital mass lesions of the chest in newborn infants that are related to anomalies of the developing foregut.**
- **Bronchopulmonary foregut malformations:** These are a group of anomalies that arise from the foregut from cells that migrate separately and caudally along the developing esophagus and lung. Conditions include the following:
  - **Esophageal duplication cysts:** These usually share a common wall with the esophagus and can be found anywhere along its length; duplications may or may not communicate with the esophageal lumen.
  - **Bronchogenic cysts:** Lined by epithelium and mucus glands, these cysts may be located centrally in the mediastinum or peripherally in the lung parenchyma, where they may communicate with the bronchial tree.
  - **Pulmonary sequestration:** This malformation of the lung usually receives its blood supply from anomalous systemic vessels; they may be intralobar (i.e., incorporated within the normal lung) or extralobar (i.e., separate from the normal lung) and do not communicate with the bronchial tree.
  - **Cystic adenomatoid malformation:** This type of lesion results from an overgrowth of the bronchial structures and may consist of large cysts, small cysts, or a solid lesion within the lung.
- **Congenital lobar emphysema:** This represents overinflation of a lobe or segment of the lung usually caused by cartilaginous deficiency of the bronchial tree, leading to distal air trapping.

DeLorimeir AA: Respiratory problems related to the airway and lung. In O'Neill JA Jr, Rowe MI, Grosfeld JL, et al (eds): Pediatric Surgery, 5th ed. St. Louis, Mosby, 1998, pp 873–897.

12. **What are the ways in which congenital mass lesions of the chest present?**
These anomalies may be asymptomatic and be discovered incidentally on an imaging study for another condition. They may produce symptoms from compression (e.g., chest pain, wheezing, dyspnea) or infection (e.g., chest pain, fever, cough, dyspnea). Increasingly, these conditions are being discovered in utero by ultrasonography.

13. **What is the treatment of congenital mass lesions of the chest?**
The treatment is almost always surgical excision, although some observers think that certain completely asymptomatic lesions may be observed.

14. **Is it always possible to differentiate the type of congenital foregut malformation a patient has preoperatively?**
No. Not only is it sometimes not possible to arrive at an exact diagnosis before surgery, but often these lesions will have histologic findings that have features of a combination of these anomalies.

ESOPHAGEAL ATRESIA AND TRACHEOESOPHAGEAL FISTULA

15. **Describe the embryologic etiology of esophageal atresia and tracheoesophageal fistulas.**
The precise etiology is unknown, but it is believed that the septation process that normally separates the foregut into the trachea and esophagus by the seventh week of gestation is incomplete. The more rapidly dividing trachea separates the upper and lower portions of the esophagus into discontinuous segments.

16. **Describe the five possible configurations of esophageal atresia and tracheoesophageal fistulas. Which is the most common?**
Esophageal atresia and tracheoesophageal fistula usually occur in combination but may occur in isolation.
- **Type A:** Isolated esophageal atresia (rare)
- **Type B:** Esophageal atresia with a proximal fistula (rare)
- **Type C:** The upper esophagus ends blindly with a fistulous connection between the distal esophagus and the trachea (by far the most common type, accounting for approximately 85% of cases)
- **Type D:** Esophageal atresia with a double fistula (rare)
- **Type E:** Isolated tracheoesophageal fistula (rare)

KEY POINTS: PATTERNS OF ESOPHAGEAL ATRESIA AND TRACHEOESOPHAGEAL FISTULA

1. Isolated esophageal atresia (5–10% of cases)

2. Esophageal atresia with a tracheal fistula to the upper esophageal segment (rare)

3. Esophageal atresia with a tracheal fistula to the lower esophageal segment (most common, in 85% of cases)

4. Esophageal atresia with tracheal fistulas to both esophageal segments (rare)

5. Isolated tracheoesophageal ("H" type) fistula (5–10% of cases)

17. **Explain the VACTERL association.**
    VACTERL is an acronym for a combination of congenital abnormalities that frequently occur together; the presence of one or more should prompt a search for the others. These anomalies may involve the following structures:
    - **V**ertebrae
    - **A**nus
    - **C**ardiac anomalies
    - **T**rachea
    - **E**sophagus
    - **R**enal anomalies
    - **L**imb

18. **How do babies born with esophageal atresia usually present? How can the diagnosis be established?**
    Infants with esophageal atresia have excessive drooling because they cannot swallow their oral secretions. If feeding is attempted, the baby will cough and choke due to the blind-ending upper esophageal pouch. An attempt should be made to pass a nasogastric tube, which will encounter resistance. A chest radiograph will demonstrate the tip of the tube lodged in the upper chest, confirming the diagnosis of esophageal atresia. Air visualized in the gastrointestinal tract indicates the presence of a fistula to the trachea, whereas a gasless abdomen implies an isolated esophageal atresia.

19. **Outline the initial management plan for a baby with esophageal atresia.**
    The prevention of aspiration is most crucial. A double-lumen tube from the nose or mouth is placed into the blind upper esophageal segment and connected to suction while the baby is maintained in a head-up position to minimize gastroesophageal reflux into the distal fistula. Intravenous fluids and broad-spectrum antibiotics are administered, and the baby is investigated for additional VACTERL abnormalities.

20. **When is a primary repair performed? When is the surgical repair done in stages?**
    If the baby is stable and the gap between esophageal segments is short, operative division of the fistula and a primary esophageal anastomosis is performed. When the infant is extremely premature, sick, or there is a long esophageal gap (as is frequent in isolated esophageal atresia without a fistula), the repair is done in stages with division of any fistula and a feeding gastrostomy as the initial procedure.

21. **List the common complications that may develop after repair of esophageal atresia.**
    Complications include anastomotic leak, stricture formation, recurrence of the tracheoesophageal fistula, and gastroesophageal reflux. These babies may also have underlying tracheomalacia.

CONGENITAL OBSTRUCTION OF THE INTESTINAL TRACT

22. **List four clinical findings that may indicate that a newborn infant has an obstruction of the intestinal tract.**
    - **Polyhydramnios:** The fetus swallows large quantities of amniotic fluid, which is absorbed in the upper intestinal tract in the latter stages of pregnancy; an obstruction in the proximal intestine will cause this fluid to back up and accumulate in excessive quantities.
    - **Bilious vomiting:** Regurgitation of feedings is common in newborn infants, but vomiting significant quantities of bile may be evidence of mechanical obstruction.

- **Abdominal distention:** Progressive abdominal distention in the first 24–48 hours after birth as the infant swallows air may indicate a relatively distal intestinal blockage.
- **Failure to pass meconium:** If there is no passage of meconium within 24–48 hours after birth, one must consider the possibility of a congenital obstruction.

Not all of these clinical manifestations may occur, and the presence of any of them may signify the presence of an obstruction.

23. **If congenital obstruction is suspected from the scenarios just mentioned, what should be done next?**

    A careful history and physical examination is the next important step. Did the mother have an antenatal ultrasound? (This often demonstrates dilated intestine proximal to an obstruction.) Was amniocentesis performed? (Down syndrome is frequently associated with duodenal atresia and less often with Hirschsprung's disease.) Is there a family history of cystic fibrosis (which may point to meconium ileus) or siblings with intestinal atresia (which may be familial)? On examination, the baby's overall condition should be noted (sepsis is in the differential diagnosis and has several similar features with obstruction). Are there features of Down syndrome? Is there abdominal distention? Is the abdominal wall red? (This may signify an antenatal perfo-ration.) Are there any palpable hernias? Is the anal opening in the normal location and patent?

KEY POINTS: SIGNS OF CONGENITAL OBSTRUCTION OF THE INTESTINAL TRACT IN NEONATES

1. Polyhydramnios

2. Bilious vomiting

3. Abdominal distention

4. Failure to pass meconium within 24–48 hours after birth

24. **Which imaging study should be performed first if congenital intestinal obstruction is suspected?**

    Plain abdominal radiographs (supine and decubitus) are most useful and should always be per-formed first. A normal gas pattern with no dilation of intestinal loops and air in the rectum very much lowers the likelihood of obstruction. A "double bubble" sign is pathognomonic for com-plete duodenal obstruction. Several dilated loops of intestine with air fluid levels and a lack of distal gas are indicative of a high intestinal obstruction. Many dilated loops of intestine suggest a distal small bowel or colonic obstruction.

25. **What is the role of contrast radiographs if congenital obstruction is suspected?**

    In some instances, contrast radiographs may be unnecessary—air is an excellent contrast medium, and if there is evidence of complete duodenal or jejunal obstruction on the plain films (*see* question 32), further imaging studies are not necessary. If there is dilated proximal intes-tine and some distal gas, suggesting a partial obstruction or a volvulus, an upper gastrointesti-nal tract contrast series is indicated. If there appears to be a distal obstruction, a contrast enema should be performed to differentiate meconium plug, meconium ileus, intestinal atresia, and Hirschsprung's disease.

26. **Name two general causes of duodenal obstruction in infants. Explain their embryologic origins.**

Duodenal obstruction is most commonly due to atresia and malrotation. Atresia may take the form of stenosis, a web, or complete separation of the duodenal segments. One cause of atresia is the failure of complete recanalization of the lumen of the duodenum after the solid phase of embryologic development, when the epithelial lining occludes the lumen; another is an annular pancreas, wherein the ventral and dorsal pancreatic buds fuse around the duodenum and compress it during development. Eighty percent of cases of duodenal atresia occur distal to the ampulla of Vater, accounting for the bilious nature of the vomiting.

Normal rotation consists of a 270-degree turning of the midgut, resulting in the duodenojejunal junction being fixed in the left upper quadrant and the cecum attached in the right lower quadrant. In malrotation, this process does not occur or is incomplete, and the small bowel hangs down in the abdomen from a narrow base like a bell clapper, allowing the bowel to develop a volvulus and become obstructed.

27. **How do patients with malrotation and midgut volvulus present?**

The most common scenario is bilious vomiting for no apparent reason in an infant who has been otherwise well and has a flat abdomen. The baby may then become jittery or listless, mottled, tachycardic, and diaphoretic. Abdominal tenderness and rectal bleeding are late and ominous signs.

28. **If an infant has bilious vomiting, what should be done?**

Unexplained bilious vomiting in an infant is a surgical emergency until proven otherwise. If no other explanation is apparent (e.g., bilious vomiting with profuse diarrhea and fever may signify a systemic infection, such as gastroenteritis), an immediate evaluation for malrotation should be performed. Plain abdominal radiographs are often nonspecific, and an urgent upper gastrointestinal tract contrast study is mandatory to determine the position of the ligament of Treitz and look for a possible twist.

29. **If the diagnosis of midgut volvulus is delayed, what are the potential consequences?**

The twist can occlude venous outflow and then arterial inflow to the bowel, resulting in ischemia, bleeding, and necrosis. Gangrene of the entire small intestine may occur within as short a period as several hours from the onset of symptoms.

30. **Differentiate the etiology of jejunal and ileal atresia from that of duodenal atresia.**

As mentioned above, duodenal atresia may arise from failure of recanalization of the lumen or from an annular pancreas. There is no similar solid phase of development of the jejunum or ileum; instead, atresia is believed to result from an intrauterine vascular accident that produces infarction. Since there are no bacteria within the intestine at this time, gangrene and bacterial peritonitis do not develop, and the involved segment atrophies, resulting in an atresia.

31. **How do the clinical presentations of proximal jejunal atresia and of distal ileal atresia differ?**

- **Jejunal atresia:** Bilious emesis and mild distention
- **Ileal atresia:** Bilious emesis and significant distention

32. **What is the optimal radiographic study for the diagnosis of jejunal atresia?**

Plain abdominal radiographs will demonstrate a few dilated small bowel loops indicative of a proximal to mid small intestine obstruction. There is no advantage to performing a gastrointestinal tract contrast study.

33. **What is the optimal imaging study in an infant with significant abdominal distention and multiple dilated intestinal loops as demonstrated on a plain abdominal radiograph?**
This pattern is consistent with ileal atresia, but meconium ileus, meconium plug, neonatal small left colon syndrome, and Hirschsprung's disease can all produce similar radiographic findings. A contrast enema will clarify the etiology of distal intestinal obstruction in most instances.

34. **How often do infants with cystic fibrosis present with meconium ileus?**
Approximately 15% of infants with cystic fibrosis have meconium ileus at the time of birth.

35. **What is the difference between simple meconium ileus and complicated meconium ileus?**
Simple meconium ileus is the mechanical blockage of the distal ileum by the sticky, inspissated meconium characteristically found in babies with cystic fibrosis. Radiographs often demonstrate a foamy appearance of the dilated meconium-filled bowel loops and a lack of air-fluid levels. A barium enema will demonstrate multiple filling defects in the distal ileum and should be followed by the administration of Gastrografin. Its high osmolarity causes fluid to pass into the bowel lumen and will often relieve the obstruction nonoperatively.
   Complicated meconium ileus refers to an in utero perforation resulting from the initial intestinal obstruction, leading to chemical peritonitis, ascites, an abdominal meconium cyst, or intestinal atresia. Infants are usually distended at the time of birth (unlike with simple meconium ileus in which distention is initially minimal and progresses over 24–48 hours) and may have erythema of the abdominal wall and calcifications on abdominal radiographs.

36. **What are the indications for surgery in patients with meconium ileus?**
Neonates with uncomplicated meconium ileus who have failed to respond to two or three therapeutic enemas require operative intervention. There is no place for attempted Gastrografin treatment of complicated meconium ileus, because urgent surgical exploration is required.

37. **What are the dangers associated with attempted Gastrografin enema treatment of simple meconium ileus?**
The hydrostatic pressure of the enema can perforate the intestine, so it is imperative that the procedure be performed by a radiologist skilled and experienced in treating newborn infants. Also, the fluid shift into the intestinal lumen from the hyperosmolar Gastrografin can render the baby hypovolemic, and it is essential that the baby be well hydrated with intravenous fluids at the time of the procedure.

38. **How do intestinal duplications produce obstruction?**
Duplications are endothelial-lined cystic or tubular structures found on the mesenteric side of the intestine that usually share a common wall. Mucous secretions or stool may accumulate in the duplication causing it to distend, which may compress the adjacent bowel and cause obstruction.

39. **Why does the zone of aganglionosis in Hirschsprung's disease always involve the rectum?**
Hirschsprung's disease results from the failure of the parasympathetic nervous system to fully invest the digestive tract. Normally, ganglion cells migrate from the esophagus to the anus during fetal development. Arrest of this process anywhere along its length results in aganglionic intestine, which is always distal to this point.

40. **How does Hirschsprung's disease cause obstruction?**
The intestine distal to the transition zone, lacking ganglion cells, is unable to relax and propagate a peristaltic wave, producing a functional obstruction.

41. **Where is the transition zone found in infants with Hirschsprung's disease?**
    Two thirds of the time the transition zone is in the rectosigmoid region, but the zone of agang-
    lionosis may involve the entire colon or even extend into the small intestine (i.e., long-segment
    Hirschsprung's disease). Although Hirschsprung's disease affects boys four times as often as
    girls, long-segment disease affects boys and girls equally.

42. **How do patients with Hirschsprung's disease typically present?**
    The typical newborn with Hirschsprung's disease fails to pass meconium in the first 24 hours
    after birth. In addition, there is a wide spectrum of presentations ranging from complete func-
    tional distal obstruction with bilious vomiting and a distended abdomen to chronic constipation
    (in which case the diagnosis is usually not made until after the newborn period). Sepsis result-
    ing from Hirschsprung's enterocolitis can occur at any time.

43. **How is the diagnosis established?**
    A contrast enema is suggestive of Hirschsprung's disease if it shows a change in the
    caliber of the colon at the transition zone. It is important that the study be delayed if the
    baby has had an enema, a digital rectal examination, or even a rectal thermometer inserted,
    because any rectal manipulation may temporarily obliterate the radiographic appearance of
    the transition zone. The diagnosis is established definitively by a rectal biopsy that typically
    demonstrates an absence of ganglion cells and hypertrophy of parasympathetic nerve fibers,
    which stain intensively for acetylcholinesterase. This biopsy can be done at the bedside in
    the neonate.

44. **What is the treatment for Hirschsprung's disease?**
    Even in instances in which there is significant abdominal distention, the proximal intestine can
    almost always be decompressed by enemas, allowing time for a diagnostic work-up. The tradi-
    tional surgical repair is a staged operation with a temporary diverting colostomy constructed
    above the transition zone, followed several months later by a "pull-through" operation in which
    the ganglionic bowel is brought down and anastomosed to the anal canal. In full-size babies
    without enterocolitis, the pull-through procedure is performed as a single operation, often with
    laparoscopic assistance.

45. **What is Hirschsprung's enterocolitis?**
    Patients with Hirschsprung's disease may develop an enterocolitis, the precise cause of which
    is not well understood, but which involves bacterial overgrowth and translocation through the
    wall of the colon. Enterocolitis may be the first recognized manifestation of Hirschsprung's
    disease and may also occur after surgery. It can be mild or severe with explosive diarrhea,
    dehydration, peritonitis, and sepsis. Enterocolitis is the most common cause of mortality from
    Hirschsprung's disease. Treatment must be immediate and consists of bowel rest, broad-
    spectrum antibiotics, and thorough colonic irrigations.

46. **Differentiate meconium ileus from meconium plug and the small left colon
    syndrome.**
    Meconium ileus, as previously described, is obstruction of the distal ileum due to thick and vis-
    cid meconium, occurring in 10–20% of neonates with cystic fibrosis. Meconium plug is caused
    by meconium blocking the left colon in otherwise healthy babies. The small left colon syndrome
    is most common in infants of diabetic mothers and produces an obstruction from a temporarily
    dysfunctional, small-caliber left colon. A contrast enema with barium is usually diagnostic as
    well as therapeutic for both meconium plug and the small left colon syndrome (through its
    mechanical effect), although subsequent testing for Hirschsprung's disease or cystic fibrosis
    may be indicated.

IMPERFORATE ANUS

47. **How is *imperforate anus* defined?**
Imperforate anus comprises a spectrum of disorders in which the rectum fails to reach its normal perineal termination. When the rectum ends above the levator muscles, the malformation is termed *high*; when it passes through these muscles, the malformation is *low*. High lesions are more common in males; low lesions are more common in females.

48. **How is imperforate anus diagnosed?**
The diagnosis is usually obvious on inspection of the perineum, which should be standard procedure for a newborn examination. Either no perineal opening is present or an external fistula is visible. In males, this fistula is usually a small opening anterior to the normal anal location in the perineum or as far forward as the scrotal raphe. Females may also have an external fistula draining into the anterior perineum, or else in the posterior vulva behind the hymen (the vaginal "fourchette"). A single perineal opening signifies a cloaca, where the rectum, vagina, and urethra all open into one common chamber.

49. **Outline the steps for the evaluation of a baby with an imperforate anus.**
Inspection and urinalysis are able to determine the anatomy in most cases. A perineal fistula always means the lesion is low and a colostomy can be avoided. If such a fistula cannot be detected initially, there should always be a 16–24-hour waiting period to allow increased luminal pressure to force meconium through a possible fistula so that it becomes visible on examination. If there is meconium in the urine, an internal fistula to the urinary tract is confirmed. If there is no visible fistula, a cross-table lateral film with the baby in the prone position can be used to measure the most distal aspect of the rectum relative to the perineal skin.

   The work-up should also include a search for other possible components of the VACTERL association (*see* question 17).

50. **When does a colostomy not need to be performed as the initial operative procedure? Is surgery always necessary?**
If there is an external fistula to the perineum, or "bucket handle" deformity in a male (i.e., a vertical raphe in the perineum with indentations on both sides), the lesion is low, and a primary anoplasty can be performed in the newborn period. Otherwise, the lesion is probably high or intermediate, and an initial colostomy is recommended, followed by a pull-through within the next several months. If there is a large fistulous opening only slightly anterior to the normal anal location ("anterior anus"), function can be normal and surgery may be unnecessary.

51. **What is the Peña procedure?**
Alberto Peña devised the *posterior sagittal anorectoplasty* in which the anal and rectal sphincter muscles are divided posteriorly in the midline; this operative approach has become the standard procedure for the pull-through due to the excellent visualization obtained. Recently, a laparoscopic pull-through operation has become feasible.

52. **What is the main determination of continence in persons who have had an imperforate anus? What should parents be told?**
Continence depends on the coordinated actions of the external sphincter, internal sphincter, and levator muscles. The levators are most important, so infants with low lesions in whom the bowel has descended normally within the levator sling have an excellent functional outlook. Children with high anomalies frequently have underdeveloped sphincter muscles, and their results are mixed, with many having at least occasional soiling. Finally, children with a flat bottom (which implies very poorly developed muscles) without a developed gluteal fold and those having sacral anomalies on radiograph have the worst prospects for normal continence. These patients require a structured bowel management program including daily enemas to achieve "functional" continence.

NECROTIZING ENTEROCOLITIS (NEC)

53. What is NEC?

NEC is a condition that most commonly affects premature infants after the institution of oral feedings, and it also occasionally occurs in term babies who have other debilitating illnesses. It is a hemorrhagic necrosis that initially affects the mucosa but may progress to involve full-thickness injury. Manifestations cover a broad spectrum, from mild abdominal distention with hematochezia to fulminant sepsis with necrosis of the entire intestinal tract.

54. List the factors considered to predispose to the development of NEC.

Although the precise etiology is unknown, three factors that seem to act in concert in promoting the development of NEC are:

1. Damage to the intestinal mucosa, which may result from ischemia due to perinatal hypoxia, low-flow states, or reperfusion injury
2. The presence of feedings in the intestinal tract, which act as a substrate for bacterial proliferation (NEC is highly uncommon among infants who have not received enteral feeds)
3. Impaired host defense mechanisms, as is the case in premature infants, allowing intestinal bacteria to invade the wall of the intestine

55. Which portion of the gastrointestinal tract is affected by NEC?

NEC may involve any portion of the gastrointestinal tract, but the ileocecal region is the most commonly affected.

56. Is there a specific type of bacteria associated with NEC?

No. Although affected patients may be clustered in place and time, no consistent agent has been isolated from all reported epidemics, and it is considered that a variety of the enteric flora may contribute.

57. How do babies with NEC typically present?

Clinical signs are initially nonspecific and may consist of lethargy, apnea, temperature instability, and feeding intolerance. Gastrointestinal manifestations follow and include vomiting, bloody stools, abdominal distention, and abdominal tenderness. Generalized sepsis may supervene.

58. How is the diagnosis of NEC established?

Although the diagnosis may be strongly suspected by the clinical findings outlined above, the presence of a lucent halo around the intestinal wall on x-ray, called *pneumatosis intestinalis*, is pathognomonic. Pneumatosis represents gas in the bowel wall produced by enteric organisms and is seen in 80% of cases of NEC. Other radiographic features may include irregularly dilated air-filled loops of bowel and the visualization of gas in the portal venous system.

59. Do all infants who develop NEC require surgery?

No. Most infants with NEC will respond to medical treatment consisting of withholding all enteral feeds, nasogastric decompression, broad-spectrum systemic antibiotics, and general supportive measures to optimize tissue oxygenation and perfusion. Frequent clinical examinations are mandatory, and serial abdominal radiographs are obtained.

KEY POINTS: INDICATIONS FOR SURGERY IN INFANTS WITH NEC

1. **Absolute indication:** Free air in the abdomen on radiograph
2. **Relative indications:** Clinical deterioration with erythema of the abdominal wall, a distended and tense abdomen, metabolic acidosis, and thrombocytopenia

60. **When is surgery indicated in an infant with NEC?**
Absolute indications for surgery include pneumoperitoneum and intestinal gangrene (as evidenced by abdominal wall erythema, a fixed mass, or paracentesis positive for dark brown fluid or bacteria on Gram stain). Relative indications include progressive clinical deterioration as evidenced by a firm, tender abdomen; metabolic acidosis; ventilatory failure; oliguria; thrombocytopenia; and portal vein gas.

61. **What type of operation is recommended when surgery is undertaken for NEC?**
Traditionally, after inspection of the entire intestinal tract, necrotic or perforated segments are resected, and an ostomy is performed. Recently, primary anastomoses have been undertaken in low-risk patients with minimal peritoneal contamination.

62. **When should the stoma be closed?**
Ideally, stomas are reversed months later, when the patient is thriving, and the procedure is very low risk. In reality, malabsorption or skin breakdown often necessitates earlier closure.

63. **Is there ever an indication for peritoneal drainage alone as the surgical treatment for NEC?**
Extremely small (weighing <1000 gm) infants with NEC-induced perforations, in whom the operative mortality would be high, have been treated successfully with the insertion of peritoneal drains performed at the bedside. If there is no significant improvement in the infant's condition within 48 hours, a formal laparotomy is then considered.

64. **If an infant who has recovered from NEC develops vomiting and abdominal distention several weeks later, what complication should be suspected?**
Approximately 10–15% of patients with NEC who do not develop full-thickness necrosis and perforation will develop an obstructive intestinal stricture from partial-thickness damage. A distal contrast study should always be obtained before reversing an ostomy to be certain there is no silent stricture in the defunctionalized bowel.

65. **Are all cases of intestinal perforation in premature infants due to NEC?**
No. There is an entity in which the small intestine develops an isolated perforation without full-blown NEC. These babies are generally younger (<1 week old) and more premature than NEC babies and often have not been fed. The exact etiology is unknown, but a very localized area of ischemia may be causative. Unlike with NEC, the surrounding bowel is not affected. Treatment consists of a localized resection with either an ostomy or possibly a primary anastomosis.

ABDOMINAL WALL DEFECTS: OMPHALOCELE AND GASTROSCHISIS

66. **Describe the different embryologic events that result in the development of an omphalocele and a gastroschisis.**
Between the fifth and tenth weeks of embryologic development, the intestine is extruded out of the umbilical ring and into the yolk sac. An omphalocele results when the lateral abdominal folds do not close and the exteriorized viscera remain in the sac. The etiology of gastroschisis is not so clear—it may be caused by an in utero perforation of the developing abdominal wall where one of the paired umbilical veins undergoes atrophy in an area of relative weakness, or it may occur from the antenatal perforation of a small omphalocele sac.

67. **How does the embryology described in question 66 account for the anatomic appearances of omphalocele and gastroschisis?**
   - **Omphalocele:** This is a centrally located defect of the umbilical ring that has not closed, and the viscera are covered with a sac composed of peritoneum and amnion (Fig. 17-2).

■ **Gastroschisis:** This defect is always lateral to the cord, usually on the right, and has no covering sac (Fig. 17-3).

The defects in the abdominal wall are generally larger in omphalocele than in gastroschisis.

68. **Which entity, omphalocele or gastroschisis, is more often associated with other syndromes?**

Babies with an omphalocele have a very high incidence of associated anomalies such as trisomy 13 and 18 syndromes, Beckwith-Wiedemann syndrome, pentalogy of Cantrell, bladder and cloacal exstrophy, and congenital cardiac abnormalities.

Gastroschisis is not associated with genetic syndromes. However, approximately 10% of these infants do have intestinal atresias, perhaps related to compression of the developing intestine against the edge of the abdominal opening.

69. **What is the importance of prenatal diagnosis?**

Detection of abdominal wall defects in utero is important for several reasons. Early parental counseling can be initiated with perinatologists, obstetricians, neonatologists, pediatric

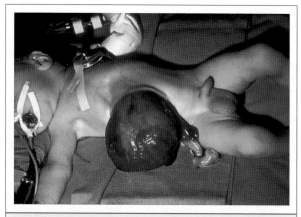

Figure 17-2. Omphalocele.

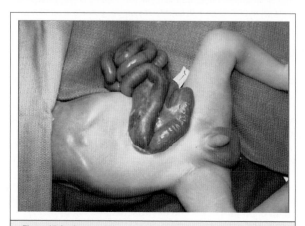

Figure 17-3. Gastroschisis.

surgeons, and ethicists. In the case of an omphalocele, associated defects can be searched for, the presence of which may affect prenatal care, timing and mode of delivery, and, in the case of multiple severe anomalies, potential termination of pregnancy.

70. **What is the best method for delivering a child with an abdominal wall defect?**
Most studies show that cesarean section provides no significant advantage over vaginal delivery. One exception is the fetus with a very large omphalocele, for which case several reports have documented dystocia and liver damage during vaginal delivery.

71. **Outline the immediate postnatal management in infants with abdominal wall defects.**
Infants born with abdominal wall defects are prone to three serious problems: hypovolemia, hypothermia, and sepsis. Exposed bowel leads to increased loss of insensible fluid as well as heat loss. Immediate management includes placing the lower half of the infant, including exposed viscera, in a plastic wrapping or moist, sterile gauze; maintaining the infant in a warmer; initiating intravenous access and fluids; and providing nasogastric decompression. Parenteral antibiotics are administered to decrease the risk of sepsis.

72. **How urgent is surgical closure? What are the surgical options?**
Babies with gastroschisis require emergency surgery because the viscera are exposed, whereas in the case of omphalocele, surgery is not so emergent, and there is time for stabilization and evaluation of potential associated anomalies.
The two surgical options are primary closure or, if there is tension that might compromise respiratory function or the viscera itself, staged closure with a silo.

73. **How does staged closure work?**
Staged closure involves placing prosthetic material, usually a reinforced Silastic silo, over the viscera and attaching it to the fascia at the edges of the defect. The silo is manually compressed daily to gradually reduce the viscera and expand the peritoneal cavity. Most infants can be closed within 7–10 days with this method.

74. **Is nonoperative treatment ever appropriate in a baby with an omphalocele?**
Yes. In cases of severe associated anomalies or prohibitive operative risks, the omphalocele sac can be painted with an antiseptic, such as silver sulfadiazine or povidone-iodine. The sac will eventually epithelialize and contract, leaving a ventral hernia (which may be quite large) that can be repaired electively if the baby survives.

ABDOMINAL MASSES

75. **What is the origin of most neonatal abdominal masses?**
More than half of all abdominal masses in neonates arise from the urinary tract.

76. **List the two most common causes of abdominal masses of urologic origin in the neonate.**
1. Hydronephrosis secondary to ureteropelvic junction (UPJ) obstruction
2. Multicystic kidney disease

77. **A pregnant woman has an antenatal ultrasound that reveals an intra-abdominal mass in the fetus. Are any special arrangements necessary for the timing and mode of delivery?**
No.

78. **How do the location and other physical examination characteristics of the common abdominal masses in newborn infants provide clues for their identification?**

    Physical examination may significantly narrow the diagnostic possibilities, even if it does not provide any absolute answer (Table 17-1). Of particular note:

    - Large masses may fill the entire abdomen, making it impossible to determine the site of origin on examination.
    - Hard, nodular masses are usually malignant tumors.
    - A highly mobile mass is usually a mesenteric cyst, a duplication, or an ovarian cyst.

79. **What is the recommended treatment for a newborn girl with an ovarian cyst that has been detected on antenatal ultrasound?**

    The management of ovarian cysts in a neonate is somewhat controversial. Most arise in response to antenatal hormonal stimulation and may subsequently resolve after birth. Potential complications such as torsion, hemorrhage into the cyst, and rupture are somewhat related to

TABLE 17-1. COMMON ABDOMINAL MASSES IN NEONATES

Mass Location	Type	Characteristics
Lateral mass	Multicystic kidney or hydronephrosis	Smooth, moderate mobility, transilluminates
	Renal tumor (Wilms' or mesoblastic nephroma)	Smooth, minimal mobility, does not transilluminate
	Neuroblastoma	Irregular contour, minimally mobile, frequently crosses the midline, does not transilluminate
Midabdominal mass	Mesenteric cyst	Smooth, mobile, transilluminates
	Gastrointestinal duplication cyst	Smooth, mobile, does not transilluminate; may be associated with obstruction
	Ovarian cyst	Smooth, mobile, transilluminates
Upper abdominal mass	Hepatic tumors	Hard, immobile, does not transilluminate
	Choledochal cyst	Smooth, immobile, does not transilluminate; may be associated with jaundice
Lower abdominal mass	Hydrometrocolpos	Smooth, immobile, does not transilluminate; may be associated with imperforate hymen
	Bladder	Smooth, fixed; associated with lower urinary obstruction
	Urachal cyst	Smooth, fixed to abdominal wall, extends to umbilicus
	Sacrococcygeal teratoma	Hard, fixed, does not transilluminate; often associated with external sacral component

the size of the cyst; the risk of malignancy depends on whether the cyst is simple (homogeneous) or complex.

Most authorities recommend carefully following up on asymptomatic cysts with serial ultrasonography for several months if they are ECHO-free and <5 cm in diameter. If the cyst causes compressive symptoms, has any solid components, or is >5 cm in diameter, it should be excised, possibly laparoscopically.

80. **What imaging studies are most useful in treating a newborn with an abdominal mass?**
A plain abdominal radiograph might reveal a mass effect or bowel obstruction, can help localize the mass, and can sometimes provide useful information about the mass itself, such as the presence of calcifications or stool. An abdominal ultrasound is extremely useful in the majority of cases because it can show whether the mass is cystic or solid, can reveal the effect on adjacent anatomic structures, and often can identify the exact anatomic location of the mass. Further information can be provided with abdominal computed tomography, magnetic resonance imaging, or urologic imaging.

81. **What is the differential diagnosis of a solid mass arising from the liver in a neonate?**
   - Hemangioma (benign)
   - Hemangioendothelioma (benign)
   - Hepatoblastoma (malignant)
Ultrasound appearance is characteristic and often diagnostic. Serum alpha-fetoprotein is usually elevated in hepatoblastoma. Small to moderate hemangiomas can be observed or treated medically with corticosteroids or alpha-interferon. Most large or symptomatic hemangiomas (causing pain, heart failure, thrombocytopenia) and all hemangioendotheliomas and hepatoblastoma require hepatic resection.

82. **What is the most common cause of bilateral abdominal masses in the neonate?**
Hydronephrosis secondary to UPJ obstruction.

83. **A newborn infant has a large mass below the spine arising from the presacral region, compressing the rectum and anus anteriorly. What is the nature of this lesion?**
Presacral teratomas are the most common congenital tumor (Fig. 17-4). They can appear alarming because of their large size and compressive effects, but 90% are benign and can be completely resected.

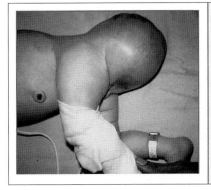

Figure 17-4. Sacrococcygeal teratoma.

HERNIAS AND CRYPTORCHIDISM

84. **What are the embryologic causes of an indirect inguinal hernia? Why are they more common in premature infants?**
When the testes descend from the abdomen during embryologic development, there is a resulting communication between the scrotum and the peritoneal cavity, the processus vaginalis, which usually becomes obliterated between the seventh and ninth weeks of gestation. Failure of this processus to close allows viscera to protrude into the groin or scrotum as an indirect inguinal hernia. Premature infants are less likely to have had time for the processus vaginalis to close.

85. **Do all inguinal hernias need to be repaired?**
Yes. Inguinal hernias will not resolve spontaneously, and there is a serious risk of incarceration (inability to be reduced), which can lead to strangulation.

86. **When should an asymptomatic inguinal hernia that is discovered in a newborn infant be repaired?**
There is some controversy over this issue. If an inguinal hernia is asymptomatic, some surgeons will wait several months until the baby is older, but most recommend repairing it before the baby's discharge from the nursery to prevent complications. If the infant is premature and has diminished respiratory reserve (e.g., BPD), the operative procedure can be done under spinal or epidural anesthesia, in most cases without having to intubate the baby.

87. **Which structure is most likely to be contained in an inguinal hernia in a girl?**
The ovary.

88. **If a newborn infant has an umbilical hernia, should operative repair be performed at this time?**
No. The vast majority of umbilical hernias will close spontaneously by 4–5 years of age. The risk of incarceration in the interim is extremely small.

89. **A newborn infant born at 34 weeks' gestation is found to have an undescended right testicle. What should be done?**
Undescended testes are very common in newborn males, especially when they are born prematurely. Observation only is indicated at this time, because most of the time the testes will descend spontaneously by 1 year of age.

UROLOGIC CONDITIONS

90. **What is the incidence of hypospadias?**
The incidence of hypospadias is approximately 1 in 300 live male births.

Ducket JW: Hypospadias. In Walsh PC, Retik AB, Vaughan ED, Wein AJ (eds): Campbell's Urology, 7th ed. Philadelphia, W.B. Saunders, 1998, pp 2093–2119.

91. **Which additional abnormalities are usually associated with classical bladder exstrophy?**
Epispadias, abnormal gait, anteriorly displaced anus, and vesicoureteral reflux.

Gerhart JP, Jeffs RD: Exstrophy-epispadias complex and bladder anomalies. In Walsh PC, Retik AB, Vaughan ED, Wein AJ (eds): Campbell's Urology, 7th ed. Philadelphia, W.B. Saunders, 1998, pp 1939–1990.

92. **Describe the embryologic events that lead to classical bladder exstrophy.**
Bladder exstrophy is caused by a persistence of the cloacal membrane after the fourth gestational week and a lack of medial migration of the lateral mesoderm.

Gerhart JP, Jeffs RD: Exstrophy-epispadias complex and bladder anomalies. In Walsh PC, Retik AB, Vaughan ED, Wein AJ (eds): Campbell's Urology, 7th ed. Philadelphia, W.B. Saunders, 1998, pp 1939–1990.

93. **What are the major components of prune belly syndrome (also known as *Eagle-Barrett syndrome*)?**
Prune belly syndrome consists of deficient abdominal wall musculature, hydronephrosis, and undescended testes.

Sutherland RS: Congenital anomalies. In Baskin LS, Kogan BA, Duckett JW (eds): Handbook of Pediatric Urology. Philadelphia, Lippincott-Raven, 1997, pp 183–199.

94. **What is the most common genitourinary malformation associated with imperforate anus?**
Renal agenesis.

Sutherland RS: Congenital anomalies. In Baskin LS, Kogan BA, Duckett JW (eds): Handbook of Pediatric Urology. Philadelphia, Lippincott-Raven, 1997, pp 183–199.

95. **What is the approximate percentage of children with spina bifida who have abnormal bladder innervation?**
90%.

Sutherland RS: Congenital anomalies. In Baskin LS, Kogan BA, Duckett JW (eds): Handbook of Pediatric Urology. Philadelphia, Lippincott-Raven, 1997, pp 183–199.

CIRCUMCISION

96. **Why should attempts to retract the foreskin in uncircumcised boys be avoided in neonates?**
The undersurface of the foreskin is fused with the glans at birth, and it is not until later in childhood that the foreskin is truly retractable.

97. **Is the American Academy of Pediatrics in favor of or against circumcision as a routine in newborn males?**
Neither. The Academy remains neutral on the subject, stating that the decision should be left to the parents, after the potential risks and benefits are explained.

98. **What are the potential advantages and disadvantages of neonatal circumcision?**
Advantages:
- Prevents phimosis
- Prevents paraphimosis (i.e., inability to pull the foreskin back over the glans after it is retracted)
- Lowers the incidence of urinary infections
- Prevents balanoposthitis (i.e., infection of the glans and foreskin)
- Prevents cancer of the penis
Disadvantages:
- Medically unnecessary in most boys
- Painful
- Risks of complications (e.g., bleeding, infection, ulcers, damage to glans)

99. **What are the contraindications to circumcision in neonates?**
Neonatal circumcision should not be performed if the baby is otherwise ill or there are congenital anomalies of the penis (in which case the foreskin may be needed for eventual reconstruction).

ACKNOWLEDGMENT

A number of the questions and answers in this chapter are adapted from an earlier publication by one of the authors:
Wolfson PJ, Poenaru D, Ledbetter DJ: Pediatric surgery: Surgical diseases of children. In Lawrence PF, Bell, RM, Dayton MT (eds): Essentials of Surgical Specialties, 2nd ed. Philadelphia, Lippincott Williams & Wilkins, 2000, pp 68–107.

INDEX

Page numbers in **boldface type** indicate complete chapters.

Streptococcus infections *(Continued)*
  sexual transmission of, 305
Streptococcus pneumoniae infections, 148, 316, 317
Streptococcus pyogenes infections, 324
Streptomycin, as congenital deafness cause, 36
Stress
  light-related, 48
  neonates' experience of, 46–47
  noise-related, 48
Stress management, in neonatal intensive care units, 46
Strokes, 361, 365
Sturge-Weber syndrome, 125, 354
Subclavian artery, aberrant right, 98
Subependymal nodules, 353
Substance abuse. *See also* Alcohol use; Drug abuse
  as contraindication to breast-feeding, 204
Succinyl coenzyme A acetoacetate coenzyme
    transferase deficiency, 150
Sucking
  evaluation of, 346
  nonnutritive, 45, 47
Sucralfate
  as eosinophilic colitis treatment, 213
  as gastroesophageal reflux treatment, 213
Sudden infant death syndrome (SIDS), 107, 153, 389,
    440–442
Sulfadiazine, 336
Sulfa drugs, hyperbilirubinemia-exacerbating effect
    of, 36
Sulfamethoxazole/trimethoprim, cardiotoxicity of, 36
Sulfite oxidase deficiency, 151
Sunlight, as hyperbilirubinemia treatment, 60, 69
Surfactant, 393, 406, 407–408
Surfactant replacement therapy, 408, 409, 412–413
  as ductus arteriosus risk factor, 75, 76
Surgery, **448–466**
  fetal, 17, 18–20
Surgical patients, analgesia in, 383
Sutures, cranial, 348, 349
Swallowing
  evaluation of, 346
  impaired, 349
Symphalangia, 377
Syncytiotrophoblast, iron transport protein
    expression on, 209–210
Syndactyly, 251, 377
Syndrome X, 195
Syndromic bile duct paucity (Alagille syndrome),
    230–234
Syphilis
  congenital, 176, 326–327
  screening for, 326
Syringomyelia, 352
Systemic lupus erythematosus, maternal, 83
  as congenital heart block cause, 108

T
Tachycardia
  magnesium deficiency-related, 134

Tachycardia *(Continued)*
  maternal Graves' disease-related, 138
  as stress response, 47
  supraventricular, 105
Tachypnea, transient, of the newborn, 405
Tactile sensory development, 44, 46
Talipes equinovarus (clubfoot), 375–376, 377
Tamponade, cardiac, warning signs of, 114
Tape sites, pustules around, 128
TAR (thrombocytopenia with absent radius)
    syndrome, 81, 273, 280, 378
Taste, development of, 10, 44, 45
Taurine, 198
Taussig, Helen, 80
Tay-Sachs disease, 247
Telangiectasia, 124
Tendon reflexes, in progressive central nervous
    system disorders, 362
Tendon stretch reflexes, 348
Teratoma
  as fetal airway obstruction cause, 418
  intrapericardial, 111
  sacrococcygeal, 19, 236, 238, 462, 463
Testes
  development of, 143
  undescended, 139, 464
Testosterone, 143
Tetany, hypocalcemic and hypocalcemic, 366
Tethered cord, 124, 350, 352
Tetracycline, teratogenicity of, 36
Tetralogy of Fallot, 92, 93
  Blalock-Taussig shunt placement in, 111
  chest x-ray findings in, 94
  DiGeorge syndrome-related, 256
  with left-to-right shunt, 89
  surgical repair of, as phrenic nerve palsy cause, 102
  tet spells associated with, 101–102
Tet spells, 101–102
α-Thalassemia, 247, 270, 271
  silent carriers of, 271
β-Thalassemia, 247
Thalassemia, as anemia cause, 265
α-Thalassemia trait, 271
Thalidomide, as congenital heart disease cause, 83
Thermal burns, 121
Thermoregulation, intrauterine growth restriction-
    related impairment of, 15
Thiamin, breast milk content of, 207
Thiazide, as hypercalcemia cause, 133
Thiouracil, as contraindication to breast-feeding, 204
Thomas, Vivien, 80
Thoracopagus twins, 32
Threonine, 198
Thrombectomy, 181
Thrombocytopenia, 279–281
  with absent radii (TAR), 81, 273, 280, 378
  alloimmune
    maternal, 281
    neonatal, 280–281